CONVERSION OF TRADITIONAL UNITS TO SI UNITS

Current unit X conversion factor = SI unit;
SI unit ÷ conversion factor = current unit.

	Current Unit	SI Unit	Conversion Factor
FactorAlbumin	g/dL	g/L	10
Aspartate aminotransferase	U/L (mU/ml)	µkat/L	0.0167
Ammonia	µg/dL	µmol/L	0.587
Bicarbonate (HCO_3)	mEq/L	mmol/L	1.0
Bilirubin	mg/dL	µmol/L	17.1
BUN	mg/dL	mmol/L	0.357
Calcium	mg/dL	mmol/L	0.25
Chloride	mEq/L	mmol/L	1.0
Cholesterol	mg/dL	mmol/L	0.026
Cortisol	µg/dL	µmol/L	0.0276
Creatinine	mg/dL	µmol/L	88.4
Creatinine clearance	mL/min	mL/s	0.0167
CSF protein	mg/dL	g/L	0.01
Folic acid	ng/mL	nmol/L	2.27
Glucose	mg/dL	mmol/L	0.0555
Iron	mg/dL	µmol/L	0.179
HDL cholesterol	mg/dL	mmol/L	0.0259
Lithium	mEq/L	µmol/L	1.0
Magnesium	mEq/L	mmol/L	0.44
Osmolality	mOsm/kg	mmol/kg	1.0
Phosphorus	mg/dL	mmol/L	0.323
Potassium	mEq/L	mmol/L	1.0
Sodium	mEq/L	mmol/L	1.0
Thyroxine (T_4)	µg/dL	nmol/L	12.9
Total protein	g/dL	g/L	10
Triglyceride	mg/dL	mmol/L	0.0113
Uric acid	mg/dL	mmol/L	0.0595
Vitamin B_{12}	ng/mL	pmol/L	0.0738
pCO_2	mm/Hg	kPa	0.133
pO_2	mm/Hg	kPa	0.133
Hemoglobin	g/dL	g/L	10
Hematocrit	vol %	none	0.01
MCV	μ^3	FL	1.0
WBC count	mm^3	10^9/L	0.001
Platelet count	mm^3	10^9/L	0.001

From Ravel R. Clinical Laboratory Medicine: Clinical Application of Laboratory Data, 6th ed. St. Louis: Mosby, in press.

WEIGHT CONVERSION CHART

lb	kg	kg	lb
1	0.454	1kg	2.204
2	0.9	2	4.4
4	1.8	3	6.6
6	2.7	4	8.8
8	3.6	5	11.0
10	4.5	6	13.2
20	9.1	8	17.6
30	13.6	10	22
40	18.2	20	44
50	22.7	30	66
60	27.3	40	88
70	31.8	50	110
80	36.4	60	132
90	40.9	70	154
100	45.4	80	176
150	68.2	90	198
200	90.8	100	220

Reprinted from Flomenbaum and Roberts: *Emergency reference guide*, New York, 1993, Cahners.

NORMAL CARDIAC INTERVALS (SEC.)

P-R	0.12-0.20
QRS	0.06-0.10

Heart Rate/Min.	Q-T
60	0.33-0.43
70	0.31-0.41
80	0.29-0.38
90	0.28-0.36
100	0.27-0.35

Reprinted from F[illegible]nbaum and Roberts: *Emergency reference guide*, [illegible]

Emergency Diagnostic Testing

Emergency Diagnostic Testing

SECOND EDITION

Neal Flomenbaum, M.D.
Associate Professor of Clinical Medicine
State University of New York at Brooklyn
Chairman of Emergency Medicine
The Long Island College Hospital
Brooklyn, New York

Lewis Goldfrank, M.D.
Associate Professor of Clinical Medicine
New York University School of Medicine
Director of Emergency Medical Services
Bellevue and NYU Medical Centers
New York, New York

Sheldon Jacobson, M.D.
Professor and Chairman of Emergency Medicine
Mount Sinai School of Medicine
New York, New York

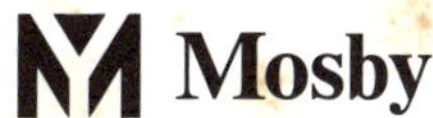

St. Louis Baltimore Berlin Boston Carlsbad Chicago London Madrid
Naples New York Philadelphia Sydney Tokyo Toronto

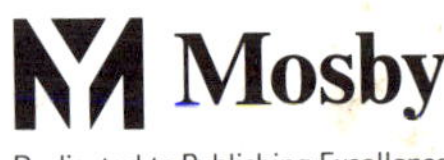

Dedicated to Publishing Excellence

Editor: Laurel Craven
Associate Developmental Editor: Wendy Buckwalter
Project Manager: Gayle Morris
Production Editor: Donna L. Walls
Manufacturing Supervisor: Karen Lewis
Cover design: GW Graphics

SECOND EDITION

Printed in the United States of America
Composition by Clarinda
Printing/binding by Maple-Vail-York

Mosby–Year Book, Inc.
11830 Westline Industrial Drive
St. Louis, Missouri 63146

Library of Congress Cataloging in Publication Data

Emergency diagnostic testing / [edited by] Neal Flomenbaum, Lewis Goldfrank, Sheldon Jacobson. — 2nd ed.
p. cm.
Rev. ed. of: Diagnostic testing in the emergency department. 1984
Includes bibliographical references and index.
ISBN 0-8151-3248-4
1. Medical emergencies—diagnosis. I. Flomenbaum, Neal,
II. Goldfrank, Lewis R. III. Jacobson, Sheldon,
IV. Diagnostic testing in the emergency department.
[DNLM: 1. Emergency Service, Hospital. 2. Diagnosis.
3. Diagnostic Tests, Routine, WX 215E5345 1994]
RC86.7.E5653 1994
616.07'5—dc20
DNLM/DLC
for Library of Congress 94-4538
CIP

94 95 96 97 98 / 9 8 7 6 5 4 3 2 1

Contributors

Jonathan Arden, M.D.
Clinical Assistant Professor of
Forensic Medicine
New York University School of Medicine and
State University of New York at Brooklyn;
First Deputy Chief Medical Examiner (Acting)
Office of Chief Medical Examiner
New York, New York

Theodore Benzer, M.D., Ph.D.
Instructor in Medicine
Harvard Medical School
Assistant in Emergency Medicine
Massachusetts General Hospital
Boston, Massachusetts

Daniel Brookoff, M.D., Ph.D.
Assistant Professor of Emergency Medicine
and Internal Medicine
University of Tennessee at Memphis
Attending Physician, Regional Medical Center
Memphis, Tennessee;
Associate Director of Medical Education
Methodist Hospitals of Memphis

Stephen V. Cantrill, M.D., F.A.C.E.P.
Associate Director,
Emergency Medical Services,
Denver General Hospital,
Denver, Colorado

Jeffrey Duchin, M.D.
Assistant Professor of Medicine
Attending Physician, Emergency Services
Hospital of the University of Pennsylvania
Philadelphia, Pennsylvania

Samuel Engel, M.D.
Clinical Assistant Professor of Medicine
Albert Einstein College of Medicine
Bronx, New York

Donald Feinfeld, M.D., FACP
Associate Professor of Medicine
State University of New York at Stony Brook
Co-Director of Nephrology
Nassau County Medical Center
East Meadow, New York

Leon Feldhamer, M.D.
Director of Ultrasonography
Maimonides Medical Hospital
Brooklyn, New York

Mark Flomenbaum, M.D., PhD.
Clinical Assistant Professor of
Forensic Medicine
New York University School of Medicine
City Medical Examiner
Office of Chief Medical Examiner
New York, New York

Neal Flomenbaum, M.D., F.A.C.P., F.A.C.E.P.
Associate Professor of Clinical Medicine
State University of New York at Brooklyn
Chairman,
Department of Emergency Medicine
The Long Island College Hospital
Consultant,
New York City and Long Island
Poison Centers
Brooklyn, New York

Stuart M. Garay, M.D., F.A.C.P., F.C.C.P.
Clinical Professor of Medicine
New York University School of Medicine
New York, New York

Lewis Goldfrank, M.D., F.A.C.P., F.A.C.E.P.
Associate Professor of Clinical Medicine
New York University School of Medicine
Director of Emergency Services
Bellevue and NYU Medical Centers
Medical Director
New York City Poison Center
New York, New York

Karen Hansen, M.D.
Associate Attending Physician
Suburban Hospital
Bethesda, Maryland

Mark C. Henry, M.D.
Associate Professor of Clinical Emergency
Medicine
Chairman of Emergency Medicine
State University of New York at Stony Brook
Stony Brook, New York

Mary Ann Howland, Pharm.D.
Clinical Professor of Pharmacy
St. John's University
Consultant
New York City Poison Center and
Bellevue Hospital Emergency Services
New York, New York

Sheldon Jacobson, M.D.
Professor and Chairman
Emergency Medicine
Mount Sinai School of Medicine
New York, New York

Gabor D. Kelen, M.D., F.A.C.E.P., F.R.C.P.
Professor and Chairman
Department of Emergency Medicine
Johns Hopkins University School of Medicine
Emergency Physician in Chief
The Johns Hopkins Hospital
Baltimore, Maryland

Itzhak Kronzon, M.D., F.A.C.P., F.A.C.C.
Professor of Medicine
New York University School of Medicine
Director, Non-Invasive Cardiology
NYU Medical Center
New York, New York

Richard Lanoix, M.D.
Assistant Director
Emergency Medicine Residency Training Program
Lincoln Hospital
Bronx, New York

Katherine Leonard, M.D.
Clinical Assistant Professor of Pediatrics
State University of New York at Brooklyn
Director, Pediatric Emergency Service
Department of Emergency Medicine
The Long Island College Hospital
Brooklyn, New York

Richard I. Levin, M.D., F.A.C.P., F.A.C.C.
Associate Professor of Medicine
New York University School of Medicine
Director
Laboratory for Cardiovascular Research
NYU Medical Center
New York, New York

Neal A. Lewin, M.D., F.A.C.P., F.A.C.E.P.
Assistant Professor of Clinical Medicine
New York University School of Medicine
Assistant Director of Emergency Services
Bellevue and NYU Hospitals
Consultant, New York City Poison Center
New York, New York

Thomas Manis, M.D.
Director, Dialysis Service
Division of Nephrology
Nassau County Medical Center
East Meadow, New York

Michelle A. Merchant, J.D.
Associate
Bower and Gardner
Health Care Law Group
New York, New York

Harold Mignott, M.D.
Assistant Professor of Emergency Medicine
University of Pennsylvania School of Medicine
Philadelphia, Pennsylvania

Wayne J. Olan, M.D.
Assistant Professor of Radiology
George Washington University Medical Center
Washington, D.C.

Harold Osborn, M.D., F.A.C.P., F.A.C.E.P.
Professor of Clinical Emergency Medicine
Acting Chairman of Emergency Medicine
New York Medical College
Chief of Service, Lincoln Hospital
Bronx, New York

Kevin Porter, J.D.
Partner
Parker Chapin Flattau & Klimpl
New York, New York

Frank Raymond, M.D.
Clinical Instructor
State University of New York at Brooklyn
Attending Physician
Department of Emergency Medicine
The Long Island College Hospital
Brooklyn, New York

Richard A. Rosen, M.D.
Associate Professor of Radiology
Albert Einstein College of Medicine
Director, Department of Radiology
Bronx-Lebanon Hospital Center
Bronx, New York

Marc R. Salzberg, M.D.
Chairman
Emergency Medicine
Baystate Medical Center
Springfield, Massachusetts

Miguel R. Sanchez, M.D.
Assistant Professor of Dermatology
New York University School of Medicine
Attending-in-Chief
Dermatology Outpatient Services
Bellevue Hospital
New York, New York

Stephen Alan Senreich, M.D., F.A.C.O.G., F.A.C.S.
Assistant Clinical Professor in Obstetrics and Gynecology
Albert Einstein College of Medicine
Bronx, New York
Attending Physician
Long Island Jewish Medical Center
New Hyde Park, New York

Harry Shamoon, M.D.
Professor of Medicine
Albert Einstein College of Medicine
Bronx, New York

Karl Verebey, Ph.D., DABFT
Director of Toxicology
New York State Institute for Basic Research

Carmen Warner, MSN, R.N., M.A.T., F.A.A.N.
Editor
Topics in Emergency Medicine
Publishing Consultant
San Diego, California

Stephen P. Waxman, M.D.
Clinical Assistant Professor of Surgery
New York University School of Medicine
Assistant Director of Emergency Services
Bellevue Hospital Center
New York, New York

William A. Weiner, D.O.
Fellow in Neuroradiology
State University of New York at Stony Brook
Stony Brook, New York

Richard Weisman, Pharm.D., A.B.A.T.
Research Associate Professor of Pediatrics
Miami University School of Medicine
Director
Florida Poison Center--Miami
Miami, Florida

TO

the physicians, nurses, physician assistants, nurse practitioners,
emergency medical technicians, paramedics and staffs
of the six hospital emergency departments
where the questions about diagnostic testing
became the basis for this book

AND TO

my wife Meredith
my son Adam
my mother Mollie Wexler Flomenbaum
and especially my father Lieutenant H. Stanley Flomenbaum USNR, (Ret.)
Without their active ongoing encouragement, this book would not have been possible

N.F.

my supportive family
who also recognizes the many ways we can improve emergency health care

L.G.

my wife Dianna
who is able to make the correct diagnosis without laboratory data and often via telephone

S.J.

Preface

Almost ten years have elapsed since the first edition of this book appeared as *Diagnostic Testing in the Emergency Department.* The strongly positive response it received, as well as the frequent requests by our students and residents to update, expand, and reissue the book, motivated us to undertake this second edition. To make the book more meaningful, we have refocused the contents, concentrating on the interpretation and use of laboratory test results available to the emergency physician, and eliminating those chapters primarily concerned with procedures and techniques. To make the book more useful as a reference guide, we have added a significant amount of illustrative material, particularly to the Urinalysis and Dermatologic Testing chapters.

Virtually all of the chapters have been significally rewritten and/or expanded, and new chapters have been added on blood chemistries (Chapter 4), gastrointestinal evaluation (Chapter 14), skin tests (Chapter 15), body fluids (Chapter 16), the random needle stick (Chapter 17), nuclear medicine (Chapter 20), interacting with the Medical Examiner (Chapter 23), and decision analysis and cost containment (Chapter 25).

We have resisted the temptation to allow the text to become more "advanced" with our own interests and experience, choosing instead to write and edit this book for all of the residents and attending physicians who would like to have a fairly comprehensive overview of currently available emergency diagnostic tests and specific advice on their indications and usefulness. We have also retained and expanded the number of cases throughout the book to make the text more relevant and more interesting.

With this edition, Sheldon Jacobson, M.D. joins us as an editor. In the 1970's Dr. Jacobson started the first emergency medicine residency in New York State and the first paramedic program in New York City. Between 1979 and 1992, he served as Director of Emergency Services at the Hospital of the University of Pennsylvania and Associate Professor of Medicine and Surgery at the University of Pennsylvania before returning to his New York City "roots."

There are only two types of contributors to this book: those who practice Emergency Medicine and those who practice with those who practice Emergency Medicine. The second group of practitioners admirably represent the generation of physicians from other specialties and subspecialties who have spent most or all of their professional lives working with emergency physicians. They have a clear appreciation of the role of the emergency physician and an equally clear understanding of the many ways we can all interact with one another in the best interests of our patients. It has been a distinct privilege and pleasure to work with each and all of the contributors to this edition and if this edition meets with the same success as the first, we promise not to wait ten more years for the next edition.

In preparing a book such as this, it is not possible to adequately thank everyone who contributed in a significant way to its appearance. Nevertheless, we would like to acknowledge the efforts of Meredith Altman RNP for reviewing parts of the manuscript, the initial efforts of James Shanahan for arranging for Mosby–Year Book to publish the second edition and the continued efforts of Laurel Craven, Lauranne Billus, Wendy Buckwalter, and Donna Walls of Mosby–Year Book for handling the myriad of technical and editorial problems as they arose. We gratefully acknowledge the invaluable assistance of Gabriel Bakcsy, Director; George Wahlert, Reference Librarian; and Maria Vega, Library Clerk of the Morgan Library of The Long Island College Hospital. Finally, we would like to thank Ida Grant, Administrative Secretary of the Department of Emergency Medicine, of The Long Island College Hospital, for faithfully transforming major portions of this manuscript into the book you have before you.

Neal Flomenbaum
Lewis Goldfrank
Sheldon Jacobson

Introduction to first edition

In Emergency Medicine, we consider careful triage, an excellent history and physical examination, and simple, rapidly available, reliable, and definitive tests the hallmarks of high quality, expeditious care. In the short amount of time we have available as emergency department providers, we must establish a strong patient bond that supports, reassures, and assists.

The Emergency Department is not impoverished for equipment, but the limited time and the extensive demands make quick and accurate clinical reflexes vital tools. This work attempts to define the technical skills that a good emergency department physician should have. It describes some of the methods of clinical assessment that are valuable in making a correct diagnosis, but it is not meant to portray the emergency department physician as bound to a particular technique or laboratory skill. Written by persons closely involved with emergency care as primary providers or consultants, this book describes thought processes and technical skills utilized in the daily practice of emergency medicine. The approaches represent sound knowledge and are not experimental or academic; the techniques are valuable or essential to practice high quality emergency care anywhere in America today.

Finally, the techniques emphasized in this book represent a technical core curriculum of sorts for achieving excellence of care by precisely defining problems in the Emergency Department. Yet, in spite of their importance, we emphasize again that the history and physical examination are the hallmarks of quality emergency care; most critical decisions must still be made through the skillful social and verbal interchange with patient and family. Although we generally regard an abnormal laboratory finding as something requiring an explanation or further investigation—even in the absence of historical or physical evidence of disease—ultimately, we are forced to recognize two basic principles of emergency care: (1) laboratory data do not define a clinical condition or quality of existence, and (2) a patient who looks sick is sick regardless of the normalcy of the laboratory data.

Contents

PART VI

MedicoLegal and Forensic Considerations

PART VII

Planning and Cost Considerations

APPENDICES

Emergency Diagnostic Testing

PART I

Emergency Diagnostic Testing

Chapter 1

Diagnostic Testing in the Emergency Department

Neal Flomenbaum, M.D.

Lewis Goldfrank, M.D.

Sheldon Jacobson, M.D.

To be useful, a diagnostic test must satisfy several criteria: the test must provide information not readily obtainable by history or physical examination alone or must confirm information not conclusively established by these means; the test must be sensitive enough to include the diagnosis and/or be specific enough to exclude one or more possibilities from the differential diagnosis; the test's performance must not subject the patient to any risk or, if there is a risk, the risk must be less than is the presumed benefit and also be otherwise unavoidable. To be useful to an *emergency physician* a diagnostic test must satisfy at least one additional criterion: the test results must be available soon enough to affect emergency department (ED) decisions. Such decisions include whether to admit the patient to the hospital and whether treatment must be started in the ED or may safely be deferred until the condition is further evaluated.

The availability of a test result within the relatively short amount of time emergency physicians have to interact with patients is what defines "emergency diagnostic testing" and what separates it from "diagnostic testing in the emergency department." Almost all of the following chapters are concerned with the selection and use of diagnostic tests that are critical to *emergency department* diagnosis and treatment. Clearly, however, considerably more diagnostic tests are initiated in the ED than are necessary for the emergency physician to function effectively. These additional tests include "routine" testing batteries, such as automated blood chemistry profiles (e.g., "SMAC", "SMA-7", "SMA-18"), "standard admission tests" for a medical service or "pre-operative" tests for a surgical service and screening tests, such as those for tuberculosis (e.g., "PPD", admission chest radiograph) or syphilis (e.g., VDRL, RPR). Lundberg [1] recorded 35 different answers to the question, "Why do physicians order laboratory tests?" (see box), and in a study by Wertman and colleagues,[2] diagnosis, monitoring, and screening were given as the most frequent reasons. Before discussing those tests which are essential to an emergency physician, it may be useful to consider briefly this larger group of tests requested for screening, monitoring, or "admission," and to examine both the extent to which they contribute to the overall care of the ED patient and the extent to which they negatively affect the care of other patients by using the limited diagnostic resources available in most EDs.

Why Do Physicians Order Laboratory Tests?*

Confirmation of clinical opinion	CYA (in Munich)
Diagnosis	Documentation
Monitoring	Personal profit
Screening	Hospital profit
Prognosis	Attempt to defraud
Unavailability of previous result	Research
Previous abnormal result	Curiosity
Question of accuracy of previous result	Insecurity
Patient-family pressure	Frustration at nothing else to do
Peer pressure	To buy time
Pressure from recent articles	Hunting (in Fresno, Cal) or fishing (in Seattle) expeditions
Personal reassurance	To establish baseline
Patient-family reassurance	To complete a data base
Public relations	Personal education
Ease of performance with ready availability	To report to an attending physician
Hospital policy	Habit
Legal requirement	Others
Medicolegal need	

*From Lundberg AD: Preservation of laboratory test ordering: a syndrome affecting clinicians, *JAMA* 1983; 249:639.

"ROUTINE" ADMISSION TESTS

When the decision to admit a patient to an adult medical service has been made on the basis of the history, the physical examination, or a particular abnormal test result(s), several other "routine" tests are almost always requested at, or soon after, admission. Whether these tests are typically initiated in the ED or after the patient arrives on the medical service or special care unit usually depends on several factors such as efficiency, overall hospital staffing, local (hospital) custom, and the effect that initiating such tests in the ED will have on other patients.

"Standard" diagnostic tests required by adult medical services typically include urinalysis, complete blood count (CBC), blood urea nitrogen (BUN), serum glucose and electrolytes, a chest radiograph (CXR), and an electrocardiogram (ECG).

Some medical services also request a prothrombin time (PT), partial thromboplastin time (PTT), erythrocyte sedimentation rate (ESR), and a serologic test for syphilis (VDRL, RPR). Except for those tests specifically indicated by the patient's complaints, routine admission tests serve either as "screening" tests or to establish baseline values for future reference, particularly when a disease or treatment is expected to alter one or more of the normal laboratory parameters. Other screening procedures routinely performed on or soon after admission include a stool guaiac test and a tuberculin skin test (PPD).

The rationale for such admission testing or screening is perhaps best expressed in the following statement:

> . . . screening tests are usually limited to simple, less expensive procedures that can detect medically significant abnormalities with a high prevalence in the general population. The blood count . . . and urinalysis . . . are done so frequently to supplement the history and physical examination, that they may be considered essential components of an initial evaluation. This type of laboratory information is considered a part of the "data base". . .[3]

Similar thoughts are expressed in other comprehensive textbooks of internal medicine,[4] although current editions of most medical texts now also emphasize the lack of a statistical basis for universal screening batteries.[5] Driven perhaps by dual concerns over the high cost of health care and numerous studies reporting no benefit from most screening tests, the current trend is to question both the usefulness and necessity of routine admission screening tests.[5]

More disturbing than the question of which (if any) admission screening tests should be obtained, is evidence demonstrating that when an unexpectedly abnormal result *is* reported on a screening battery, physicians tend to pay little attention to it and so such an abnormality results in a diagnosis only infrequently.[6,7]

Another disadvantage of routinely obtaining admission screening tests in the ED is the assumption by the in-service physicians and staff that the tests were done even if circumstances in the ED did not allow for it in a particular patient. When this occurs, a test that should have been done soon after admission may *not* be done until its absence becomes problematic. Few charts *reliably* indicate tests *not* done, and many clinicians assume charting may not accurately reflect all of the tests which were initiated in the ED.

There are many valid reasons for not obtaining routine screening tests in the ED, nevertheless, in most hospitals the quickest and, in some cases, even the most efficient means of obtaining tests is from the ED. If this is true, requesting those tests which predictably may be necessary during admission *in the ED* may have significant benefits with respect to timely diagnosis, treatment, and overall length of stay. An ECG obtained in the ED on a middle-aged or elderly patient admitted early Friday afternoon and interpreted by the cardiologist later in the day may identify a significant but unexpected or contributing problem before the weekend instead of afterwards, when the ECG technician obtains a routine "admission" ECG Monday morning.

PREOPERATIVE ADMISSION TESTS

When a patient is admitted from the ED for urgent or emergent surgery such as an appendectomy or herniorraphy, which laboratory tests should be requested in the ED in the absence of any specific indications for those tests? Very few answers to this question are currently available in either the emergency medicine literature or the surgery and anesthesiology literature and, at best, some extrapolation from currently available data is necessary.

Most current textbooks of surgery and anesthesiology recommend that patients have the following preoperative tests: UA, CBC (with platelets), BUN, glucose and electrolytes, CXR, and, for patients over 45 years of age, an ECG. Additionally, many texts suggest clotting tests, a PT, and a PTT.[8] As in the case of routine admission tests, however, there is no scientific justification or substantiation for most of these recommendations.[8]

The following criteria have been suggested for selecting appropriate routine preoperative tests: (1) the condition must significantly affect the morbidity or mortality associated with surgery or must represent significant risk to those associated with the patient's care, and (2) preoperative diagnosis must be more beneficial to management than would be a diagnosis established in the perioperative or postoperative periods.[8] However, these criteria may be too broad to be applicable to the individual patient. Moreover, in some cases, using diagnostic testing to assess significant risk to those associated with the patient's care may be *technically* possible but *legally* impossible or impractical—whereas testing a patient for tuberculosis out of concern for the resurgence of the disease, and particularly the appearance of resistant strains, can be accomplished without restrictions almost anywhere, it is generally not possible to routinely test a patient for HIV infection without specific consent from the patient and without instituting extensive precautions to protect the patient's confidentiality.

Numerous studies may be cited to demonstrate the lack of usefulness of routine preoperative laboratory screening in otherwise healthy patients.[9–12] However, most patients admitted for surgery *from the ED* are not healthy. In a recent review article on preoperative laboratory testing, subtitled "Should Any Tests be Routine before Surgery?," Macpherson[9] carefully differentiated between elective and emergency surgery, noting that "the decision to order preoperative tests in patients before *emergency* surgery is different from elective surgery as abnormalities in patients undergoing emergency procedures are likely common, making routine testing more justifiable."

Middle-aged or elderly patients in this country are at a significant risk for undiagnosed coronary artery disease. In certain areas of the country, tuberculosis and/or HIV infection may be prevalent; a very high percentage of patients who are victims of all forms of trauma (e.g., blunt, penetrating, motor-vehicle–related) have substantial exposure to alcohol or drugs that may significantly affect management. Ultimately, routine preoperative admission testing standards for a particular ED and hospital must take all of these variables into consideration.

SPECIFIC TESTS

Radiologic Evaluations

Of all the routine tests questioned during the past few decades, none has received more attention than have radiologic evaluations, particularly plain film evaluations of the chest, abdomen, and skull. The reasons for this attention are understandable: radiologic studies are more expensive and more time-consuming; they interfere with ongoing care of the patient; and they may delay care of other patients. Finally, because they are not completely "noninvasive" from a teratogenic or carcinogenic perspective, risk-benefit arguments become applicable as well. Many of the more recent studies on the role of routine radiologic examinations appear in the emergency medicine literature and therefore include the variables that define patients who are evaluated and treated in the ED setting.

Routine Chest Radiographs

In a 1986 review examining the literature on admission and preoperative chest radiography, Tape and Mushlin[13] noted that historically, the major reason for obtaining routine CXRs on all hospital admissions was to identify patients with clinically silent pulmonary tuberculosis. The authors presented evidence that such routine radiography was not indicated for either admission or preoperative evaluation. However, some cities in this country are currently experiencing epidemics of tuberculosis, in some cases involving strains resistant to all previously effective antimicrobials. For this reason and also because many patients with clinically inapparent tuberculosis or pneumocystis pneumonia are infected with HIV but cannot be tested directly for HIV (see above), routine admission CXRs may once again be indicated in some hospitals.

Even apart from the issues raised by HIV, the situation is still not straightforward: the authors of two studies conducted in Veterans Administration (VA) hospitals in the 1980s appeared to reach opposite conclusions with respect to the usefulness of admission CXRs: in a 1981 study[14] of routine chest films obtained on 113 patients admitted to general medical wards, 46% (52 films) revealed abnormal acute and chronic findings, suggesting to the authors that routine admission chest radiography was necessary for hospitals with a prevalence of patients with intrathoracic disease. However, 4 years later, in another VA study[15] involving patients admitted to a medical service from the ED, although 106 abnormalities on 294 routine films were found, only 12 resulted in a change of therapy. Of those 12, only 4 were not identified by history or physical examination. These authors concluded that the effect of routine admission CXRs on patient care is very small, even in a population with a high prevalence of cardiopulmonary disease. They recommended not ordering CXRs solely because of admission.[15]

In a study of 125 consecutive hospital admissions for acute bronchospasm, Aronson and colleagues[16] found that routine admission CXRs in people with uncomplicated asthma may be unnecessary. People with uncomplicated asthma were defined as those with no known history of underlying conditions such as recent fever or chills, immune suppression, cancer, IV drug use, previous thoracic surgery, cardiac disease, or other pulmonary disease. All other cases of asthma were considered complicated. By categorizing asthmatic patients in this manner, the authors were able to isolate all admission CXRs affecting management (13 of 44) to the group with complicated asthma.

Applying the same criteria *prospectively* to adult ED patients admitted with obstructive airway disease, the group[17] again demonstrated that the use of a simple clinical strategy could safely reduce the number of chest radiographs in patients with uncomplicated acute exacerbations of obstructive airway disease, thereby decreasing both health care costs and exposure to ionizing radiation.

In his review of preoperative laboratory testing, Macpherson[9] summarized the findings of 17 studies of preoperative chest radiography, "Although the relationship between chest radiograph findings and perioperative morbidity is not well-defined, unanticipated findings are common, especially in the elderly." Macpherson[9] recommended a preoperative chest radiograph for all patients 60 years of age or older and for those under 60 with evidence of likely chest disease from history or physical examination.

The need for chest radiography in evaluating ED patients for pneumonia (regardless of whether or not they are admitted) has been examined in several recent studies, also with mixed conclusions by the authors. Gennis and colleagues[18] again attempted to identify sensitive clinical criteria for diagnosing pneumonia in a prospective study of 308 adult patients, of whom 118 were considered to have pneumonia. Although no single symptom or sign reliably predicted pneumonia, abnormal vital signs—a temperature of more than 37.8° C (100° F), a pulse above 100/min, or respirations greater than 20/min—were 97% sensitive for detecting pneumonia. After a retrospective chart review of 464 chest roentgenograms of adult patients demonstrating 129 cases of pneumonia and 45 other abnormalities, Heckerling[19] concluded that no symptom, sign, or laboratory finding evaluated could reliably predict the presence of pneumonia, but that the absence of abnormal auscultatory findings on lung examination excluded pneumonia with greater than 95% certainty. By stratifying adults with acute respiratory complaints without CHF on the basis of clinical variables, Heckerling[19] also concluded that patients with acute asthma do not routinely require roentgenograms because they rarely have pneumonia, but that patients *with dementia and a history suggesting respiratory infection require roentgenograms.* Almost 76% of such patients had pneumonia in the study.

To compare physicians' judgement regarding the necessity of obtaining CXRs to four "decision rules" (including the two above), Emerman and colleagues[20] prospectively studied 290 adult patients, of whom 21 had pneumonia. They concluded that physicians' diagnostic and therapeutic decisions were characterized by high sensitivity but lower specificity for ordering chest radiographs to diagnose pneumonia. The sensitivity of physician judgement, as expected, exceeded all four decision rules, but the higher specificity and accuracy of two of the decision rules—those of Gennis and colleagues[18] and Heckerling[19]—suggested to the authors that they may have a role in patient evaluation.

Finally, after reviewing 5000 ED CXRs of patients 16 years old or greater, Buenger[21] found that they revealed serious disease in 35% of patients with chest symptoms, 18% of patients with noncardiorespiratory symptoms, and 27% of all patients examined. Asthma (14%) and trauma (5%) presented the *lowest* incidence of significant findings. He concluded that, "the chest radiograph continues to be a significantly important examination in the diagnosis of disease, the prevention of overtreatment and the redirection of clinical investigation in the acute care emergency department unit."[21]

Considering all of these studies, it appears that the pendulum has swung back somewhat from the extreme position advocated by many a decade ago of trying to eliminate virtually all routine admission and preoperative chest radiographs. Increasing numbers of elderly and immunocompromised patients (as well as psychotic, demented, homeless, and uncooperative patients) of all ages certainly make routine admission ED chest radiography more reasonable now in the absence of specific indications. However, one other factor should always be considered in deciding whether or not to obtain a routine chest radiograph and that is the interval since the last CXR was obtained. For example, an asthmatic seen frequently for exacerbations does not need a CXR with each visit.

Electrocardiograms

Physicians usually obtain ECGs in the ED for one of three reasons: (1) to aid in the diagnosis of an acute problem under consideration, such as a myocardial infarction or dysrhythmia; (2) as a routine admission test to screen for silent cardiac disease; or (3) to establish a baseline for routine ECG comparisons when, for example, chest pain develops in the future or if a patient is to be started on cyclic antidepressants, phenothiazines, or lithium.

According to Hoffman and Igarashi,[22] neither current nor comparison ECGs altered the ultimate decision of whether or not to admit to a coronary care unit a patient who sought treatment for chest pain or chest pain equivalents such as neck, jaw, or arm pain. The authors prospectively studied 100 consecutive adult patients triaged to a monitored unit between 8 AM and 8 PM because of these complaints. Of the 84 patients analyzed, 39 were admitted to the CCU, 37 were discharged, and 8 were admitted to an ICU or ward. Of the patients admitted to the CCU, a current ECG influenced *house officers* to favor admission of only two patients whom they had previously planned to discharge. No physician altered a decision to admit a patient on the basis of comparison ECGs. Of the patients who were discharged, this decision was the result of a current ECG only once in the case of a *resident* who initially favored admission. A comparison ECG also influenced the decision to discharge a patient once. The opinions of the triage nurses following only a brief evaluation and without ECGs were 83% sensitive and 76% specific, with a positive predictive value of 75% and a negative predictive value of 85% when compared with the ultimate decision. Although the authors concluded that an ECG need not be obtained in many patients with acute chest pain or when the clinical likelihood of acute myocardial ischemia or infarction is small, they cautioned against over-extending the results of their study. Specifically, they point out that ECGs are *necessary* for certain scoring systems to predict prognosis, for determining the need for specific interventions such as thrombolytic therapy, and for ultimately establishing the diagnosis (using serial ECGs) when enzyme findings are equivocal.[22]

An earlier retrospective review[23] of the value of baseline ECGs in the evaluation of acute cardiac complaints revealed that 195 out of 236 patients seeking treatment for chest pain had clinical or ECG findings sufficiently diagnostic that the baseline ECG could not have affected the decision to hospitalize or discharge the patient, and that in only 11 cases would a baseline ECG have helped to avoid an unnecessary admission *if it had been available*. Thus, the routine ECG had little value as a baseline for future comparison when patients later developed chest pain.

The usefulness of routine admission ECGs was evaluated in a prospective study of 1410 patients admitted to a general medical service from the emergency department, clinics, and other hospitals.[24] Of the 1410 patients, 775 had no indication for an ECG by history or physical examination. Fifty-two admission ECGs (8 of those with no indication) added new information to what was already known from the history and physical examination. Of the 31 new diagnoses established by the ECGs, 28 involved a change in management. Additionally, 21 ECGs suggested a new diagnosis, of which 13 proved correct. A routine ECG on admission added information that was usually diagnostic and beneficial in 4% of patients. The yield ranged from 8.4% in patients over 45 years with evident cardiac abnormalities to 0.4% in patients under 45 with no evidence of cardiac abnormalties. The increased yield of the ECG in patients older than 45 years of age was of only borderline statistical significance when adjusted for the presence of a cardiac abnormality. Among patients without cardiac abnormalities, ECG yield was 1.0% overall. The authors[24] concluded that an admission ECG infrequently added new information but was useful when it did, and that admission ECGs are as cost effective as many accepted medical practices.

A similar recent retrospective study[25] examining routine admission ECGs exclusively in patients admitted from an ED, and including patients admitted to intensive care settings, reported similar findings in that only 3 (1.5%) of the 202 ECGs obtained without identifiable indication resulted in a change of management, and none affected the outcome. Also, none of the 45 patients who did not have any indication for an admission ECG and, in fact, did *not* have an admission ECG taken, experienced an identifiable adverse consequence during hospitalization.

The study by Moorman and colleagues[24] also reviewed the literature on routine preoperative ECGs and concluded that the ECG was frequently abnormal but that it was unclear whether the ECG either added information not previously known or affected management. In his review of preoperative laboratory testing, Macpherson[9] summarized the data from six studies of preoperative ECG abnormalities. He concluded that ECG abnormalities are both common and age related and, because some abnormalties have been shown to be related to important perioperative morbidity, recommended a routine ECG before elective surgery in all patients over 40 years of age.

Admission Urinalysis

Of 123 urinalyses (UAs) ordered for no recognizable medical indications on patients admitted to the internal medicine wards of a university teaching hospital, 42 produced abnormal results and led to additional testing in 20 cases.[26] However, the results of 17 of the repeat UAs were normal, and the abnormal findings (pyuria) resulted in a change in therapy for only 3 patients; moreover, 2 of the changes were considered to be probably unnecessary. When the UA was ordered for diagnostic purposes as opposed to routinely, the percentage of abnormalities detected was much higher (80% versus 34%). The authors[26] of this retrospective study concluded that there was little justification for routinely ordering this test on admission.

Kroenke and colleagues[27] reviewed 1607 admission UAs, of which 746 were considered routine. Only 45 of the routine UAs revealed abnormalities that led to diagnostic action and of those 45 urines, 18 were normal on repeat testing and 17 were considered insignificant. Again, pyuria represented the largest number of abnormalities affecting therapy (eight of ten), and six of the eight cases of "pyuria" (defined as three or more WBCs per high-power field) proved to be asymptomatic *bacteriuria*.[27]

Complete Blood Count and Leukocyte Differential Count

Shapiro and Greenfield[28] considered the evidence that the CBC and leukocyte differential count (DIF) contribute to patient care in four clinical situations, including (1) case findings on admissions to the hospital, and (2) testing for suspected abnormalities. They concluded that the CBC and DIF are clearly indicated when a patient is admitted for surgery that may involve more than minor blood loss or if an infection or hematologic disorder is suspected. They suggest that the tests are not necessary for otherwise well patients undergoing surgical procedures associated with minimal blood loss or as an admission test for nonsurgical patients when the probability of an abnormality is very low and if the information obtained will not affect diagnosis or therapy.[28] However, the authors note that no study has evaluated the tests adequately as routine admission tests for patients hospitalized on nonsurgical services.

In testing for suspected abnormalities, Shapiro and Greenfield[28] recommended a CBC when there are clinical findings suggestive of anemia (e.g., fatigue, conjunctival pallor, or peripheral neuropathy), abnormal bleeding, polycythemia, or another primary hematologic disorder.

After reviewing the records of 172 patients with abnormal white blood counts (WBCs), Callaham[29] found that the total leukocyte count, the neutrophil count, and the band (immature polymorphonuclear leukocyte) count did not reliably distinguish between bacterial, nonbacterial, and noninfectious disease. He concluded that the WBC does not reliably predict either the severity or the cause of disease in acutely ill adults, and its use as a screening test in that setting probably should be abandoned. The predictive value for bacterial disease was 26% for a WBC equal to or over 12,500/mm^3 and 39% for bands equal to or over 1000/mm^3. As the author notes, an acutely ill adult in the study with an elevated WBC and a shift to the left was still more likely to have a viral or noninfectious disease then a bacterial disease.[29] Similar low benefits from WBCs and DIFs have been found in many clinical series. A study of preoperative cases that included 610 CBCs and 390 DIFs yielded only 2 abnormal CBC results and 1 abnormal DIF among the tests done without specific indications; none of the abnormal findings had any clinical consequences.[10] In a retrospective review of 475 outpatient (not ED) DIFs ordered without an apparent clinical indication, none of the 63 abnormal DIFs resulted in the discovery of any clinically apparent disease.[30]

Admission Prothrombin Times

Erban and colleagues[31] examined how commonly and for what reason the PT and APTT tests were requested routinely for admission to the medical service of a major teaching hospital. They found that 81% of all patients admitted had a PT and APTT test requested and that at least 70% of the tests were not clinically indicated according to modified guidelines developed by the Blue Cross and Blue Shield Association and endorsed by the American College of Physicians. Of the 72% of patients admitted *via the ED* who had a PT and APTT requested, few had invasive procedures performed during their hospitalizations, and the authors concluded that the pattern of high use in the ED was probably "due to habit."[31]

The use of the PT and APTT as a means of detecting occult liver disease, based primarily on rapid turnaround time when compared with other LFTs, probably accounts for the high percentage of tests ordered in the ED in the study by Erban and colleagues.[31] However, in an earlier study, Eisenberg and Goldfarb[32] determined that of 107 prothrombin screening tests, only 1 was abnormal, and even in 73 patients with a history of alcoholism, only 1 PT was abnormal. They too concluded that routine PTs should not be used as a screening test to detect occult liver disease or coagulation defects.

Erythrocyte Sedimentation Rate

When an ESR is requested in the ED, it is frequently for one of two reasons: (1) as a routine admission test to help determine how sick an *admitted* patient is, and (2) as a means of helping to determine whether an ED patient with equivocal findings requires admission (e.g., attempting to differentiate between acute and chronic illness or bacterial and viral infection). During the 1980s and 1990s the ESR received considerable attention in the clinical literature,[33–38] and almost all authors found the test not useful as a screening test for the presence of disease in asymptomatic patients. As Bedell and Bush[33] concluded, because the sensitivity is low or unknown for most infectious, inflammatory, and malignant conditions, judicious clinicians would not use the ESR as a screening test or a test to rule out a disorder.

Although not useful as a diagnostic test because of its low sensitivity and because of the large number of different diseases associated with a markedly elevated value, the ESR may be useful as a "sickness index."[33] When used as a sickness index, the specificity of an ESR of 100 mm/hr or more was greater than 99% (i.e., 877 of 881), and the positive predictive value was 90% (i.e., only 10%, or 4 of 42 patients had no identifiable cause) according to Fincher and Page.[36]

The problem with trying to use the ESR as a general sickness index in the ED is that the prevalence of ESR values greater than 100 is low—1 to 2 for every 100 determinations.[33] Thus, even though the cost per test is low, requesting the test indiscriminantly will make the cost per positive result extremely high. However, the ESR can be useful in certain situations that occur in the ED:

1. Diagnosing bacterial endocarditis. In this instance the sensitivity is known to be high—93%, according to Bedell and Bush.[33]
2. Diagnosing temporal arteritis and monitoring treatment response.[34]
3. Diagnosing metastases in a patient with known cancer. When the ESR is more than 100 mm/hr, metastases are usually present, but a normal or low ESR does not exclude either cancer or metastases.[34]
4. Identifying serious illness in IV drug users with fevers. An ESR equal to or more than 100 mm/hr had a specificity of 96% in 106 IV drug users aged 18 or over with fevers at or above 37.8°C[38]; in the study the ESR was the only variable consistently associated with illness severity, and the frequency of serious disease among febrile IV drug users was 72%. In this setting, the ESR could only be used to help identify serious disease, *never* to exclude it.[38]
5. Identifying a high or low likelihood of new disease in clinically ill, elderly patients with a decline in health status. The ESR was most useful among patients in whom the probability of disease was moderate following the initial history and examination.[35]

Outpatient Blood Cultures

Because of the frequent attempts by hospital utilization review committees, peer review organizations, and government and private insurers to reduce or eliminate unnecessary admissions, much pressure is often brought to bear on emergency physicians to not admit patients for the purpose of excluding or "ruling out" particular diseases. Myocardial infarctions and such bacterial infections as endocarditis, bacteremia, and sepsis are common clinical problems that often cannot be diagnosed during the time the patient is in the ED. The role of routine, or base-line, ECGs in the ED was discussed on pages 6 and 7. The role of outpatient blood cultures is considered here.

When Eisenberg and colleagues[39] examined the use of routine blood cultures to detect bacteremia in febrile outpatients in the 1970s, they found that bacteremia was present in only 1 of the 123 patients who were not admitted to the hospital, compared with its presence in 9 of 86 patients who were admitted. Because positive cultures were found so infrequently, the authors concluded that obtaining routine blood cultures to screen febrile adult outpatients was unnecessary. However, in 1987 when Sklar and Rusnak[40] assessed the value of adult blood cultures by a retrospective chart review of 411 cases, they found that bacteremia was subsequently identified in 5 of the 86 patients who were not admitted. Three (or four) of the five had endocarditis, one of whom was an intravenous (IV) drug user and these authors concluded that blood cultures are helpful in detecting endocarditis and other bacteremic conditions before obvious signs develop.

The increased positive yield in the second study compared to the one published a decade earlier may reflect the above considerations (that is, a higher incidence of obtaining outpatient blood cultures on patients who previously would have been admitted), more discriminate use of blood cultures in outpatients, or both. The role of outpatient blood cultures in the management of febrile children has been more clearly defined in the past decade and is further discussed in Chapter 16. In adults, outpatient blood cultures may, in fact, be helpful in avoiding unnecessary admissions of some asymptomatic febrile patients with risk factors for endocarditis, but wider use may be problematic for several reasons:

First, it may be impossible to recall the patient because of difficulties establishing contact—a particular concern with respect to febrile IV drug users. Second, by the time contact is established, a patient may be partially or fully treated with the correct antibiotic(s), and so the physician may be faced with the choice of admitting a well patient or of drawing yet another set of outpatient blood cultures. For example, if a urinary tract infection is diagnosed, blood cultures are obtained, and afterwards the patient is deemed well enough (and reliable enough) to take oral antibiotics at home, what should be done if the blood cultures are later reported to be positive when the patient is improving and back at work? (This consideration arose in one of Sklar's five blood culture–positive outpatients.[40]) Perhaps one may argue that obtaining blood cultures before antibiotic therapy is begun is beneficial for a patient who does not respond fully to treatment because antibiotic therapy may significantly affect blood culture positivity.[41] However, the enormous costs and low yields would make this practice prohibitive in all but the most serious clinical situations.

A third problem with obtaining outpatient blood cultures is the occurrence of false positive results because of accidental contamination. The study by Sklar and Rusnak[40] included 20 contaminants (4.9%) of the 411 blood cultures drawn from both admitted patients and outpatients. In another study[42] of 8467 culture specimens collected in the emergency department of a large urban teaching hospital, 421 (4.97%) were considered to be contaminated (6.25% when povidine-iodine was used as a skin antiseptic and 3.74% when iodine tincture was used). The difficulties and expense of dealing with such false positives in an outpatient population is easy to envision.

More problematic than these three factors, however, is deciding on the selection criteria for the appropriate use (if any) of outpatient blood cultures. On the one hand, three different groups concluded that physicians' judgment could not reliably distinguish bacteremic from nonbacteremic adults[40] or symptomatic IV drug users with endocarditis from those without endocarditis.[43,44] In addition, Young and colleagues[44] concluded that attempts to prospectively use total WBCs and DIFs to discriminate between the two groups of IV drug users will not succeed, and Marantz and colleagues[43] concluded that all IV drug users appearing in an ED with fever need to be hospitalized.

Conversely, if one firmly believes that there is no role for outpatient blood cultures, then how does one prevent this belief from becoming a self-fulfilling prophecy? In other words, if all patients for whom blood cultures are indicated should be admitted, then by definition no one who is considered well enough to go home should have cultures drawn and if this is the case, how many patients sent home are in fact bacteremic? Perhaps only a prospective study requiring blood cultures of all patients with fevers in the ED over a period of time can begin to answer this question.

Electrolytes

Requesting an electrolyte panel such as an SMA-6 consisting of BUN, glucose, sodium, potassium, chloride, and bicarbonate (or CO_2 content), or an SMA-7, which also includes creatinine, is so common an ED practice that adult patients are rarely admitted to an internal medicine service without one.[45] Nevertheless, the percentage of routine admission or screening electrolyte tests revealing a clinically significant abnormal value is exceedingly small.[45–49]

A recent study[49] strongly challenges the inclusion of electrolyte determinations as a screening test in ED patients. Lowe and colleagues[49, 50] tested the predictive value of a set of previously developed criteria[50] for detecting clinically significant electrolyte abnormalities.[49] The 10 criteria evaluated were poor oral intake, vomiting, chronic hypertension, diuretic use, seizure activity, muscle weakness, age of or more than 65, alcoholism, abnormal mental status, and a recent history of electrolyte abnormality. Although 730 out of 982 patients had 1 or more electrolytes out of the normal range for the laboratory, only 143 had what the authors considered to be clinically significant electrolyte abnormalities. The 10 clinical criteria predicted 135 of the clinically significant abnormalities, for a sensitivity of 94.4% and a specificity of 27.8%. None of the eight clinically significant abnormalities that were not predicted affected clinical outcome. The authors noted that use of the criteria would have avoided unnecessary testing in 233 patients. The most common abnormality was a high chloride level, but the most common *clinically significant* abnormalities were abnormal carbon dioxide content (78 patients) and potassium levels (59 patients). Of the 143 clinically significant abnormalities, 81 affected both diagnosis and therapy, 38 affected diagnosis, and 24 affected therapy. Cebul and Beck[48] recommended that screening and routine preadmission biochemical profiles be abandoned because their use is not supported by studies examining their effect on patient care, hospital costs, or length of stay. But, after analyzing individual component tests, they found that periodic screening is warranted for serum glucose, cholesterol, and possibly BUN and creatinine.

In the study by Kaplan and colleagues[10] of the usefulness of preoperative laboratory screening, a third of the 514 panels (Na, K, Cl, CO_2, BUN, creatinine) examined were considered to be unindicated and 1 (0.2%) was abnormal. Of the 464 glucose determinations, 25 were abnormal, including 4 in patients for whom there were no indications for performing that test. The authors felt that only 2 determinations were clinically significant. Macpherson[9] concluded that no rationale can be constructed for base-line electrolyte investigations and that routine electrolyte and glucose determinations are unnecessary for *elective* surgery.

CONCLUSIONS AND RECOMMENDATIONS

In contributing to a book such as this, there is a strong tendency to become an advocate for the subject—diagnostic testing. For this reason we have attempted to provide the reader with an appropriate perspective on the different types and purposes of diagnostic testing conducted in the ED. Most, but not all, of the studies reviewed in the previous sections conclude that the test being examined is either not indicated as a routine test, an admission test, or a screening test, or that the test may be ordered more selectively and more appropriately by applying certain clinical criteria. However, there are problems in widely applying the results of some of these studies: (1) clinical criteria in some cases have been developed *retrospectively* for the particular patient-population being examined; (2) the abnormal results of those tests which would not have been requested by applying the criteria are then deemed to be "clinically insignificant" because they did not change the diagnosis, the therapy, or both; and (3) the "gold standard" used to diagnose the abnormality and render the test unnecessary, may itself be a diagnostic test. For example, a CXR confirming clinical findings and demonstrating pneumonia may make a WBC and a DIF "unnecessary" by the study criteria (or vice versa). However, in reality the positive test result may not be as definitive as required. In this example, when the infiltrate on CXR could be either old or new, the WBC and/or DIF may further define the nature of the infiltrate.

More importantly, one has to consider how reliable and reproducible are the *clinical findings* that are used to negate the necessity of obtaining a diagnostic test. This is especially true under adverse ED conditions (i.e., a junior house-officer examining a patient at 3 AM while simultaneously managing another patient in acute pulmonary edema and a third with a serious gunshot wound): Under such circumstances, a certain amount of redundancy may be desirable in the interest of diagnosing and treating patients accurately and rapidly—an argument substantiated by the findings of Murata and colleagues.[47]

In a sense, then, we have presented a worst-case scenario for diagnostic testing in the ED, one that will undoubtedly satisfy those interested solely in cost containment or maximizing positive yields for tests. But one does not need to be so rigid in adhering to various suggested guidelines to reduce unnecessary tests or contain costs. Instead, in addition to considering such guidelines, one should consider the following questions before requesting a test:

- Is the sensitivity, specificity, and predictive value of the test adequate to provide clinically useful information?
- Will results of this test change the diagnosis, prognosis, or therapy?
- Will the results of this test provide a better understanding of the disease process in this patient?
- What am I looking for and why? Will the patient benefit if I find it?[51, 52]

These questions apply to all physicians. In the ED the following considerations can be added:

- Will requesting a series of tests soon after the patient arrives accelerate patient care in the ED without generating an unacceptable number of unnecessary tests?
- Given the number and variety of possible testing errors, will receiving a broad range of normal test results give me a false sense of security and cause me to overlook a serious condition or a seriously ill patient?
- Which diagnostic tests are necessary for this patient's overall care by my colleagues?

THE FUTURE OF EMERGENCY DIAGNOSTIC TESTING

Point of Source Testing

Point of source testing (POST) is a relatively new concept that has evolved with the development of new microdiagnostic technologies.[53, 54] This development allows many of the stat laboratory tests to be performed at the bedside with turn-around times ranging from 1 to 7 minutes. Examples of POST systems currently available are the ISTAT Pocket Doc®, manufactured by ISTAT, and the Gem Premier®, by Mallinkrodt Co. The Pocket Doc® device is a hand-held instrument the size of a pocket cellular telephone that uses less than 1 mL of blood to determine the NA^{+}, K^{+}, glucose, BUN, and hemoglobin. The Gem Premier® is approximately the size of a portable monitor-defibrillator and determines the following analytes: Na^{+}, K^{+}, ionized Ca^{++}, blood gases, and hemoglobin. Still another system, the Vision® analyzer by Abbott, currently has a menu of 15 or more analytes, including liver function tests, total CPK, and anticonvulsants, which are determined by individual cassettes. Test results are available in approximately 7 minutes. All systems use disposable cartridges and require less than an hour for the average medical professional to learn how to use them. Each system is self standardizing, can store data, and can transfer information via infrared interface or can be "hard-wired" to the laboratory mainframe.

The new automated blood cell counters are quite compact and, although not quite in the same microminiature state as the ISTAT system, are portable enough to use as part of a POST system.

In addition to the devices described above, many systems designed to measure one analyte or process are commercially available. Monodiagnostic POST systems are available for determining CPK-MB (both isozymes and isomorphs), prothrombin time, aminophylline, cocaine, phenobarbital, phenytoin, acetaminophen, and digoxin. Of course, the standard dipstick tests of blood and urine can also be considered POST systems.

The vast array of POST equipment already approved and on the market can be clustered together with a minimal space requirement to form a POST stat laboratory. The test results are available in several minutes because of both the speed of the equipment and the elimination of the time delay necessary for transporting the samples to the laboratory, as well as for accessioning and processing.

One drawback to this revolution is the cost per test, which is usually 10 to 20 times that of conventionally performed tests. However, cost-saving features that are intrinsic to POST testing include the following: the actual testing may not require laboratory personnel; the rapid turnaround of test results decreases patient "throughput" times, the need for repetitious testing is decreased; and lost specimens and the cost of specimen transportation to a central laboratory are markedly reduced or eliminated.

The rapid availability of test results is the paramount and overriding benefit of POST systems. The prompt return of results expedites patient diagnosis and ongoing clinical patient management. If rapid patient disposition is the essence of emergency care, POST devices will have a major affect on helping achieve these goals. Additionally, the availability of POST will make it easier to differentiate between those tests necessary for the emergency physician to effectively diagnose and treat patients in the ED and those diagnostic tests requested for routine or screening purposes. Whether POST is used for both purposes or exclusively for emergency diagnostic testing remains to be seen.

• • •

Exercising appropriate clinical judgement in the ED is based on an accurate history and a properly performed physical examination supplemented by selective use of diagnostic tests. Clinical judgement should also take into account what is best for the patient after the patient leaves the ED, rather than considering only what is necessary during the time that the patient remains in the ED and is the direct responsibility of the emergency physician.

The most effective way of dealing with the issues raised in this chapter in a *prospective* manner is by organizing and/or participating in a hospital diagnostic testing committee similar in purpose to the hospital pharmacy and therapeutics (P & T) committee. A diagnostic testing committee with strong input from the ED can (1) consider the advisability of obtaining various routine screening tests based on the prevalence of particular diseases in that hospital or ED population; (2) monitor the results of various tests and modify the test-requesting protocols accordingly; and (3) implement new technologies such as POST and integrate the newer tests with existing facilities in the hospital. Such a committee can effectively deal with issues involving both *emergency diagnostic testing* and *diagnostic testing in the emergency department.*

REFERENCES

1. Lundberg AD: Preservation of laboratory test ordering: a syndrome affecting clinicians. *JAMA* 1983; 249:639.
2. Wertman BG, Sostrin SV, Paulova Z, et al: Why do physicians order laboratory tests? A study of laboratory test request and use patterns. *JAMA* 1980; 243:2080-2082.
3. Johns RJ, Fortuin NJ, Wheeler PS: The collection and evaluation of clinical information. In Harvey AM, Johns RJ, McKusick VA, et al, eds: *The principles and practice of medicine,* ed 22, p. 18, Norwalk, 1988, Appleton-Lange.
4. Isselbacher KJ, Braunwald E, Wilson JD, et al, eds: The practice of medicine. In *Harrison's principles of internal medicine,* ed 13, p. 2, New York, 1994, McGraw-Hill.
5. Wyngaarden JB: The use and interpretation of laboratory-derived data. In Wyngaarden JB, Smith LH Jr, Bennett JC, eds: *Cecil's textbook of medicine,* ed 19, p. 73, Philadelphia, 1992, WB Saunders.
6. Schneiderman LJ, DeSalvo L, Baylor S, et al: The "abnormal" screening laboratory results—its effect on physician and patient, *Arch Intern Med* 129:88–90, 1972.
7. Korvin CC, Pearce RH, Stanley J: Admission screening: clinical benefits, *Ann Intern Med* 83:197–203, 1975.
8. Robbins JA, Mushlin Al: Preoperative evaluation of the healthy patient, *Med Clin North Am* 63:1145–1156, 1979.
9. Macpherson DS: Preoperative laboratory testing: should any tests be routine before surgery? *Med Clin North Am* 77:289–308, 1993.
10. Kaplan EB, Sheiner LB, Boeckmann AJ, et al: The usefulness of preoperative laboratory screening, *JAMA* 253:3576–3581, 1985.
11. Narr BJ, Hansen TR, Warner MA: Preoperative laboratory screening in healthy Mayo patients: cost-effective elimination of tests and unchanged outcomes, *Mayo Clin Proc* 66:155–159, 1991.
12. Velanovich V: The value of routine preoperative laboratory testing in predicting postoperative complications: a multivariate analysis, *Surgery* 109:236–243, 1991.
13. Tape TG, Mushlin AL: The utility of routine chest radiographs, *Ann Intern Med* 104:663–670, 1986.
14. Fink DJ, Fang M, Wyle FA: Routine chest x-ray films in a veterans' hospital, *JAMA* 245:1056–1057, 1981.
15. Hubbell FA, Greenfield S, Tyler JL, et al: The impact of routine admission chest x-ray films on patient care, *N Engl J Med* 312:209–213, 1985.
16. Aronson S, Gennis P, Kelley D, et al: The value of routine admission chest radiographs in adult asthmatics, *Ann Emerg Med* 18:1206–1208, 1989.
17. Tsai TW, Gallagher EJ, Lombardi G: Guidelines for the selective ordering of admission chest radiography in adult obstructive airway disease, *Ann Emerg Med* 22:1854–1858, 1993.
18. Gennis P, Gallagher EJ, Falvo C, et al: Clinical criteria for the detection of pneumonia in adults: guidelines for ordering chest roentgenograms in the emergency department, *J Emerg Med* 7:263–268, 1989.
19. Heckerling PS: The need for chest roentgenograms in adults with acute respiratory illness. Clinical predictors, *Arch Intern Med* 146:1321–1324, 1986.
20. Emerman CL, Dawson N, Speroff T: Comparison of physician judgement and decision aids for ordering chest radiographs for pneumonia in outpatients, *Ann Emerg Med* 20:1215–1219, 1991.

21. Buenger RE: Five thousand acute care/emergency department chest radiographs: comparison of requisitions with radiographic findings, *J Emerg Med* 6:197–202, 1988.
22. Hoffman JR, Igarashi E: Influence of electrocardiographic findings on admission decisions in patients with acute chest pain, *Am J Med* 79:699–707, 1985.
23. Rubenstein LZ, Greenfield S: The baseline ECG in the evaluation of acute cardiac complaints, *JAMA* 244:2536–2539, 1980.
24. Moorman JR, Hlatky MA, Eddy DM, et al: The yield of the routine admission electrocardiogram: a study in a general medical service, *Ann Intern Med* 1203:590–595, 1985.
25. Garland JL, Wolfson AB: Routine admission electrocardiography in emergency department patients, *Ann Emerg Med* 23:275-280, 1994.
26. Akin BV, Hubbell FA, Frye EB, et al: Efficacy of the routine admission urinalysis, *Am J Med* 82:719–722, 1987.
27. Kroenke K et al: The admission urinalysis: impact on patient care, *J Gen Intern Med* 1:238–242, 1986.
28. Shapiro MF, Greenfield S: The complete blood count and leukocyte differential count, *Ann Intern Med* 106:65–74, 1987.
29. Callaham M: Innacuracy and expense of the leukocyte count in making urgent clinical decisions, *Ann Emerg Med* 15:774–781, 1986.
30. Rich EC, Crowson TW, Connelly DP: Effectiveness of differential leukocyte count case finding in the ambulatory care setting, *JAMA* 249:633–636, 1983.
31. Erban SB, Kinman JL, Schwartz JS: Routine use of the prothrombin and partial thromboplastin times, *JAMA* 262:2428–2432, 1989.
32. Eisenberg JM, Goldfarb S: Clinical usefulness of measuring prothrombin time as a routine admission test, *Clin Chem* 22:1644–1647, 1980.
33. Bedell SE, Bush BT: Erythrocyte sedimentation rate. From folklore to facts, *Am J Med* 78:1001–1009, 1985.
34. Sox HC, Liang MH: The erythrocyte sedimentation rate. Guidelines for rational use, *Ann Intern Med* 104:515–523, 1986.
35. Tinetti ME, Schmidt A, Baum J: Use of the erythrocyte sedimentation rate in chronically ill, elderly patients with a decline in health status, *Am J Med* 80:844–884, 1986.
36. Fincher RME, Page MI: Clinical significance of extreme elevation of the erythrocyte sedimentation rate, *Arch Intern Med* 146:1581–1583, 1986.
37. Haber HL, Leavy JA, Kessler PD, et al: The erythrocyte sedimentation rate in congestive heart failure, *N Engl J Med* 324:353–358, 1991.
38. Gallagher EJ, Gennis P, Brooks F: Clinical use of the erythrocyte sedimentation rate in the evaluation of febrile intravenous drug users, *Ann Emerg Med* 22:776–780, 1993.
39. Eisenberg JM, Rose JD, Weinstein AJ: Routine blood cultures from febrile outpatients used in detecting bacteremia, *JAMA* 236:2863–2865, 1976.
40. Sklar DP, Rusnak R: The value of outpatient blood cultures in the emergency department, *Am J Emerg Med* 5:95–100, 1987.
41. Pazin GJ, Scott S, Thompson ME: Blood culture positivity. Suppression by outpatient antibiotic therapy in patients with bacterial endocarditis, *Arch Intern Med* 142:263–268, 1982.
42. Strand CL, Wajsbort RR, Sturmann K: Effect of iodophor vs. iodine tincture skin preparation on blood culture contamination rate. *JAMA* 1993; 269:1004-1006.
43. Marantz PR, Linzer M, Feiner CI, et al: Inability to predict diagnosis in febrile intravenous drug abusers. *Ann Intern Med* 1987; 106:823-882.
44. Young GP, Hedges JR, Dixon L, et al: inability to validate a predictive score for infective endocarditis in intravenous drug users. *JEM* 1993; 11:1-7.
45. Rucker L, Hubbell A, Akin BV, et al: Electrolyte blood urea nitrogen and glucose level screening in medical admissions: impact on patient management, *West J Med* 147:287–291, 1987.
46. Belliveau RE, Fitzgerald JE, Nickersen DA: Evaluation of routine profile chemistry screening of all patients admitted to a community hospital, *Am J Clin Pathol* 53:497–451, 1970.
47. Murata GH, Muranaka E, Ellrodt AG: Laboratory testing on admission to a teaching service: expectations and outcomes for serum electrolytes, *Mt Sinai J Med* 51:141–147, 1984.
48. Cebul RD, Beck JR: Biochemical profiles: applications in ambulatory screening and preadmission testing of adults, *Ann Intern Med* 106:403–413, 1987.

49. Lowe RA, Arst HF, Ellis BK: Rational ordering of electrolytes in the emergency department, *Ann Emerg Med* 20:35–40, 1991.
50. Lowe RA, Wood AB, Burney RE, et al: Rational ordering of serum electrolytes: department of clinical criteria, *Ann Emerg Med* 16:260–269, 1987.
51. Krieg AF, Gambino R, Gaten RS: Why are clinical laboratory tests performed? When are they valid: *JAMA* 233:76–78, 1975.
52. Lacombe MA: A six-point test ban treaty for house staff, *Res Staff Physician* 19:47–48, 1973.
53. Beasley R, Baer D, Sewell D: Laboratory test analysis near the patient: opportunities for improved clinical diagnosis and management, *JAMA* 255:775–786, 1986.
54. Salem M, Chermow B, Burke R, et al: Bedside diagnostic blood testing: its accuracy, rapidity, and utility in blood conservation, *JAMA* 266:382–389, 1991.

PART II

Tests Frequently Requested in the Emergency Department

Chapter 2

Throat Culture and Antigen Testing for Pharyngitis

Jeffrey S. Duchin, M.D.

CASE 2–1

An 18-year-old college sophomore returns home from school during winter recess and is brought to the emergency department by his mother with complaints of a sore throat, fever, malaise, and headache of several days' duration. Physical examination reveals a temperature of 101.5° F, an erythematous posterior pharynx with white exudate on both tonsillar pillars, and tender anterior cervical adenopathy. There is no history of rheumatic fever. A rapid streptococcal test is negative. What is the best course of action?

OVERVIEW

The clinical approach to diagnostic testing for acute pharyngitis is straightforward. There are currently two widely used satisfactory diagnostic techniques available: throat culture and direct rapid antigen testing of pharyngeal swabs. The two methods differ in turnaround time, sensitivity, and cost. In addition, depending on the specific type of rapid antigen test (RAT) kit employed, ease of use may be an additional consideration.

The RAT is a good first test when quick results are desirable despite the increased cost of rapid testing. *All negative rapid test results must be confirmed with a conventional throat culture.* Thus there are a limited number of diagnostic choices in a patient with acute pharyngitis.

The first decision is whether to do any diagnostic test at all. If acute group A streptococcal (GAS) pharyngitis is a consideration and determining the cause of the infection will alter the treatment plan, the answer is yes. Understanding the epidemiologic factors and clinical features of the various types of pharyngitis will help the clinician decide when the likelihood of GAS infection is high.

The next step is to decide whether rapid antigen testing would be useful. In general, rapid testing is most useful when follow-up is not possible or probable and the clinician does not want to initiate treatment without confirmation of infection. With a positive rapid test result, treatment can be initiated immediately. In patients with severe symptoms, a positive rapid test result will be useful if it allows the clinician to initiate treatment sooner rather than waiting for the culture results. However, if the decision to treat has already been made on the basis of severe symptoms or concern for the risk of rheumatic heart disease, rapid antigen testing adds nothing to conventional throat culture.

Likewise, in those patients in whom follow-up is likely, treatment can be initiated and then stopped or continued depending on the culture result. If immediate treatment is not indicated, infection with GAS is considered less likely, or the clinician wants to avoid potentially unnecessary antibiotics, treatment may be deferred until culture results are available.

Careful attention to technique in obtaining the throat swab is critical to ensure reliable results from either test. In addition, neither rapid antigen testing nor throat culture is sufficiently sensitive to be relied upon in a partially treated patient.

INTRODUCTION

Acute pharyngitis, one of the most common conditions for which ambulatory patients seek medical care, accounts for over 40 million visits by adults and up to 5% of visits to pediatricians annually in the United States.[1–3] It has been estimated that 11% of all school-age children consult a physician each year with complaints of sore throat.[4]

Although viruses are responsible for most cases of pharyngitis, recent reports of a resurgence of rheumatic fever in the United States and northern Europe make accurate diagnosis of GAS pharyngitis mandatory.[5,6]

Accurate and prompt identification of the cause of the infectious pharyngitis allows for effective therapy when indicated and avoidance of antimicrobial use when a treatable cause is ruled out. Clinicians may significantly overestimate the likelihood of disease due to GAS and prescribe unnecessary antibiotic regimens.[7]

Treatment of GAS pharyngitis has been shown to reduce duration of symptoms; prevent suppurative complications including peritonsillar abscess, retropharyngeal abscess, and cervical lymphadenitis; and prevent the nonsuppurative sequela of acute rheumatic fever.[8–12] Additionally, prompt treatment may minimize secondary spread of infection by eradication of the infecting organism.[12,13] However, immediate penicillin treatment may be associated with an increased incidence of subsequent GAS infections.[14]

ETIOLOGY OF PHARYNGITIS

Organisms causing pharyngitis are listed in Table 2–1. A number of infective agents produce a clinical syndrome indistinguishable from GAS pharyngitis.[15] Viruses are the most common microbial agents causing pharyngitis. *Mycoplasma pneumonia* and *Chlamydia pneumonia* are common pathogens in adults.[16] *Corynebacterium haemolyticum* is a cause of pharyngitis often associated with a scarlatiniform rash in adolescents and young adults.[17,18] The precise role of non-GAS organisms including groups C and G is undefined; however, nonsuppurative sequelae do not occur. *Neisseria gonorrhoeae* and *Corynebacterium diphtheriae* should be recognized in the appropriate clinical setting. Pharyngitis may be the initial complaint in early human immunodeficiency virus (HIV) infection[19] and secondary syphilis.[20] Pharyngitis should be distinguished from early epiglottitis.

Noninfectious causes of acute pharyngitis include low humidity; exposure to environmental irritants including air pollution, cigarette smoke, or chemicals; and neoplasm.[21]

Table 2–1. Microbial Causes of Acute Pharyngitis

Cause	Syndrome/Disease	Estimated Importance*
Viral		
Rhinovirus (89 types and 1 subtype)	Common cold	20
Coronavirus (4 or more types)	Common cold	≥5
Adenovirus (types 3, 4, 7, 14, 21)	Pharyngoconjunctival fever, ARDS†	5
Herpes simplex virus (types 1 and 2)	Gingivitis, stomatitis, pharyngitis	4
Parainfluenza virus (types 1–4)	Common cold, croup	2
Influenza virus (types A and B)	Influenza	2
Coxsackievirus A (types 2, 4–6, 8, 10)	Herpangina	<1
Epstein-Barr virus	Infectious mononucleosis	<1
Cytomegalovirus	Infectious mononucleosis	<1
Human immunodeficiency virus (HIV)	Primary HIV infection	<1
Bacterial		
Streptococcus pyogenes (group A β-hemolytic streptococcus)	Pharyngitis, tonsillitis, scarlet fever	15–30
Mixed anaerobic infection	Gingivitis, pharyngitis (Vincent's angina)	<1
	Peritonsillitis/peritonsillar abscess (quinsy)	<1
Neisseria gonorrhoeae	Pharyngitis	<1
Corynbacterium diphtheriae	Diphtheria	≥1
Corynbacterium ulcerans	Pharyngitis, diphtheria	<1
Corynebacterium haemolyticum (Arcanobacterium haemolyticum)	Pharyngitis, scarlatiniform rash	<1
Yersinia enterocolitica	Pharyngitis, enterocolitis	<1
Treponema pallidum	Secondary syphilis	<1
Chlamydial		
Chlamydia psittaci	ARDS, pneumonia	Unknown
Chlamydia pneumonia		
Mycoplasmal		
Mycoplasma pneumoniae	Pneumonia/bronchitis/pharyngitis	<1
Mycoplasma hominis (type 1)	Pharyngitis in volunteers	Unknown
Unknown		40

Modified with permission from Mandell GL, Douglas RG, Bennett JE, editors: *Principles and Practice of Infectious Diseases*, ed 3, New York, 1990, Churchill Livingstone, p. 494.
*Estimated percentage of cases of pharyngitis due to indicated organism in civilians of all ages.
†*ARDS*, adult respiratory distress syndrome.

DIAGNOSIS OF PHARYNGITIS

The classic "textbook" signs and symptoms of GAS pharyngitis include fever, tonsillar or pharyngeal exudate, swollen tender anterior cervical adenitis, pain on swallowing, headache, and more commonly in children, abdominal pain, nausea, and vomiting.[10, 13, 22, 23] Unfortunately, this symptom complex is neither sensitive nor specific enough to be relied on without further diagnostic confirmation.[12, 23–25] In addition, mild or inapparent infection can lead to nonsuppurative sequelae.[23, 25] As noted above, GAS pharyngitis may have different signs and symptoms in adults and children.[25, 26] Scoring systems have been developed that may help identify a group of children at low risk of acute infection.[26]

The inability of experienced clinicians to accurately diagnose GAS infections on clinical grounds alone is well documented.[7, 24, 27, 28] However, awareness of epidemiologic factors can be important in correctly diagnosing GAS pharyngitis. The infection is most common in school-age children 5 to 15 years of age and is seen with decreasing frequency in adolescents, adults, and children under 3 years of age.[3, 29, 30] The disease occurs year-round in temperate climates, with a peak incidence in late winter and early spring.[12, 13] Person-to-person spread by airborne droplet transmission is enhanced in closed communities with crowded living conditions such as dormatories, military barracks, and overcrowded dwellings. In epidemic conditions the attack rate of rheumatic fever is approximately 3%, whereas in the endemic condition more commonly encountered in medical practice it is thought that the incidence of rheumatic fever is significantly lower.[23, 27] The epidemic state is characterized by rapid spread of infection and the emergence of highly virulent organisms rich in M protein.[31, 32]

Lewis W. Wannamaker, the eminent streptococcologist, summarized the ideal diagnostic approach to streptococcal pharyngitis[8]:

> Epidemiologic, clinical and cultural findings are all important. By neglecting any one of them—by necessity or by deliberate choice—we must recognize that we are operating in semidarkness. The diagnosis of streptococcal infection requires the use and careful evaluation of all available clues and pieces of evidence.

The Streptococcal Carrier State

The streptococcal carrier state may be defined as recovery of GAS from the nasopharynx in the absence of a streptococcal antibody response. Fewer than half of the patients with acute pharyngitis in whom GAS colonies grow on throat culture demonstrate a rise in antistreptococcal antibody titers indicating true infection.[25, 33] Thus in a large proportion of patients with acute pharyngitis the presence of GAS on throat culture may indicate previous infection or a chronic carrier state. Throat cultures cannot discriminate between active infection with GAS and concurrent infection with another organism in a GAS carrier. In contrast to those with acute infection, in carriers of GAS sequelae or dissemination of the organism is unlikely.[23]

During convalescence from acute infection, 97% of untreated patients can carry the organism for 4 months or longer; however, the number of bacteria and the virulence of the strain as manifested by synthesis of M protein and contagiousness decrease with time.[13] Carrier rates in children during the school year vary from 10% to 40%.[25] The carrier rate is lower in infants and adults; thus, a positive throat culture can be a better indicator of infection in these groups.[25]

Although carriers may harbor fewer organisms leading to low colony counts on culture, there is no reliable correlation between the degree of positivity of the throat culture and true infection as indicated by subsequent serologic response.[12, 25, 33] One third of patients with fewer than 10 colonies of β-hemolytic organisms per plate demonstrate a significant antibody response.[33]

The American Heart Association does not recommend routine identification or treatment of GAS carriers.[23] At this time there is no accurate and convenient method for the clinician to distinguish the GAS carrier state from acute infection.

Gram Stain

Although one group of investigators found Gram-stained smears of pharyngeal secretions to be more accurate than a clinical algorithm for the early diagnosis of GAS pharyngitis,[34] the technique is generally considered to be of little use or reliability.[30, 35]

Throat Culture

Use of the blood agar throat culture to diagnose GAS pharyngitis was first reported in a pediatric office practice by Breese and Disney in 1954.[28] Despite a delay of 18 to 48 hours before results are known, an estimated 28 to 36 million throat cultures are processed yearly in the United States.[36] American Heart Association guidelines for prevention and treatment of rheumatic fever state that GAS is virtually always found on throat culture during acute infection.[23, 37]

Meticulous collection of the specimen for culture is crucial to maximize the sensitivity of the test.[38–40] Proper technique for obtaining a culture specimen includes vigorous swabbing with a cotton or Dacron swab under strong illumination. The posterior of the pharynx, tonsils or tonsillar fossa, and any exudate should be sampled while avoiding the lips, tongue, and buccal mucosa. Sheep blood agar (SBA) is the preferred culture medium for the growth of GAS because of the ease with which hemolytic patterns are visualized and the inhibition of confounding hemolytic *Haemophilus* species.[41] The specimen should be plated as soon as possible since a delay in plating the swab or methods such as broth tubes that dilute, select, or enrich organisms make accurate quantitation of organism burden difficult.[37, 38, 41] Other factors affecting the colony count on the culture plate include the presence of competing oral flora, the technique used in obtaining the specimen and inoculating the specimen onto the culture plate, the culture medium itself, and the atmosphere used for incubation.[42]

The culture plate must be streaked properly with the swab to ensure even distribution of organisms and allow for well-isolated colonies with observable subsurface hemolysis.[37] The proper method for streaking the culture plate is as follows[30, 37, 38]: the primary inoculum streaks are applied to SBA plates by firmly rolling the swab onto and across one sixth of the plate. With a sterile loop the secondary inoculum is made by streaking 10 to 20 times through the primary inoculum site. The final inoculum is done without reentering the primary site and is followed by several stabs into the agar to produce subsurface colonies demonstrating enhanced hemolysis. The plate is incubated at 37° C for a minimum of 24 hours, and preferentially for 48 hours[43] (Fig. 2–1).

Members of the genus *Streptococcus* are catalase-negative, gram-positive cocci that are facultative anaerobes. The organisms can appear gram-negative if the culture is old or antibiotics have been administered before culturing. Preliminary identification is based on colony morphology and the hemolytic pattern of colonies. Colony

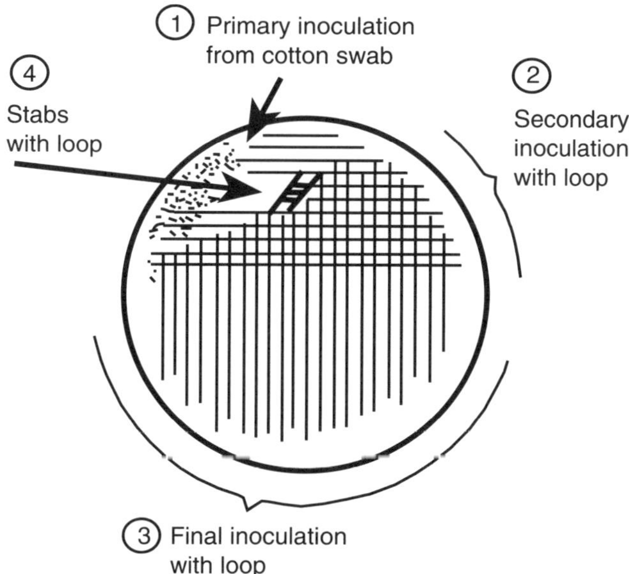

Fig. 2–1. The proper method for inoculation of a blood agar plate to identify group A β-hemolytic streptococci. (With permission from Kaplan E: *Conn Med* 37:45–48, 1973.)

morphology varies with the conditions of incubation. A zone of clear hemolysis surrounding the colony represents β-hemolysis, and partial and no hemolysis represents α- and γ-hemolytic organisms, respectively. Organisms are best isolated in pure subculture for study of colony morphology and hemolysis patterns.

There is a lack of concensus in the literature on the ideal method of processing throat cultures.[44] Variables in throat culture technology include inhibitory vs. noninhibitory media (trimethoprim-sulfamethoxazole [SMX]-containing vs. nonsupplemented media) and the duration and atmosphere of incubation (CO_2 enrichment vs. nonenriched, aerobic vs. anaerobic).[45] There is probably no single optimal throat culture method, and no single medium-atmosphere combination will provide 100% recovery.[44, 46] It seems prudent for each laboratory to do its own evaluation of the selected throat culture procedure.[47] However, the following methods should detect 90% to 95% of GAS from symptomatic patients if processed meticulously: SBA incubated anaerobically for 48 hours or aerobically without CO_2 and with a cover glass over the primary inoculum to reduce oxygen tension, SBA with SMX incubated aerobically in 5% to 10% CO_2 for 48 hours, and SBA-SMX incubated anaerobically for 48 hours.[45] A two-plate culture method using SBA incubated aerobically and SBA-SMX incubated anaerobically has been proposed to maximize sensitivity.[48] The American Society for Microbiology recommends 5% defibrinated SBA plates incubated anaerobically with 5% to 10% CO_2 and 85% to 90% N_2 but also states that normal aerobic incubation may be done with very little loss in recovery of GAS.[49]

GAS organisms may be distinguished from non–group A species in several ways. The *Lancefield capillary precipitation method* is the reference standard. The most sensitive and specific technique, it is also complex and time-consuming. The assay detects group A–specific cell wall antigen by reacting cell wall extract with type-specific antisera. *Fluorescent antibody (FA) techniques* are used to group streptococci after isolation on blood agar plates. Although the technique can be used to detect GAS from throat swabs, a 4-hour incubation period is required. The technique is complicated and requires expensive fluorescent microscopy equipment. FA techniques may be employed in epidemiologic studies of patients with poststreptococcal sequelae; however, they are not widely used to detect GAS directly from throat swabs.[50] The *bacitracin disk test* is the most common screening test used to differentiate GAS from non–group A organisms. It involves placing a 0.02- or 0.04-unit, commercially available bacitracin disk on a subcultured isolate of β-hemolytic colonies. This concentration is intended to inhibit GAS but not other streptococci. Sensitivity and specificity are decreased when the disk is placed on the primary plate, although under some circumstances this may be acceptable.[46] Inhibition of growth by the bacitracin disk characterizes most GAS organisms; however, 5% to 20% of non-GAS species are susceptible, and 2% to 5% of GAS species may be resistant.[37, 38, 44] In a study at the Centers for Disease Control Streptococcal Laboratory, 12,560 strains were tested over a 5-year period. The bacitracin disk test failed to correlate with the Lancefield precipitin test in 4.2% of isolates.[51] The *PYR test* detects L-pyrrolidonyl amino peptidase activity in isolated colonies on the primary plate or a pure subculture. Although slightly more complex than the bacitracin disk test, it is equal in sensitivity and has greater specificity.[42, 52] The test is not suitable for detection of GAS directly from throat swabs.[52, 53]

Throat cultures are approximately 90% sensitive for the presence of GAS in the pharynx; thus, 10% of patients may be missed with a single culture.[13, 28, 35, 38] Other authors report even lower sensitivities and note that office cultures show variable results when compared with bacteriology laboritories.[44]

To maximize sensitivity of throat cultures the following components are necessary: meticulous specimen collection and plating of inoculum; inspection of plates at 18 hours and if negative again at 24 and 48 hours; thorough training and supervision of individuals processing and reading cultures; and quality control of the medium, incubator, and reagents.[45]

Serologic diagnosis of GAS infection is possible with commercially available latex and whole red blood cell (RBC) agglutination tests that assay for antistreptococcal antigens including antistreptolysin O, anti-DNAase B, antistreptokinase, and antihyaluronidase. Serologic methods are based on demonstrating rising antibody titers, which take several weeks to develop.

OTHER CAUSES OF PHARYNGITIS

In patients with suspected pharyngeal *N. gonorrhoeae* infection the specimen is processed on modified Thayer-Martin media under aerobic incubation with 5% to 10% supplemental CO_2 for 24 to 48 hours. Cultures should also be obtained from rectal, urethral, and cervical sites. *N. gonorrhoeae* will not be detected in specimens processed for GAS.

In an unvaccinated patient with a clinical picture consistent with *C. diptheriae* infection, the pharyngeal swab is inoculated onto an enrichment medium and selective plate and processed according to standard methods.[40] *C. diphtheriae* will not be detected in specimens processed for GAS.

Viral culture of the nasopharynx may be indicated in infants and immunocompromised patients.

DIRECT ANTIGEN DETECTION TEST KITS

A rapid test to detect GAS would obviate the 18- to 48-hour delay required to process throat cultures. Rapid diagnosis of infection would allow prompt administration of antibiotic therapy. Patients could then benefit from the advantages of early therapy, and noncompliance and unnecessary or empirical antibiotic treatment could be avoided. It has been suggested that a rapid test with high sensitivity and specifity would substantially reduce throat culture use and unnecessary antibiotic exposure in children.[54] The use of a rapid test as an adjunct to throat culture has been shown to result in an increased treatment rate in children with GAS pharyngitis and decreased antibiotic use in those patients without infection.[55]

RATs are based on the detection of specific GAS cell wall polysaccharide antigen directly from Dacron- or rayon-tipped throat swabs. The rapid streptococcal test technology is based on the fundamental work done by Rebecca Landsfield in the 1930s on immunologic typing of streptococcal species.[56] The basic technology involved in rapid streptococcal testing has been described and is summarized below.[56] All available techniques involve extraction or solubilization of group A carbohydrate and some method of making the target antigen accessible to antibody. *Latex agglutination (LA) tests* use antistreptococcal antibody bound to latex particles that are reacted with extract from the clinical specimen; an agglutination reaction is visible in the presence of streptococcal antigen. Multiple control tests are necessary to provide a reference comparison for interpreting results. An *enzyme-linked immunosorbent assay* (ELISA or EIA) or sandwich immunoassay is easier to interpret than an LA test, but it is more complex and generally costlier. In the ELISA test the multivalent streptococcal antigen is bound to a capture antibody fixed to a solid surface. A second labeled antibody termed conjugate or detection antibody is then added to combine with exposed epitopes. Unreacted labeled conjugate is washed away. The label may be enzymes with the capacity for signal amplification (that convert a colorless substrate to a col-

Table 2–2. Methods of Identifying Group A Streptococci

Methods	Turnaround Time* (hr)	Complexity (No. of Steps)	Sensitivity (%)	Specificity (%)
Lancefield grouping	42–48	10–15	99	99
Bacitracin				
Subculture	42–48	3–4	99	75
Primary plate	18–24	2	75	50
PYRase†				
Group A only	18–24	5–6	98	99
Complete identification	42–48	6–8	98	99
Latex or coagglutination	18–24	5–10	95–98	99
Fluorescent antibody	4–6	5–8	95	99
Direct antigen	5–70 min	3–8	60–90	98

From Facklam RD: Group A streptococcal pharyngitis, ASCP Microbiology Check Sample, MB 87–3, Chicago, 1987, American Society of Clinical Pathologists.
*Time required for swabbing the throat to final identification.
†*PYRase,* pyrrolidonylarylamidase.

ored dye) or a particulate dye containing conjugates (such as prepared liposomes). The liposome assay eliminates the need to add a substrate for the antibody-antigen complex to generate a signal.[57] Most rapid tests can be done in 10 to 15 minutes, with a range of 5 to 70 minutes.

The majority of clinical studies cited by the manufacturers of RAT kits have not been published in peer review journals.[58] In addition, most studies of the RAT have been done under laboratory conditions, and performance is often poorer in the primary care setting.[59–61]

Sensitivities reported in peer review journals have generally ranged from 60% to 95% when compared with blood agar culture, whereas specificities have remained high at 90% to 100%.[62–64] An in vitro comparison of 8 RAT kits demonstrated up to 100-fold differences in the highest dilution of organisms detectable.[65] A study of 18 RAT kits under laboratory conditions demonstrated specificities ranging from 78% to 100% and sensitivities of 44% to 100%. The same investigators noted difficulty in interpreting end points on slide agglutination tests.[66] In general, colorimetric end points are easier to interpret than agglutination reactions.[58, 62, 66]

Sensitivities of the kits tend to increase with increasing positivity of the throat culture; therefore the majority of false-negative results occur when there are low colony counts on culture.[63, 67] Kits with high reported sensitivities may have been evaluated by considering low-growth cultures negative. As noted above, the colony count on throat culture is not a reliable indicator of infection. Thus, almost half of the children with false-negative RAT results have true GAS infection.[68] Interpretation of reports of RAT performance must be made with a detailed understanding of the culture method used as a reference standard. Variations in culture technique may account for a broad range of reported sensitivities.[67]

The accuracy of rapid tests has been shown to vary with the clinical setting and the personnel performing the test.[64] The importance of determining the accuracy of the RAT in the clinical setting in which it will be used is evident. Ideally the test should demonstrate reproducible accuracy in a variety of clinical settings.[65] No single rapid test has been shown to be clearly superior.[58, 62] Neither LA nor EIA kits are able to accurately detect GAS in the pharynx after partial antibiotic treatment[69] (Table 2–2).

PATIENT MANAGEMENT

Acute pharyngitis due to β-hemolytic GAS remains a challenge to accurately diagnose. Although methods with sufficiently high sensitivity are available to detect the presence of GAS, there is no test to indicate whether the organism represents acute infection or the carrier state. Physical examination, epidemiologic factors, and laboratory tests must all be considered before arriving at a clinical diagnosis.

RATs offer convenience, prompt results, and high specificity. However *the sensitivity remains too low to reliably rule out GAS infection on the basis of a negative test result.* The cost of the rapid test materials is significantly higher than the cost of the blood agar culture.[62] Additional costs result when negative rapid test results must be followed by conventional culture. Carefully performed and interpreted throat cultures therefore remain the gold standard for diagnosis, especially in areas experiencing a resurgence of rheumatic fever.[34, 36, 46, 58]

A reasonable approach in selected populations in which the benefit of rapid results may outweigh the additional cost of testing is to initially employ a rapid test with a low false-positive rate to detect and treat positive cases and follow negative results with a standard blood agar culture. This approach would minimize false-negative results and the consequences of untreated GAS infection while subjecting an undefined number of symptomatic carriers of GAS to antibiotic therapy.

Consideration of epidemiologic factors and physical examination will help reduce the number of patients exposed to unnecessary therapy.[46] At this time it seems prudent to err on the side of overtreating potential cases of acute GAS pharyngitis.

Since the prevention of rheumatic fever can be accomplished by appropriate therapy within 9 days of the onset of pharyngitis,[13, 70] in those patients with reliable follow-up and good compliance the additional cost of the rapid tests may not be justified. In those patients with a high probability of GAS and poor follow-up or questionable compliance, diagnosis (if possible) and treatment at the time of initial evaluation would be preferable.

CASE 2–1 CONTINUED

Because the rapid streptococcal test was negative, the student was just beginning his winter recess, and he and his family appeared to clearly understand the consequences of treating streptococcal infections, the decision was made to culture the pharynx and send the patient home with a prescription for oral penicillin. They were told to fill the prescription and that the student should take the full course of antibiotics only if they were notified that the culture was positive for streptococci. They were also given a telephone number to call for results in 3 days if they did not hear from the hospital. Subsequently, the throat culture was negative, and the family was told to destroy the prescription.

REFERENCES

1. Hedges JR, Lowe RA: Approach to acute pharyngitis, *Emerg Med Clin North Am* 5:335–351, 1987.
2. Huovinen P: Causes, diagnosis, and treatment of pharyngitis, *Compr Ther* 16:59–65, 1990.
3. Mandel JH: Pharyngeal Infections—causes, findings and management, *Postgrad Med* 77:187–199, 1985.
4. Klein MD: Streptococcal pharyngitis in children, *Pediatr Emerg Care* 5:259–261, 1989.
5. Veasy LG, Wiedmeier SE, Orsmond GS et al: Resurgence of acute rheumatic fever in the intermountain area of the United States, *N Engl J Med* 316:421–426, 1987.
6. Herold AH: Group A β-hemolytic streptococcal toxic shock from a mild pharyngitis, *J Fam Pract* 31:549–551, 1990.
7. Poses RM, Cebul RD, Collins M, Fager SS: The accuracy of experienced physicians' probability estimates for patients with sore throats, *JAMA* 254:925–929, 1985.
8. Markowitz M: The decline of rheumatic fever: role of medical intervention, *J Pediatr* 106:545–550, 1985.

9. Randolph MF, Gerber MA, DeMeo KK, Wright L: Effect of antibiotic therapy on the clinical course of streptococcal pharyngitis, *J Pediatr* 106:870–875, 1985.
10. Lowe R, Hedges JR: Early treatment of streptococcal pharyngitis, *Ann Emerg Med* 13:440–448, 1984.
11. Krober MS, Bass JW, Michels GN: Streptococcal pharyngitis. Placebo controlled double-blind evaluation of clinical response to penicillin therapy, *JAMA* 253:1271–1274, 1985.
12. Gerber MA: Group A streptococcal infections. In Balows A et al, editors: *Laboratory diagnosis of infectious diseases, principles and practice,* ed 6, New York, 1988, Springer-Verlag.
13. Peter G, Smith AL: Group A streptococcal infections of the skin and pharynx, *N Engl J Med* 297:365–370, 1977.
14. Pichichero ME, Disney FA, Talpey WB: Adverse and beneficial effects of immediate treatment of group A beta-hemolytic streptococcal pharyngitis with penicillin, *Pediatr Infect Dis J* 6:635–643, 1987.
15. Glezen WP, Clyde WA, Senior RJ et al: Group A streptococci, mycoplasmas, and viruses associated with acute pharyngitis, *JAMA* 202:119–122, 1967.
16. Huovinen P, Lahtonen R, Ziegler T et al: Pharyngitis in adults: the presence and coexistence of viruses and bacterial organisms, *Ann Intern Med* 110:612–616, 1989.
17. Miller RA, Brancato F, Holmes KK: *Corynebacterium hemolyticum* as a cause of pharyngitis and scarlatiniform rash in young adults, *Ann Intern Med* 105:867–872, 1986.
18. Banck G, Nyman M: Tonsillitis and rash associated with *Corynebacterium haemolyticum, J Infect Dis* 154:1037–1040, 1986.
19. Kessler HA, Blaauw B, Spear J et al: Diagnosis of human immunodeficiency virus infection in seronegative homosexuals presenting with an acute viral syndrome, *JAMA* 258:1196–1199, 1987.
20. Wilson JD, Braunwald E, Isselbacher KJ et al, editors: *Harrison's principles of internal medicine,* ed 12, New York, 1991, McGraw-Hill.
21. Loos GD: Pharyngitis, croup and epiglottis, *Prim Care* 17:335–344, 1990.
22. Dillon HC: Streptococcal pharyngitis in the 1980's, *Pediatr Infect Dis* 6:123–130, 1987.
23. Dajani AS, Bisno AL, Chung KJ et al: Prevention of rheumatic fever. A statement for health professionals by the Committee on Rheumatic Fever, Endocarditis and Kawasaki disease of the Council on Cardiovascular Disease in the Young, the American Heart Association, *Circulation* 78:1082–1086, 1988.
24. Gerber MA: Diagnosis of group A beta-hemolytic pharyngitis, *Diagn Microbiol Infect Dis* 4(suppl):5–15, 1986.
25. Wannamaker LW: Perplexity and precision in the diagnosis of streptococcal pharyngitis, *Am J Dis Child* 124:352–358, 1972.
26. Shulman ST: Streptococcal pharyngitis: clinical and epidemiologic factors, *Pediatr Infect Dis J* 8:816–819, 1989.
27. Siegel AC, Johnson EE, Stollerman GH: Controlled studies of streptococcal pharyngitis in a pediatric population. 1. Factors related to the attack rate of rheumatic fever, *N Engl J Med* 265:559–566, 1961.
28. Breese BB, Disney FA: The accuracy of diagnosis of beta streptococcal infections on clinical grounds, *J Pediatr* 44:670–673, 1954.
29. Klein JO: Diagnosis of streptococcal pharyngitis: an introduction, *Pediatr Infect Dis J* 8:813–815, 1989.
30. Mandell GL, Douglas RG, Bennett JE, editors: *Principles and practice of infectious diseases,* ed 3, New York, 1990, Churchill Livingstone.
31. Stollerman GH: Factors that predispose to rheumatic fever, *Med Clin North Am* 44:17–28, 1960.
32. Massell BF, Chute CG, Walker AM, Kurland GS: Penicillin and the marked decrease in morbidity and mortality from rheumatic fever in the United States, *N Engl J Med* 318:280–285, 1988.
33. Kaplan EL, Top FH, Dudding BA, Wannamaker LW: Diagnosis of streptococcal pharyngitis: differentiation of active infection from the carrier state in the symptomatic child, *J Infect Dis* 123:490–501, 1971.
34. Crawford G, Brancato F, Holmes KK: Streptococcal pharyngitis: diagnosis by Gram stain, *Ann Intern Med* 90:293–297, 1979.

35. Kaplan EL: The rapid identification of group A beta-hemolytic streptococci in the upper respiratory tract, current status, *Pediatr Clin North Am* 35:535–542, 1988.
36. Gerber MA: Culturing of throat swabs: end of an era? *J Pediatr* 107:85–88, 1985.
37. Wannamaker LW: A method for culturing beta-hemolytic streptococci from the throat, *Circulation* 32:1054–1058, 1965.
38. Kaplan E: The throat culture: its techniques, pitfalls, limitations and meaning, *Conn Med* 37:45–48, 1973.
39. Koneman EW, Allen SD, Donell VR et al: *Color atlas and textbook of diagnostic microbiology,* ed 3, Philadelphia, 1988, JB Lippincott.
40. Howanitz JH, Howanitz PJ, editors: *Laboratory medicine: test selection and interpretation,* New York, 1991, Churchill Livingstone.
41. Wannamaker LW, Matson JM, editors: *Streptococci and streptococcal diseases; recognition, understanding and management,* New York, 1972, Academic Press.
42. Baron EJ, Finegold SM: *Bailey and Scott's diagnostic microbiology,* ed 8, St Louis, 1990, Mosby Inc.
43. Schaub IG, Mazeika I, Lee R et al: Ecologic studies of rheumatic fever and rheumatic heart disease. Procedure for isolating beta-hemolytic streptococci, *Am J Hyg* 67:46–56, 1957.
44. Centor RM, Meier FA, Dalton HP: Throat cultures and rapid tests for diagnosis of group A streptococcal pharyngitis, *Ann Intern Med* 105:892–899, 1986.
45. Kellogg JA: Suitability of throat culture procedures for detection of group A streptococci and as reference standards for evaluation of streptococcal antigen detection kits, *J Clin Microbiol* 28:165–169, 1990.
46. Gerber MA: Comparison of throat cultures and rapid strep tests for diagnosis of streptococcal pharyngitis, *Pediatr Infect Dis J* 8:820–824, 1989.
47. Kurzynski TA, Van Holten CM: Evaluation of techniques for isolation of group A streptococci from throat cultures, *J Clin Microbiol* 13:891–894, 1981.
48. Wegner DL, Witte DL, Schrantz RD: Insensitivity of rapid antigen detection methods and single blood agar plate culture for diagnosing streptococcal pharyngitis, *JAMA* 267:695–697, 1992.
49. Lennette EA, editor: *Manual of clinical microbiology,* ed 4, Washington, DC, 1985, American Society for Microbiology.
50. Ayoub EM, Wannamaker LW: Identification of group A streptococci. Evaluation of the use of the fluorescent antibody technique, *JAMA* 187:908–913, 1964.
51. Moody MD: Old and new techniques for rapid identification of group A streptococci. In Wannamaker LW, Matson JM, editors: *Streptococci and streptococcal diseases; recognition, understanding, and management,* New York, 1972, Academic Press.
52. Facklam RD: *Group A streptococcal pharyngitis,* ASCP Microbiology Check Sample, MB 87-3 (MB-164), Chicago, 1987, American Society of Clinical Pathologists.
53. Gerber MA, Randolph MF, Tilton RC: Enzyme fluorescence procedure for rapid diagnosis of streptococcal pharyngitis, *J Pediatr* 108:421–423, 1985.
54. Berwick DM, Gorss E, Macone AB et al: Impact of rapid antigen tests for group A streptococcal pharyngitis on physician use of antibiotics and throat cultures, *Pediatr Infect Dis J* 6:1095–1102, 1987.
55. Lieu TA, Fleisher GR, Schwartz JS: Clinical evaluation of a latex agglutination test for streptococcal pharyngitis: performance and impact on treatment rates, *Pediatr Infect Dis J* 7:847–854, 1988.
56. Berke CM: Development of rapid strep technology, *Pediatr Infect Dis J* 8:825–828, 1989.
57. Drulack M, Bartholomew W, la Scolea L et al: Evaluation of the modified Visuwell Strep-A enzyme immunoassay for detection of group-A streptococcus from throat swabs, *Diagn Microbiol Infect Dis* 14:281–285, 1991.
58. Radetsky M, Solomon JA, Todd JK: Identification of streptococcus in the office laboratory: reassessment of new technology, *Pediatr Infect Dis J* 6:556–563, 1987.
59. Hoffmann S: Detection of group A streptococcal antigen from throat swabs with five diagnostic kits in general practice, *Diagn Microbiol Infect Dis* 13:209–215, 1990.
60. Huck W, Reed BD, French T, Mitchell RS: Comparison of the Directigen 1–2–3 Group A Strep Test with culture for detection of group A beta-hemolytic streptococci, *J Clin Microbiol* 27:1715–1718, 1989.

61. Hasin M, Furst A: Sore throat in family practice: comparison of throat culture with a rapid enzyme immunoassay test for diagnostic purposes, *J R Coll Gen Pract* 39:332–334, 1989.
62. Rapid diagnostic tests for group A streptococcal pharyngitis, *Med Lett* 33:40–41, 1991.
63. DuBois D, Ray VG, Nelson B, Peacock JB: Rapid diagnosis of group A strep pharyngitis in the emergency department, *Ann Emerg Med* 15:86–88, 1986.
64. Macknin ML, Indioh N, Ezsley KA et al: Comparison of two rapid diagnostic tests for group A streptococcus, *Pediatr Infect Dis J* 7:735–736, 1988.
65. White CB, Lieberman MM, Morales E: An in vitro comparison of eight rapid streptococcal antigen detection tests, *J Pediatr* 113:691–693, 1988.
66. Facklam RR: Specificity study of kits for detection of group A strep directly from throat swabs, *J Clin Microbiol* 25:504–508, 1987.
67. Kellog JA, Manzella JP: Detection of group A streptococci in the laboratory or physicians office—culture vs antibody methods, *JAMA* 255:2638–2642, 1986.
68. Gerber MA, Randolph MF, Chanatry J et al: Antigen detection kits for streptococcal pharyngitis: evaluation of sensitivity with respect to true infections, *J Pediatr* 108:654–657, 1986.
69. Beach PS, Balfour LC, Lucia HL: Group A streptococcal rapid test—antigen detection after 18–24 hours of penicillin therapy, *Clin Pediatr (Phila)* 28:6–10, 1989.
70. Catanzaro FJ, Stetson CA, Morris AJ et al: The role of the streptococcus in the pathogenesis of rheumatic fever, *Am J Med* 17:749–756, 1954.

Chapter 3

Urinalysis and Urine Cultures

Richard Lanoix, M.D.

Harold H. Osborn, M.D.

CASE 3–1

A 38-year-old male was brought to the emergency department with complaints of numbness of his right foot of several hours duration. He stated that he had fallen asleep in a chair while watching television the night before and had awakened with a feeling of pain and tingling in the affected extremity. He denied any previous medical history, hospitalizations, or operations and stated that he was not taking any medications.

On physical examination he had a blood pressure of 130/80 mm Hg, a heart rate of 100/min, a respiratory rate of 18/min, and a temperature of 99.0° F. His physical examination was unremarkable. Neurologic examination revealed decreased sensation over the dorsum of the right foot and an absent Achilles reflex on the right. Plantar flexion and dorsiflexion of the right ankle were weak, and the foot was not warm, red, or tender to touch. Pulses were difficult to palpate in the right foot but were present by Doppler examination.

Laboratory evaluation included a complete blood count (CBC) with a white blood cell (WBC) count of 12,000/mm^3 and a hematocrit of 34%. The chemistry profile was normal. Urinalysis revealed a large amount of blood on the urine dip stick. Microscopic urine examination revealed 0 to 2 red blood cells (RBCs) per high-power field (HPF), 0 WBC/HPF, and occasional granular casts.

Because of the positive test for blood by urine dipstick and the negative microscopic evaluation for RBCs, a diagnosis of myoglobinuria was entertained. A creatine phosphokinase (CPK) level was ordered, and the result was 20,000 ng/mL. A urine myoglobin level was sent to confirm the diagnosis. The serum was centrifuged for the presence of a pink color, and a smear was examined to rule out hemolysis. The hematocrit remained stable, and there was no evidence of hemolysis. Rhabdomyolysis and compartment syndrome were diagnosed.

The patient was questioned again and this time admitted to snorting heroin and drinking a pint of blackberry brandy before falling asleep in the chair.

URINE

Urine is composed of free water and various metabolic end products: urea and ammonium from deaminated amino acids, uric acid from the breakdown of purines, creatinine from muscle breakdown, and porphyrins and their precursors from heme synthesis. Other end products are derived from the catabolism of hormones, drugs, and foreign chemicals.

Normally urine should *not* contain glucose (unless the maximum rate at which glucose can be reabsorbed [transport maximum, or T_{max}] is exceeded. The T_{max} is normally 320 mg/min.), free amino acids, albumin in excess of 10 mg per 24 hours, myoglobin, or hemoglobin. Certain proteins (β-microglobulins and Tamm-Horsfall protein) are secreted into the urine but are usually undetectable. Proteinuria over 150 mg per 24 hours is always abnormal and implies a pathologic derangement.

The formation of urine begins with filtration of the blood plasma through glomerular capillaries. In normal adults, 25% of the cardiac output, or more than a liter of blood, perfuses both kidneys each minute, and an ultrafiltrate of the plasma passes through each glomerular capillary tuft into Bowman's capsule to produce a glomerular filtration rate of 120 mL/min. Modification of this filtrate to produce excreted urine occurs in the tubules and collecting duct of each nephron. Final concentrations depend on the state of hydration. Normally the total glomerular filtrate volume of about 180 L in 24 hours is reduced to 1 or 2 L, and water and sodium are conserved. The final product, urine, passes from the collecting ducts into the kidney, pelvis, ureters, bladder, and urethra to be voided. In disease states, this fluid is altered chemically and cytologically.

URINE COLLECTION METHODS

The diagnostic value of urinalysis, including microscopic examination, depends on the quality of the specimen obtained. It is therefore essential to obtain a urine specimen as free as possible from periurethral contamination.

Infants Less Than 1 Year Old

Urine collected with a perineal bag is useful only for chemical analysis and microscopic examination. Because of the high rates of contamination, cultures obtained by this method are often unreliable.[1–3] If a urinary tract infection (UTI) is suspected, the urine should be collected by catheter or suprapubic aspiration. In male infants an alternative method is to use the primitive Perez reflex as described by Boehm and Haynes.[4] The infant is held in the prone position, with the collection cup held under the penis. Stroking the back along the midline will cause the infant to reflexly arch his back and urinate. If the infant is uncircumcised, the foreskin may be retracted, but only as far as it will go without meeting resistance.

In infants less than 1 year old, suprapubic aspiration is a safe procedure and the most aseptic method for obtaining a urine specimen.[1, 5–7] Suprapubic aspiration of urine was first introduced in 1959 by Pryles et al.[6] but has not gained widespread use. The intraabdominal location of the bladder in this age group makes it particularly accessible by this route.

The abdomen should be prepared with an antiseptic solution. A 1½-in, 22-gauge needle for children and a 1-in, 25-gauge needle for infants is attached to a 10 mL syringe and the needle inserted with negative pressure, midline, into the suprapubic area approximately 1 in above the symphysis pubis at a 10- to 15-degree angle cephalad. Because contamination should be virtually nonexistent with this technique, any bacteria seen on Gram stain and/or any number of colonies on culture should be considered significant.

Complications of the suprapubic technique (i.e., bowel puncture, hemorrhage, and bacteremia) have been reported, although they rarely cause significant problems.[8–11] By using aseptic technique, a gentle touch, ensuring that the bladder is full with a bottle of glucose solution, and avoiding the method when the abdomen is distended or the child is uncooperative, complications may be minimized. Furthermore, the use of ultrasound-guided suprapubic aspiration has been demonstrated to increase the success of the procedure and reduce the complication rate.[12]

Children

In older children, sterile midstream urine can be collected. If the voided specimen is free of epithelial cells, it is probably acceptable for analysis. If not, it is appropriate to catheterize the patient.

Adult Females

In women, there are a variety of collection methods. With regard to a midstream voided specimen, the major concern is perineal contamination. One study has shown that in up to 50% of women with sterile bladder urine 1000 to 100,000 bacteria/mL grew from a midstream-catch specimen.[13] This figure assumes major significance in the emergency department (ED) where accurate, initial supportive evidence for the diagnosis of urinary infection is important. However, a properly collected specimen containing no or few epithelial cells is as accurate as urine obtained by catheterization. Female patients should be instructed to remove their underwear, sit facing the back of the toilet, spread the labia with one hand, cleanse from front to back with povidone-iodine swabs or liquid soap, pass a small amount of urine into the toilet, and then urinate into a sterile cup.

If the patient cannot void spontaneously or is ill, immobilized, extremely obese, or unable to provide a sample free of epithelial cells, catheterization is indicated.

Catheterization is safe and relatively atraumatic and carries a small risk of infection (1% to 3% in most series). This risk increases to 20% if the patient is elderly or debilitated.[14] However, because of this risk, albeit small, of introducing infection, routine catheterization is not indicated.

Adult Males

In men, a clean-catch, midstream voided specimen should be obtained. A recent study has demonstrated that the specimen is not affected significantly by lack of cleansing or by the timing of specimen collection.[15, 16] The study suggests that the time and effort spent instructing adult males in the proper technique of cleansing and collecting a midstream specimen is simply not necessary. Nor is it usually necessary to catheterize males simply for the purpose of obtaining a urine specimen.

URINALYSIS

A complete urinalysis consists of a description of the physical appearance, a determination of specific gravity, dipstick analysis, microscopic examination, and Gram stain if indicated. Indications for a complete urinalysis include the following:

- Suspicion of UTI
- A febrile patient without a recognizable source for the fever
- Suspicion of systemic disease with renal manifestations
- Hypertension

In children and elderly adults, it may not be possible to elicit an adequate history. Therefore the physician must have a high degree of suspicion and be capable of recognizing the signs and symptoms of UTIs in patients at the extremes of age (see the accompanying box).

At times, a urine specimen is obtained for specific reasons and only a partial urinalysis is indicated (Table 3–1).

Signs and Symptoms of Urinary Tract Infections in Children

Failure to thrive
Anorexia, poor feeding
Nausea, vomiting or diarrhea
Lethargy or irritability
"Sepsis"
Hyperbilirubinemia
"Colic"
Hypothermia
Unexplained fever
Discolored or malodorous urine
Urgency, frequency, dysuria, tenesmus
Abdominal or flank pain
Enuresis or daytime incontinence
Shaking chills

Physical Characteristics

Color

The yellow color of urine is due largely to the pigment, urochrome, and to small amounts of urobilins and uroerythrin. The color varies with the specific gravity and is influenced by a variety of metabolic products, foods, drugs, and pigments. A comprehensive listing is given in Tables 3–2 and 3–3. On standing, urine darkens because of oxidation of the colorless urobilinogen to colored urobilin.

Table 3–1. Indications for Partial Urinalysis

- Dipstick for blood
  - Abdominal, flank, back, or perineal trauma
  - Abdominal or pelvic mass
  - Coagulopathy
  - Suspicion of hemoglobinuria or myoglobinuria
- Protein
  - Patient with edema, including periorbital swelling
  - Suspicion of glomerular disease
  - Pregnancy
- Specific gravity
  - Dehydration or clinical condition predisposing to dehydration (vomiting, diarrhea)
  - Assessment of concentrating ability
- Glucose and ketones
  - Suspicion of diabetic ketoacidosis
- pH
  - To monitor alkalinity or acidity of urine to aid in the diagnosis of renal tubular acidosis and nephrolithiasis and in the treatment of drug overdose
- Ketones
  - Assessment of pregnant female with hyperemesis
  - Suspicion of diabetic ketoacidosis, salicylate overdose, or isopropyl alcohol ingestion
- Ferric chloride test
  - Suspicion of ingestion of salicylate or phenothiazine

Table 3–2. Appearance and Color of Urine

Appearance	Cause	Remarks
Colorless	Very dilute urine	Polyuria, diabetes insipidus
Cloudy	Phosphates, carbonates	Soluble in dilute acetic acid
	Urates, uric acid	Dissolves at 60° C and in alkali
	Leukocytes	Insoluble in dilute acetic acid
	Red cells ("smoky")	Lyses in dilute acetic acid
	Bacteria, yeasts	Insoluble in dilute acetic acid
	Spermatozoa, prostatic fluid	Insoluble in dilute acetic acid
	Mucin, mucous threads	May be flocculant
	Calculi, "gravel" clumps, pus, tissue	Phosphates, oxalates
	Fecal contamination	Rectovesical fistula
	Radiographic dye	In acid urine
Milky	Many neutrophils (pyuria)	Insoluble in dilute acetic acid
	Fat	
	Lipiduria, opalescent	Nephrosis, crush injury—soluble in ether
	Chyluria, milky	Lymphatic obstruction—soluble in ether
	Emulsified paraffin	Vaginal creams
Yellow	Acriflavine	Green fluorescence
Yellow-orange	Concentrated urine	Dehydration, fever
	Urobilin in excess	No yellow foam
	Bilirubin	Yellow foam if sufficient bilirubin
Yellow-green	Bilirubin-biliverdin	Yellow foam
Yellow-brown	Bilirubin-biliverdin	"Beer" brown, yellow foam
Red	Hemoglobin	Reagent strip positive for blood
	Erythrocytes	Reagent strip positive for blood
	Myoglobin	Reagent strip positive for blood
	Porphyrin	May be colorless
	Fuscia, aniline dye	Foods, candy
	Beets	Yellow alkaline, genetic
	Menstrual contamination	Clots, mucus
Red-purple	Porphyrins	May be colorless
Red-brown	Erythrocytes	Reagent strip positive for blood
	Hemoglobin on standing	Reagent strip positive for blood
	Methemoglobin	Acid pH
	Myoglobin	Muscle injury
	Bilifuscin (dipyrrole)	Result of unstable hemoglobin
Brown-black	Methemoglobin	Blood, acid pH
	Homogentisic acid	On standing, alkaline alkaptonuria
	Melanin	On standing, rare
Blue-green	Indicans	Small intestine infections
	Pseudomonas infections	
	Chlorophyll	Mouth deodorants

With permission from Henry JB: *Clinical diagnosis and management by laboratory methods,* ed 18, Philadelphia, 1991, WB Saunders, p 394.

Odor

The normal odor of urine may be modified by the presence of acetone, which imparts a fruity odor. Malodorous urine may be caused by bacterial decomposition in the presence of leukocytes, which produces an ammoniacal odor. However, malodorous urine may also be caused by diet (e.g., garlic and asparagus), medication (e.g., menthol), and metabolic disorders and is therefore not a reliable sign of infection. Urine odors associated with disorders of amino acid metabolism are listed in Table 3–4. In addition, there are a variety of drugs that can alter the odor as well as the other characteristics of urine (Table 3–5).

Clarity

Freshly voided urine is clear and moderately transparent depending on its concentration.

Table 3–3. Urine Color Produced by Various Substances

Substance	Colors Produced in Urine
Acetanilid	Yellow to red
Acetophenetidin (metabolite)	Yellow (dark brown wine color)
Alcohol	Lightens color
Aloin	Red-brown to yellow-pink (alkaline urine), yellow-brown (acid urine)
Aminopyrine	Red-brown
Aminosalicylic acid (paraamino-salicylic acid)	Discoloration (no distinctive color)
Amitriptyline	Blue green
Anisindione	Orange (alkaline urine), pink to red-brown
Anthraquinone laxatives	Reddish (alkaline urine)
Anticoagulants (indandione derivatives)	Orange
Antipyrine	Yellow to red-brown
Azuresin	Blue or green
Beets	Red
Benzene	Red-brown
Carbon tetrachloride	Red-brown
Carrots	Yellow
Cascara	Yellow-brown (acid urine), yellow-pink (alkaline urine), darkens to brown to black on standing
Chloroquine	Rust-yellow to brown
Chlorzoxazone	Orange to purple-red
Cinchophen	Red-brown
Creosote	Dark green
Cresol	Dark color on standing
Danthron	Pink to red
Deferoxamine mesylate	Reddish (in presence of free iron)
Dihydroxyanthraquinone	Pink to orange (alkaline urine)
Dinitrophenol	Red-brown
Dithiazanine hydrochloride	Blue
Doans' kidney pills	Greenish blue
Emodin (in cascara)	Pink to red to red-brown (alkaline urine)
Ethoxazene	Orange to red
Ethylene glycol	Fluorescent with Wood's light
Ferrous salts	Black
Fluorescein (intravenous)	Yellow-orange
Furazolidone (metabolite)	Brownish or rust-yellow
Indandiones	Orange (alkaline urine)
Indomethacin	Green (biliverdinemia)
Iron sorbitex	Dark to black on standing
Lead	Red-brown
Levodopa	Dark
Mercury	Red-brown
Methocarbamol	Dark brown, black or green on standing
Methyldopa	Dark (red to black) on standing
Methylene blue	Greenish blue to blue
Metronidazole	Dark brown
Naphthol	Dark color on standing
Nitrobenzene	Dark color on standing
Nitrofurantoin and derivatives	Brown or rust-yellow
Phenacetin (see acetophentidin)	
Phenazopyridine	Orange-red to red-brown (HNO_3 turns orange to pink)
Phenindione	Reddish brown to pink, orange in alkaline urine
Phenolphthalein	Pink to red to magenta (alkaline urine), yellow-brown (acid urine)
Phenolsulfonphthalein	Red (alkaline urine)
Phenol	Dark green to brownish black (darkens on standing)
Phenothiazines	Pink to red-brown
Phensuximide	Pink to red to red-brown

Modified with permission from Martin EW: *Hazards of medication,* Philadelphia, 1978, JB Lippincott, pp 188–189.

Table 3–3. Urine Color Produced by Various Substances—cont'd

Substance	Colors Produced in Urine
Phenyl salicylate	Dark green
Phenytoin	Pink to red-brown
Picric acid	Yellow to red-brown
Porphyrins	Burgundy red, darkens on standing
Primaquine naphthosate	Rust-yellow or brown
Primaquine phosphate	Rust-yellow to brown
Pyrogallol	Brown to black (darkens on standing)
Quinacrine hydrochloride	Yellow (deep yellow upon acidification)
Quinine and derivatives	Brown to black
Resorcinol	Dark green to greenish blue, darkens on standing
Rhubarb	Yellow-brown (acid urine), yellow-pink (alkaline urine), darkens on standing
Riboflavin	Yellow
Rifampin	Red to orange
Salicylazosulfapyridine	Orange-yellow (alkaline urine)
Salol	Dark color on standing
Santonin	Bright yellow (NaOH changes to pink or scarlet)
Senna	Yellow-brown (acid urine), yellow-pink (alkaline urine), darkens on standing
Sulfonamides	Rust-yellow or brown
Sulfasalazine	Orange-yellow
Sulfonethylmethane	Red
Sulfonmethane	Red-brown
Tetrahydronaphthalene (Tetralin)	Greenish blue
Thiazosulfone	Pink to red
Thymol	Greenish blue
Tolonium (Blutene)	Blue-green
Trinitrotoluene (TNT)	Red-brown
Triamterene	Bluish color (pale blue fluorescence)
Warfarin sodium	Orange

Causes of Turbidity

Temperature and pH.—Diffuse clouding or a sediment may form normally on standing because of changes in pH and temperature. For this reason, about 50% of normal urine specimens received in the laboratory are cloudy.

Amorphous Phosphates and Carbonates.—These are soluble in acid urine but may precipitate in alkaline urine. They dissolve on addition of 5% to 10% acetic acid (amorphous phosphates *without*, and carbonates *with* gas formation).

Urates.—Urates are soluble in neutral or alkaline urine but may precipitate in acid urine. They are often pink and dissolve on heating. If protein is present, the cloudiness may increase on heating.

Oxalates.—Clearing is produced by 12% hydrochloric acid.

Table 3–4. Urine Odors Associated with Amino Acid Metabolism

Condition	Specific Odor
Isovaleric acidemia and glutaric acidemia	Sweaty feet
Maple syrup urine disease	Maple syrup
Methionine malabsorption	Cabbage, hops
Phenylketonuria	Mousy
Trimethylaminuria	Rotting fish
Tyrosinemia	Rancid

Table 3–5. Drugs That Influence Routine Results of Urinalysis

- Odor
  - Antibiotics
  - Paraldehyde
  - Vitamins
- Increased specific gravity
  - Dextran
  - Glucose
  - Radiopaque contrast media
  - Albumin
- Decreased pH
  - Ammonium chloride
  - Ascorbic acid
  - Diazoxide
  - Methenamine
  - Metolazone
- Increased pH
  - Acetazolamide
  - Amphotericin B
  - Mafenide
  - Sodium bicarbonate
  - Potassium citrate
- True proteinuria or false-positive results
  - Penicillin in large doses (except with Ames Reagent strips); however, some penicillins cause true proteinuria
  - Sulfonamides (sulfosalicylc acid method)
- False-positive result for glycosuria
  - Aminosalicylic acid (Benedict's test)
  - Ascorbic acid (Clinistix, Diastix, or Tes-Tape)
  - Ascorbic acid in large doses (Clinitest tablets)
  - Cephalosporins (Clinitest tablets)
  - Chloral hydrate (Benedict's test)
  - Chloramphenicol (Benedict's test for Clinitest tablets)
  - Isoniazid (Benedict's test)
  - Levodopa (Clinistix, Diastix, or Tes-Tape)
  - Levodopa in large doses (Clinitest tablets)
  - Methyldopa (Tes-Tape)
  - Nalidixic acid (Benedict's test or Clinitest Tablets)
  - Nitrofurantoin (Benedict's test)
  - Penicillin G in large doses (Benedict's test)
  - Phenazopyridine (Clinistix, Diastix, or Tes-Tape)
  - Probenecid (Benedict's test or Clinitest tablets)
  - Salicylates in large doses (Clinitest tablets, Clinistix, Diastix, or Tes-Tape)
  - Streptomycin (Benedict's Test)
  - Tetracycline (Clinistix, Diastix, Tes-Tape)
  - Tetracyclines, because of ascorbic acid buffer (Benedict's test or Clinitest tablets)
- True glycosuria
  - Ammonium chloride
  - Asparaginase
  - Carbamazepine
  - Corticosteroids
  - Dextrothyroxine
  - Lithium carbonate
  - Nicotinic acid (large doses)
  - Phenothiazines (long term)
  - Thiazide diuretics
- Increased white blood cell count
- False-positive result for proteinuria
  - Acetazolamide (Combistix or Labstix)
  - Aminosalicylic acid (sulfosalicylic acid method)
  - Nafcillin (sulfosalicylic acid method)
  - Cephalothin in large doses (sulfosalicylic acid method)
  - Sodium bicarbonate (all methods)
  - Tolbutamide (sulfosalicylic acid method)
  - Tolmetin (sulfosalicylic acid method)
- True proteinuria
  - Amikacin
  - Amphotericin B
  - Bacitracin
  - Gentamicin
  - Gold preparations
  - Kanamycin
  - Neomycin
  - Netilmicin
  - Phenylbutazone
  - Polymyxin B
  - Streptomycin
  - Tobramycin
  - Trimethadione
- Hematuria
  - Amphotericin B
  - Coumarin derivatives
  - Methenamine in large doses
  - Methicillin
  - Paraaminosalicylic acid
  - Phenylbutazone
  - Sulfonamides
- False-positive results for ketonuria
  - Levodopa (Ketostix or Labstix)
  - Phenazopyridine (Ketostix, Gerhardt's reagent strip shows atypical color)
  - Phenolsulfonphthalein (Rothera's test)
  - Phenothiazines (Gerhardt's reagent strip shows atypical color)
  - Salicylates (testing with Gerhardt's reagent strip shows reddish color)
  - Sulfobromophthalein (Bili-Labstix)
- True ketonuria
  - Ether (anesthesia)
  - Isoniazid (intoxication)
  - Isopropyl alcohol (intoxication)
  - Insulin (excessive doses)
- Casts
  - Amphotericin B
  - Aspirin toxicity
  - Bacitracin
  - Ethacrynic acid
  - Furosemide
  - Gentamicin
  - Griseofulvin
  - Isoniazid
  - Kanamycin
  - Neomycin
  - Penicillin
  - Radiographic agents
  - Streptomycin
  - Sulfonamides

Modified from *Clinical laboratory tests: values and implications,* Springhouse Corp, 1992, pp 651–652.
**NSAIDs,* nonsteroidal antiinflammatory drugs.

Table 3–5. Drugs That Influence Routine Results of Urinalysis—cont'd

Allopurinol	Crystals (if urine is acidic)
Ampicillin	Acetazolamide
Salicylates and NSAIDs*	Aminosalicylic acid
Kanamycin	Ascorbic acid
Methicillin	Nitrofurantoin
	Theophylline
	Thiazide diuretics
	Ethylene glycol

Cells.—Leukocytes, erythrocytes, and epithelial cells may be present in urine. About 200 leukocytes/mm^3 or 500 erythrocytes/mm^3 produce turbidity.

Bacteria.—Bacteria are not removed by filtration through filter paper unless some inert substance such as kaolin is added first; even then the results are not always satisfactory.

Lipuria.—Fat globules impart a milky appearance to the specimen but may be removed and cleared by extraction with ether.

Chyle.—Chyluria may be parasitic (filarial) or nonparasitic (as in thoracic duct obstruction, trauma, and tumor) in origin and imparts a cream color to the urine. Obstructed lymph vessels may force chylous fluid and cholesterol into the excretory urinary apparatus and the urine. Shaking the specimen with ether will clear the urine sample.

Specific Gravity

Specific gravity is defined as the ratio of the weight of a fixed volume of solution to that of the same volume of water at a specified temperature, usually 20° C. For most chemical substances, an increase in the amount dissolved in a fixed volume of water causes an almost linear increase in the specific gravity of the solution. Specific gravity is a measure of the total amount of material dissolved in urine and thus a measure of the concentrating and excreting power of the kidneys. Urea (20%), sodium chloride (25%), sulfate, and phosphate contribute most of the specific gravity of normal urine.

Normal adults with normal diets and fluid intake will produce urine of specific gravity 1.016 to 1.022 during a 24-hour period, whereas in infants, normal specific gravity values are 1.002 to 1.006. In adults, if a random specimen of urine has a specific gravity of 1.023 or more, concentrating ability can be considered normal. After taking no fluids for 12 hours, urine specific gravity should be about 1.022, and after 24 hours, it should be approximately 1.026. After a standard water load minimum specific gravity should be less than 1.003.

Low specific gravity ($<$1.005) may be caused by exaggerated oral or intravenous fluid intake, administration of diuretics, hypothermia, diabetes insipidus, acute tubular necrosis, and pyelonephritis. Fixed specific gravity (isosthenuria) in which values remain at approximately 1.010 (the specific gravity of plasma) regardless of fluid intake occurs in chronic glomerulonephritis with severe renal damage and medullary necrosis. High specific gravity (greater than 1.020) may be caused by nephrotic syndrome (proteinuria), adrenal insufficiency, acute glomerulonephritis, congestive heart failure, dehydration, shock, radiologic contrast media, and chemical urinary preservatives[17, 18] such as mineral acids, asorbic acid, boric acid, benzoic acid, phenols, thymol, toluol, chloroform, formaldehyde, and mercury compounds used to prevent bacterial growth or to preserve cells. The specific gravity may be determined by means of a urinometer or a refractometer.

Methods

Urinometer

A urinometer is a hydrometer adapted to measure the specific gravity of urine at room temperature. The urinometer vessel is filled three-fourths full with urine. The minimum volume of urine required is about 15 mL. The urinometer is inserted with a spinning motion to make sure that it is floating freely. When reading the urinometer, one should be sure that it is not touching the sides or bottom of the cylinder. Care should be taken to avoid surface bubbles, which obscure the meniscus. The correct value is that number of the urinometer on a level with the bottom of the meniscus.

Because temperature affects the specific gravity, urine samples should be allowed to come to room temperature before a reading is made, or a correction of 0.001 should be added for each 3° C above or subtracted for each 3° C below the calibration temperature indicated on the urinometer (usually 20° C). For accurate determinations, corrections should also be made for protein or glucose. One should subtract 0.003 for every 1% of protein and 0.004 for every 1% of glucose.[19]

There are several disadvantages of using the urinometer: (1) mass-produced urinometers are often inaccurate and should be checked against solutions of known specific gravity, and the appropriate corrections should be applied to all measurements; (2) at least 15 mL of urine is required to float the instrument; and (3) turbid urine may make reading of the scale difficult.

Refractometer

The refractive index of a solution is the ratio of the velocity of light in air to the velocity of light in a solution and varies with the concentration of dissolved solids present. The commercial hand refractometers are convenient, accurate, and easy to use. They require only a few drops of urine, and the measurement takes only a few seconds. The instrument also has a built-in temperature compensator so that corrections for temperature are not necessary in the usual room temperature range of 20 to 30° C. However, as with the urinometer, one should make a correction for glucose and protein in the urine. For glucose, the same correction may be used as with the urinometer. For protein, a slightly higher correction of 0.004 is probably more accurate.

REAGENT STRIPS

Urine reagent strips can be used to determine pH, protein, glucose, ketones, bilirubin, urobilinogen, blood, nitrites, and leukocyte esterase. These strips, which provide colorimetric chemical assays, offer a quick, inexpensive method for performing an urinalysis. However, these tests must be used and interpreted carefully because the many agents that alter urine color (see Tables 3–2 and 3–3) can also interfere with color development on the reagent pad.

pH

The test for urinary pH uses a double indicator—methyl red and bromothymol blue—in order to give clearly distinguishable colors over the pH range from 5 to 9.

Urine pH can be helpful in the diagnosis and treatment of UTIs, urinary calculus disease, and certain drug overdoses (e.g., salicylate overdose).

An alkaline urine in patients with presumed urinary tract infection suggests infection with an organism, most commonly *Proteus mirabilis* or *Klebsiella*, which splits urea to ammonia. These patients are likely to have struvite calculi because these inorganic salts (magnesium, ammonium, and phosphate) are less soluble in alkaline urine. Other causes of alkaline urine are Fanconi's syndrome, renal tubular acidosis, metabolic or respiratory alkalosis, diets high in certain fruits and vegetables (especially citrus fruits), dairy products, sodium bicarbonate, potassium citrate, and acetazolamide.[17, 19]

Acid urine may be produced by a diet high in meat protein and some fruits such as cranberries, by starvation, metabolism of fat, metabolic and respiratory acidosis, ammonium chloride, methionine, methenamine mandelate, acid phosphate, renal tuberculosis, pyrexia, phenylketonuria (PKU), and alkaptonuria. It may be a sign of nephrolithiasis in patients with uric acid or cystine stones.[17, 19]

Protein

A normal kidney excretes less than 20 mg of protein daily, and approximately half of this is albumin. Over 95% of filtered protein is reabsorbed in the proximal tubules. Reagents strips are saturated with tetrabromphenol blue or a combination of tetrachlorophenol and tetrabromosulfophthalein and turn green or blue in the face of proteinuria. They react more to albumin than to globulins, Bence Jones protein, and mucoprotein. They are sensitive to approximately 10 mg/dL or less. Therefore normal urine should not turn the strip positive for protein.

There are several factors that produce false-positive reactions for protein: basic urine specimens (pH > 9), phenzopyridine (Pyridium and Azo Gantrisin) usage, polyvinylpyrrolidone (infusions of blood substitutes), contact with disinfectants (chlorhexidine on the skin or ammonium cleansers in the container), and urine specimens obtained following prostatic massage. High urine specific gravity, hematuria, or prolonged immersion of the dipstick in the urine can also cause color changes and lead to false-positive results. False-negative results are seen with dilute urine.

The "gold standard" for urinary protein analysis is the sulfosalicylic acid test, which is equally sensitive for albumin as well as the other urinary proteins at levels as low as 5 mg/dL.

The test is performed by adding 2.5 mL of supernatant urine to 7.5 ml of 2% sulfosalicylic acid. Any precipitate is indicative of proteinuria. False-positive results may be caused by radiologic contrast agents, large doses of penicillin, paraaminosalicylic acid and tolbutamide metabolites.[19] Overall, the advantages of the sulfosalicylic acid test over dipstick analysis are greater accuracy and sensitivity, an ability to detect Bence Jones protein, and fewer false-positive results.

Urobilinogen and Bilirubin

These tests provide information concerning bile pigment circulation and liver function and can occasionally explain altered urine color. Bilirubin detection is based upon the binding reaction of bilirubin to a diazonium salt in an acid medium. Urobilinogen determination has classically been performed by the Ehrlich aldehyde reaction with a dimethylaminobenzaldehyde reagent. Subsequently, other methods using diazonium salts have been developed.

Since the unconjugated bilirubin-albumin complex cannot be filtered, it is therefore not found in the urine, whereas 1% of the conjugated bilirubin-glucuronyl albumin complex is excreted by glomerular filtration. Normally, no bilirubin is found in the urine on the reagent strip because only amounts greater than 0.4 mg/dL are measured. Approximately 1 to 40-mg/day of urobilinogen is normally excreted in the urine. Urobilinogen is formed by the catabolism of conjugated bilirubin in the gut by normal intestinal bacteria and then excreted in the feces or is reabsorbed into the plasma, where it is taken up by the liver and reexcreted into the bile. The small amount that avoids hepatic uptake is then excreted by the kidney into the urine. Hemolytic anemias increase urobilinogen excretion. Hepatocellular diseases that interfere with enterohepatic circulation, such as hepatitis and cirrhosis, can lead to increased urinary urobilinogen, whereas interruption of intrahepatic circulation of bile pigments (common bile duct obstruction) or antibiotic usage that alters intestinal flora can stop the excretion of urinary urobilinogen. Causes of increases in urine bilirubin are listed in the accompanying box.

Ascorbic acid in amounts as low as 2-mg/dL lowers the sensitivity of this test and can cause false-negative results. Phenazopyridine can also cause false-positive results because it colors the urine and turns it red in an acid medium.

Glucose and Ketones

Small amounts of glucose are normally excreted in the urine. However, these amounts are usually below the sensitivities of urine reagent strip tests (40 to 75 mg/dL). Therefore, any positive findings are abnormal and should be evaluated.

Glucose detection is based upon a double sequential enzymatic reaction. In the initial reaction, glucose oxidase is required for the oxidation of glucose into gluconic acid and hydrogen peroxide. Subsequently, peroxidase catalyzes the reaction of hydrogen peroxide with an indicator chromogen, thereby causing a color change by oxidation of the chromogen.

The dipstick test is specific for glucose; other sugars such as lactose, galactose, and fructose do not cross-react. The test is less reliable with increased specific grav-

Causes of Conjugated Hyperbilirubinemia

- Defective excretion
  - Intrahepatic obstruction
    - Familial syndromes
      - Dubin-Johnson
      - Rotor
    - Drugs (i.e., chloramphenicol, methyltestosterone)
    - Benign recurrent cholestasis
    - Recurrent jaundice of pregnancy (third trimester)
  - Extrahepatic obstruction (tumors, stone, stricture of the bile duct)
- Hepatocellular disease
  - Hepatitis (viral or drug induced)
  - Cirrhosis
- Impaired hepatocellular function
  - Halothane anesthesia
  - Drugs (i.e., oral contraceptive agents, chlorpromazine, erythromycin estolate, phenytoin, isoniazid, sulfonamides)
  - Shock, hypotension, hypoxemia (with resultant hepatocellular necrosis)
  - Sepsis

Modified with permission from Wilson JD, Braunwald E, Isselbacher KJ, editors, et al: *Harrison's principles of internal medicine,* ed 12, New York, 1991, McGraw-Hill.

ity and increased temperature. Ascorbic acid (>50 mg/dL) or ketones (>30 mg/dL) in the urine can cause a false-negative result when urinary glucose is in the range of 100 mg/dL. The enzyme glucose oxidase may also be affected by many different substances (see accompanying box).

Ketones are usually not found in urine. However, fasting, starvation diets, postexercise states, pregnancy, diabetic ketoacidosis, alcoholic ketoacidosis, salicylate overdose, and isopropyl alcohol ingestion can all produce ketones in the urine.

The sodium nitroprusside method for determining ketones in urine identifies acetone and acetoacetate at levels of 5 to 10 mg/dL but not β-hydroxybutyric acid. β-Hydroxybutyrate (the reduced form of acetoacetate) is technically not a ketone and does not participate in the sodium nitroprusside reaction. The ratio of acetoacetate to β-hydroxybutyrate depends on the redox potential. In the setting of diabetic ketoacidosis, the usual ratio of acetoacetate to β-hydroxybutyrate is 1:2.8. However, this ratio may be as high as 1:30 (particularly in alcoholic acidosis), in which case the urine strip does not reflect the true level of ketosis. When ketones are in the form of β-hydroxybutyrate, the urine strip test may uncommonly reveal a trace or negative reaction in spite of significant ketosis. False-positive determinations can be caused by

Substances Interfering with Glucose Oxidase Tests

False-positive tests

- Chloride
- Glucose hypochlorite

False-negative tests

- Alcaptonuria
- Ascorbic acid
- Aspirin
- Bilirubin
- Catalase
- Catechols
- Cysteine
- 3,4-Dihydroxyphenylacetic acid
- L-Dopamine
- Epinephrine
- Ferrous sulfate (Feosol)
- Gentisic acid
- Glutathione
- Homogentisic acid
- Hydrogen peroxide
- 5-Hydroxyindole acetic acid
- 5-Hydroxytryptamine
- 5-Hydroxytryptophan
- Levodopa
- Meralluride injection
- Methyldopa (Aldomet)
- Peroxide
- Sodium bisulfate
- Tetracycline (Tetracyn, Achromycin) with vitamin C
- Uric acid

With permission from *Contemp Pharm Pract* 3:224, 1980.

very acidic urine with high specific gravity as seen in dehydration, abnormal urine color, levodopa metabolites, 2-mercaptoethane sulfonate sodium, and other sulfhydryl-containing compounds.[20]

SCREENING TESTS FOR URINARY TRACT INFECTIONS

Since up to 80% of "routine" urine cultures may be negative and the cost of skilled technicians to perform microscopic examinations and process urine cultures is significant, many hospitals use a variety of screening tests for UTIs (Figs. 3–1 and 3–2). The most widely used chemical reagent strip tests measure leukocyte esterase and nitrites. According to most laboratory protocols, a urine that is reagent strip negative for leukocyte esterase and nitrites is not subsequently examined microscopically.

Nitrites

Normal urine does not contain nitrites. However, many species of gram-negative bacteria can convert nitrates to nitrites, thereby enabling this simple test (Griess test) to identify bacteriuria.[21]

The specificity of the nitrite reagent test for detection of bacteriuria is high, between 92% and 100%.[22] However, the sensitivity of the test varies from 35% to 85% depending on the population tested, the manner in which the specimen is collected, and the criteria used for defining a UTI or significant bacteriuria.[23] In specimens containing fewer than 10^5 colonies on culture, the strip test for nitrites is less accurate.[24]

The only major cause of a false-positive finding is specimen contamination. Common causes of a false-negative result are presence of non–nitrate-reducing organisms such as *Staphylococcus saprophyticus*, presence of organisms that further reduce nitrites to ammonia, frequent voiding (bladder dwell time of less than 4 hours), not using the first morning specimen (the use of a random specimen identifies only 50% to 60% of patients with UTIs), dilute urine (low concentration of bacteria), acidic urine (pH < 6), large dietary intake of ascorbic acid ($>$25 mg/dL), and the presence of abnormal amounts of urobilinogen.

Currently available data suggest that a positive strip test for nitrites is significant and an indication of bacteriuria. However, a negative result does not indicate that significant bacteriuria is not present. Therefore, if your institution screens urine with a strip before performing microscopic examination, a mandatory microscopic examination should be requested when the clinical situation is suggestive of a UTI.

Leukocyte Esterase

Leukocyte esterase is an enzyme produced by neutrophils. This enzyme can catalyze the hydrolysis of an indoxylcarbonic acid ester to an indoxyl. The indoxyl formed then oxidizes a diazonium salt chromogen to produce a color change. This reagent test correlates well with chamber counts for urinary leukocytes, is highly specific for detecting pyuria, and is not affected by the presence of bacteria or erythrocytes ($<$1000/dL).[25] However, screening for a UTI with a test that assesses pyuria may not be entirely reliable. Studies have shown that 50% to 66% of patients with bacteriuria may not have pyuria, depending on the definition of pyuria.[26–28] Two WBCs/HPF is commonly accepted as the cutoff for significant pyuria.[29–31] Even at this level, many patients with bacteriuria do not have pyuria, and therefore leukocyte esterase findings are negative. Initial reports of high sensitivity supported use of a leukocyte esterase dipstick test as a screening tool for pyuria. However, in an ED setting, Propp et al. demonstrated an unacceptable rate of false-negative results for low-level pyuria (6 to

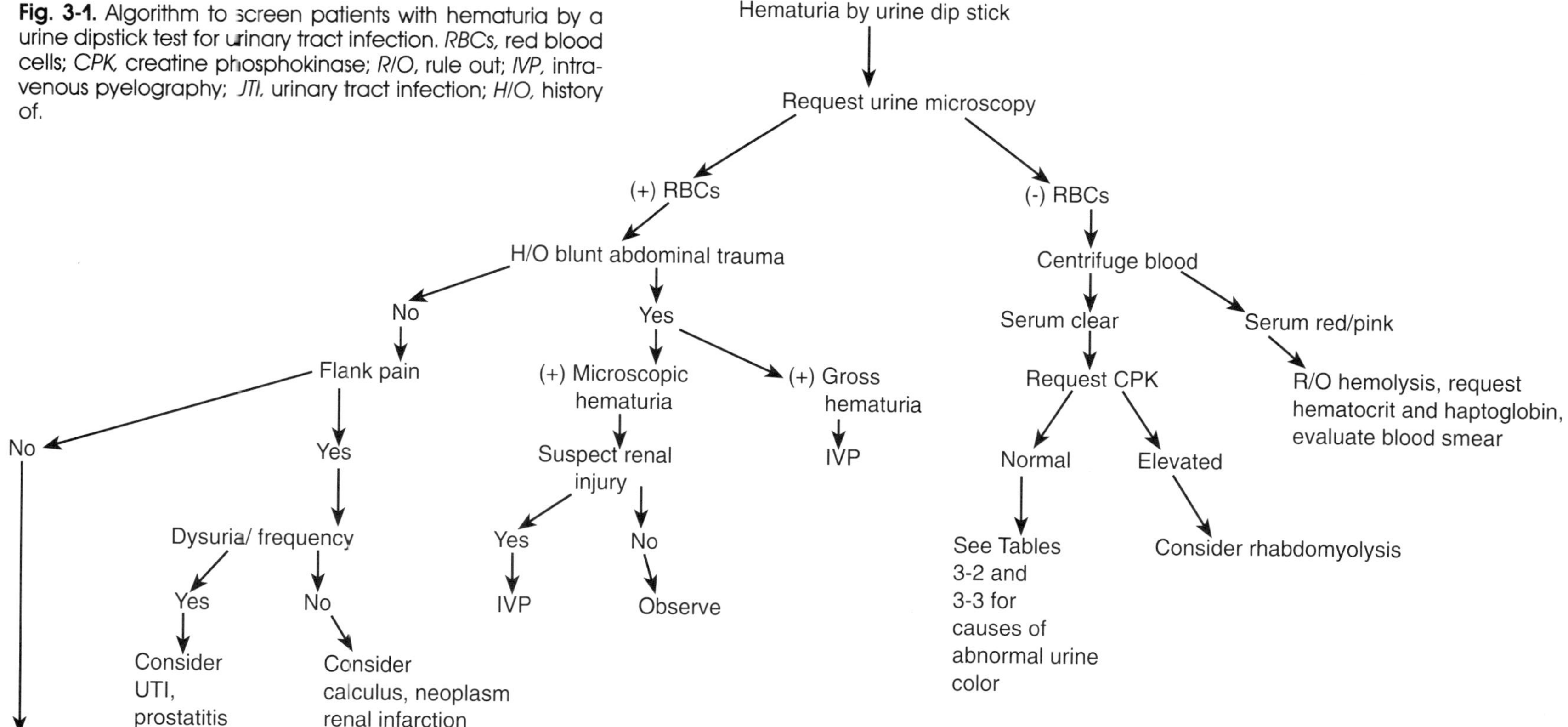

Fig. 3-1. Algorithm to screen patients with hematuria by a urine dipstick test for urinary tract infection. *RBCs,* red blood cells; *CPK,* creatine phosphokinase; *R/O,* rule out; *IVP,* intravenous pyelography; *UTI,* urinary tract infection; *H/O,* history of.

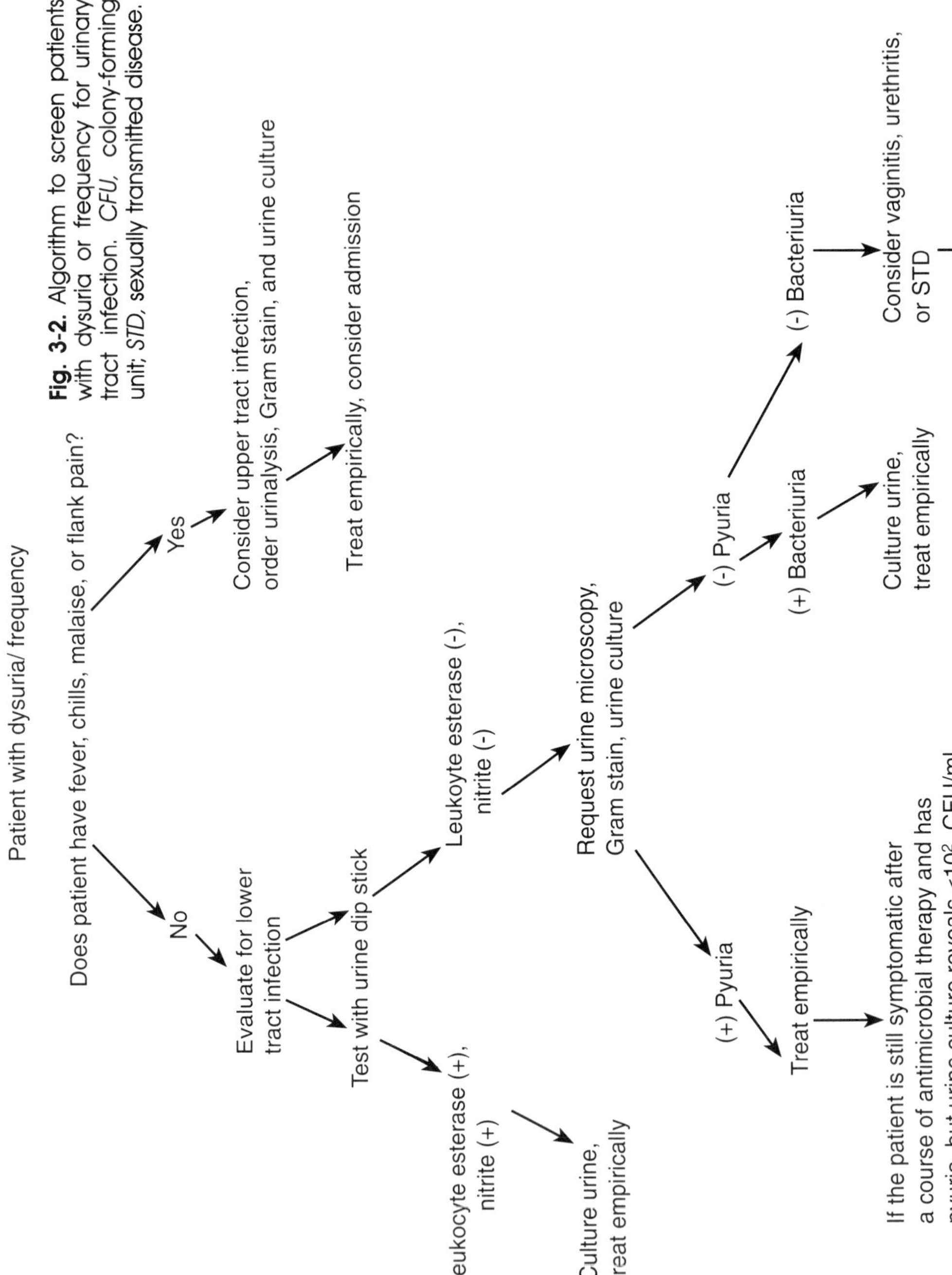

Fig. 3-2. Algorithm to screen patients with dysuria or frequency for urinary tract infection. *CFU,* colony-forming unit; *STD,* sexually transmitted disease.

20 WBCs/HPF).[32] Overall, leukocyte esterase strips have a sensitivity that varies from 72% to 97% and a specificity ranging from 64% to 83%.[33–36]

The predominant cause of a false-positive strip test result is specimen contamination. False negatives can occur because of increased specific gravity, glycosuria, the presence of urobilinogen, medications that alter urine color (refer to Tables 3–2 and 3–3), and a large intake of ascorbic acid.[22]

Reagent strip testing is acceptable as a screening method for bacteriuria in asymptomatic adults and may be justified in women over age 60 and in diabetics. However, the test is not adequate for pregnant women because of the serious potential consequences of untreated bacteriuria, which include pyelonephritis, abortion, and low-birth-weight babies. These patients require standard urine cultures. Acutely symptomatic patients with clinical symptoms that suggest a UTI should have a microscopic examination performed despite a negative leukocyte esterase determination in order to detect clinically significant pyuria.

Additionally, since "low-count infections" (less than 10^5 or 100,000 colonies per milliliter) are present in 30% to 40% of acutely symptomatic women, the screening test will be less useful in this group.[37] In summary, a microscopic examination should always be performed despite a negative reagent strip test result in acutely symptomatic patients and in all pregnant females.

BLOOD

The urinary reagent strip for blood measures intact erythrocytes, free hemoglobin from lysed erythrocytes, and myoglobin. Chemical detection of blood in urine is based on the peroxidase-like activity of hemoglobin. When in contact with an organic peroxide substrate, hemoglobin and myoglobin catalyze the oxidation of a chromogen indicator, which changes color according to the degree and amount of oxidation. The amount of color change and oxidation is directly related to the amount of hemoglobin or myoglobin present in the specimen. Most strips demonstrate colored dots as well as field color changes. Free hemoglobin and myoglobin produce a field change color effect, whereas intact erythrocytes produce a dot color change. The greater the number of intact erythrocytes in a specimen, the greater the number of dots that will appear on the strip. When there are more than 250 erythrocytes per milliliter, a coalescence of the dots occurs.

If the urine reagent strip demonstrates a positive test for blood but urine microscopy is negative for erythrocytes, myoglobinuria should be suspected and the patient evaluated further for rhabdomyolysis. Destruction of striated muscle, regardless of the cause, liberates myoglobin. Because of its relatively small size, myoglobin (molecular weight, 17,000 Da) unlike hemoglobin, is filtered by the glomerulus rapidly, appears quickly in the urine, and imparts a burgundy red color to it. The serum is effectively cleared and retains its normal color. In contrast, hemolysis results in free hemoglobin (molecular weight, 68,000 Da) that is cleared more slowly from the serum by the glomerulus. Thus, whereas the urine turns red, the serum retains a pink color because of the high renal threshold. Myoglobinuria should thus be suspected when the urine is deep red and the serum normal in color (Table 3–6).

Myoglobinuria occurs only in the presence of rhabdomyolysis; however, rhabdomyolysis can occur without the detection of myoglobin in the urine. Myoglobin will not appear in the urine until serum levels exceed 1.5 mg/dL.[38] Once this critical serum level is reached, there are several factors that affect the degree of myoglobinuria present: its plasma concentration, the glomerular filtration rate, the extent of myoglobin binding in plasma, and the urine flow rate. Furthermore, as a result of the rapid

Table 3–6. Differential Diagnosis of Positive Reagent Strip Test for Blood

Diagnosis	Reagent Strip	Microscopic	Serum
Hematuria	Positive	RBCs	Normal
Hemoglobinuria	Positive	Negative	Pink
Myoglobinuria	Positive	Negative	Normal

excretion of myoglobin from urine, a significant number of patients with rhabdomyolysis will have negative strip test results.

Measurement of CPK levels is a more sensitive method to detect the presence of rhabdomyolysis. It is an excellent marker for this entity because it is easily measured, is present in the serum immediately after muscle injury, and is not rapidly cleared from the serum. In general, peak CPK levels occur within 24 to 36 hours from the time of muscle injury. Most experts consider CPK levels of five times normal or greater to indicate the presence of rhabdomyolysis.[39–43]

False-positive reagent strip determinations for blood in females are most commonly due to contamination of the specimen with menstrual blood. High specific gravity can also cause false-positive results because of the altered concentration of erythrocytes and elevated concentrations of hemoglobin. Normal individuals excrete between 5000 and 8000 erythrocytes per milliliter of urine.[44,45] Therefore, using a concentrated specimen such as the first morning voided specimen increases the likelihood of a false-positive result. Other causes of false-positive results are dehydration, exercise, and various vitamins and food products containing high concentrations of oxidants. False-negative results are caused by high dietary intake of ascorbic acid, which interferes with the strip test, and contamination of the specimen with formalin.

The sensitivity of reagent strips for identifying hematuria, with microscopy as the "gold standard," is over 90%,[46–48] whereas the specificity is more variable and reported to be 65% to 99.3%.[48–50]

URINARY SEDIMENT

Complete urinalysis should include microscopic examination of a wet mount of the centrifuged specimen under high dry power (×40) and with stain under an oil immersion field (×100). Ten to 12 mL of fresh, well-mixed urine should be poured into a test tube and centrifuged at 2000 to 2500 rpm for 5 minutes. The supernatant should be decanted and the sediment resuspended by tapping the tube in the drop of urine that is left. The ideal volume of urinary sediment to be obtained is between 0.01 and 0.02 mL, which is the maximum that will fit under a standard 22 mm^2 cover glass. A second slide should be similarly prepared for staining.

Microscopic analysis of the urinary sediment should be performed with both low power (×10) and high power (×40). Under low power, the whole specimen should be scanned, with particular attention to the coverslip edges where casts and other elements tend to concentrate. The following components should be searched for at this magnification: erythrocyte casts, cellular casts, oval fat macrophages, trichomonads, leukocyte clumps, and crystals.

Erythrocyte casts represent glomerulonephritis, whereas leukocyte casts reflect interstitial disease (Fig. 3-3). Although fat-laden histiocytes (oval fat macrophages) are frequently associated with nephrotic syndrome and heavy proteinuria, they can be seen in most nephropathies as well as in a substantial proportion of patients with nonglomerular renal disease (Fig. 3-4). Trichomoniasis is a frequent cause of vaginal discharge in females and occasionally urethritis in males. Most commonly, trichomonads are an incidental finding on microscopy. Identification of large cells moving suddenly is indicative of a trichomonad adjacent to it; identification of rapidly moving flagella under high power confirms the diagnosis (Fig. 3-5).

Urate, phosphate, and oxalate crystals can be seen in the urine of stone formers

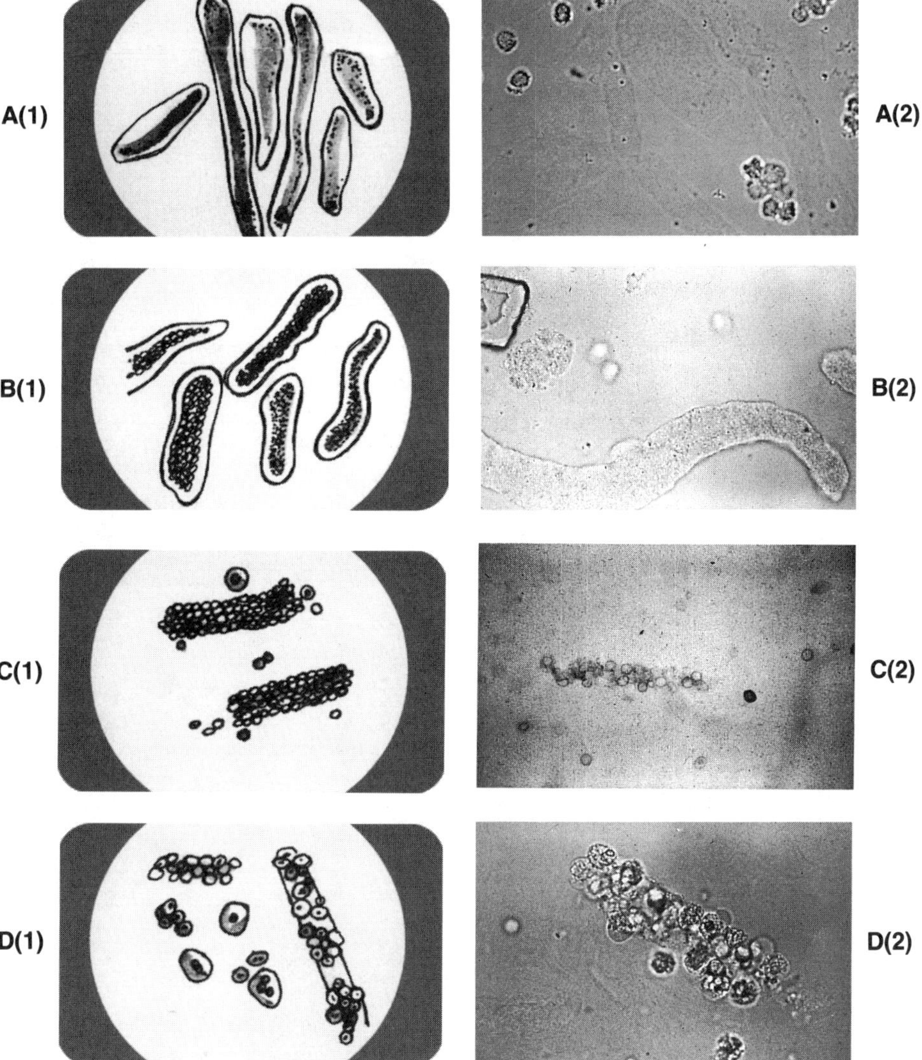

Fig.3-3. A, Hyaline casts are formed from a protein gel in the renal tubule. Hyaline casts may contain cellular inclusions. Hyaline casts will dissolve very rapidly in alkaline urine. Normal urine sediment may contain one to two hyaline casts per low power field (LPF). **B,** Granular casts are casts with granules present throughout the cast matrix. They are quite refractile. If the granules are small, the cast is defined as a finely granular cast. If granules are large, it is termed a coarsely granular cast. Granular casts can appear in urine in normal or abnormal states. **C,** RBC casts are pathologic, and their presence usually indicates severe injury to the glomerulus. Rarely, transtubular bleeding may occur, forming RBC casts. RBC casts are found in acute glomerulonephritis, lupus, bacterial endocarditis, and septicemias. "Blood" casts are granular and contain hemoglobin from degenerated RBCs. **D,** WBC casts occur when leukocytes are incorporated within the cast matrix. WBC casts will usually indicate an infection, most commonly pyelonephritis. They may also be seen in glomerular diseases. WBC casts may be the only clue to pyelonephritis. With permission from: *Atlas of urine sediment,* Elkhart, Indiana, 1991, Miles Incorporated, Diagnostics Division.

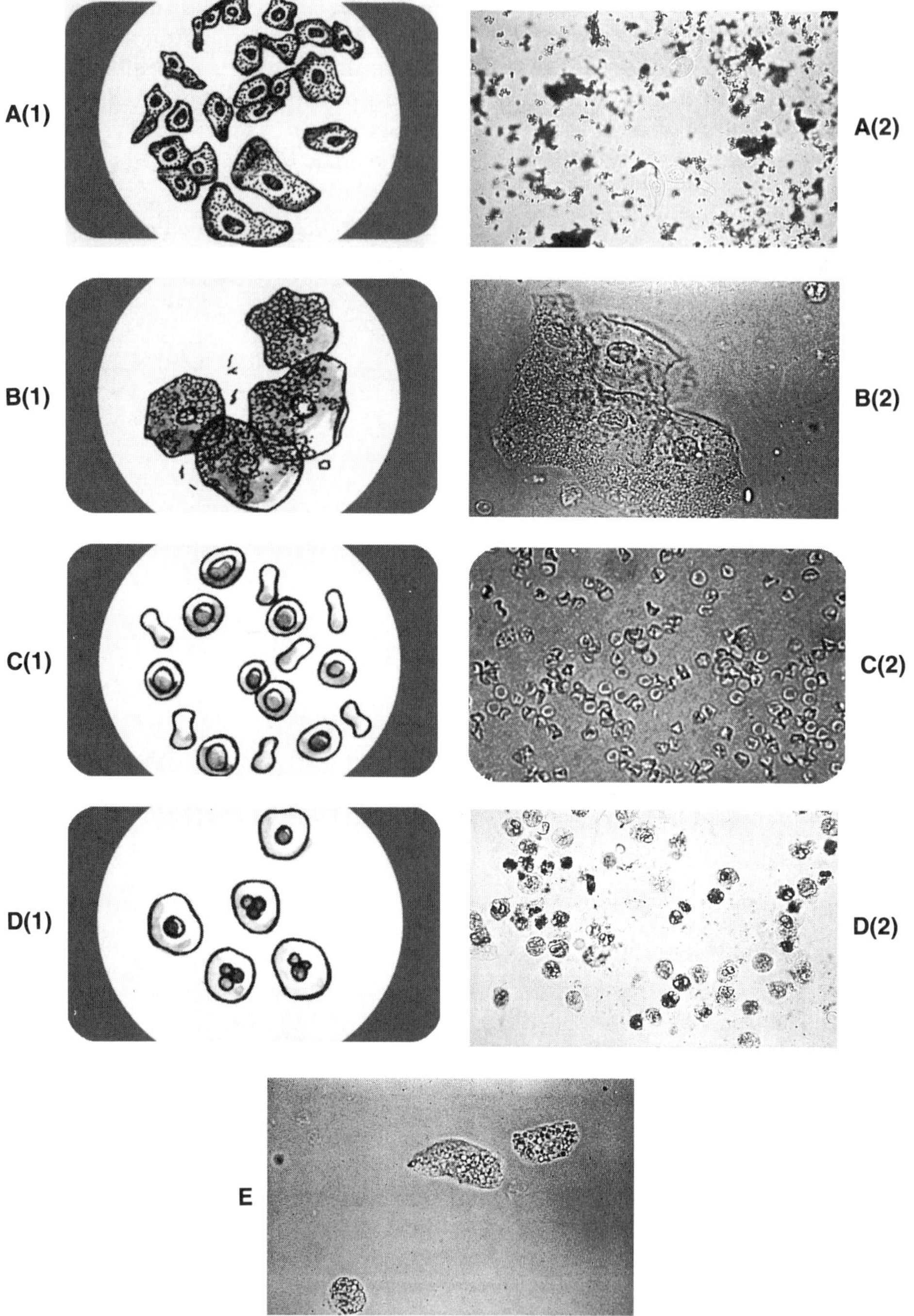

Fig 3-4. A and **B,** Three types of epithelial cells may appear in urine sediment: renal tubular, transitional, and/or squamous. Other types of cells may appear in urine but are difficult to identify because of morphologic changes caused by urine. Tubular cells are approximately ⅓ larger than white blood cells. Transitional epithelial cells may arise from the renal pelvis, ureters, bladder, or urethra. They tend to be pear-shaped. Squamous cells are large and flat with a prominent nucleus. They originate in the urethra. **C,** Red blood cells may originate from any part of the renal system. Large numbers of RBCs in the urine suggest conditions such as infection, trauma, tumors, and renal calculi. However, the presence of one or two RBC/HPF in the urine sediment , or blood in the urine from menstrual contamination, should not be considered abnormal. **D,** WBCs in the urine (pyuria) may originate from any part of the renal system. The presence of more than five WBCs/HPF may suggest infection, cystitis, or pyelonephritis. **E,** Fat

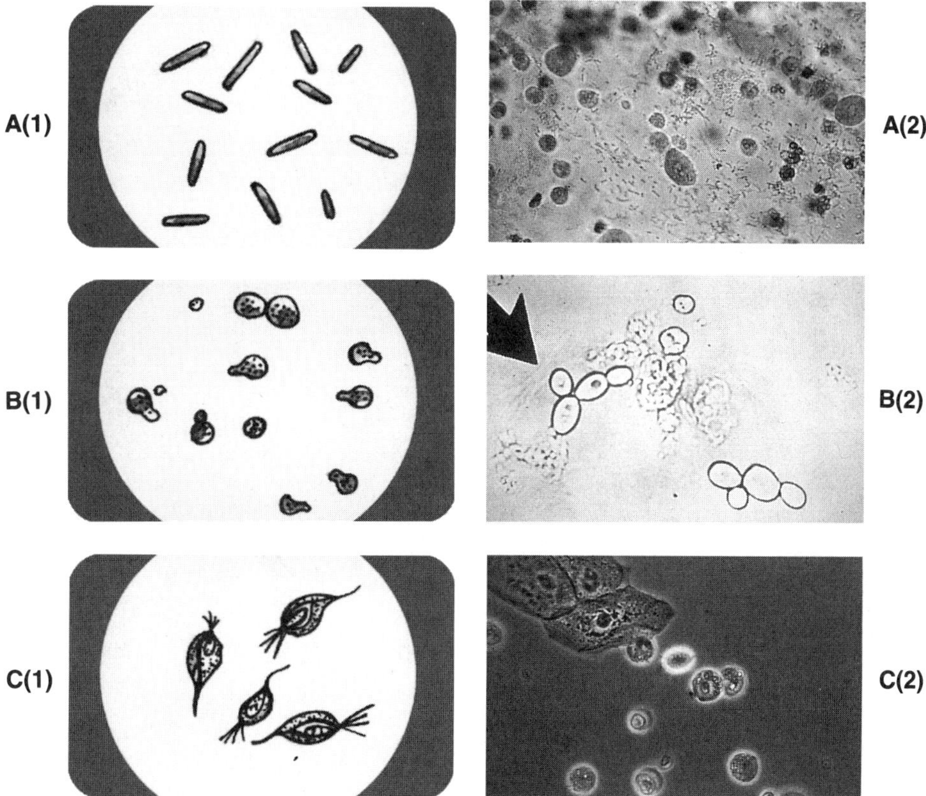

Fig. 3-5. A, Bacteria in the urine (bacteriuria) can result from contaminants in collection vessels, from periurethral tissues, the urethra, or from fecal or vaginal contamination as well as from true urinary infection. **B,** Yeast cells vary in size, are colorless, ovoid, and are often budding. They are often confused with RBCs. *Candida albicans* is often seen in diabetes, pregnancy, obesity, and other debilitating conditions. **C,** Trichomonas vaginalis is a flagellate protozoan that affects both males (urethritis) and females (vaginitis). With permission from: *Atlas of urine sediment,* Elkhart, Indiana, 1991, Miles Incorporated, Diagnostics Division.

and normal patients (Figs. 3-6, 3-7, & 3-8). However, the appearance of cystine crystals (hexagon shaped) occurs only in those with cystinuria and is therefore diagnostic of this condition (see Fig. 3-6). Also, in an intoxicated, stuporous, or comatose patient with metabolic acidosis and a history of unknown ingestion, calcium oxalate crystals are highly suggestive of ethylene glycol ingestion (see Figs. 3-6 & 3-7).

USE OF HIGH-POWER MAGNIFICATION

The purpose of high-power examination is to identify bacteria, yeast (see Fig. 3-5), casts (see Fig. 3-3), and cells (see Fig. 3-4). The standard high-power examination should cover 10 to 15 fields.

---

may be present in urine as free droplets or globules within degenerating cells or incorporated in a cast. Oval fat bodies are renal tubular cells that contain highly refractile fat droplets. Lipids may appear in the urine as free fat droplets. These droplets frequently vary in size because fat globules can coalesce together. Anisotrophic fat globules that manifest the "Maltese-cross" formation under polarized light are termed *doubly refractile fat bodies.* Fat is frequently found in nephrotic syndrome. It may be present in diabetes mellitus, eclampsia, toxic renal poisoning, and chronic glomerulonephritis. With permission from: *Atlas of urine sediment,* Elkhart, Indiana, 1991, Miles Incorporated, Diagnostics Division.

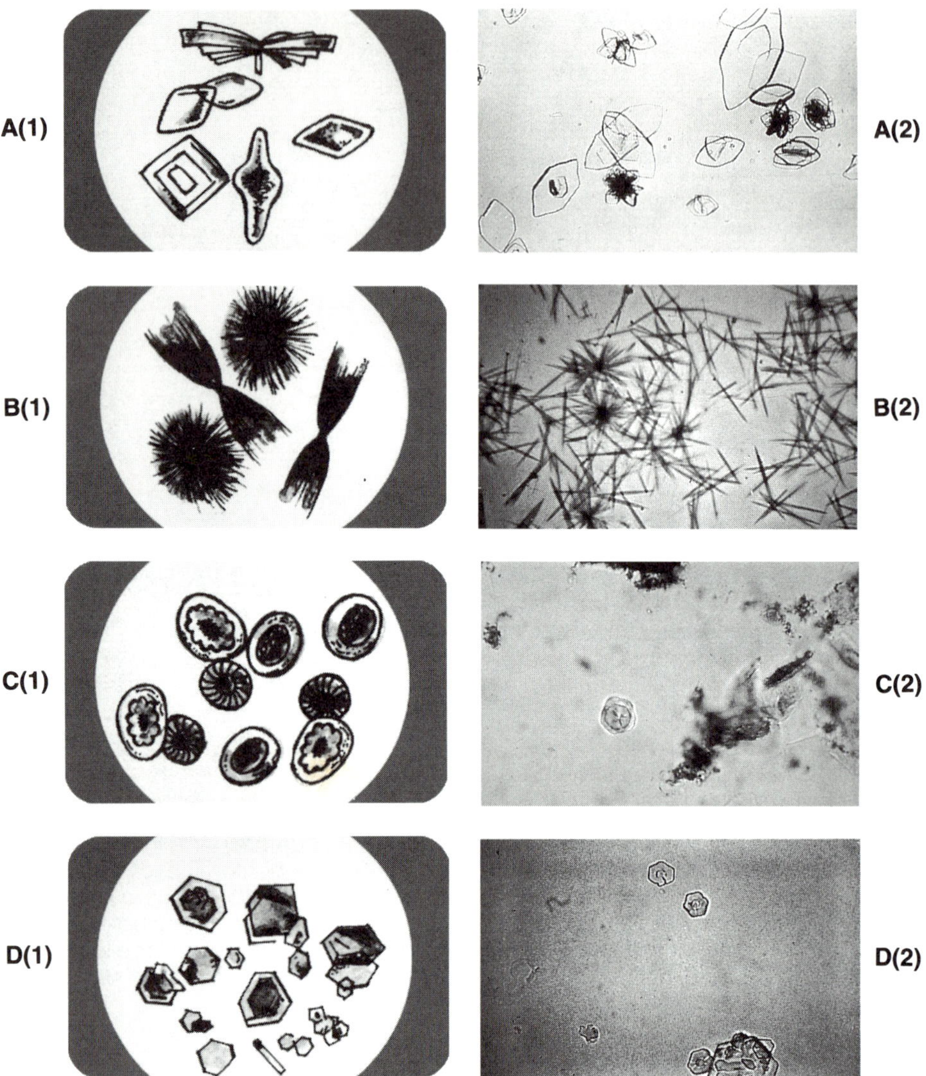

Fig. 3-6. A, Uric acid has birefringent characteristics; therefore, it polarizes light, giving multicolors. Uric acid crystals are found in acid urine. Uric acid may assume various forms (e.g., rhombic, plates, rosettes, small crystals). The color may be red-brown, yellow, or colorless. Although increased in 16% of patients with gout, and in patients with malignant lymphoma or leukemia, the presence of such crystals does not usually indicate a pathologic condition or increased uric acid concentrations. **B,** and **C,** Leucine and tyrosine are amino acids that crystallize and often appear together in the urine of patients with severe liver disease. Tyrosine usually appears as fine needles arranged as sheaves or rosettes and appear yellow. Leucine is usually yellow, oily-appearing spheres with radial and concentric striations. **D,** Cystine crystals are thin, hexagonal-shaped (6-sided) structures. They appear in the urine as a result of a genetic defect. Cystine crystals and stones will appear in the urine in cystinuria and homocystinuria. Cystine crystals are frequently confused with uric acid crystals. Cystine crystals do not polarize light. With permission from: *Atlas of urine sediment,* Elknart, Indiana, 1991, Miles Incorporated, Diagnostics Division.

Exact criteria for what constitutes an abnormal number of erythrocytes and leukocytes have not been established. As approximate guidelines, some authorities consider more than five erythrocytes or more than two leukocytes per HPF of *centrifuged* urine to be significant,[51–53] although others feel strongly that only criteria based on unspun urine are reliable enough to establish or exclude the diagnosis of UTI.

Although examination of the urine is the means by which a clinician makes a pre-

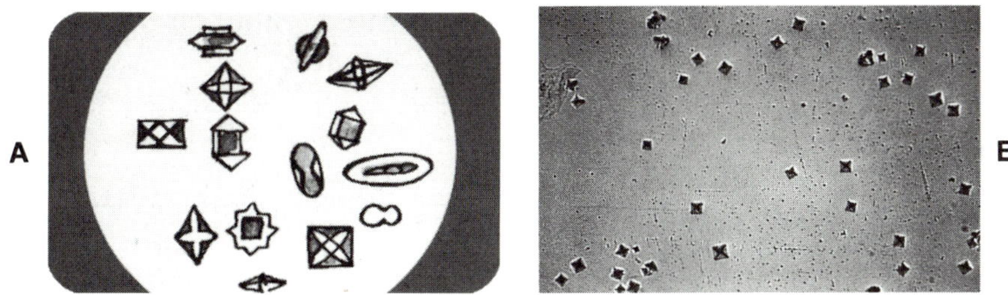

Fig 3-7. Calcium oxalate crystals most frequently have an "envelope" shape and appear in acid, neutral, or slightly alkaline urine. They appear in the urine after the ingestion of certain foods (e.g., cabbage, asparagus) and ethyleneglycol. With permission from: *Atlas of urine sediment,* Elkhart, Indiana, 1991, Miles Incorporated, Diagnostics Division.

sumptive diagnosis of UTI, the limitations of the procedure are substantial. The finding of bacteriuria or pyuria may be affected by a number of factors: false-positive results can occur with nonbacterial inflammatory disorders or vulvovaganial contamination during collection. The frequency of voiding, the rate of urine flow, the growth rate of bacteria in the urine, variability in the methods of urine centrifugation and slide preparation, severe dehydration, fever, trauma, stones, and foreign bodies will also affect the extent of bacteriuria and pyuria.

Despite these limitations, the most useful test for a presumptive diagnosis of UTI remains the identification of bacteria on microscopic examination. The finding of bacteria in unspun urine correlates highly with a colony count of greater than 10^5 colonies per milliliter.[54–58] (In a centrifuged, unstained urine sample, greater than 10 organisms per HPF is significant.[54–58])

Any study of the urine must be done immediately after collection. Urine specimens that are allowed to sit become alkaline with subsequent dissolution of the cellular elements and multiplication of bacteria and provide the clinician with markedly

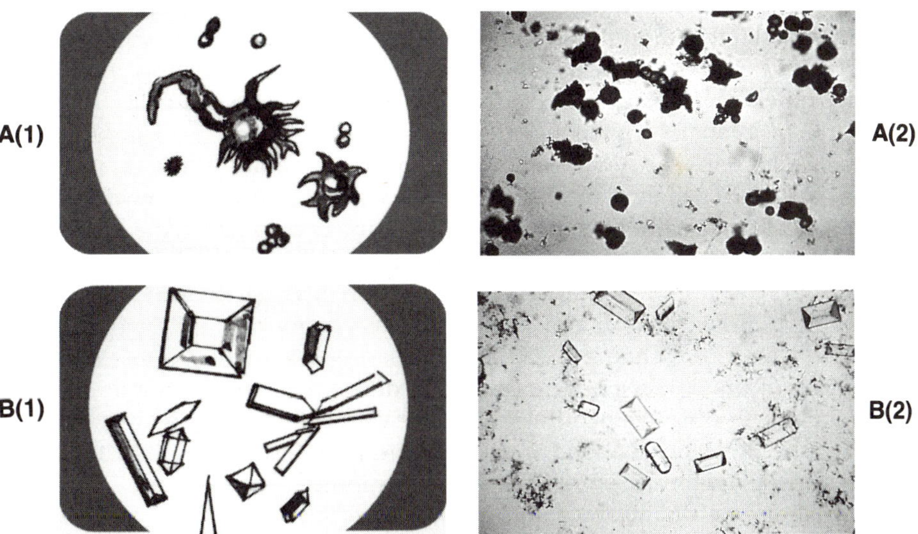

Fig. 3-8. A, Ammonium urates are yellow-brown in appearance and occur in urine as spheres or spheres with spicules ("thorny apples"). Both forms are frequently seen together. They appear in urine when there is ammonia formation in the urine present in the bladder. They are considered to have little clinical significance. **B,** Triple phosphate crystals are common in urine sediment. They have a "coffin-lid" shape, are colorless, and appear in alkaline urine. The ingestion of fruit may cause triple phosphate to appear in urine. With permission from: *Atlas of urine sediment,* Elkhart, Indiana, 1991, Miles Incorporated, Diagnostics Division.

unreliable results. If the specimen cannot be cultured within 30 minutes of collection, it should be refrigerated and plated within 24 hours.[59–63]

Urine Staining

A complete urinalysis may include examination of a stained specimen. The stain, whether the traditional Gram stain or methylene blue stain, will aid in differentiating leukocytes and epithelial cells as well as in identifying bacteria. If examination of the wet mount under high, dry power is negative, examination of a stained specimen is unnecessary.

Triple-strength methylene blue is an excellent and rapid stain to use in the ED. The sediment is fixed on the slide with heat and is then flooded with dye for 10 to 20 seconds, rinsed, and dried with mild heat or gentle blotting with a tissue. The sediment may then be examined under an oil immersion field.

Physicians should remember that the Gram stain can confirm infection but cannot rule it out. A Gram-stained urine may be negative in patients with low-count bacterial infection ($<10^5$ colony-forming units [CFUs]/mL), as in the case of infections caused by *S. saprophyticus* and *Chlamydia*.

Urine Culture

The gold standard for significant bacteriura (UTI) is the quantitative urine culture. Since the landmark studies of Kass and Sanford a quantitative culture of midstream urine containing 10^5 CFUs per milliliter or greater has been the criterion generally used to establish a diagnosis of UTI.[64–67] They found that 95% of infected women lack greater than 10^5 CFUs/mL and that this number of colonies on culture would reliably distinguish contamination from true infection. It is important to note that these studies compared symptomatic women with acute pyelonephritis to asymptomatic controls and did not include women with infections of the lower genitourinary tract.

More recently, Stamm and others[68, 69] have used simultaneous suprapubic tap and midstream urine collection to document infection in symptomatic women with pyuria and midstream colony counts less than the traditional 10^5 CFUs/mL. As many as 30% to 50% of women with dysuria and pyuria will have midstream urine colony counts less than 10^5 of a single organism (often *Staphylococcus saphrophyticus, S. albus,* or *Chlamydia trachomatis*) and will respond to appropriate antibiotic therapy.[70–74] This syndrome, variously called "acute urethral syndrome," "dysuria-pyuria syndrome," or "symptomatic abacteriuria," has created significant problems in the standard definition of UTIs. Multiple studies have now demonstrated that a midstream colony count over 10^2/mL in symptomatic women with pyuria is a sensitive and specific indicator of infection.[69, 70] Since many hospital laboratories do not routinely work up or report urine cultures with less than 10^5 CFUs/mL, it is important to request a culture with determination of sensitivities on the urine of women with symptomatic pyuria regardless of the colony count. The positive predictive value of a relatively lower colony count improves as the prevalence of UTI increases, and an arbitrary cutoff of 10^5 CFUs/mL is no longer appropriate in a symptomatic population.

The dipslide method of urine culture compares favorably with more conventional laboratory techniques (such as the pour-plate or calibrated-loop methods) in its ability to detect significant bacteriuria.[75–78] This technique employs a plastic paddle coated on each side with agar-based medium. A variety of media can be used depending on the selectivity for specific organisms desired. In general, the dipslide will have eosin–methylene blue or MacConkey's medium on one side, which will support the growth of most gram-negative organisms, whereas the opposite side will have nutrient agar or cystine-lactose-electrolyte–deficient (CLED) agar medium, which is more selective for gram-positive organisms. After the media are coated with urine, the paddle is placed in a self-contained cover and then incubated.

The dipslide technique offers a number of advantages especially suitable for an ED:

- It eliminates lengthy transit times of specimens to a central laboratory, thus preventing bacterial overgrowth and mixed culture growth.
- It allows the clinician to start therapy immediately if a UTI is suspected with the knowledge that a reliable result may be available within 18 to 24 hours.
- It increases recovery of staphylocci while decreasing the recovery of gram-positive commensals.
- It can be performed by any emergency personnel with a minimum of training.

MISCELLANEOUS TESTS

Phenistix

This test was originally created to detect PKU in newborns. The Phenistix turns brownish purple when either salicylates or phenothiazines are in the urine or serum, as opposed to the typical gray-green to blue color change when PKU is present. Adding a drop of 50% sulfuric acid to the strip bleaches out the color in the case of salicylates but not in the case of phenothiazines.[79] Color resulting from phenothiazines will intensify to brilliant pink or purple. A single 325 mg tablet of salicylate can produce a positive urine Phenistix reaction. Therefore, salicylate *intoxication* can be excluded when the urine is Phenistix-negative. However, a positive reaction indicates only that salicylates have been used, not necessarily salicylate intoxication.

Ferric Chloride

This is an extremely sensitive and useful qualitative indicator for the presence of salicylates. The test is performed by adding 2 to 3 drops of 10% ferric chloride solution to 1 mL of urine. A violet-to-purple color indicates salicylate ingestion 30 minutes (or longer) earlier. Again, a negative test result is strong evidence against salicylate *ingestion*, but a positive test result does not necessarily imply an *overdose*, since the ingestion of a single tablet will result in a positive reaction.

Ketone bodies can give a false-positive ferric chloride reaction but can be removed by acidifying and boiling the urine before adding the ferric chloride. False-positive results may also be produced by phenylpyruvic acid, diflunisal, isoniazid, coal tar dyes, and phenothiazines, although the latter tend to give more of a brown color.[80] This test is extremely useful because there are no false negatives. Roberts et al. compared ferric chloride with Phenistix in 48 healthy volunteers and found that ferric chloride was superior in sensitivity and specificity.[81]

Deferoxamine

When a normotensive patient is suspected of having a significant iron overdose, deferoxamine, a highly specific chelator of free iron, may be administered intramuscularly. If the patient is hypotensive, 15 mg/kg (up to 1 g) may be given intravenously over a 1-hour period. If free iron is present in the serum, this will chelate with the deferoxamine to form ferrioxamine, which is excreted renally and will cause the urine to become a *vin rose* or orange color. Because the first urine may reflect residual urine present in the bladder before the administration of deferoxamine, the bladder should be emptied and all subsequent voidings saved for comparison. A positive change in urine requires only that free iron be present in the serum and therefore does not imply toxicity in an otherwise asymptomatic patient.

REFERENCES

1. Aronson AS, Gustafen B, Svenningsen NW: Combined suprapubic aspiration and clean-voided urine examination in infants and children, *Acta Pediatr Scand* 62(4):396-400, 1973.
2. Hardy, JD, Furnell PM, Brumfitt W: Comparison of sterile bag, clean catch, and suprapubic aspiration in the diagnosis of urinary infection in early childhood, *Br J Urol* 48:279–283, 1967.
3. Crain EF, Gershel JC: Urinary tract infection in febrile infants younger than eight weeks of age, *Pediatrics* 86:363–367, 1990.
4. Boehm JJ, Haynes JL: Bacteriology of "midstream catch" urines, *Am J Dis Child* 3:366–369, 1966.
5. Huze LB, Beeson PB: Observations on the reliability and safety of bladder catheterization for bacteriologic study of the urine, *N Engl J Med* 255:474, 1956.
6. Pryles CV, Atkin MD, Morse TS et al: Comparative bacteriologic study of urine obtained from children by percutaneous suprapubic aspiration of the bladder, *Pediatrics* 24:983–988, 1959.
7. Hildebrand WL, Schreiner RL, Stevens DC et al: Suprapubic bladder aspiration in infants, *Am Fam Physician* 23:115–118, 1981.
8. Stamey TA: *Pathogenesis and treatment of urinary tract infections,* Baltimore, 1980, Williams & Wilkins.
9. Mustonen A, Uhari M: Is there bacteremia after suprapubic aspiration in children with urinary tract infection? *J Urol* 119:822, 1978.
10. Weuthers WT, Wenzl JE: Suprapubic aspiration. Perforation of the viscus other than the bladder, *Am J Dis Child* 117:590, 1969.
11. Pass RF, Waldo, FB: Anaerobic bacteremia following suprapubic bladder aspiration, *J Pediatr* 94:748–750, 1979.
12. O'Callaghan C, McDougall PN: Successful suprapubic aspiration of urine, *Arch Dis Child* 62:1072–1073, 1987.
13. Stamm WE, Wagner KF, Amsel R et al: Causes of the acute urethral syndrome in women, *N Engl J Med* 303:409, 1980.
14. Terndrkup TE, McCabe JG: Urinary tract infections in women. In Harwoood-Nuss A, editor: *The clinical practice of emergency medicine,* Philadelphia, 1991, JB Lippincott.
15. Lipsky BA, Inui TS, Plorde JJ et al: Is the clean-catch midstream void procedure necessary for obtaining urine culture specimen from men? *Am J Med* 76:257, 1984.
16. Lipsky BA, Fihn SD, Hackett R et al: Diagnosis of bacteriuria in men: specimen collection and culture interpretation, *J Infect Dis* 15:847, 1987.
17. *Clinical laboratory tests: values and implications,* Philadelphia, *1991, Springhouse Corp, pp 646–648.*
18. Baner JD: *Clinical laboratory methods,* ed 9, St Louis, 1982, Mosby Inc.
19. Henry JB: *Clinical diagnosis and management by laboratory methods,* ed 18, Philadelphia 1991, WB Saunders, pp 397–403.
20. Csako G: False positive results for ketone with the drug MESNA and other free-sulhydryl compounds, *Clin Chem* 33:289, 1987.
21. Waltmann O: Method for the simple detection of UTI, *Wein Med Wochenschr* 72:618, 1922.
22. Pels RJ, Bor DH, Woolhandler S et al: Dipstick urinalysis screening of asymptomatic adults for urinary tract disorders. II Bacteriuria, *JAMA* 262:1221, 1989.
23. Bank CM, Codrington JF, Van Dieijan-Viss MP et al: Screening urine specimen populations for normality using different dipsticks: evaluation of parameters influencing sensitivity and specificity, *J Clin Chem Clin Biochem* 25:299, 1987.
24. Kellogg JA, Manzella JP, Shaffer SN et al: Clinical relevance of culture versus screens for the detection of microbial pathogens in urine specimens, *Am J Med* 83:739, 1987.
25. Scheer DW: The detection of leukocyte esterase activity in urine with a new reagent strip, *Am J Clin Pathol* 87:86–93, 1987.

26. Kass EH: Asymptomatic infections of the urinary tract, *Trans Assoc Am Physicians* 69:56, 1956.
27. Freedman LR, Phair JP, Seki M et al: The epidemilogy of UTI in Hiroshima, *Yale J Biol Med* 37:262, 1965.
28. Kunin CM, Southall I, Paquin AJ: Epidemiology of UTI: a pilot study of 3057 school children, *N Engl J Med* 263:817, 1960.
29. Brumfitt W: Urinary cell counts and their value, *J Clin Pathol* 18:850, 1965.
30. Kusumi RF, Grover PJ, Kunin CM: Rapid detection of pyuria by leukocyte esterase activity, *JAMA* 245:1653, 1981.
31. Stansfeld JM: The measurement and meaning of pyuria, *Arch Dis Child* 37:257, 1962.
32. Propp DA, Weber D, Ciesla ML: Reliability of a urine dipstick in emergency department patients, *Ann Emerg Med* 18:560–563, 1989.
33. Doern GV, Saubolle MA, Sewell DL: Screening for bacteriuria without the LN strip test, *Diagn Microbiol Infect Dis* 4:355, 1986.
34. Jones EA, Berk PD: Chemical and immunological tests in the evaluation of liver. In Brown SS, Mitchell FL, Young DS, editors: *Chemical diagnosis of disease,* Amsterdam, 1979, Elsevier, pp 525–662.
35. Pfaller MA, Koontz FP: Laboratory evaluation of LE and nitrite tests for the detection of bacteriuria, *J Clin Microbiol* 21:840, 1985.
36. Males BM et al: LE-nitrate and bioluminescence assays: a urine screen, *J Clin Microbiol* 22:531, 1985.
37. Nachamkin I, editor: *Diagnostic testing alert,* Philadelphia, 1984, International Thomson Medical Information.
38. Kagen LJ: *Myoglobin biochemical, physiological and clinical aspects,* New York, 1973, Columbia University Press.
39. Roberts R, Sobel BE: Isoenzymes of CPK and diagnosis of myocardial infarction, *Ann Intern Med* 79:741–742, 1973.
40. Dawson DM, Fine IH: CK in human tissues, *Arch Neurol* 16:175–180, 1967.
41. Brody SL et al: Predicting the severity of cocaine-associated rhabdomyolysis, *Ann Emerg Med* 19:1137–1143, 1990.
42. Welch RD, Todd K, Krause GS: Incidence of cocaine-associated rhabdomyolysis, *Ann Emerg Med* 20:155–157, 1991.
43. Ward MM: Factors predictive of acute renal failure in rhabdomyolysis, *Arch Intern Med* 148:1553–1556, 1988.
44. Kesson AM, Talbott JM, Gyory AZ: Microscopic examination of urine, *Lancet* 2:809, 1978.
45. Kincaid-Smith C: Hematuria and exercise related hematuria, *BMJ* 285:1595, 1982.
46. Herne CR, Donnell MG, Fraser CG: Assessment of new urinalysis dipstick, *Clin Chem* 26:170, 1980.
47. Mariani AJ, Luangphinith S, Loo S et al: Dipstick chemical urinalysis: an accurate cost effective screening test, *J Urol* 132:64, 1984.
48. Messing EM, Young TB, Hunt VB et al: The significance of asymptomatic microhematuria in men 50 or more years old: findings of a home screening study using urinary dipsticks, *J Urol* 137:919, 1987.
49. Loo SYT, Scottolini AG, Luangphinith S et al: Urine screening strategy employing dipstick analysis and selective culture: an evaluation, *Am J Clin Pathol* 81:634, 1984.
50. Shaw ST, Pan SY, Wong ET: Routine urinalysis: is the dipstick enough? *JAMA* 253:1956, 1985.
51. Vehaskari VM, Chang CT, Stevens JK et al: Microscopic hematuria in school children: epidemiology and clinicopathologic evaluation, *J Pediatr* 95:676–684, 1979.
52. Lieberman E: Work up of the child with hematuria. In Lieberman E, ed: *Clinical pediatric nephrology,* Philadelphia, 1976, JB Lippincott, pp 12–26.
53. Stansfeld JM, Webb JK: Observations on pyuria in children, *Arch Dis Child* 28:386–391, 1953.
54. Kunin CM: The quantitative significance of bacteria visualized in the unstained urinary sediment, *N Engl J Med* 265:589–590, 1961.
55. Littlewook JM, Jacobs SI, Ramsden CH: Comparison between microscopical examination of unstained deposits of urine and quantitative culture, *Arch Dis Child* 52:894–896, 1977.

56. Robins DG, Rogers KB, Shite RHR: Urine microscopy as an aid to detection of bacteriuria, *Lancet* 1:476–478, 1975.
57. Stamm WE: Recent developments in the diagnosis and treatment of UTI's, *West J Med* 137:215–220, 1982.
58. Jenkins RD, Fenn JP, Matsen JM: Review of urine microscopy for bacteriuria, *JAMA* 255:3397–3403, 1986.
59. Asscher AW, Sussman M, Waters WE et al: Urine as a medium for bacterial growth, *Lancet* 2:1037–1041, 1966.
60. Aurelius G: Bacterial growth in urine, *Acta Pathol Microbiol Scand* 55:201–208, 1962.
61. Kass EH: Asymptomatic infections of the urinary tract, *Trans Assoc Am Physicians* 69:56–64, 1956.
62. Stamm WE: Interpretation of urine cultures, *Clin Microbiol Newslett* 5:15–17, 1983.
63. Pollock HM: Laboratory techniques for detection of urinary tract infections and assessment of value, *Am J Med* 75:79–84, 1983.
64. Kass EH: Chemotherapeutic and antibiotic drugs in the management of infections of the urinary tract, *Am J Med* 18:764–781, 1955.
65. Kass EH, Finland M: Asymptomatic infections of the urinary tract, *Trans Assoc Am Physicians* 69:56–64, 1956.
66. Kass EH: Bacteriuria and the diagnosis of infections of the urinary tract, with observations on the use of methionine as a urinary antiseptic, *Arch Intern Med* 100:709–714, 1957.
67. Sanford JP, Favour CB, Mao FH et al: Evaluation of the "positive urine culture: an approach to positive differentiation of significant bacteria from contaminants," *Am J Med* 20:88–93, 1956.
68. Stamm WE, Wagner KF, Amsel R et al: Causes of the acute urethral syndrome in women, *N Engl J Med* 303:409–415, 1980.
69. Stamm WE, Counts GW, Running KQ et al: Diagnosis of coliform infection in acutely dysuric women, *N Engl J Med* 307:463–468, 1982.
70. Komaroff A: Acute dysuria in women, *N Engl J Med* 310:368–375, 1984.
71. Stamm WE, Hooton TM, Johnson JR et al: Urinary tract infections: from pathogenesis to treatment, *J Infect Dis* 159:409, 1989.
72. Johnson JR, Stamm WE: Urinary tract infections in women: diagnosis and treatment, *Ann Intern Med* 111:906, 1989.
73. Stamm WE: Protocol for diagnosis of urinary tract infection: reconsidering the criterion for significant bacteriuria, *Urology* 32(suppl B):6, 1988.
74. De Vrie C: Hemorrhagic cystitis: a review, *J Urol* 143:1, 1990.
75. Cohen SN, Kass EH: A simple method for quantitative urine culture, *N Engl J Med* 277:176–180, 1967.
76. Edwards PD, Burke EA, Wear JB: A new method for out patient culture and sensitivity of urine, *J Urol* 109:689–691, 1973.
77. Guttman D, Naylor GRE: Dip-slide: an aid to quantitative urine culture in general practice, *BMJ* 3:343–345, 1967.
78. Ellner ED, Papachristos T: Detection of bacteriuria by dipslide. Routine use in a large general hospital, *Am J Clin Pathol* 63:516–521, 1975.
79. Johnson PK, Free HM, Free AH: A simplified screening test for salicylate intoxication, *J Pediatr* 63:949–953, 1962.
80. Trinder P: Rapid determination of salicylate in biological fluids, *Biochem J* 57:301–303, 1954.
81. Roberts JR, Chabot J, Lundberg T: A comparison of methods to screen urine for the presence of small amounts of salicylates. Paper presented to the AAPCC/AACT/ABMT annual scientific meeting, Sante Fe, NM, Sep 1986.

Chapter 4

Blood Chemistries

Donald A. Feinfeld, M.D.
Thomas Manis, M.D.

Blood chemistry studies are frequently requested for patients seen in the emergency department (ED) as well as patients admitted to the hospital from the ED. Blood chemistry tests reveal a great deal about a patient's state of metabolism, fluid balance, and acid-base status. Disorders of blood chemistry may provide important clues to the cause of nonspecific complaints or findings when a patient's problem is not elucidated by the history or physical examination. Such nonspecific abnormalities include alterations of mental status and muscular or neural function and general feelings of malaise or fatigue. Blood test results may also disclose an asymptomatic disorder.

Although blood tests are often obtained on a routine basis, it is nevertheless important for the physician to understand when such testing is indicated. Abnormal findings on blood chemistry examination may require emergent intervention or close follow-up and repetition of the determinations. It is therefore vital for emergency physicians to develop skills in evaluating these data in order to logically plan for the patient's care.

In modern laboratories, many of these blood chemistry tests are obtained as a group. For example, all four electrolytes (Na^+, K^+, Cl^-, HCO_3^-) are invariably obtained together, often with blood glucose (to be covered in a separate chapter), blood urea nitrogen (BUN), and creatinine. Nevertheless, in this chapter, the individual determinations will be discussed separately, and their relative costs listed separately. When relevant, of course, interpretation of two or more members of the group will be discussed together, for example, Na^+ and K^+ or BUN and creatinine. The relative cost of the blood chemistry tests is shown in Table 4–1.

SERUM ELECTROLYTES (NA^+, K^+, Cl^-, CO_2)

Disorders of serum electrolytes are common, especially in patients with diarrheal, renal, and metabolic disorders. Abnormalities of individual electrolytes and of the group as a whole need to be addressed whenever they are uncovered by laboratory results.

Table 4–1. Relative Cost of Blood Chemistries

Test	Dollars
Na^+	14
K^+	14
Cl^-	13
CO_2	13
BUN	12
Creatinine	15
SMA-7 (all the above + serum glucose)	23
Ca^{++}	15
$PO_4^{\equiv}$	14
Mg^{++}	35

Sodium (Na^+)

CASE 4–1

A 76-year-old man was sent to the ED from a local nursing home. He had a previous history of heart failure and cerebrovascular accidents and had been treated with hydrochlorothiazide. According to the nursing home staff, he had been coughing for weeks and had been febrile for 4 days despite antibiotic treatment. He had also been anorexic and had been able to tolerate only sips of water and ginger ale orally. Examination revealed fever, bibasilar pulmonary rales, greater at the right base, an S_4 gallop, and left hemiparesis. Serum Na^+ was 124 mEq/L.

The major role of sodium ion in the body is to hold water in the extracellular fluid space. Sodium thus acts as the major extracellular osmole.[1] Body sodium content is normally regulated by the kidneys in response to hormonal, neural, and vascular signals reflecting intravascular fluid volume.

Until a few years ago, serum sodium was determined by flame photometry. In this test, a small aliquot of serum was vaporized in a flame, and the intensity of the spectrophotometric pattern of sodium measured, calibrated with standards, and calculated as a ratio per liter of serum based on the aliquot volume. This technique, however, sometimes led to a spuriously low measured sodium level in blood samples in which severe hyperlipidemia or hyperproteinemia lowered the water content of the serum. Since sodium is not distributed in either lipid or protein layers, the amount of sodium per aliquot would be perceived as reduced even though the amount of sodium dissolved in water was perfectly normal. This condition, known as *pseudohyponatremia,*[2] is no longer seen when serum sodium is determined with the ion-selective electrode, the method used by most laboratories today. This ion-selective electrode is placed in contact with an aliquot of serum, and since the membrane is selective for sodium, changes in the flow of ions across the membrane can be directly calibrated with the sodium concentration in the aqueous phase of serum.

Alterations in serum sodium concentration invariably mean abnormalities of *osmolality* (see Chapter 5). With one exception (see below) the relationship is direct: hyponatremia implies hypoosmolality, and hypernatremia implies hyperosmolality. Since the capillary interface between extracellular and intracellular fluid is freely permeable to water, changes in extracellular osmolality generally imply an identical change in intracellular osmolality unless the extracellular change has been too rapid for equilibration to occur. Abnormal serum sodium values reflect an altered ratio of sodium to water, or of body osmoles to water. *Since the body has different mechanisms for handling sodium and water, serum sodium levels tell absolutely nothing about total-body sodium balance:* hypernatremia[3] or hyponatremia[4] may develop with high, normal, or low total-body sodium.

The only major exception to the direct relationship between the serum sodium concentration and osmolality results from the condition known as *hypertonic hyponatremia.* In this situation, an additional extracellular osmotically active substance accumulates that is not measured by standard electrolyte determinations. The presence of large amounts of this osmole in the extracellular fluid causes water to shift from the intracellular to the extracellular space, thus lowering the actual sodium concentration. Because of the unmeasured osmole, however, the measured extracellular osmolality will be increased.

Only two osmotically active substances can generally appear in the extracellular fluid in large enough amounts to cause a significant lowering of the serum sodium level. The most common one is glucose when present in a diabetic with severe hyperglycemia. The second substance is mannitol that has been injected by a physician but, because of renal disease, has not been excreted by the kidneys. Hyponatremia due to severe hyperglycemia is almost always immediately apparent because blood glucose and electrolytes are usually determined together on the same blood specimen. Blood glucose levels of 400 mg/dL or more coupled with a low serum sodium value should make one think of this possibility. In order to determine whether the fall in serum sodium is solely due to the hyperglycemia, a "correction" should be made: for each increase in serum glucose of 100 mg/dL, serum sodium activity will fall by about 1.6 mEq/L.[5] Therefore, in order to correct the serum sodium upward, the physician should first subtract 100 from the reported value of the serum glucose, (100 being the normal serum glucose value), next divide the remainder by 100, then multiply the result by 1.6, and add that figure to the actual measured blood sodium. If the result is in or close to the normal serum sodium range, the hyponatremia is due entirely to the hyperglycemia. Hyponatremia due to unexcreted mannitol can usually be elucidated by a careful review of the patient's treatment, medication record, and a comparison of initial and subsequent serum sodium levels.

Hyponatromia

Hypotonic hyponatremia is the most common situation when the serum sodium concentration is low. As it is impossible to lose large quantities of hypertonic fluid, hypoosmolality invariably results from the intake of water in excess of the body's ability to excrete it. Occasionally, as in psychogenic polydipsia or the rapid consumption of large quantities of beer, the body's water excreting ability is normal but has been temporarily exceeded by massive water intake. When this occurs, urine osmolality will be low (>100 mOsm/kg). Most commonly, however, hyponatremia is caused by a combination of the intake of water coupled with a reduced renal water-excreting capacity and urine osmolality will be greater than 200 mOsm/kg, implying an antidiuretic hormone (ADH) effect (see box).

Essentially three processes may limit water-excreting capacity.[6] First, anything

Causes of Hyponatremia

- With normal water-excreting capacity
  - Psychogenic polydipsia
  - Massive beer drinking
- Impaired water-excreting capacity and intake of dilute fluids
  - Volume depletion (gastrointestinal loss, diuresis, bleeding, etc.)
  - Edematous states (heart failure, cirrhosis)
  - Renal failure
  - Loss of cortisol (adrenal insufficiency, hypopituitarism)
  - Hypothyroidism (severe)
  - Syndrome of inappropriate antidiuretic hormone secretion

that decreases effective renal perfusion, such as volume depletion, congestive heart failure, hypotension, or cirrhosis, will cause a marked enhancement of proximal tubular salt and water absorption and result in decreased delivery of salt and water to the segment of the nephron where a dilute tubular fluid is made. Second, anything that interferes with diluting segment function—such as diuretics, lack of thyroxine or cortisol, or tubulointerstitial renal disease—will interfere with renal water-excreting ability. Finally, whenever there is release of ADH in the face of low plasma osmolality, such as in the syndrome of inappropriate ADH secretion or with a decrease in effective intravascular volume, any free water made in the tubules will be reabsorbed back into circulation.

When a patient is found to be a hyponatremic, it is therefore important that the examining physician look for underlying conditions that limit water-excreting capacity. The history should include a detailed list of the patient's medications, including over-the-counter preparations; conditions that lead to volume depletion such as vomiting or diarrhea; a history of cardiac, hepatic, or renal disease; endocrine disorders; or severe infection. The physical examination should be geared toward assessing intravascular volume as well as looking for stigmata of endocrine diseases and cardiac dysfunction. Measurement of urinary sodium on a random specimen is often helpful in distinguishing disorders where the primary problem is renal hypoperfusion (urine Na^+ usually less than 20 mEq/L) from disorders where renal perfusion is normal (urine Na^+ usually greater than 30 mEq/L). It is also extremely important to begin limiting the administration of free water as soon as a hyponatremic state is uncovered. Continued administration of hypotonic solutions in the presence of hyponatremia will only make the electrolyte abnormality worse.

CASE 4–1 CONTINUED

The patient in Case 4–1 had decreased water excretion due to heart failure and diuretics; he had replaced his salt and water losses with dilute fluids.

Hypernatremia

Hypernatremia always means hyperosmolality. In hypernatremia, the ratio of osmoles to water is too high. Hypernatremia invariably comes from the loss of water in excess of sodium or other osmoles.

Although osmoles such as Na^+ cannot be lost without a concomitant water loss, it is certainly possible for the body to lose free water (with no osmolar content). The average adult loses approximately 500 ml of free water by evaporation and respiration every day. It is also possible to lose hypotonic fluid and thus become hyperosmolar. Failure to replace hypotonic fluid loss invariably leads to hypernatremia.

The body primarily defends against free water loss by limiting urinary water excretion. Maximum urine osmolality normally runs between 800 and 1200 mOsm/kg. This response is effected by ADH, which is normally released in a linear proportion to the extracellular osmolality after the osmolality rises above 283 mOsm/kg. Coupled with the release of ADH, thirst centers in the brain are generally stimulated by extracellular osmolalities in excess of 290. As water is lost then, ADH is released, and if this fails to minimize the water loss, the individual becomes thirsty and generally replaces the water losses.

The most common cause of hypernatremia is therefore, no access to water or a blunted thirst sensation. The latter cause has been shown to be extremely common in the elderly: the sensation of thirst is substantially decreased in people over 65 years of age.[7] Less common causes of hypernatremia are situations where the body is unable to produce ADH (neurogenic or "central" diabetes insipidus) or failure of the kidney to respond to appropriate amounts of ADH (nephrogenic diabetes insipidus) (see

Causes of Hypernatremia

Failure to replace insensible water loss (fever, hyperthermia, diaphoresis, or diminished thirst sensation)
Excessive insensible loss of water (burns, sustained hyperventilation)
Neurogenic diabetes insipidus (failure to secrete antidiuretic hormone)
Nephrogenic diabetes insipidus (failure of the kidney to respond to antidiuretic hormone)
Osmotic diuresis (sustained glycosuria, mannitol, prolonged very high protein intake)

box at right). Determination of urine osmolality is often helpful in distinguishing failure to replace water losses on the one hand from the two forms of diabetes insipidus on the other. Urine osmolality of less than 100 mOsm/kg implies no ADH effect. Additionally, patients with diabetes insipidus often complain of polyuria and polydipsia.

Potassium (K^+)

CASE 4–2

A 54-year-old woman with long-standing diabetes mellitus and heart failure secondary to ischemic heart disease was brought to the ED with weakness and lethargy. Examination showed mild, generalized muscle weakness, and the patient made monosyllabic responses to questions. Blood chemistry studies revealed K^+, 6.9 mEq/L; Na^+, 135 mEq/L; glucose, 214 mg/dL; BUN, 30 mg/dL; and creatinine, 1.6 mg/dL.

Potassium plays a role in the intracellular space analogous to that of sodium in the extracellular space, that is, it is the major intracellular cation and osmole. The intracellular potassium content is approximately 50 times that of its extracellular fluid content. However, because it is impractical to examine intracellular fluid, we are forced to rely on extracellular measurements of potassium, i.e., serum potassium, in estimating body K^+ balance.

As with sodium, serum potassium was once routinely determined by flame photometry. However, ion-selective electrodes for potassium are now also available and have become the method of choice for determining potassium levels. The methodology is similar to that for serum sodium determinations (see above).

As the vast majority of body potassium is intracellular but potassium entering and leaving the body does so by way of the extracellular space, the physician must keep in mind that there are two forms of potassium balance: *external balance,* or the entry and excretion of potassium into and out of the body, and *internal balance,* or the distribution of potassium between extracellular and intracellular spaces.[8] Measured abnormalities in serum potassium levels may be due to a disturbance in either of these balances or both.

Hyperkalemia

Hyperkalemia is a potentially life-threatening electrolyte abnormality. The upper limit of normal is usually considered to be 5 mEq/L. Levels between 5.0 and 6.0 mEq/L should be noted but do not require specific action, particularly in patients with chronic tubulointerstitial renal disease. Levels between 6.0 and 7.0 should be thoroughly investigated and treated. Levels above 7.0 constitute a true electrolyte emergency because severe hyperkalemia may lead to imminent cardiac arrest.

Table 4–2. Electrocardiographic Changes in Electrolyte Disorders

Disorder	Changes
Hyperkalemia (progression)	Peaked T waves (precordial leads)
	Widened PR and QRS intervals
	Flattening and loss of P waves
	"Sine wave"*
Hypokalemia	Appearance of U waves
	Flat or inverted T waves
	ST depression
	Decreased QRS voltage
	Increased AV conduction time*
Hypercalcemia	Shortened QT interval
Hypocalcemia	Prolonged QT interval
	Nonspecific T-wave changes
Hypermagnesemia	Prolonged PR interval
	Prolonged QRS interval
Hypomagnesemia	Prolonged QT interval

*The absence of these findings does not exclude a significant electrolyte disturbance.

Two factors must be considered when significant hyperkalemia is reported:

1. Electrocardiographic (ECG) abnormalities. Whenever hyperkalemia is found, an ECG should be done immediately. The usual progression of ECG abnormalities due to hyperkalemia is peaking of T waves, particularly in the medial precordial leads, widening of the QRS complex, loss of P waves, loss of discrete T waves, sine wave abnormality, and finally cardiac arrest (Table 4–2). Finding any of these abnormalities on ECG warrants the immediate use of measures to prevent cardiac arrest. *However, the absence of ECG abnormalities in a patient with hyperkalemia does not necessarily mean that elevated potassium levels are not present or can be ignored.*

2. Factitiously elevated potassium levels. Because serum potassium is measured in blood, which contains a large number of circulating cells, and since, as noted above, cells constitute the major body storehouse of potassium, it follows that any breakdown of blood cells during collection or storage of blood samples may factitiously elevate measured blood potassium levels in the absence of true hyperkalemia. Hemolysis of blood during or after collection and breakdown of red cells during collection (if too small a needle is used) are the most common causes of factitious hyperkalemia. Serum potassium levels may also be spuriously elevated if potassium is released from extraordinarily high numbers of platelets or white blood cells. For this to happen, the platelet count usually has to be greater than 500,000/mm^3 (as in thrombocythemia) or the white blood cell count greater than 100,000/mm^3 (leukemia).[1] If there is a question of factitious hyperkalemia, plasma potassium should be measured from a sample drawn through a large-bore needle (20 gauge or larger) and anticoagulated with powdered heparin (green top).

Hyperkalemia may reflect a failure to excrete the normal daily K^+ intake (about 100 mEq) or the movement of K^+ from intracellular to the extracellular space (see top box on pg. 65).[10] Often, both internal and external balance are affected simultaneously.

CASE 4–2 CONTINUED

In this case the patient's hyperkalemia was found to be caused by a combination of chronic renal insufficiency and hyporeninemic hypoaldosteronism, which

Causes of Hyperkalemia

External balance
- Massive intake of potassium
- Decreased urinary potassium excretion (renal failure of any cause, hypoaldosteronism, decreased urine flow)

Internal balance (K^+ shift from intracellular to extracellular fluid)
- Metabolic acidosis (particularly inorganic acidosis)
- Massive tissue breakdown (e.g., rhabdomyolysis)
- Absolute insulin deficiency
- β-Adrenergic antagonism
- Severe digitalis poisoning
- Hyperkalemic periodic paralysis
- Succinylcholine administration

decreased renal potassium excretion, and hyperchloremic metabolic acidosis, which caused potassium to move into the extracellular fluid.

Hypokalemia

When assessing hypokalemia, the physician must decide whether there has actually been a loss of potassium from the body or merely a shift of potassium from the extracellular to the intracellular space (see box below). External potassium balance is important in hypokalemia for two reasons. First, the urinary potassium concentration cannot be lowered below 10 to 15 mEq/L, so there is always some urinary potassium loss. Therefore, failure to ingest any potassium over a period of time will lead to a significant loss of body potassium. Second, although the gastrointestinal tract, under normal circumstances, is not a major route of potassium excretion, under certain circumstances such as diarrhea, it may be responsible for a substantial quantity of potassium loss.

Causes of Hypokalemia

External balance
- Excessive kaliuresis
  - Hyperaldosteronism
  - Diuretics, including osmotic diuretics
  - Renal tubular acidosis
  - Vomiting
  - Administration of unreabsorbable anion (penicillin, carbenicillin, sulfate)
  - Magnesium deficiency (e.g., due to alcohol abuse)
  - Prior therapy with aminoglycoside antibiotics or cisplatin
- Gastrointestinal loss
  - Diarrhea
  - Laxative abuse
  - Villous adenoma
  - Intestinal fistula

Internal balance (K^+ shift from extracellular to intracellular fluid)
- Alkalemia
- β-Adrenergic stimulation (e.g., albuterol, epinephrine)
- Hypokalemic periodic paralysis

Hypokalemia is generally a less life-threatening abnormality than hyperkalemia, except for patients taking digitalis preparations, in which case hypokalemia may precipitate a fatal dyrhythmia. As with hyperkalemia, hypokalemia should always be evaluated by ECG to look for the U wave characteristic of low K^+ levels or, in the case of a patient taking digitalis, to look for dyrhythmias. However, as with hyperkalemia, the absence of characteristic ECG findings in a hypokalemic patient does not mean that significant hypokalemia is not present. In contrast to hyperkalemia, however, it is generally not urgent to restore serum K^+ levels to normal immediately, except in patients taking digitalis.

Chloride (Cl^-)

CASE 4–3

A 68-yr-old woman was brought to the ED because of a 4-day history of progressive irritability, confusion, and weakness. The family related the history that the patient had been taking "nerve pills." Physical examination revealed normal vital signs, disorientation to time, generalized mild weakness, slurred speech, and a mild, nonintentional tremor. Blood chemistry values were BUN, 18 mg/dL; creatinine, 12 mg/dL; Na^+, 143 mEq/L; K^+, 4.1 mEq/L; Cl^-, 118 mEq/L; CO_2, 24 mEq/L; and glucose, 113 mg/dL.

The major role of chloride in the body is to serve as the anionic accompaniment to sodium. Since the vast majority of body sodium is in the extracellular space, it follows that the same is true for chloride ion. There is no evidence for active transport of chloride in the human body[11]; changes in the serum chloride concentration generally reflect changes in the extracellular content of other anions, particularly bicarbonate. Abnormalities of serum chloride levels associated with changes in bicarbonate concentration will be discussed in Chapter 5.

Serum chloride is now generally measured by exposing an aliquot of serum to an ion-specific electrode, similar to the method for measuring sodium and potassium. As with the cations, flame photometry is no longer widely used in chloride determination. However, the anion-selective electrode used for chloride determination is equally permeable to all of the halogens. Therefore, an excess of another halogen ion, such as Br^-, will be measured by the electrode as an increase in Cl^-, thereby resulting in a factitiously elevated serum chloride value.

CASE 4–3 CONTINUED

In bromide poisoning, such as in this case, the abnormally and factitiously high serum chloride measurement coupled with the patient's physical findings made the physicians suspicious of bromide poisoning. A serum bromide level was ordered and determined to be 9 mEq/L, thus accounting for the rise in measured "serum chloride."

Normal values for serum Cl^- are apparently equipment specific. With the use of new, ion-specific Cl^- electrodes, a slightly higher measured Cl^- value as compared with one to two decades ago has been reported. Since the "anion gap" depends on Cl^- measurement, the "anion gap" may now be lower in normal settings and a slightly elevated gap may appear to be normal by the old standards (see Chapter 5). Physicians need to establish familiarity with the values at their own institutions.[12]

Carbon Dioxide Combining Power (CO_2) ("HCO_3^-")

Serum carbon dioxide combining power (usually abbreviated as serum CO_2) is generally used on standard electrolytes as a substitute for the measurement of bicarbonate (HCO_3^-). Serum CO_2 actually measures bicarbonate plus carbonic acid in the serum.

By the Henderson-Hasselbalch equation,

$$pH = 6.1 + \log \frac{[HCO_3^-]}{[H_2CO_3]}.$$

At pH 7.4,

$$7.4 = 6.1 + \log \frac{[HCO_3^-]}{[H_2CO_3]}.$$

$$1.3 = \log \frac{[HCO_3^-]}{[H_2CO_3]}.$$

Since the antilogarithm of 1.3 is 20 (base 10), at normal pH 7.4, the ratio of bicarbonate to carbonic acid is 20 to 1.[1] Therefore, serum CO_2 is normally about 5% higher than the actual serum bicarbonate concentration. This ratio is useful to emergency physicians: whenever measurements of serum electrolytes and arterial blood gases are done, the CO_2 level on the electrolytes should be slightly higher than the bicarbonate calculated from the blood gas values. If this is not the case, one (or both) of the determinations is probably erroneous or the two blood samples were not obtained simultaneously.

Serum CO_2 is measured by a coupled enzymatic reaction. Bicarbonate plus the bicarbonate released from carbonic acid reacts with phosphoenolpyruvate in the presence of the enzyme phosphoenolpyruvate carboxylase to produce oxaloacetate and release phosphate. The oxaloacetate reacts with reduced nicotinamide-adenine dinucleotide (NAD) in the presence of the enzyme malic dehydrogenase to produce malate NAD^+. To perform a serum CO_2 determination, an aliquot of serum is mixed with specific amounts of phosphoenolpyruvate, phosphoenolpyruvate carboxylase, reduced NAD (NADH), and malic dehydrogenase. The formation of NAD^+, via the coupled reaction, is measured in a spectrophotometer at 376 nm. The increase in absorbance, signaling the production of NAD^+, is directly proportional to the concentration of actual or available CO_2 in the sample.

Bicarbonate ion is the major buffer of the extracellular space. Abnormalities in levels of plasma bicarbonate therefore invariably represent disorders of acid-base balance, as discussed in Chapter 5. Changes in the relative levels of chloride and bicarbonate on the standard electrolyte "panel" (the "anion gap") are also discussed in Chapter 5 since their primary use is in the differentiation of metabolic acidoses.

Magnesium (Mg^{++})

CASE 4–4

A 35-year-old man with a history of chronic alcoholism was brought to the ED with complaints of muscle cramps and twitching. The physical examination was remarkable for mild lethargy and positive Chvostek and Trousseau signs with hyperreflexia. Laboratory studies revealed Na^+, 135 mEq/L; K^+, 3.2 mEq/L; Cl^-, 100 mEq/L; CO_2, 31 mEq/L; BUN, 8 mg/dL; creatinine, 1.1 mg/dL; and glucose, 85 mg/dL. Subsequent blood studies revealed Ca^{++}, 6.2 mEq/L; PO_4, 2.1 mEq/L; Mg^{++}, 0.8 mEq/L; and albumin, 3 g/dL.

As with potassium, only 2% of total-body magnesium is found in the extracellular fluid.[13] Although we measure magnesium in serum, this may not be a good parameter of actual body magnesium balance. The largest store of body magnesium is in bone, where it is complexed with apatite. The remaining body magnesium is found primarily in the intracellular fluid, particularly in striated muscle cells and erythrocytes where it serves as the second most abundant intracellular cation and as a cofactor in many enzymatic reactions. Adequate amounts of magnesium have been found to be necessary for both the production and release of parathyroid hormone (PTH).

Magnesium is measured in serum by using a dye called calmagite. In the presence of potassium cyanide, magnesium ion forms a violet complex with calmagite. To perform the test, an aloquot of serum is mixed with a known quantity of calmagite and CKN and then placed in a spectrophotometer. The absorbance of light at 546 nm is directly proportional to the concentration of Mg^{++} in the specimen.

The major determinants of body magnesium balance are intake, intestinal absorption, and renal excretion. Magnesium is found in most foodstuffs and in medications such as antacids and some cathartics. The main conditions that affect intestinal magnesium absorption are diarrhea, steatorrhea, and uremia. All of these conditions depress Mg^{++} absorption. Many factors alter renal magnesium excretion: loop diuretics, osmotic diuretics, phosphate depletion, alcohol ingestion, and toxic drugs, including cisplatin and aminoglycoside antibiotics, may increase magnesium in the urine, and hyperparathyroidism, hypothyroidism, hypocalcemia, and alkalemia will decrease urinary magnesium.

Hypomagnesemia

Hypomagnesemia is a common finding in many medical conditions. The physician needs to evaluate the hypomagnesemic patient's intake and the condition of the gastrointestinal tract. However, most clinical magnesium depletion is due to excessive renal loss of this ion. Causes of hypomagnesemia are shown in the accompanying box. The ECG change resulting from hypomagnesemia is a prolonged Q-T interval.

Causes of Hypomagnesemia

- Decreased intake of magnesium
- Decreased magnesium absorption
  - Diarrhea
  - Steatorrhea
- Urinary loss of magnesium
  - Diuretics (loop or osmotic)
  - Toxic drugs (cisplatin, aminoglycoside antibiotics)
  - Hyperaldosteronism
  - Alcoholism
  - Hyperthyroidism
  - Syndrome of inappropriate antidiuretic hormone secretion
  - Chronic volume expansion

Causes of Hypermagnesemia

Renal failure
Administration of massive doses of magnesium
Adrenal insufficiency

CASE 4–4 CONTINUED

In case 4–4, the patient's hypomagnesemia is probably due to both decreased intake (alcoholics often ingest very little besides alcohol) and the renal magnesium wasting caused by high alcohol intake. The hypocalcemia and hypokalemia seen in this case are common complications of magnesium depletion. The hypocalcemia is due to impairment of parathyroid function (see above) and the hypokalemia to the tendency of magnesium depletion to cause urinary potassium wasting.

Hypermagnesemia

Hypermagnesemia in contrast to hypomagnesemia, is a relatively uncommon problem. When it occurs, most of the time it is in the setting of severe renal failure. Most patients with renal failure have mild hypermagnesemia; for this reason, magnesium-containing salts should never be given to such patients. Rarely, massive administration of magnesium salts or adrenal insufficiency may cause hypermagnesemia in individuals with normal renal function. Hypermagnesemia causes prolonged PR and QRS intervals (see box).

CALCIUM Ca^{++}

The human body normally contains about a kilogram of elemental calcium, almost all (about 99%) of which is in the skeleton in the form of hydroxyapatite, a complex of calcium, phosphate, and hydroxide. About 10 g of bone calcium is readily exchangeable with the extracellular pool of calcium, which is about 1 g. The calcium contained in normal diets varies widely from 200 to 2000 mg and averages about 1 g of calcium per day. Net absorption is about 150 to 200 mg/day and is balanced by renal excretion into the urine. About 500 mg leaves bone and is replaced daily in the course of normal remodeling. Despite all of these shifts and major dietary swings, the serum calcium level remains remarkably constant at about 10 mg/dL (2.5 mM or 5.0 mEq/L). Normal ranges for laboratories vary slightly but are generally about 8.6 to 10.6 mg/dL. A remarkable system of three hormones, vitamin D, PTH, and calcitonin, is responsible for this homeostasis. Derangement of serum calcium levels threatens many vital cell functions including muscle contraction, nerve excitation, cell membrane integrity, and various intracellular reactions.

The almost universal availability of the autoanalyzer has enabled emergency physicians to determine a patient's serum calcium level whenever it is useful or necessary. The serum calcium level reported is almost invariably the total serum calcium, as opposed to the ionized and biologically active fraction (normally about 45% of the total). The development of calcium selective electrodes has made automated measurements of calcium levels possible, but this technique is not currently used in most laboratories for routine "screening panel" determinations. Consequently, to meaningfully interpret reported calcium values, physicians must be familiar with all of the factors that influence the total calcium determination. Some factors affect the ionized (active) calcium level and represent disorders of calcium metabolism. Others factors are merely "artifacts" resulting from other conditions in the patient. These factors include diet, renal excretion, serum protein levels, blood pH, and at least three hormonal systems (PTH, calcitonin, and activated vitamin D), all interacting in turn with the major bone reservoir. The hormonal factors all normally influence and in turn are regulated by the ionized calcium level. The nonhormonal factors may or may not alter the ionized calcium level and are not feedback related (diet, protein levels, pH) or only indirectly feedback related (renal excretion).

Factors that alter the measured serum calcium level do not necessarily affect the ionized fraction. About half of circulating calcium is free, ionized, and physiologically active.[14] Another 5% to 10% is complexed to phosphate, citrate, bicarbonate, and other anions. The remaining 40% to 45%, circulates bound to serum proteins, particularly albumin. Any condition that increases or decreases serum protein levels to a significant extent will also affect the total calcium level. A change of 1 g/dL of albumin (from a baseline normal value of 4 g/dL) will move the total calcium about 0.8 mg/dL in the same direction by increasing or decreasing the amount of bound calcium, thereby leaving the ionized calcium level the same. Calcium levels that have been adjusted in this proportion to account for changes in serum albumin levels are referred to as "corrected" calcium levels, although no formula has proved completely reliable in predicting the actual ionized calcium level.[15] Since albumin levels as low as 1.0 g/dL are not rare in severely malnourished patients, the correction factor for total calcium (3 g/dL × 0.8 mg/dL = 2.4 mg/dL correction) in such an instance can be greater than the normal range of total calcium (8.5 to 10.6, that is, greater than 2.1 mg/dL); thus an uncorrected "low" total calcium value in a severely hypoalbuminemic patient could in fact represent hypercalcemia!

Further complicating matters is the fact that the protein-binding effect is pH dependent. The number of calcium-binding carboxyl groups on albumin increases as the pH rises and decreases as the pH falls, increasing or decreasing binding sites per unit of albumin. The 0.8 correction factor for albumin changes is accurate only when blood pH is in the normal range. The ionized calcium level will be decreased (more of the total calcium will be bound and less ionized) in the presence of alkalosis, which accounts for the signs of tetany accompanying severe hyperventilation syndrome and acute respiratory alkalosis with a normal serum calcium level. Conversely, the ionized calcium level will be increased by acidosis (minimizing the effect of the hypocalcemia associated with untreated chronic renal failure and metabolic acidosis).

CASE 4–5

A 69-year-old man with known carcinoma of the lung was seen in the ED because of somnolence. He was barely responsive but had no focal neurologic signs. Other than marked cachexia and evidence of dehydration, no remarkable findings were noted on the remainder of the examination. His laboratory data included a total calcium of 14 mg/dL and a serum albumin of 1.4 g/dL.

Hypercalcemia

Hypercalcemia is most often an incidental finding on chemical screening of the blood. It may be suspected and a serum calcium level specifically requested for this reason, but its signs are nonspecific despite their potentially serious nature: depressed neuromuscular function (emotional problems, fatigue, weakness, lethargy), dehydration due to polyuria (hypercalcemia causes resistance to the action of ADH), and low fluid intake due to nausea and vomiting. Most patients with hypercalcemia are asymptomatic. Finding a short QT interval on ECG, the most common ECG manifestation of hypercalcemia, might also lead one to check the serum calcium level.

The list of causes of hypercalcemia is long but relatively well known (see box). Most of the diagnostic possibilities are readily explored by a good history and physi-

Causes of Hypercalcemia

Hyperparathyroidism
Malignancy
Thiazide diuretics
Immobilization
Vitamin D intoxication
Multiple myeloma
Granulomatous disease (sarcoid, tuberculosis)
Thyrotoxicosis
Paget's disease
Milk-alkali syndrome
Adrenal insufficiency

cal examination. The first two causes listed, primary hyperparathyroidism and malignancy, account for more than 90% of cases, with primary hyperparathyroidism somewhat more common. When hypercalcemia results from cancer, it is usually a late finding in patients with extensive disease rather than an early marker of occult disease. Breast cancer and multiple myeloma are the tumors that most commonly cause hypercalcemia by forming osteolytic metastases, although almost any malignancy metastatic to bone can be responsible by causing local activation of osteoclasts. Alternatively, tumors not metastatic to bone may elaborate a humoral factor that stimulates osteoclastic bone resorption. Such tumors are most commonly squamous cell cancers of the head, neck, lung, or esophagus; renal and bladder cancers; and ovarian carcinoma. Recently parathyroid hormone–related protein (PTHrP) has been identified as at least one of the humoral factors responsible.[16] PTHrP resembles PTH in its initial amino acid sequence and can be measured with commercially available assays. However, tests routinely available to the emergency physician are in general not particularly helpful in differentiating the two prime diagnoses. For example, alkaline phosphatase levels are commonly elevated in both hyperparathyroidism and malignant hypercalcemia.

Mild hypercalcemia does not require quick treatment, but patients who are symptomatic and have calcium levels of 13 mg/dL (corrected) or higher require urgent treatment.[17] Infusion of normal saline at a rate of 3 to 5 L per 24 hours should be given along with furosemide if any evidence of fluid overload is seen. Hemodialysis is the only measure that will never fail to lower the calcium level within a few hours after initiating the treatment and can be used to "buy time" for slower, less predictable therapies to take effect when dealing with a patient who is obtunded from extremely high calcium levels.

CASE 4–5 CONTINUED

Intravenous hydration with normal saline was begun in the ED while computed tomographic (CT) examination of the head was performed. CT findings were normal, but when the patient returned from the radiology department after receiving 1 L of saline intravenously, he was tachypneic and appeared to be in congestive heart failure.

Comment.—Appropriate management at this time would begin with intravenous furosemide. Since his coma is almost certainly due to severe hypercalcemia (corrected calcium, about 16 mg/dL) and because he tolerated intravenous hydration poorly, immediate consideration of hemodialysis for acute lowering of the serum calcium level is also indicated. Note that in a patient with far-advanced malignancy, a decision *not* to use an aggressive measure like hemodialysis may be appropriate, particularly if the patient has provided advanced directives in this regard.

Hypocalcemia

True hypocalcemia, that is, after correction for hypoproteinemia, is quite unusual except in patients with chronic renal failure.[18] In that setting, it is seen as a consequence of two major factors: phosphate retention due to failure of renal excretion and deficiency of active 1,25-dihydroxyvitamin D due to failure of the kidney to hydroxylate the 25-hydroxy precursor. Untreated patients characteristically have high serum phosphate levels and prolongation of the QT interval on ECG, which is characteristic of hypocalcemia. Clinical findings attributable to low calcium levels such as carpopedal spasm, tetany, paresthesias, confusion, or seizures rarely occur in this setting. The importance of calcium homeostasis in patients with declining renal function is widely recognized, and therefore most diagnosed patients are routinely given active vitamin D and phosphate binders. Most such patients will have normal calcium and phosphate levels. The phosphate binder of choice is calcium carbonate (to avoid the long-term accumulation of aluminum). Calcium citrate, a commonly available over-the-counter calcium supplement, is dangerous: citrate enhances intestinal aluminum absorption and has produced aluminum dementia syndrome.[19] Other causes of hypocalcemia are listed in the accompanying box.

Clinical manifestations of hypocalcemia generally occur when levels remain below 7 mg/dL and include increased neuronal irritability. The earliest manifestations of such neuronal irritability are positive Chvostek and Trousseau signs, with perioral paresthesias, followed by carpopedal spasm and rarely laryngospasm. Seizures may develop and represent a generalized tetanic state, with characteristic electroencephalographic findings. Long-standing hypocalcemia may be associated with a variety of organic brain syndromes, cataracts, calcification of the basal ganglia, and papilledema with increased cerebrospinal fluid pressure (pseudotumor cerebri). The ECG will show prolongation of the QT interval.

Most patients with hypocalcemia do not require emergency treatment, but those displaying clinical signs of neuromuscular irritability or seizures may require urgent therapy. First, arterial blood gas studies and the levels of potassium and magnesium should be obtained and appropriate supportive measures provided. Alkalosis, if present, should be corrected to increase the ionized calcium level. Calcium replacement is empirical since the body deficit cannot be calculated. Most commonly, calcium gluconate is given by intravenous infusion, 10 to 20 mL of a 10% solution containing 90 mg calcium per 100 mL. The infusion rate should not exceed 2 mL/min,

Causes of Hypocalcemia

- Renal failure
- Hypoparathyroidism
- Acute pancreatitis
- Vitamin D deficiency
  - Dietary
  - Malabsorption
  - Anticonvulsants
  - Chronic liver disease
- Hypomagnesemia
- Malignancy

and ECG monitoring is required for digitalized patients because calcium may precipitate digitalis intoxication. PTH and vitamin D levels should also be obtained to help determine the cause.

PHOSPHATE

As is the case with calcium, the major store of body phosphorus (85%) is in bone. Of the remainder, 14% is in soft tissues where it performs major roles as a component of cell membranes and genetic material and in energy metabolism. Only 1% is present in the blood, and of that, 70% is in organic form. The clinical laboratory measures and reports the remaining 30% (i.e., 30% of 1%) of circulating phosphorus as serum inorganic phosphate. Normal values range between about 2.5 and 4.5 mg/dL (or 0.81 to 1.45 mmol/L in SI units). Inorganic phosphate serves as an important buffer in blood and urine but is a weak indicator of body phosphate stores.

Normal phosphate intake varies widely, between 800 and 1500 mg/day. Blood levels respond to the same hormone systems—PTH, vitamin D, and calcitonin—that regulate calcium. Phosphate levels are not as closely controlled as calcium and tend to vary significantly in a particular individual. Gastrointestinal absorption is considerably affected by such nondietary factors as antacid intake; all the commonly used antacid agents (calcium, magnesium, and aluminum) form insoluble phosphate complexes. Excess phosphate is excreted by the kidneys; in the urine, phosphate serves as an important buffer and is needed for normal acid excretion.

Hypophosphatemia

Hypophosphatemia may result from decreased absorption of dietary phosphate, shifting of phosphate into cells, or increased urinary losses. The most common causes of hypophosphatemia are listed in the accompanying box.

Overt symptoms of phosphate depletion are unusual with serum levels over 1.0

Causes of Hypophosphatemia

- Increased urine losses
  - Alcohol abuse
  - Uncontrolled diabetes
  - Primary hyperparathyroidism
  - Vitamin D deficiency
  - Drug-induced (steroids, diuretics, calcitonin, bicarbonate)
  - Renal tubular dysfunction
- Decreased gastrointestinal absorption
  - Antacids
  - Vitamin D deficiency
  - Starvation
  - Malabsorption
  - Chronic diarrhea
- Intracellular shifting
  - Hyperalimentation without PO_4
  - Respiratory alkalosis
  - Leukemia in crisis
  - Alcohol withdrawal

mg/dL. Manifestations of phosphate depletion include skeletal and cardiac muscle dysfunction, sensorimotor neuropathy, impaired tissue oxygenation (due to depletion of 2,3-diphosphoglycerate (2,3-DPG), and platelet and white blood cell dysfunction. In urgent situations, cautious repletion with intravenous potassium or sodium phosphate (2.5 to 5.0 mg/kg) over a 6-hour period may be indicated. There is no accurate means of estimating the body deficit, and repletion is empirical.

Hyperphosphatemia

Hyperphosphatemia is usually the result of acute or chronic renal failure (glomerular filtration rate [GFR] less than 20% of normal) (see box). Much less commonly, massive release of intracellular phosphate may be responsible (tumor lysis after therapy or rhabdomyolysis). Self-treatment with phosphate enemas or laxatives can directly cause exogenous hyperphosphatemia. Excess vitamin D intake can indirectly cause hyperphosphatemia.

The most important acute effect of hyperphosphatemia is depression of the serum calcium level with consequent tetany. Chronic hyperphosphatemia, mainly in patients with renal failure, causes secondary hyperparathyroidism and soft tissue calcification.

Treatment of hyperphosphatemia centers on correction of the primary cause. Urgent therapy in the form of saline diuresis or hemodialysis is almost never required.

BLOOD UREA NITROGEN, CREATININE, AND TESTS OF RENAL FUNCTION

Normal kidneys are endowed with a considerable degree of "excess" function in the sense that symptoms of renal failure are unusual until 80% to 90% of function has been lost. As a consequence, mild to moderate degrees of renal impairment are undetectable without the help of the laboratory. In the ED the physician will have urinalysis and serum creatinine and BUN levels available to assess the status of the kidneys. It is essential to point out that half of normal renal function

Causes of Hyperphosphatemia

- Renal failure (glomerular filtration rate, <20 mL/min)
  - Acute or chronic
- Increased tubular reabsorption
  - Hypoparathyroidism
  - Hyperthyroidism
  - Acromegaly
  - Diphosphonate therapy
- Phosphate load
  - Endogenous
    - Cell destruction
      - Tumor lysis
      - Rhabdomyolysis
      - Hyperthermia
      - Acute hepatitis
      - Acute leukemia
  - Exogenous
    - Phosphate enemas or laxatives
    - Vitamin D overdose

may be lost before either the BUN or creatinine level rises above the normal range. For this reason, urinalysis is the most sensitive indicator of renal disease in most cases (see Chapter 2). A completely normal urinalysis (no proteinuria, no abnormal sediment) will rarely be seen in the presence of clinically significant kidney disease. Even with a loss of function sufficient to elevate the BUN and creatinine levels, examination of the urine still provides vital guidance in ascertaining the nature of the renal disease.

CASE 4–6

A 78-year-old man was brought to the ED by his family because of progressive confusion over a 3-day period. The confusion began after a fall that resulted in a contusion on his forehead and a fracture of his left wrist. The patient had been evaluated immediately after the fall, and at that time, normal neurologic and CT findings were noted. His fracture was reduced and casted in the ED, and he had been sent home on a regimen of acetaminophen, 650 mg, and codeine, 30 mg, every 4 hours for pain.

On neurologic examination, the patient was now somewhat lethargic and disoriented to place and time and his memory was markedly impaired, but there were no focal neurologic findings. A bruise on the forehead was noted, his abdomen was obese, and he had a moderately enlarged, smooth prostate gland.

CASE 4–7

A 67-year-old woman with a long history of hypertension was brought to the ED because of a 5-day history of productive cough, fever, and progressive shortness of breath. She stated that she had been taking her usual antihypertensive medications as prescribed, including clonidine and a diuretic. Her appetite had been poor since becoming ill. A review of body systems was positive for intermittent vaginal bleeding of several months' duration. On physical examination she was febrile to 102° F and had findings consistent with right lower lobe infiltrates. She refused to allow a pelvic examination.

Blood Urea Nitrogen

The BUN should more correctly be termed the SUN (serum urea nitrogen) since the test is almost never performed on whole blood. According to the SI system for reporting laboratory values, results should be reported as urea alone in millimoles per liter; by convention, however, we express results as units of urea nitrogen (two nitrogen atoms, atomic weight 28, per urea molecule, atomic weight 60). The normal range for BUN is about 6 to 20 mg/dL, or 2.1 to 7.1 mmol/L. The wide range of normal values reflects the fact that the BUN level is influenced by several independent parameters, only one of which is renal function. In a recently published textbook of nephrology,[20] the BUN is not even discussed in the chapter on renal function testing. The BUN reflects major effects exerted by dietary protein, liver disease, tissue breakdown, and reduced renal blood flow of whatever cause, in addition to disease of the kidney itself.

A brief review of the basic processes involved in the body's handling of urea is helpful in understanding and incorporating what follows into everyday practice. Urea (molecular weight, 60 Da) has the following chemical structure:

$$\begin{array}{c} NH_2 \\ | \\ C = 0 \\ | \\ NH_2 \end{array}$$

With two amino groups per carbon atom, urea is an efficient end product for disposal of unneeded protein nitrogen. The body normally produces about 12 to 14 g of urea per day in the liver through the urea cycle. Urea is distributed through the total-body water, intracellularly as well as extracellularly. It is excreted almost completely by the kidneys and represents about half of all urinary solutes; 80% to 90% of all urinary nitrogen is in the form of urea. Large amounts of urea (about 70 g/day) enter the bowel in various secretions. Wherever urea-splitting microorganisms are present (primarily in the colon), urea is degraded into carbon dioxide and ammonia. Ammonia is freely diffusible and returns to the liver via the portal circulation where it is then converted back to urea and once again returned to the circulation. In the presence of advanced liver disease, ammonia passes unaltered into the systemic circulation where it may contribute to hepatic coma. In the past, therapy for hepatic coma included neomycin to destroy the intestinal flora responsible for degrading urea (which itself has no clearly defined toxicity). More recently, oral lactulose (a nonabsorbed disaccharide) syrup has been used. Rather than killing the bacteria, lactulose is metabolized by the colonic flora into acidic products that are thought to convert ammonia into nondiffusable ammonium ion, which is then carried out in the diarrhea produced by the lactulose, an osmotic cathartic. Theoretically, the bowel could be used to eliminate nitrogen as a treatment for uremia, but a practical means to trap and eliminate clinically significant amounts of urea nitrogen remains to be found. Thus the kidney remains the only significant route of excretion for nitrogenous wastes, of which urea is quantitatively if not toxicologically the most significant.

Urea is freely diffusable across the glomerular membrane. There is no proven active transport mechanism for urea; moreover, its handling by the nephron can be accounted for by passive mechanisms alone. Urea is a small molecule that is highly permeable across cell membranes and thus can follow the movement of water out of the nephron, with nearly half of the filtered urea being reabsorbed in the proximal tubule. What happens to the remaining urea is highly dependent on the rate of urine flow. When diuresis is high, urea excretion is high as well, and the BUN concentration falls. When flow in the nephron is slowed, urea is reabsorbed much more efficiently, and the BUN concentration rises. Remarkably, the kidney can achieve very high degrees of urea concentration in the urine despite the permeability of this substance, mainly because of the relative impermeability of some cells to urea in the absence of ADH and the countercurrent blood flow pattern of the renal medulla that prevents the washout of high urea concentrations deep within that area.

As noted above, the reason for BUN's lack of value as a renal function test is the fact that so many common nonrenal variables affect its levels. On the other hand, our common practice of analyzing BUN by considering both its absolute value and its relation to serum creatinine (a more accurate parameter of GFR) can provide valuable information about the patient's status. Certainly the combination of values is far more useful to us than either parameter alone might be.

Prerenal Azotemia

It is common clinical practice to categorize azotemic (high BUN) states into "prerenal," "renal," and "postrenal." The term *prerenal* refers to inadequate renal perfusion of any cause. If the underperfusion is sufficient to reduce glomerular filtration significantly, this will soon be reflected by an increase in both BUN and creatinine levels. There will be an additional increase in the BUN, however, because of slowed urine flow through the kidney (increased sodium and water retention is the kidney's normal response to underperfusion). Consequently, the BUN:creatinine ratio, normally 10 to 15:1, will rise. Common causes of prerenal azotemia include congestive heart failure and hypotension of any cause (for example, sepsis, myocardial infarction, blood loss, overtreatment with diuretics). It must be kept in mind that circumstances that increase urea production, which have nothing to do with renal perfusion or urine flow rate, can also elevate the BUN while not changing the creatinine level, thus simulating the chemical picture of prerenal azotemia resulting from renal hypoperfusion. Common among such masqueraders is excessive protein intake. This may be exogenous, in the form of dietary protein; occasionally this is unwittingly iatrogenic, in the form of hyperalimentation. Since patients receiving hyperalimentation are commonly in precarious hemodynamic condition, it can be crucial to recognize the difference between dietary factors and a significant drop in renal blood flow because the treatment options are dramatically different. Gastrointestinal bleeding is often associated with a prerenal picture, in part because of digestion and absorption of blood proteins but primarily because of lowered blood volume. Another iatrogenic situation rather commonly encountered is the use of high-dose steroids, which have an antianabolic effect and can dramatically increase urea production and hence the BUN concentration. In the context of treating fulminant systemic lupus erythematosus or severe renal transplant rejection with "pulse" doses of 500 to 1000 mg of methylprednisolone, BUN:creatinine ratios of 50:1 are not unusual. This must be appreciated in the ED where it is not unusual to encounter patients taking significant doses of oral steroids. The BUN:creatinine ratio cannot be interpreted simplistically under such circumstances.

Renal azotemia is a much less commonly used term and indicates that the retention of urea is due to kidney disease with consequent loss of renal function. Under these circumstances, the BUN:creatinine ratio is expected to be "normal," about 10 to 15:1. Deviations from this range suggest that extrarenal factors should be sought and corrected if practical. It is important to remember that any combination of factors may exist in the same patient.

Postrenal Azotemia

The blood chemistry profile of postrenal azotemia, which is related to obstruction of the urinary tract or very rarely to its perforation with extravasation of urine, is the same as that of the prerenal form, that is, a high BUN:creatinine ratio. The slowing of urine flow by the backpressure of obstructive disease permits significantly increased reabsorption of urea to occur. It is important to appreciate the difference between a structural problem and a hemodynamic one as soon as practical. One of the clinical hallmarks of urinary obstruction (but only in certain cases) is intermittency resulting in wide swings in urine volume; few "medical" renal problems are characterized by oliguria alternating with regular urine output. Oliguria, however, is not common in obstruction until the last stages. Rather, normal and even high urine volumes (due to loss of concentrating ability) are typical to the end. A high index of suspicion is therefore necessary when treating any patient known by history or otherwise to be at increased risk for obstruction, and the BUN:creatinine ratio should be particularly scrutinized. All older male patients are at risk for prostatic obstruction. Patients with a history of stone disease or urologic surgery in the past, those known or suspected to have pelvic malignancy, and those with diabetic neuropathy (and perhaps a neurogenic bladder) are also prime candidates for obstruction. If bladder outlet obstruction is suspected, placement of a urinary catheter in the ED may establish the diagnosis immediately and allow for appropriate treatment. Never forget to record the volume found in the bladder! The absence of a high BUN:creatinine ratio does not exclude obstructive disease when other factors suggest it. Just as a high-protein diet can independently elevate the BUN concentration, sick, anorectic, or vomiting patients and those who are not ingesting much protein may all have low BUN levels. In addition, patients with advanced liver disease cannot make urea at a normal rate (hence the observation that patients with BUN values less than 10 are either starving or have serious liver disease). Commonly encountered clinical circumstances or a combination of circumstances can "distort" the BUN value in either direction. Often an aberrant or unexpectedly abnormal BUN will cause the emergency physician to consider a problem that at first was unclear or invisible.

Creatinine

Of the commonly available blood chemistry determinations, serum creatinine provides the single best clinical test for renal function. Normal values are 0.9 to 1.5 mg/dL in men and 0.6 to 1.2 mg/dL in women by the less specific total chromogen method (SI 88 μmol/L = 1 mg/dL). An increase from baseline values provides an approximation of the loss of renal glomerular filtration: doubling of the creatinine level indicates that half of the original renal function is lost. Unlike urea, creatinine values are not significantly influenced by diet, liver disease, or medications. Oddly, although the chemical structure of urea is readily recognized (see pg. 75), the somewhat larger creatinine molecule (molecular weight, 109 Da) is unfamiliar to most physicians:

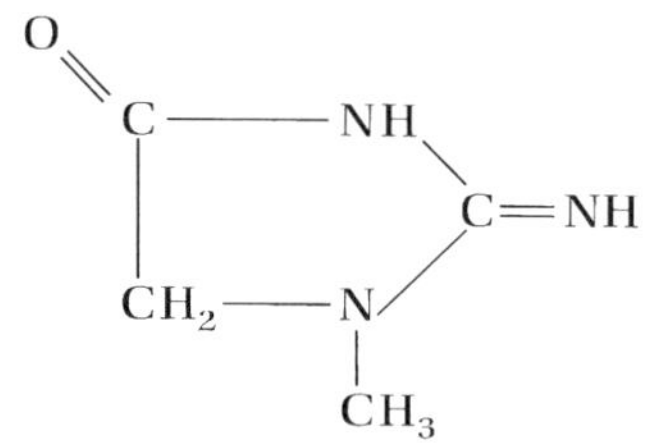

O
C — NH
C=NH
CH_2 — N
CH_3

Creatinine is the end product of metabolism of creatine, a substance produced in the liver and transported via the bloodstream to muscle tissue, which contains 98% of the body stores. There creatine provides a storage form for high-energy phosphate in the form of phosphocreatine. Because of muscle cell metabolism, about 1 g/day of the 100-g creatine pool is converted to creatinine, an end product whose only major route of excretion is in the urine. Dietary meat contains less than a gram of creatine and does not significantly affect creatinine production. Interestingly, prolonged boiling, but not other forms of cooking, apparently converts creatine into creatinine and can raise the serum creatinine level by as much as 1 mg/dL for several hours after a meal; this has been termed the "goulash effect."[21] Creatinine production and hence excretion is remarkably constant and in proportion to total-body muscle mass. Other characteristics that make creatinine a useful naturally occurring substance for measuring GFR are free filterability, relative ease and reliability of measurement, and lack of reabsorption metabolism or secretion—the last condition partly met by creatinine. Creatinine is usually determined by exposing serum to alkaline picrate (the Jaffe reaction) to produce an orange-red product. Unfortunately, this reaction is not totally specific for creatinine, and other substances, or chromogens, can react similarly. Glucose is the most variable and significant of these; glucose also interferes with a commonly used enzymatic method for determining creatinine. Partly because high glucose levels may produce aberrantly high creatinine results and partly because dehydration reduces the GFR, a significant decrease ("improvement") in the serum creatinine level typically occurs with appropriate fluids and other treatment of hyperglycemic diabetics. Various cephalosporin antibiotics may also be "read" as creatinine, depending on the assay. Other more specific tests for creatinine are available and less susceptible to interference; the physician should ascertain which method is in use in the hospital laboratory and which substances interfere with accurate determinations.

As noted above, creatinine is partly subjected to tubular secretion, which tends to increase significantly as advanced renal insufficiency develops. Thus the rise in creatinine levels due to poor renal function will be less than expected. Several drugs including cimetidine (but not ranitidine), the potassium-sparing diuretics (triamterene, spironolactone and amiloride), trimethoprim, and probenecid are able to block tubular secretion of creatinine and cause a rise in the serum creatinine concentration and an *apparent* loss of renal function. Although these phenomena are frustrating to renal physiologists, emergency physicians can nevertheless make excellent use of the creatinine level.

The decision to perform dialysis treatment for renal failure, whether acute or chronic, is made primarily on clinical grounds. If an azotemic patient is becoming ill in ways that may be uremic in origin, dialysis must be considered no matter what the absolute level of the creatinine (or BUN). A young, otherwise healthy man with renal disease may tolerate a creatinine level of 20 mg/dL with minimal signs and symptoms, but a level of 6 to 8 mg/dL from acute renal failure is not well tolerated and usually requires treatment. The rate of rise and the general condition of the patient (age, underlying diseases) are the important determinants of the levels at which azotemia (which is a laboratory value) becomes uremia (which is a clinical illness requiring immediate therapy). When an elevated creatinine level is recorded, the emergency physician is often faced with deciding the initial directions to be taken. Does an elevated creatinine level represent a new problem or worsening of prior disease? Previous data if available will be extremely helpful. Is the hematocrit unexpectedly high relative to the creatinine level? Assuming no replacement therapy, erythropoietin levels reflect renal mass; when the creatinine level rises to 4 mg/dL, the hematocrit typically begins to drop, eventually becoming 40% of normal in end-stage renal disease. Can a rising creatinine concentration (with a normal hematocrit) be due to factors other than progression of renal disease, and can they be reversed? Is the patient dry? Check weights, clinical status, diuretic history, fever, diarrhea, and the clinical examination. Is the patient too wet? Evidence of congestive heart failure and edema should be sought. Is the patient obstructed? A careful history and a high index of suspicion are required. A dry, wet, or obstructed patient will typically but not always have a "prerenal picture." If no treatable component is apparent, are the values high enough to justify dialysis? Remember: an elderly frail woman with chronic, slowly progressive renal failure may decompensate when the creatinine level reaches 4 to 5 mg/dL. Also, the fact that some patients may tolerate extremely high creatinine levels does not justify risk taking by the physician: even an otherwise healthy young patient may decompensate acutely at a less than predicted level. Acute decompensation from chronic renal failure is commonly seen in the ED but is much easier to prevent than to treat. After excluding or correcting obvious, promptly remediable extrarenal problems such as dehydration, prostatic obstruction, and hemodynamic instability, many nephrologists will initiate dialysis for creatinine levels of approximately 10 to 12 mg/dL even in asymptomatic patients. Whatever the numbers may represent in terms of the GFR, they should alert the physician to impending decompensation, which is easy to prevent but hard to reverse.

Complicated medical situations may require time to resolve. When a patient comes to the ED with azotemia and obtundation, the possibility of uremia may be easily confirmed or ruled out. If hemodialysis is provided, clinical improvement will indicate uremia as an important cause of the obtundation, whereas lack of improvement indicates that the explanation lies elsewhere. With the understanding that hours will pass between evaluation by a nephrologist and the time that hemodialysis can be started, initiation of the consultation process by the emergency physician will save valuable time.

A clearly uremic patient, obtunded with no other cause, perhaps convulsing or infected as well, should be promptly evaluated for immediate hemodialysis even if dehydrated or obstructed with the expected BUN-to-creatinine ratio. Potential reversibility does not always prove to be actual or promptly achievable, whereas dialysis is quick and effective. The BUN and creatinine levels will unfailingly decrease by half or more in an efficient, aggressive first treatment.

CASE 4–6 CONTINUED

A repeat CT scan of the head showed no new findings. Naloxone was administered intravenously without effect. A complete blood count and blood chemistry studies were unremarkable except for a BUN of 85 mg/dL and creatinine of 2.8 mg/dL. A Foley catheter was inserted and 1600 ml of clear urine obtained.

Comment.—Acute bladder outlet obstruction commonly develops in previously compensated prostatic enlargement when the patient becomes bedridden or receives opioids. Obviously, men are at highest risk, but women (especially diabetics with neuropathic bladders) are also at risk.

CASE 4–7 CONTINUED

Chest radiography confirmed the presence of an infiltrate. Her white blood cell count was 13,400; hematocrit, 28%; BUN, 125 mg/dL; and creatinine, 6.4 mg/dL.

Comment.—A patient with an acute febrile illness and continued diuretic therapy might well be expected to have prerenal azotemia, and indeed, this patient had an increased BUN:creatinine ratio (about 20:1). However, we should not leap to accept the most obvious explanation when clear-cut clues invite further consideration. The level of creatinine observed is rarely seen in simple dehydration, except in patients with preexisting renal disease. The clearly low hematocrit is consistent with chronic renal insufficiency. Three diagnostic possibilities must be considered: (1) the patient is a known long-term hypertensive and may have renal disease on that basis, (2) older age and azotemia with disproportionate anemia are a common triad in multiple myeloma, and (3) obstructive renal disease must be considered in an elderly woman with a history suggesting a possible pelvic malignancy. Simple differential points can be pursued: a myeloma patient may have rouleaux formation on peripheral blood smears as well as hypercalcemia and/or Bence Jones proteinuria (positive precipitation test for urine protein with a negative dipstick for albumin). The patient should be reapproached regarding the importance of a pelvic examination to seek evidence for or against a pelvic mass or malignancy. The examination is now essential for her evaluation and treatment.

REFERENCES

1. Rose BD: *Clinical physiology of acid-base and electrolyte disorders,* New York, 1977, McGraw-Hill.
2. Albink MJ, Hald PM, Man EB: The displacement of serum water by the lipid of hyperlipemic serum, *J Clin Invest* 34:481, 1955.
3. Berl T, Anderson RJ, McDonald KM et al: Clinical disorders of water metabolism, *Kidney Int* 10:117, 1976.
4. Berl T, Schrier RW: Water metabolism and the hypo-osmolar states, *Contemp Issues Nephrol* 1:1, 1978.
5. Katz MA: Hyperglycemia-induced hyponatremia. Calculation of expected serum sodium depression, *N Engl J Med* 289:843, 1973.
6. Goldberg M: Hyponatremia, *Med Clin North Am* 65:251, 1980.
7. Miller PD, Krebs RA, Neal BJ et al: Hypodipsia in geriatric patients, *Am J Med* 73:354, 1982.
8. Sterns RH, Cox M, Feig PU et al: Internal potassium balance and the control of the plasma potassium concentration, *Medicine (Baltimore)* 60:339, 1981.
9. Welt LG: Regulation of the intracellular environment; potassium and other salts. In

Bricker NS, editor: *The sea within us,* New York, 1975, Science and Medicine Publishing, p 27.

10. Cox M: Potassium homeostasis, *Med Clin North Am* 65:363, 1981.
11. Smith H: *Principles of renal physiology,* New York, 1956, Oxford University Press, p 96.
12. Winter SD, Pearson R, Gabow PA et al: The fall of the serum anion gap, *Arch Intern Med* 150:311, 1990.
13. Dirks JH, Alfrey AC: Normal and abnormal magnesium metabolism. In Schrier RW, editor: *Renal and electrolyte disorders,* ed 3, Boston, 1986, Little, Brown, pp 331–359.
14. Auerbach GD, Marx SJ, Spiegel AM: Parathyroid hormone, calcitonin, and the calciferols. In Wilson JD, Foster DW, editors: *Williams textbook of endocrinology,* ed 8, Philadelphia, 1992, WB Saunders, pp 1397–1476.
15. Ladenson JH, Lewis JW, Boyd JC: Failure of total calcium corrected for protein, albumin, and pH to correctly assess free calcium status, *J Clin Endocrinol Metab* 46:986–993, 1978.
16. Insogna KL: Humoral hypercalcemia of malignancy. The role of parathyroid hormone–related protein, *Endocrinol Metab Clin North Am* 18:779–807, 1989.
17. Ritch PS: Treatment of cancer-related hypercalcemia, *Semin Oncol* 17(suppl 5):26–33, 1990.
18. DeRubertis FR: Recognition and reversal of hypocalcemia. *Hosp Med* 1990:26:125–148.
19. Molitoris BA, Fremont DH, Mackenzie TA et al: Citrate: a major factor in the toxicity of orally administered aluminum compounds, *Kidney Int* 36:949–953, 1989.
20. Cameron JS: Renal function testing. In Cameron S et al, editors: *Oxford textbook of clinical nephrology,* Oxford, England, 1992, Oxford University Press, pp 24–49.
21. Jacobsen FK, Christensen CK, Mogensen CE et al: Evaluation of kidney function after meals, *Lancet* 1:319, 1980.

Chapter 5

Testing for Acid-Base Disturbances

Neal Flomenbaum, M.D.
Donald Feinfeld, M.D.

Arterial blood gas (ABG) determinations play a unique role in the evaluation of a patient in the emergency department (ED): ABGs provide important data for managing both medical and surgical catastrophes, application of these data requires specific knowledge not necessarily related to a particular medical specialty, and the results of an arterial sample sent for blood gas analysis are generally available immediately and long before most other laboratory test results. The three "real numbers" (pH, pO_2, and pCO_2) and the one or two calculated numbers (O_2 saturation and HCO_3^-) enable the physician to assess oxygenation, ventilation, and acid-base status. The first two considerations are dealt with in Chapter 10; the latter is considered here. Since acid-base disturbances invariably involve fluid and electrolyte considerations as well, the reader is advised to treat Chapters 4 and 5 as a unit. Definitions of commonly used terms in discussing acid-base disturbances are included at the end of this chapter.

ADVERSE EFFECTS OF ACID-BASE DISTURBANCES

Acid-base disturbances are common and require careful investigation, even when the cause appears obvious. The adverse consequences of acid-base disorders may be catastrophic (Table 5–1). *Metabolic acidosis* can compromise cardiac function, either by causing lethal dysrhythmias[1] (directly or by exacerbating hyperkalemia) or by decreasing ventricular contractility.[2] It may also cause decreased mentation and even coma.[3] Chronic metabolic acidosis mobilizes calcium from bone and may lead to severe osteopenia.[4] *Metabolic alkalosis* worsens hypokalemia,[5] with attendant muscle weakness and loss of urinary concentrating ability. It may also decrease ionized calcium[6] and cause tetany and paresthesias. *Respiratory acidosis* may cause CO_2 narcosis,[3,7] which begins as headache, blurred vision, and weakness and may proceed to dementia, delirium, or obtundation. At its worst, it may also produce cardiac dysrhythmias[8] or shock.[9] *Respiratory alkalosis* is even more likely than the metabolic variety to produce neurologic symptoms, including obtundation, paresthesias, muscle cramping, and carpopedal spasm.[10] Phosphate depletion may also accompany respiratory alkalosis.[10]

Table 5–1. Systemic Effects of Acid-Base Disturbances

Metabolic acidosis
Compromised cardiac function
Dysrhythmias
Hyperkalemia
Decreased ventricular contractility
Loss of arterial tone
Decreased mentation or coma
Calcium mobilization from bone and osteopenia (if chronic)
Metabolic alkalosis
Hypokalemia
Muscle weakness
Loss of urinary concentrating ability
Decreased ionized calcium
Paresthesias
Tetany
Respiratory acidosis
CO_2 narcosis
Early: headache, blurred vision, weakness
Late: dementia, delirium, obtundation
Cardiac dysrhythmias
Shock
Respiratory alkalosis
Neurologic symptoms
Obtundation
Paresthesias
Muscle cramps/carpopedal spasm
Phosphate depletion

REGULATION OF ACID-BASE BALANCE

The hydrogen ion concentration in the extracellular space is normally controlled to within $\pm 2.5 \times 10^{-9}$ mol/L. This pinpoint control is possible because of the extensive buffer system that modulates any change in pH when an acid or alkaline challenge occurs. Although buffering takes place both inside and outside cells and via many different buffer pairs, the isohydric principle dictates that all buffers be in equilibrium with each other; hence by studying one buffer, we know the state of all the others. We usually look at the HCO_3^-/H_2CO_3 system, the most important extracellular buffer.

The HCO_3^-/H_2CO_3 buffer system reflects acid-base metabolism via changes in HCO_3^- and pCO_2. An increase in HCO_3^- (or total CO_2 on standard electrolytes) is an increase in buffer base: either primary metabolic alkalosis or as a response to the CO_2 retention of respiratory acidosis. A decrease in HCO_3^- reflects loss of base from buffering of a metabolic acidosis or as a response to the CO_2 loss of respiratory alkalosis.

This buffer pair is particularly useful because it is an open system with dual control[11]: HCO_3^- is regulated by the kidneys and H_2CO_3, which depends on pCO_2, is regulated by the lungs. Renal dysfunction is often accompanied by failure of the kidney to maintain a normal HCO_3^- concentration. Hyperventilation from whatever cause depletes CO_2, and hypoventilation or obstructive pulmonary disease may increase pCO_2 outside the normal range. Thus, acid-base disturbances obligate us to examine the functions of the renal and respiratory systems. The relationships between HCO_3^-, H_2CO_3, and pH are usually defined by the Henderson-Hasselbalch equation:

$$\text{pH} = \text{pK}\,(6.1) + \log\frac{[HCO_3^-]}{[H_2CO_3]}$$

However, since ABG measurements usually give pH, pco_2, and plasma $[HCO_3^-]$, we may eliminate the logarithms; thus:

$$[H^+] = \frac{24(pCO_2)}{[HCO_3^-]}$$

Since pH and $[H^+]$ are roughly linear but go in opposite directions at physiologic pH, one can estimate changes in one parameter with measurement of the others. At pH 7.40, $[H^+]$ is 40 nEq/L. A pH of 7.50 corresponds to an $[H^+]$ of 30, a pH of 7.30 to an $[H^+]$ of 50, and so on.

CLINICAL EVALUATION OF ACID-BASE DISTURBANCES

To adequately evaluate a patient's acid-base status, a physician must be able to accurately identify the acid-base disturbance(s) and then provide a rational explanation for the disorder(s) by taking into account the history and physical examination together with the numbers on the ABG report. A physician who attempts to use shortcuts in identifying the problem (e.g., "eyeballing the numbers") rather than solving the Henderson-Hasselbalch and other equations for a given pH-pCO_2 combination runs a high risk of ignoring or missing a primary disturbance in the setting of a mixed acid-base disturbance. In other words, when the direction of the pH, pCO_2, and HCO_3^- changes together *seem* to be appropriate for a single primary disturbance with its expected physiologic compensation, there is a tendency to try to see the combination as a simple acid-base disturbance with physiologic compensation or "partial compensation" (Table 5–2). In reality, the patient may have a *mixed* disturbance consisting of two separate primary disturbances (each with its own physiologic compensation) that *appear* to be offsetting each other and returning the resultant pH value toward normal.

Rigorous application of the Henderson-Hasselbalch and other equations each time the results of a blood gas determination are analyzed will avoid this type of mistake but presents the emergency physician with another problem: how to find the time to solve unfamiliar or complicated mathematical equations with a patient or patients *in extremis.* An alternative method of rapidly accomplishing the same result is by using an acid-base map to clearly identify the acid-base disturbance(s). Once the possible disturbances are identified, the physician's efforts can then be applied to determining the cause of the disturbance(s) and diagnosing the responsible medical condition(s).

Table 5–2. Normal Variations in pH, pCO_2, and HCO_3^- That Characterize Single, Primary Acid-Base Disorders*

Condition	pH	pCO_2	HCO_3^-	Example
Metabolic acidosis	↓ Decreased	↓ Decreased†	↓ Decreased‡	DKA§
Respiratory acidosis	↓ Decreased	↑ Increased‡	↑ Increased†	COPD§
Metabolic alkalosis	↑ Increased	↑ Increased†	↑ Increased‡	Protracted vomiting; diuretic use
Respiratory alkalosis	↑ Increased	↓ Decreased‡	↓ Decreased†	Hyperventilation

*In primary *metabolic* disturbances, the pH and pCO_2 move in the same direction (↓ ↓ or ↑ ↑). In primary *respiratory* disturbances, the pH and pCO_2 move in opposite directions (↓ ↑ or ↑ ↓). HCO_3^- and pCO_2, which are the numerator and denominator respectively in the Henderson-Hasselbalch equation, always move in the same *direction:* one represents the primary disturbances; the other represents the compensatory change.
†Refers to the secondary or compensating disturbance.
‡Refers to the primary disturbance.
§*DKA,* diabetic ketoacidosis; *COPD,* chronic obstructive pulmonary disease.

THE ACID-BASE MAP

A grid may be constructed consisting of all the pH values compatible with life along the ordinate and all the pCO_2 values compatible with life along the abscissa. It is then possible to solve the Henderson-Hasselbalch and other equations for all pH and pCO_2 combinations on the grid, thereby constructing a graph of primary acid-base disturbances. Acid-base diagrams calculated in this way are currently available.[12] Alternatively, one can examine actual patients known to have a particular type of (single) primary disturbance who are free of other medical problems, plot their pH and pCO_2 coordinates on a similar grid, and then draw a band around all or most such values. Since the data are obtained from actual patients, such a band would *already incorporate the body's normal physiologic compensatory mechanism* if no other medical disorder interfered with compensation. For example, if a large group of diabetics with ketoacidosis, normal pulmonary function, and normally functioning brain stems is studied, a metabolic acidosis band could be constructed around the pH and pCO_2 values that would incorporate the physiologic compensatory respiratory alkalosis. In fact, such a band has been constructed to include 95% of such values.[13]

Similar "95% confidence bands" have been constructed for each of the primary acid-base disorders. Again, each band incorporates the body's physiologic compensation. The acute respiratory alkalosis band was constructed by studying the pH-pCO_2 combinations in anesthetized patients undergoing various elective surgical procedures in whom hyperventilation was used as an adjunct to general anesthesia.[14] The acute respiratory acidosis band was constructed by determining the pH values when human volunteers were acutely exposed to enough CO_2 to raise arterial pCO_2 as high as 90 mm Hg.[15] Bands for metabolic alkalosis,[16, 17] chronic respiratory alkalosis,[18] and chronic respiratory acidosis[19] were also constructed. (Dogs rather than humans were used for the chronic respiratory acidosis band.) Finally, in 1973 Goldberg and colleagues assembled all of this in vivo data, added their own accumulated experience from the Hospital of the University of Pennsylvania, and published an acid-base map displaying 95% confidence bands for each of the primary acid-base disturbances.[20]

The usefulness of this in vivo map to an emergency physician should be readily apparent (Fig. 5–1). For example, when a patient who appears to be suffering only from diabetic ketoacidosis (DKA) has pH and pCO_2 values that lie within the metabolic acidosis confidence band, the most likely description of the acid-base abnormality is (the expected) "metabolic acidosis, with the appropriate compensatory respiratory alkalosis." In contrast, a patient who *appears* to be suffering only from DKA but whose pH and pCO_2 values lie *outside* the metabolic acidosis band has a 95% probability of having an additional (clinically unsuspected) primary (not compensatory) acid-base disturbance. Cases 5–1 to 5–5 demonstrate the value of using the acid-base map in analyzing a patient's acid-base problems. A diagnostic algorithm for evaluating a patient with metabolic acidosis is provided in Fig. 5–2. One must bear in mind, however, that even when a pH-pCO_2 combination falls within a confidence band, there is no absolute guarantee that only a simple disturbance exists. Case 5–2 makes this point apparent.

CASE 5–1

A 59-year-old diabetic woman had a 2-day history of diarrhea, weakness, polyuria, and lethargy. She had been treated for diabetes mellitus for 10 years, most recently with 60 units of NPH insulin daily; however, she had omitted taking insulin the previous day because of nausea and vomiting. Physical examination revealed a temperature of 36.1° C, blood pressure of 100/70 mm Hg, and a respiratory rate of 18/min. The patient was lethargic and hyperpneic with an acetone odor on her breath; she was also dehydrated and had skin pallor. Laboratory findings disclosed

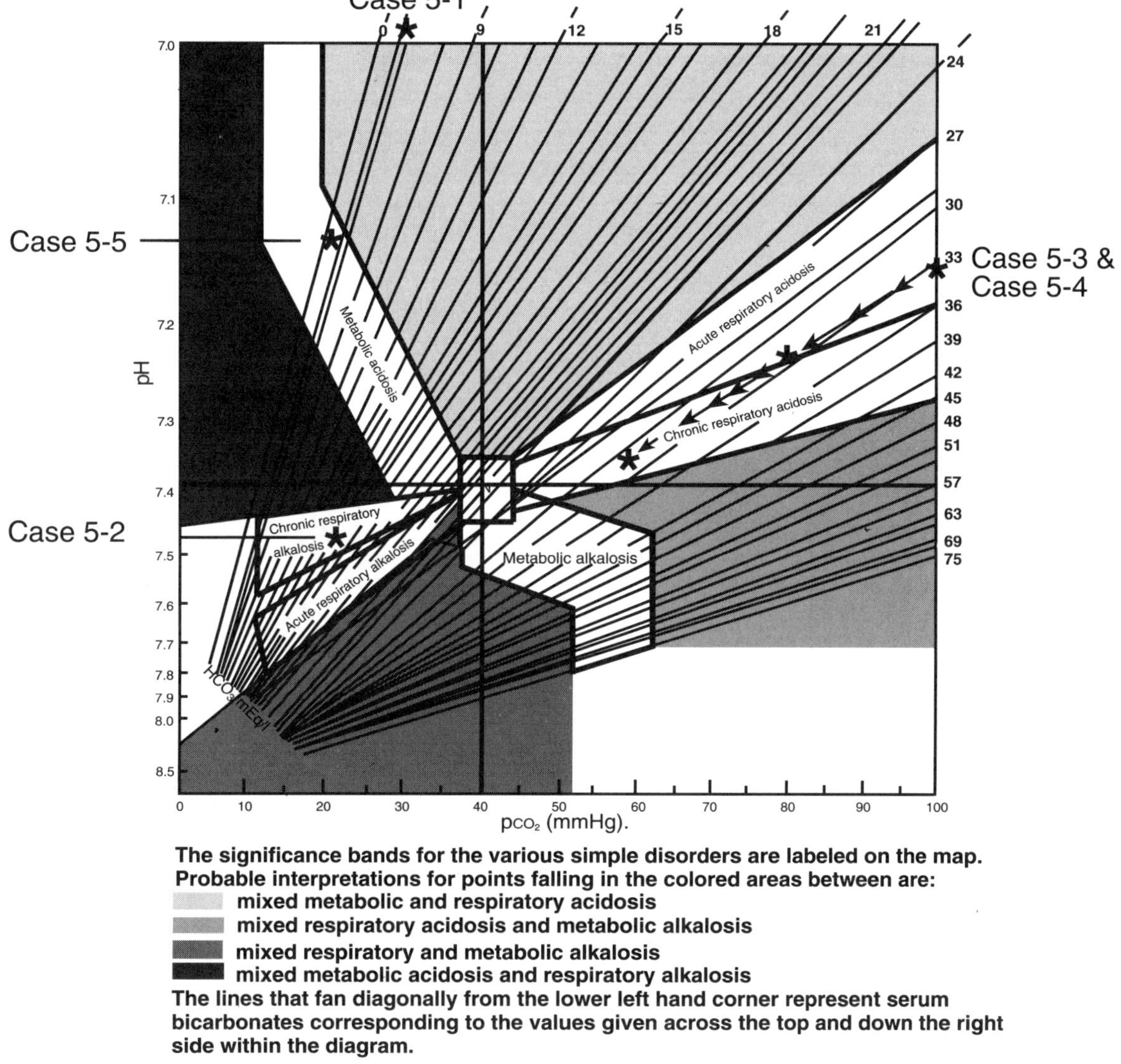

Fig. 5–1. Acid-base map. (Modified from Goldberg M et al: *JAMA* 223:269–275, 1973.)

the following values: hematocrit, 38%; urine, 4+ sugar and "large" ketones; blood urea nitrogen (BUN), 80 mg/dL; glucose, 1250 mg/dL; Na^+, 123 mEq/L; K^+, 6.6 mEq/L; Cl^-, 84 mEq/L; and serum acetone, 4+ at a 1:1 dilution. During nasal oxygen administration ABG values were pH, 6.97; pCO_2, 30 mm Hg; pO_2, 152 mm Hg; and SaO_2, 99%.[21]

Comment.—This patient obviously has diabetic ketoacidosis, but unless one is rigorous in examining the ABG data, another *primary* acid-base disturbance may be missed entirely. Although it may *appear* that the pCO_2 is appropriately low as a compensatory response for the clinically obvious metabolic acidosis, plotting the pH-pCO_2 coordinates on the acid-base map (Fig. 5–1) reveals that the coordinates do not lie in the metabolic acidosis band. Instead, the coordinates lie to the *right* of the metabolic acidosis band, that is, *between* the metabolic acidosis band and another band labeled "acute respiratory acidosis." This fact alone suggests that the patient has a mixed acid-base disturbance, that is, at least two primary acid-base disturbances, one of which is metabolic acidosis. Is it possible to be hypocapneic—as this patient is—with a pCO_2

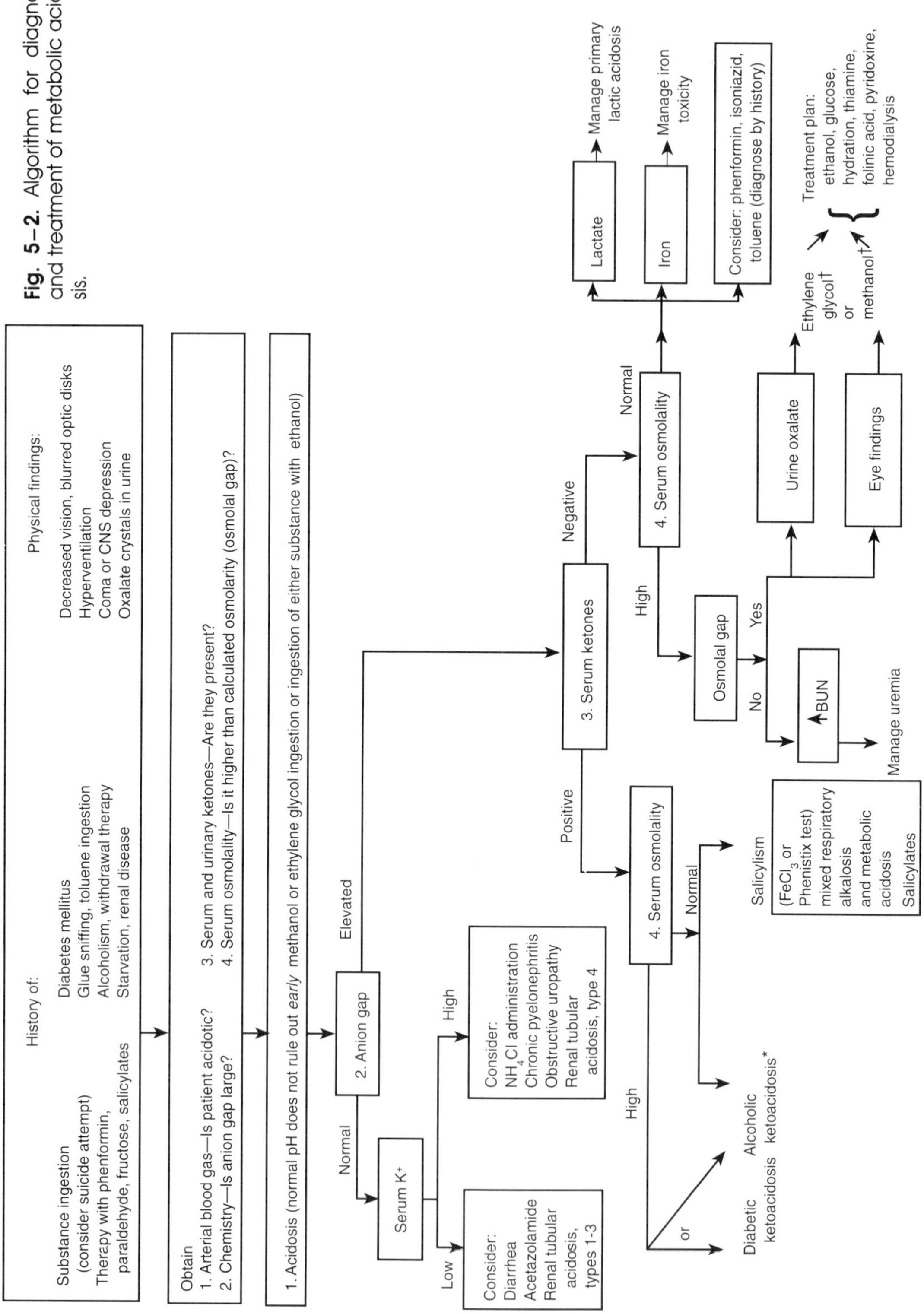

Fig. 5–2. Algorithm for diagnosis and treatment of metabolic acidosis.

History of:
Substance ingestion (consider suicide attempt)
Therapy with phenformin, paraldehyde, fructose, salicylates
Diabetes mellitus
Glue sniffing, toluene ingestion
Alcoholism, withdrawal therapy
Starvation, renal disease

Physical findings:
Decreased vision, blurred optic disks
Hyperventilation
Coma or CNS depression
Oxalate crystals in urine

→

Obtain
1. Arterial blood gas—Is patient acidotic?
2. Chemistry—Is anion gap large?
3. Serum and urinary ketones—Are they present?
4. Serum osmolality—Is it higher than calculated osmolarity (osmolal gap)?

→

1. Acidosis (normal pH does not rule out *early* methanol or ethylene glycol ingestion or ingestion of either substance with ethanol)

→ 2. Anion gap

Normal → Serum K⁺
- Low → Consider: Diarrhea, Acetazolamide, Renal tubular acidosis, types 1-3
- High → Consider: NH_4Cl administration, Chronic pyelonephritis, Obstructive uropathy, Renal tubular acidosis, type 4

Elevated → 3. Serum ketones
- Positive → 4. Serum osmolality
  - High → Diabetic ketoacidosis or Alcoholic ketoacidosis*
  - Normal → Alcoholic ketoacidosis*; Salicylism (FeCl$_3$ or Phenistix test) mixed respiratory alkalosis and metabolic acidosis Salicylates
- Negative → 4. Serum osmolality
  - Normal → Lactate → Manage primary lactic acidosis; Iron → Manage iron toxicity; Consider: phenformin, isoniazid, toluene (diagnose by history)
  - High → Osmolal gap
    - No → ↑BUN → Manage uremia
    - Yes → Urine oxalate → Ethylene glycol†; Eye findings → or methanol† → Treatment plan: ethanol, glucose, hydration, thiamine, folinic acid, pyridoxine, hemodialysis

*In alcoholic ketoacidosis, the strength of the positive acetest determination is milder than would be expected from the degree of acidosis seen on ABGs. Also note that isopropyl alcohol produces ketosis *without* metabolic acidosis.

†Start ethanol at once, even if toxicology results are not yet available.

of 30 mm Hg and yet have a (relative) respiratory *acidosis?* The answer is yes. And whether you describe this patient's combined acid-base disturbances as a "mixed metabolic and respiratory acidosis" or as a "metabolic acidosis without the appropriate respiratory compensation," the fact remains that the pCO_2 of 30 mm Hg is inappropriately high for such a severe metabolic acidosis. In other words, something is interfering with the patient's ability to appropriately compensate for the metabolic acidosis by hyperventilating fully. It is not accurate to describe this condition as merely "partial compensation" because such a description does not adequately take into account the fact that there is a respiratory problem.

Of what use is it to the emergency physician to know in this case that this patient has a respiratory acidosis? If the patient has an *acute* respiratory acidosis (which is the closest band to the right), then in addition to the obvious DKA, she may also have a thus far clinically unsuspected severe pneumonia precipitating the episode of DKA and causing the respiratory depression and consequent respiratory acidosis. Alternatively, this diabetic patient may have been psychiatrically depressed and have taken an overdose of a central nervous system (CNS) depressant causing hypoventilation and acute respiratory acidosis in addition to the DKA; or perhaps she may have had a CNS catastrophe (related or unrelated to the diabetes) causing hypoventilation and respiratory acidosis.

There is still another possibility: although we are fairly certain, based on the information available (history, blood chemistry, and urinalysis), that this patient has DKA, we are merely *hypothesizing* an acute respiratory acidosis based only on the blood gas data. However, in analyzing the pH and pCO_2 coordinates on the map, if we ignore the acute respiratory acidosis band, the patient's coordinates will then appear to lie between the metabolic acidosis band on the left and the *chronic* respiratory acidosis band on the right (the chronic respiratory acidosis band lies slightly to the right of the acute respiratory acidosis band on the map). Could this patient be a diabetic in ketoacidosis and also have chronic obstructive pulmonary disease (COPD) causing chronic respiratory acidosis? Yes, after she recovered from the episode of ketoacidosis and when she was finally able to provide a history herself, the patient told of heavy cigarette smoking for 30 years. When she fully recovered from the DKA, pulmonary function studies were performed and confirmed the diagnosis of COPD. Forced expiratory volume in 1 second (FEV_1)/vital capacity (VC) was 0.57 (0.75 is normal). Maximum midexpiratory flow (MMF) was 0.6 L/min (1.8 L/min is normal) and the diffusing capacity of carbon dioxide (DCO) was 7.2 (19.3 is normal). Undoubtedly, the COPD impaired her ventilatory response to the acute metabolic acidosis and gave her a superimposed "relative" (chronic) respiratory acidosis.[21] Awareness of the possibility of COPD at the time this patient was comatose would have alerted the staff to possible respiratory complications from administering too much oxygen which, based on the po_2 of 152 mm Hg, clearly was not necessary in the first place.

CASE 5–2

A 28-year-old woman ingested an unknown number of over-the-counter cold remedy tablets because of an argument with her mother. Physical examination revealed a blood pressure of 120/70 mm Hg, a pulse rate of 96 beats per minute, regular "deep" inspirations of 16/min, and a rectal temperature of 37.2° C. She had 5 mm reactive pupils, was mentally alert, and had no focal neurologic findings. Blood was drawn for toxicologic testing and BUN, glucose, and electrolytes determination. An ABG specimen was drawn and revealed the following values: pH 7.46; pCO_2, 22 mm Hg; pO_2, 116 mm Hg; O_2 saturation, 99% and fraction of inspired oxygen (FIO_2), 21%.

Comment.—There are two possible explanations for this patient's pH and pCO_2 values (see Fig. 5–1). Because her pH-pCO_2 coordinates clearly fall in the confidence band for chronic respiratory alkalosis (i.e., chronic respiratory alkalosis with a compensatory metabolic acidosis), this possibility must be considered first. The problem here is that there is no history of a chronic disorder. By disregarding the chronic respiratory alkalosis band, however, the patient's pH-pCO_2 coordinates appear to lie *between* two other bands: the metabolic acidosis band (above) and the acute respiratory alkalosis band (below). Thus the alternative explanation for this patient's acid-base problem is that she is suffering from a *mixed* disorder consisting of a primary metabolic acidosis and a primary respiratory alkalosis. Does this second explanation fit the clinical data? Yes, the typical acid-base disturbance characteristic of an early adult salicylate overdose is a mixed respiratory alkalosis and metabolic acidosis with a resultant arterial pH that is normal or high.[22, 23]

An understanding of the acid-base disturbances seen with salicylate poisoning is essential because there is a poor correlation between the serum salicylate level and its toxicity unless the blood pH is taken into account: as the blood pH drops, salicylate leaves the blood and enters the brain and liver where it causes the most severe damage. Alkalinization of *both* the blood and urine is important. In order to achieve ion trapping and urinary excretion of salicylate, urinary alkalinization must be accomplished with sodium bicarbonate ($NaHCO_3$) and not acetazolamide (Diamox) because bicarbonate will produce both systemic alkalemia and urinary alkalosis whereas acetazolamide causes systemic *acidemia* with the urinary alkalosis. In one series of dog experiments, the lethality of a salicylate overdose was doubled or tripled by administering acetazolamide alone to the dogs.[24]

CASE 5–3

An elderly man with a history of COPD was brought to the ED with fever and increased sputum production. Initial ABG values were pH 7.16; pCO_2, 100 mm Hg; and pO_2, 30 mm Hg. The patient was admitted and treated; 24 hours later, while receiving O_2, the patient's pH was 7.25; pCO_2, 80 mm Hg; and pO_2, 80 mm Hg. One week later, breathing room air, the patient's pH was 7.35; pCO_2, 60 mm Hg; and pO_2, 50 mm Hg.

Comment.—Taking into account the ABG determination and the fact that this elderly patient had a history of COPD, the most likely explanation for the pH-pCO_2 combination is a *mixed acute and chronic respiratory acidosis*—perhaps caused by an acute pneumonia superimposed on his COPD (see Fig. 5–1). Antibiotic treatment as well as ventilatory support and controlled oxygenation helped return this patient to his baseline pH-pCO_2 values, which were characteristic of COPD, that is, a chronic respiratory acidosis (pH 7.35; pCO_2, 60 mm Hg; and pO_2, 50 mm Hg).

CASE 5–4

An 18-year-old previously healthy male with a history of vomiting for 3 days was brought to the ED. His mother tried to feed him a bowl of lentil soup, but he immediately vomited the contents and began choking on it. He arrived in the ED in severe distress, choking, and dyspneic. His ABG values were pH 7.16; pCO_2, 100 mm Hg; and pO_2, 30 mm Hg (note the initial values of case 5–3 above!).

Comment.—Does this patient also have COPD and pneumonia? Unlikely. Another explanation for these same values is much more plausible: this man had protracted vomiting causing a metabolic alkalosis and then aspirated vomitus resulting in an aspiration pneumonia and a superimposed acute respiratory acidosis. The combination of the two disturbances would result in a predominant acute respiratory acidosis and a metabolic alkalosis. Is it possible to correctly separate and identify the two widely differing causes of the pH and pCO_2 combinations in cases 5–3 and 5–4 based on the HCO_3^-? No, the Henderson-Hasselbalch equation, which involves the three variables pH, pCO_2, and HCO_3^-, tells us that if two of the three variables are the same for the two patients, the third variable, i.e., HCO_3^-, must also be the same!

CASE 5–5

A known alcoholic appeared in the ED apparently intoxicated and complaining of abdominal pain and an inability to see clearly. There was no odor of alcohol on his breath. His pupils were dilated and sluggishly responsive to light; the retinas were edematous and the optic disks hyperemic. ABG determinations revealed the following values: pH 7.14; pCO_2, 20 mm Hg; pO_2, 96 mm Hg; and O_2 saturation, 99%. There were no ketones in the blood, but undiluted urine was 2+ for glucose and 2+ for ketones. One hour later, a BUN, glucose, and electrolyte (SMA-6) determination revealed an extremely widened anion gap.

Comment.—This patient's pH and pCO_2 values clearly lie in the metabolic acidosis confidence band (see Fig. 5–1). When this information is recognized together with the presence of a large anion gap, the physician must consider several important disorders remembered by the mnemonic *MUD PILES: M*ethanol ingestion, *U*remia, *D*iabetic and alcoholic ketoacidosis, *P*araldehyde ingestion, *I*ron and *I*NH (isoniazid) poisoning, *L*actic acidosis, *E*thylene glycol ingestion, and *S*alicylate poisoning. This group comprises almost the entire differential diagnosis for a widened anion gap metabolic acidosis (see Fig. 5-2).

Diabetic ketoacidosis (and probably salicylate poisoning) can be ruled out by the negative serum ketones. *Alcoholic ketoacidosis* is unlikely because of the absence of *any* serum ketones. The hallmark of alcoholic ketoacidosis is less than expected but present ketones by the standard Acetest (nitroprusside) tablet or strip-test reaction because of an increased ratio of β-hydroxybutyrate to acetoacetate: only the acetoacetate reacts with nitroprusside. *Uremia* is ruled out by a normal BUN, *paraldehyde* ingestion is accompanied by a characteristic odor, and the metabolic acidosis of *salicylate* poisoning is accompanied by a respiratory alkalosis until very late in the course. *Salicylates* may also be further eliminated by a negative bedside $FeCl_3$ test or, if the $FeCl_3$ test is positive, a *negative* or extremely low serum salicylate level. However, relatively low serum salicylate levels in the presence of a low blood pH may be an ominous finding of late severe salicylate poisoning. Iron poisoning severe enough to cause a metabolic acidosis is usually associated with a severely ill patient and also hematemesis; a high serum iron level and possibly radiopaque tablets on abdominal radiography will further help establish this diagnosis.

Ultimately, the physician may be left with the possibilities of methanol or ethylene glycol poisoning and lactic acidosis in the differential diagnosis. However, by comparing the measured serum osmolality with the predicted osmolarity, lactic acidosis could *theoretically* be eliminated because both the predicted and the measured serum values should be the same (normal) for lactate whereas in the case of ethylene glycol and methanol, as well as ethanol and isopropyl alcohol, the calculated osmolarity should be normal and *lower* than the actual measured serum osmolality. In other words, for the alcohols there is an osmolal gap in addition to an anion gap (see Fig. 5–2 and the Definitions section).[25, 26]

One recent paper, however, has challenged the idea that there is no osmolal gap in lactic acidosis,[27] whereas another has questioned the reliability of the osmolal gap in methanol and ethylene glycol poisoning.[28] The increasing availability of serum lactate levels should enable the physician to more accurately diagnose lactic acidosis, and although a small osmolal gap (<25) may be problematic, a large gap (>25) in the appropriate setting (including a negative or very low serum ethanol level) certainly suggests a toxic alcohol such as methanol or ethylene glycol.

Having eliminated lactic acidosis from the differential diagnosis, the physician is then left with the possibilities of methanol and ethylene glycol poisoning. The ophthalmalogic findings in this case are highly suggestive of acute methanol poisoning, but such findings in a comatose patient may not always be clinically apparent. Ethylene glycol poisoning is characterized by calcium oxalate or hippurate crystals in the urine (see Chapter 3); however, when renal shutdown occurs, the crystals may be absent. Methanol levels can be determined by most routine hospital toxicology laboratories, but ethylene glycol levels are not routinely available. Ultimately, differentiating methanol from ethylene glycol poisoning is not therapeutically critical because the treatment for both is currently the same: intravenous administration of adequate ethanol to saturate alcohol dehydrogenase activity in the liver, thereby blocking methanol or ethylene glycol metabolism (methanol and ethylene glycol are not toxic, only their metabolites are), and hemodialysis as soon as possible after the administration of ethanol.

SUMMARY

The use of an acid-base map derived from in vivo pH and pCO_2 values can simplify the identification of mixed acid-base disturbances for the emergency physician. Once all of the possible disorders have been identified, the physician must still consider various explanations for the disturbance(s) by taking into account both the ABG results as well as all of the initial clinical data. (A list of differential diagnoses is provided in Table 5–3.)

The immediate complete identification of serious acid-base disturbances enables the emergency physician to act decisively. Similarly, the recognition of "appropriately abnormal" combinations of pH and pCO_2—such as the respiratory alkalosis seen in a hyperventilating patient with carpopedal spasm or the metabolic acidosis from lactate that characteristically follows a grand mal seizure[29, 30]—enables the physician to function efficiently in the ED without wasting valuable time or unnecessarily duplicating laboratory tests.

DEFINITIONS

Some of the terms used in this chapter are listed below and defined for convenience and clarification.

Acidosis, alkalosis. These terms refer to physiologic processes that tend to cause gain or loss of H^+, bicarbonate, or CO_2 from the body. These terms do not describe the blood pH level, only the direction in which the pH would change if the abnormality were simple and uncompensated.

Acidemia, alkalemia. These terms refer to deviation of blood pH level beyond the normal range of approximately 7.35 to 7.45. Note that it is possible for a patient to have both a primary acidosis and a primary alkalosis—with their respective compensatory responses—and to be either acidemic or alkalemic or have a normal pH level.

$paCO_2$, pCO_2. These terms refer to the partial pressure of CO_2 determined by a CO_2 electrode during an arterial blood gas (ABG) determination. Hypocapnia and hypercapnia refer to deviations of the pCO_2 value beyond the normal range of 38 to

Table 5–3. Differential Diagnosis for Acid-Base Disturbances

CAUSES OF METABOLIC ACIDOSIS

- **Normal anion gap (8–12 mEq/L)**
  - "hyperchloremic" acidosis
  - GI loss of HCO_3^-
    - Diarrhea
    - Small-bowel or pancreatic drainage of fistula
    - Ureterosigmoidostomy, long or obstructed ileal loop conduit
    - Anion-exchange resins
    - Ingestion of $CaCl_2$, $MgCl_2$
  - Renal loss of HCO_3^-
    - Carbonic anhydrase inhibitors
    - Renal tubular acidosis
    - Hyperparathyroidism
    - Hyperaldosteronism
  - Miscellaneous
    - Dilutional acidosis
    - Addition of HCl or its congeners
    - Parenteral alimentation acidosis
    - Sulfur ingestion
- **Increased anion gap metabolic acidosis (>12 mEq/L)**
  - Increased acid production
    - Diabetic ketoacidosis
    - Lactic acidosis
    - Starvation ketoacidosis
    - Alcoholic ketoacidosis
    - Nonketotic hyperosmolar coma
    - Inborn errors of metabolism
  - Ingestion of toxic substances
    - Salicylate overdose
    - Paraldehyde poisoning
    - Methanol ingestion
    - Ethylene glycol ingestion
    - Toluene inhalation
  - Failure of acid excretion
    - Acute renal failure
    - Chronic renal failure

CAUSES OF RESPIRATORY ACIDOSIS

- **Acute**
  - Neuromuscular abnormalities
    - Brain stem injury
    - High cord injury
    - Guillain-Barré syndrome
    - Myasthenia gravis
    - Botulism
    - Opioid, sedative-hypnotic, or other CNS depressant overdose
  - Airway obstruction
    - Foreign body
    - Aspiration of vomitus
    - Laryngeal edema
    - Severe bronchospasm
  - Thoracic-pulmonary disorders
    - Flail chest
    - Pneumothorax
    - Severe pneumonia
    - Smoke inhalation
    - Severe pulmonary edema

CAUSES OF RESPIRATORY ACIDOSIS—cont'd

- **Acute—cont'd**
  - Vascular disease
    - Massive pulmonary embolism
- **Chronic**
  - Neuromuscular abnormalities
    - Chronic opioid or sedative ingestion
    - Primary hypoventilation
    - Pickwickian syndrome
    - Poliomyelitis
    - Diaphragmatic paralysis
  - Thoracic-pulmonary disorders
    - COPD
    - Kyphoscoliosis
    - End-stage interstitial pulmonary disease

CAUSES OF METABOLIC ALKALOSIS

- **Sodium chloride responsive (U_{Cl} < 10 mmol/L)**
  - GI disorders
    - Vomiting
    - Gastric drainage
    - Villous adenoma of the colon
    - Chloride diarrhea
  - Diuretic therapy
  - Correction of chronic hypercapnia
  - Cystic fibrosis
- **Sodium chloride resistant (U_{Cl} > 20 mmol/L)**
  - Excess mineralocorticoid activity
  - Hyperaldosteronism
  - Cushing's syndrome
  - Bartter's syndrome
  - Excess licorice intake
  - Profound potassium depletion
- **Unclassified**
  - Alkali administration
  - Milk-alkali syndrome
  - Nonparathyroid hypercalcemia
  - Massive blood transfusion
  - Glucose ingestion after starvation
  - Large doses of carbenicillin or penicillin

CAUSES OF RESPIRATORY ALKALOSIS

- Central stimulation of respiration
  - Anxiety
  - Head trauma
  - Brain tumors or vascular accidents
  - Salicylates
  - Fever
  - Pain
  - Pregnancy
- Peripheral stimulation of respiration
  - Pulmonary emboli
  - Congestive heart failure
  - Interstitial lung diseases
  - Pneumonia
  - "Stiff lungs" without hypoxemia
  - High altitude
- Uncertain
  - Hepatic insufficiency
  - Gram-negative septicemia
- Mechanical hyperventilation

Modified with permission from Schrier RW: *Renal and electrolyte disorders*, ed 2, Boston, 1980, Little, Brown, pp 122, 146, 163, 164, 169.

42 mm Hg. Because the pCO_2 value is directly proportional to the amount of dissolved CO_2 or H_2CO_3 (carbonic acid) in the blood, which is the denominator or "lung" part of the Henderson-Hasselbalch equation, it can be used with the pH to calculate the serum bicarbonate (HCO_3^-) value, which is the numerator or "kidney" part of the Henderson-Hasselbalch equation. This calculation may be performed by using the equation itself,

$$pH = pK' + \log \frac{HCO_3^- \text{ (mEq/L)}}{0.03\ paCO_2 \text{ (mm Hg)}} = \text{Constant} + \frac{\text{"Kidneys"}}{\text{"Lungs"}},$$

or by plotting the pH and the pCO_2 coordinates on the acid-base map used in this chapter, which does the calculation for you and displays serum bicarbonate [HCO_3^-] values for various pH and pCO_2 combinations.

HCO_3^-. This chemical symbol for serum bicarbonate and the phrases "total CO_2 content," and "CO_2 combining power" refer to the amount of bicarbonate in the serum or to the ways of determining or approximating it. Most autoanalyzers in use today ("SMA-6," etc.) determine the total CO_2 content. This value is an excellent approximation of HCO_3^- because the ratio of HCO_3^- to total CO_2 (total CO_2 = HCO_3^- + $H_2CO_3^-$ + CO_2) is 19:20, that is, 95% of the total CO_2 is HCO_3^-. However, when the HCO_3^- is calculated from the Henderson-Hasselbalch equation by using the pH and pCO_2 obtained from an ABG determination, this calculated HCO_3^- will actually be slightly more accurate than the HCO_3^- results on the electrolyte panel. Most ABG equipment in use today will solve the equation for you and give you the (calculated) HCO_3^- with the pH, pCO_2, pO_2, and O_2 saturation.

Anion gap ("delta"). In actuality, there is no anion gap because the body maintains electrical neutrality. However, when one looks only at the ions obtained by measuring routine serum electrolytes (by SMA-6 determination, for example), one finds that subtracting the anions Cl^- and HCO_3^- from the cations Na^+ and K^+ will normally yield 12 to 20 mEq/L more cations than anions. This normal anion gap results from the fact that more (but not all) cations than anions are routinely measured. Again, if all the cations and anions *could* be measured, there would be no gap between the two groups. To simplify the anion-gap equation, the potassium value may be dropped because it varies over a very small range. Thus

Anion gap = $NA^+ - (HCO_3^- + Cl^-)$ = 8–16 mEq/L ("old") or 3–11 mEq/L ("new").[31]

When an unmeasured acid such as lactate, phosphate, citrate, β-hydroxybutyrate, or acetoacetate (but not HCl) is generated by the cells or added to serum, the amount of unmeasured anion obviously goes up while the measured anion goes down and the gap widens. In the case of a metabolic acidosis, as predicted by the low HCO_3^- value of the serum electrolyle determination but confirmed only by the pH and $paCO_2$ of the ABG determination, the presence or absence of a widened anion gap further defines the type of metabolic acidosis. Metabolic acidosis with a widened anion gap should alert the physician to the possibility of several acute and potentially devastating "emergency department types" of acidosis such as salicylate intoxication; ketoacidosis; methanol, ethylene glycol, or paraldehyde ingestions; lactic acidosis; or uremia (see Fig. 5–2). Newer types of automated equipment now in widespread use yield higher chloride levels than previously. Consequently, the normal anion gap may now be 3 to 11 mEq/L or less, with most normal individuals having a serum anion gap of 6 mEq/L or less—unless chloride calibration is deliberately altered.[31] If you are not familiar with the normal values and ranges in use in your own laboratory, you may miss a widened gap.

Serum osmolality. The term refers to osmotic concentration and is defined as the number of osmols of a solute per *kilogram of solvent (water).* Serum osmol*arity* is defined as the number of osmols of a solute per *liter of solution.* The osmol*ality* of a given solution is numerically equal to the molality of an ideal solution of a nonelectrolyte having the same freezing point depression. Normal serum osmolality is 280 to 295 mOsm.

Serum osmolality can be measured in most clinical laboratories by determining the freezing point depression. Serum osmolarity can also be calculated or predicted from the following formula:

$$2Na^+ + BUN/2.8 + glucose/18.$$

If, however, an osmotically active substance such as ethanol, isopropyl alcohol, methanol, or ethylene glycol is present, the formula for calculating osmolarity will not take it into account and the calculated value will therefore be erroneously low.

Osmolal gap. If the measured total serum osmolality is both higher than normal and more than 10 mOsm greater than the calculated osmolarity, the presence of an osmotically active substance such as ethanol, isopropyl alcohol, methanol, or ethylene glycol is suggested. If the measured total serum osmolality is normal but the calculated value is low, a decrease in serum water content is likely.[25]

REFERENCES

1. Stewart JSS, Stewart WK, Gillies HG: Cardiac arrest and acidosis, *Lancet* 2:964, 1962.
2. Mitchell JH, Wildenthal K, Johnson RL Jr: The effects of acid-base disturbances on cardiovascular and pulmonary function, *Kidney Int* 1:375, 1972.
3. Posner J, Plum F: Spinal fluid pH and neurologic complications in systemic acidosis, *N Engl J Med* 277:605, 1967.
4. Barzel U: The effect of excessive acid feeding on bone, *Calcif Tissue Res* 4:94, 1969.
5. Needle MA, Kaloyanides GJ, Schwartz WB: The effects of selective depletion of hydrochloric acid on acid-base and electrolyte equilibrium, *J Clin Invest* 43:1836, 1964.
6. Luetscher JA: Primary aldosteronism: observations in six cases and review of diagnostic procedures, *Medicine (Baltimore)* 43:437, 1964.
7. Kilburn K: Neurologic manifestations of respiratory failure, *Arch Intern Med* 116:409, 1965.
8. Sideris DA, Katsadoros DP, Valianos G, Assioura A: Types of cardiac dysrhythmias in respiratory failure, *Am Heart J* 89:32, 1975.
9. Downing SE, Mitchell JH, Wallace AG: Cardiovascular response to ischemia, hypoxia, and hypercapnia of the central nervous system, *Am J Physiol* 204:881, 1963.
10. Saltzman H, Heyman A, Sieker HO: Correlations of clinical and physiological manifestations of sustained hyperventilation, *N Engl J Med* 268:1431, 1963.
11. Madias NE, Cohen JJ: Acid-base chemistry and buffering. In Cohen JJ, Kassirer JP, editors: *Acid-Base,* Boston, 1982, Little, Brown pp 3–24.
12. Davenport HW: *The ABC's of acid-base chemistry,* ed 6, Chicago, 1974, University of Chicago Press.
13. Albert MS, Dell RB, Winters RW: Quantitative displacement of acid-base equilibrium in metabolic acidosis, *Ann Intern Med* 66:312–322, 1967.
14. Arbus GS, Herbert LA, Levesque PR et al: Characterization and clinical application of the "significance band" for acute respiratory alkalosis, *N Engl J Med* 208:117–123, 1969.
15. Brackett NC Jr, Cohen JJ, Schwartz WB: Carbon dioxide titration curve of normal man: Effect of increasing degrees of acute-hypercapnia on acid-base equilibrium, *N Engl J Med* 272:6–12, 1965.
16. Kassirer JP, Schwartz WB: The response of normal man to selective depletion of hydrochloric acid: factors in the genesis of persistent gastric alkalosis, *Am J Med* 40:10–18, 1966.

17. Goldring RM, Cannen PJ, Heinemann HO et al: Respiratory adjustment to chronic metabolic alkalosis in man, *J Clin Invest* 47:188–202, 1968.
18. Winters RW, Engel, K, Dell RB: *Acid-base physiology in medicine,* Westlake, Ohio, 1967, London Company, pp 257–264.
19. Schwartz WB, Brackett NC Jr, Cohen JJ: The response of extracellular hydrogen ion concentration to graded degrees of chronic hypercapnia: The physiologic limits of the defense of pH, *J Clin Invest* 44:291–301, 1965.
20. Goldberg M, Green SB, Moss ML et al: Computer based instruction and diagnosis of acid-base disorders, *JAMA* 223:269–275, 1973.
21. Fulop M: Unpublished case report, 1975.
22. Proudfoot AT, Brown SS: Acidemia and salicylate poisoning in adults, *BMJ* 2:547–550, 1969.
23. Gabow PA, Andersen RJ, Potts DE et al: Acid-base disturbances in the salicylate-intoxicated adult, *Arch Intern med* 138:1481–1484, 1978.
24. Hill JB: Current concepts: salicylate intoxication, *N Engl J Med* 288:1110–1113, 1973.
25. Smithline N, Gardner KD: Gaps—anionic and osmol, *JAMA* 236:1594–1597, 1976.
26. Goldfrank L, Flomenbaum N, Lewin N et al: The liquid time bomb, *Hosp Physician* 19:38–60, 1982.
27. Schelling JR, Howard RL: Increased osmolal gap in alcoholic ketoacidosis and lactic acidosis, *Ann Intern Med* 113:580–582, 1990.
28. Hoffman RS, Smilkstein MJ et al: Osmol gaps revisited: normal values and limitations, *J Toxicol—Clin Toxicol* 3:81–93, 1993.
29. Orringer CE, Eustace JC, Wunsch CD et al: Natural history of lactic acidosis after grand-mal seizures, *N Engl J Med* 297:796–799, 1977.
30. Aminoff MJ, Simon RP: Status epilepticus—causes, clinical features and consequences in 98 patients, *Am J Med* 69:657–666, 1980.
31. Winter SD, Pearson R et al: The fall of the serum anion gap, *Arch Intern Med* 150:311–313, 1990.

SUGGESTED READINGS

Emmett M, Narins RG: Clinical use of the anion gap, *Medicine (Baltimore)* 56:38–54, 1977.

Narins RG, Emmett M: Simple and mixed acid-base disorders: a practical approach. *Medicine (Baltimore)* 59:161–187, 1980.

Chapter 6

Microbiologic Staining Techniques

Neal A. Lewin, M.D.

CASE 6–1

A 20-year-old man came to the emergency department with complaints of a penile discharge. The patient stated that he was sexually active and did not use condoms. Physical examination revealed a scant penile discharge; Gram stain revealed many leukocytes with gram-negative intracellular diplococci consistent with *Neisseria gonorrhoeae* (Fig. 6–1).

CASE 6–2

A 24-year-old woman came to the emergency department with fever, chills, and left flank pain. The patient stated that she had dysuria and frequency for several days. A urine sample was obtained under sterile conditions. Gram stain revealed white cell casts and clumps of gram-negative rods consistent with *Escherichia coli* (Fig. 6–2).

CASE 6–3

A 40-year-old man with known acquired immunodeficiency syndrome (AIDS) came to the emergency department with complaints of chills, headache, and photophobia. His physical evaluation was remarkable for a rectal temperature of 105° F and nuchal rigidity. A lumbar puncture was immediately performed and revealed a pleocytosis; Gram stain revealed gram-positive diplococci consistent with *Streptococcus pneumoniae* (Fig. 6–3).

Subsequent cultures on all of the above patients confirmed the clinician's impression from the Gram stain. As a result of the Gram stain the patients were all immediately treated with the appropriate antibiotic for the causative bacterial type.

Had Gram stains not been done, broad-spectrum antibiotics with their additional potential for adverse reactions and cost would have been necessary to "cover" the diagnostic possibilities.

Almost a century ago Hans Christian Gram, a Danish physician, discovered a bacterial staining method while working in Berlin's city morgue. Since his discovery, modifications of the technique have been few. In brief, a slide with the body fluid to be examined is heat-fixed. Gentian violet, Gram's iodine, ethanol, and safranin red are used to stain the specimen. Gram-positive refers to the purple-staining bacteria, and gram-negative refers to the red-staining bacteria. A detailed description is found later in the text.

To appreciate the clinical aspects of the Gram stain, the reader may need a brief

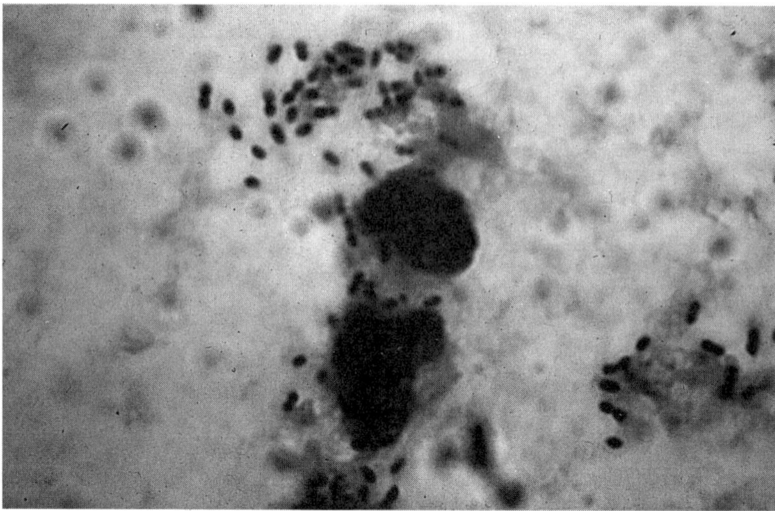

Fig. 6–1. Gram stain reveals gram-negative intracellular diplococci compatible with *N. gonorrhea.*

review of general bacterial structure. Bacteria have a rigid cell wall surrounding the cytoplasmic membrane. The cell wall, which protects the bacteria from osmotic rupture and damage, is responsible for many of the taxonomically significant features of bacteria: shape, antigenic specificities, and "gram-negativity or gram-positivity." The difference between gram-negative and gram-positive bacteria is in the cell wall structure. Salton, cited in Provine and Gardner,[1] showed that the gram-positive cell wall is not stained itself but presents an impermeable barrier to elution of the violet dye–iodine complex by alcohol solvent. The reason for this reaction is that cell walls of gram-positive bacteria contain less lipid than cell walls of gram-negative bacteria and are therefore less permeable to organic solvents. Gram-positive bacteria thus retain the violet dye–iodine complex, whereas this component is leached out of gram-negative bacteria by the alcohol solvent. In the presence of a violet gram-positive color, gram-negative bacteria appear the color of the counterstain, which is usually (safranin) red.

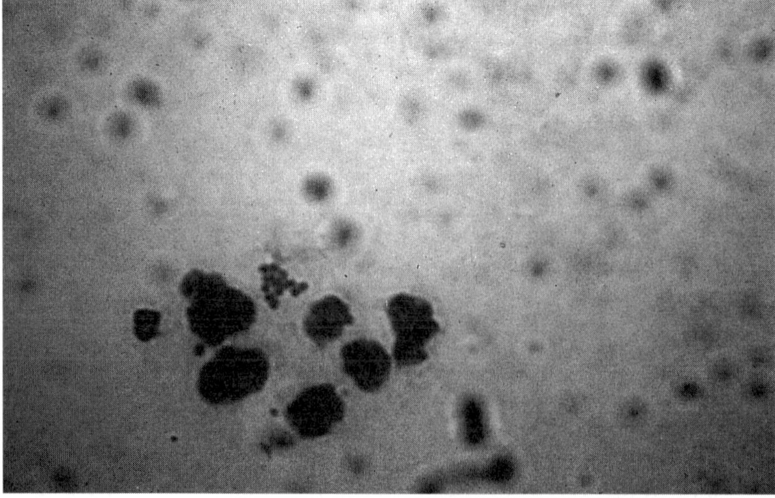

Fig. 6–2. Gram stain reveals gram-negative rods compatible with *E. coli.*

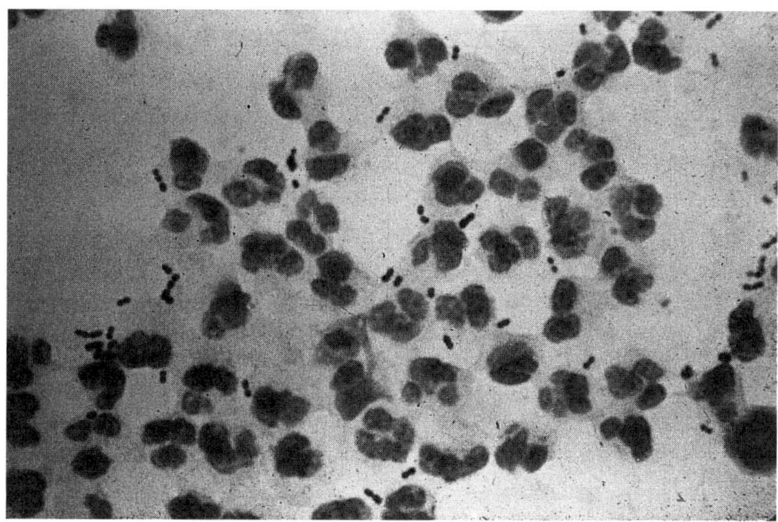

Fig. 6–3. Gram stain reveals gram-positive diplococci compatible with *S. pneumoniae.*

HOW THE GRAM STAIN IS PERFORMED

If a specimen is collected carelessly, the information obtained from a Gram stain will be misleading. The Gram stain smear is critical in classifying the morphology and the taxonomy of bacteria. Primary care providers should collect, stain, and examine the specimen themselves without delegating any of these steps to a technician. As always, the practitioner should be vigilant in adhering to universal precautions and always wear gloves!

The slide should first be cleaned with alcohol or acetone and allowed to air-dry before use (Fig. 6–4). To prepare the smear, use a sterile swab to make a thin film of the specimen on the slide. The smear should then be air-dried. Next, heat-fix the slide without making the slide hot enough to burn skin. The specimen will then be ready for staining. There are four steps in performing proper Gram stains. Each step is followed by a *gentle* tap water rinse.

1. Cover the smear with gentian or crystal violet for 10 seconds; rinse with tap water. (Use a dropper to flood the slide so that the specimen is not washed off under the full blast of a running water tap.)
2. Cover the slide with Gram's iodine for 10 seconds; rinse with water as described above.
3. Decolorize the slide by flooding it with 95% ethanol. The slide should then be rocked back and forth until a "swelling" or rising of the purple stain can be seen and then quickly washed with water. Ethanol-acetone can be used, but it decolorizes the smear so rapidly that the specimen may then be "overdecolorized" and lack the proper amount of the purple stain. This step is the most difficult and critical step because there is no precise number of seconds that the decolorization process should take.
4. Flood the slide with the counterstain safranin red for 10 seconds and then rinse with water. Blot the slide with bibulous paper or lens paper. Basic fuchsin instead of safranin has been used by some examiners to define cellular detail and fusospirochetal flora when doing throat smears, but either counterstain is acceptable.

After drying, the slide should be examined by the primary health care provider. The bacteria that retain the violet-iodine complex are seen as purple and are gram-

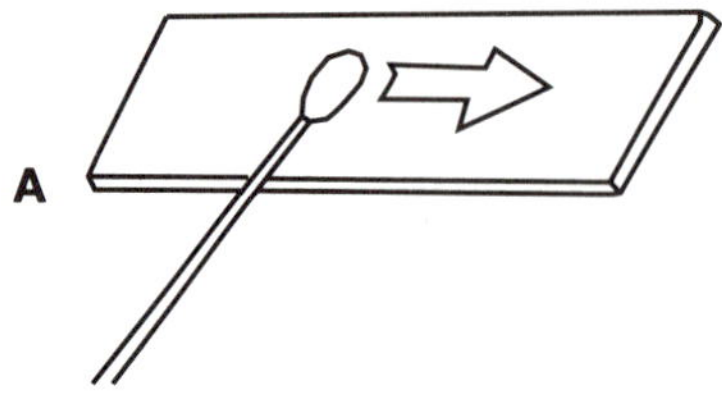

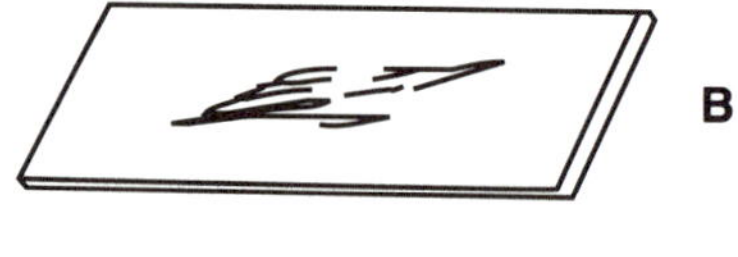

Make a thin film of the specimen on a clean slide.

Air dry.

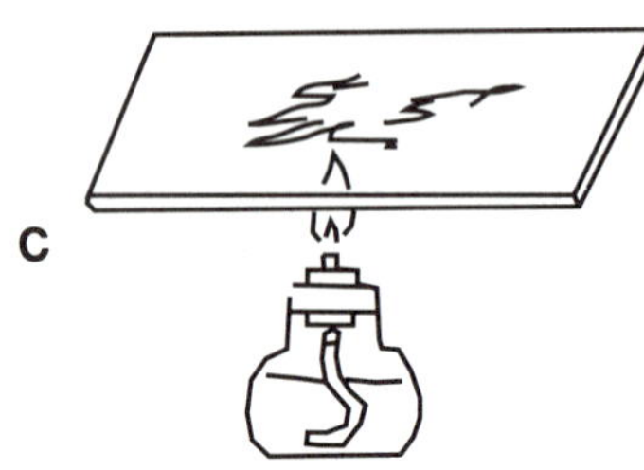

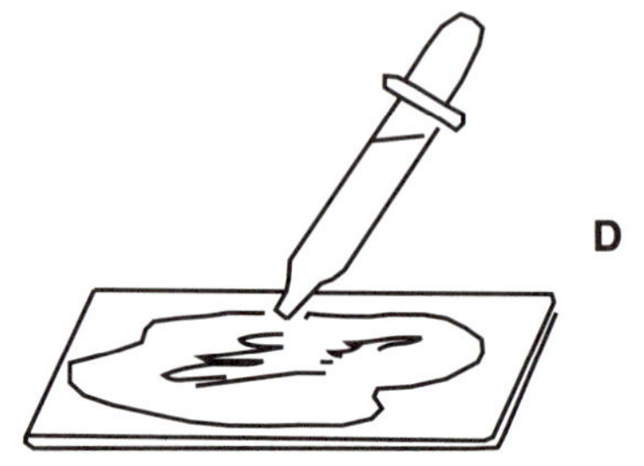

Heat fix without making the slide hot enough to burn your skin.

Cover with crystal violet for 10 seconds; rinse with tap water.

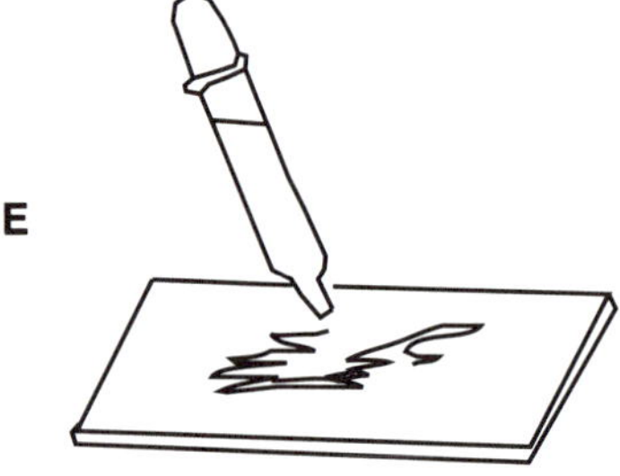

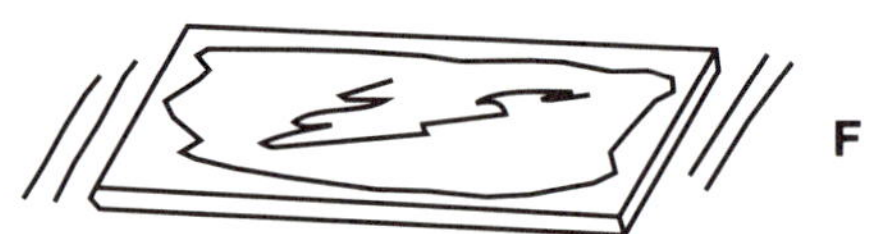

Cover with Gram's iodine for 10 seconds; rinse with tap water; decolorize with 95% ethanol.

Rock slide until "swelling" of purple is seen-this is the most difficult and critical step!

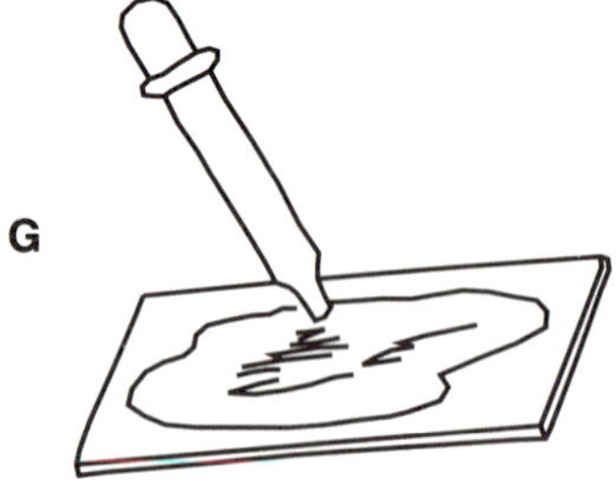

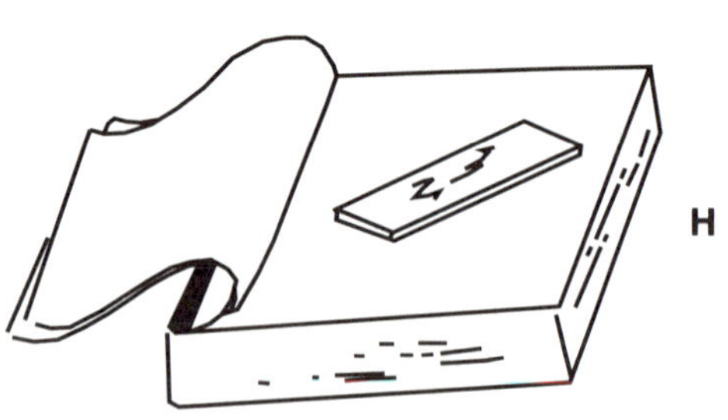

Counterstain with safranin red for 10 seconds; wash with water.

Blot with bibulous paper or lens paper.

Note: Remember, the nuclei of PMNs should be red in color if Gram stain is performed correctly!

Fig. 6–4. Gram stain technique.

positive; the organisms that lose the violet-iodine complex take up the red counterstain and are gram-negative.

Special situations that may alter one's approach have been described by Provine and Gardner.[1] If cerebrospinal fluid (CSF) is being examined, the fluid should be spun down first and the *sediment* examined because few organisms may be present despite central nervous system (CNS) infection.[2] If a specimen is bloody, it may be difficult to interpret the smear. Therefore, after air drying and heat fixing, cover the slide with water for several minutes to lyse the red blood cells and then rinse the slide.

In examining the smear, one should first use low magnification and look for polymorphonuclear leukocytes. The nuclei of these cells are red. Polymorphonuclear neutrophils are usually present in bacterial infections with the exception of neutropenic patients or infections complicated by toxins that destroy polymorphonuclear cells. Fungi, epithelial cells, and red blood cells can also be seen with the low-power lens. Next, switch to the oil immersion lens (×100), and use the maximum light available to properly interpret the colors.

REASONS TO PERFORM A GRAM STAIN

Approximately 30% of patients admitted to a general hospital are infected. Most of the infections are bacterial in nature. In addition to identifying the causative bacteria type, a Gram-stained smear can also tell the physician immediately whether the specimen is contaminated or inadequate. For example, when examining sputum, if the physician sees mostly epithelial cells rather than polymorphonuclear leukocytes, it is known that culture of this specimen is going to yield oral flora and will be misleading. On the other hand, a Gram stain of a good sputum specimen is generally more useful and more cost-effective than a sputum culture because it allows the clinician to rationally choose antibiotic therapy before contaminants and clinically insignificant organisms grow on the culture medium.[3] This growth occurs inevitably after several hours to several days.

Boerner and Zwadyk[4] found that the sputum Gram stain was a sensitive and reliable indicator to guide therapy and predict outcome in adults with community-acquired pneumonia. More than half of the patients with community-acquired pneumonia had sputum Gram stains suggestive of pneumococcal pneumonia. These patients responded dramatically to specific antimicrobial therapy. Conversely, another large subgroup with no predominant organism on sputum Gram stain responded more slowly to antibiotics, which suggests that a more reliable approach for the clinician would have been to collect sputum cytologic specimens and consider transtracheal aspiration (and also consider the possibility of atypical pneumonia).

A prospective study to determine the ability of a sputum Gram stain to predict the cause of community-acquired bacterial pneumonia by Gleckman et al.[5] looked at 59 bacteremic patients who expectorated what appeared to be a true sputum sample. Ninety-four percent of the time, physicians could select appropriate antibiotic monotherapy to treat pneumonia. This study is a confirmation of the experience of Boerner and Zwadyk.[4]

Smith et al.[6] reported four cases of pulmonary strongyloidiasis in steroid-treated patients with chronic lung disease who came from an area where strongyloidiasis was endemic. In every case routine Gram stain of their sputum was used for diagnosis. Larvae were demonstrated in the sputum, although the sensitivity of the Gram stain in this setting is unknown. The presence of the pathogen substantially changed the clinician's management.

Finally, Farrington and French[7] emphasized the fact that *Legionella pneumophila* can be seen on a Gram-stained smear of sputum as gram-negative bacilli. Some authors have suggested that the use of 0.05% carbolfuchsin as the counterstain in lieu of safranin will enhance the results. Since the management of Legionnaire's disease is quite specific, namely, erythromycin, it is another example of how one can avoid the use of broad-spectrum coverage as a result of using the Gram stain.

Thus in many cases, examination of a Gram-stained smear from an infected site enables the clinician to begin treatment immediately without awaiting culture results and to choose a narrow-spectrum antimicrobial agent rather than using a "shotgun" antibiotic technique. Furthermore, the Gram stain may lead the physician to do cultures in a highly specific manner. For example, the discovery of slender gram-negative rods suggests a gram-negative anaerobe such as *Bacteroides fragilis*. Once the laboratory personnel are alerted to this possibility, they can be more rigorous in performing anaerobic cultures. If spores or hyphae are seen, then fungal cultures and KOH preparations can be specifically requested. Inasmuch as fungal cultures are not routine laboratory procedures, the failure to request the appropriate test may ultimately cause the laboratory to miss the specific organism.

The Gram stain can be used semiquantitatively in patients with symptoms of urinary tract infection. If a Gram-stained smear of an uncentrifuged urine specimen reveals one organism per oil immersion field, a clinically significant bacterial concentration of 100,000/mL is probably present and antibiotic therapy is indicated (see Chapter 3).

In a study by Olson et al.,[8] a slide centrifuge Gram stain procedure was performed to screen for bacteriuria in over 4,000 urine specimens in men. Specimens were placed in a disposable slide centrifuge chamber, centrifuged at 2000 rpm for 5 minutes in a slide centrifuge (Cytospin), and then heat-fixed and Gram-stained. The slides were scanned in 12 consecutive oil immersion fields. The presence of the same organism in six or more fields was considered positive for infection. Urine cultures were performed on these samples. When 100,000 or more colony-forming units per milliliter was used as a reference for comparison, the screen had a sensitivity of 98%, a specificity of 90%, a negative predictive value of 99%, and a positive predictive value of 65%. This study concluded that the slide centrifuge Gram stain is very sensitive.

A positive Gram stain of a body fluid that is ordinarily sterile may enable a clinician to diagnose a serious condition, even in the absence of other expected positive laboratory test results. In a retrospective study by Fishbein et al.,[2] 7 of 50 consecutive cases of acute bacterial meningitis revealed six or fewer white blood cells (WBCs) in the CSF; however, bacteria were present on Gram stain in each case. All 7 patients were either elderly, had Hodgkin's disease, or had severe alcoholism. Although bacterial meningitis is usually characterized by CSF leukocytosis, increased protein, and decreased glucose, occasionally in severely debilitated hosts only the Gram stain is positive, thus indicating the need for antibiotic therapy without the need to wait for culture results.

BODY FLUIDS THAT SHOULD BE GRAM-STAINED

CSF, sputum, effusions (joint, chest, abdominal, and wound site), urine, and penile and vaginal (cervical) discharges should all be Gram-stained whenever infection is considered possible. As a rule, stool, blood (buffy coat), and pharyngeal smears are of limited value, and cultures are usually more beneficial to the clinician (see section on stool specimens). In a study by Reik and Rubin,[9] 599 blood samples were studied to evaluate their buffy coat smears for bacteria. Although useful on occasion, the buffy coat smear was not of substantial clinical benefit. The minimum concentration of organisms necessary to make a positive buffy coat smear is so great (1×10^5) that a positive smear virtually forecasts the patient's death.

OTHER STAINS THAT CAN BE USED IN THE OUTPATIENT SERVICES

Tuberculosis—both typical and atypical—has recently reemerged as a major health problem. When appropriate, the acid-fast stain should be used to help make a diagnosis that may take up to 6 weeks to establish by culture. Mycobacteria do not take up Gram stain well[10]; occasionally they appear as small weakly gram-positive beaded rods. Inasmuch as mycobacteria are not adequately identified with Gram staining, a stronger dye, carbolfuchsin, is used as the initial stain. In addition, mycobacteria alone among bacterial organisms are "acid-fast," that is, they retain the dye despite attempts to decolorize them with acid alcohol. The theory of acid fastness is that the dye binds to the lipid-rich cells. Other bacteria initially pick up the carbolfuchsin but are decolorized by the acid alcohol, so the acid-fast myocbacteria light up "like a red light in a field of blue."

Acid-Fast (Kinyoun Carbolfuchsin) Stain

The Kinyoun carbolfuchsin method is used to prepare the acid-fast stain as follows:

1. Wearing gloves and a mask, or working under a hood, if possible, make a thin film smear as with the Gram stain method.
2. Air-dry and heat-fix, being careful not to inhale the potentially infectious specimen.
3. Flood the slide with Kinyoun carbolfuchsin stain for 5 minutes.
4. Decolorize thoroughly with acid alcohol. Decolorize the specimen until all the color disappears and then wash with tap water.
5. Counterstain with either brilliant green or methylene blue for 2 minutes and wash off completely.

Acid-fast bacilli (so-called red snappers) stain red, whereas the background cellular elements and other bacteria are the color of the counterstain (green or blue). In examining the smear, use the oil immersion lens and the maximum light available. *Mycobacterium tuberculosis* is a slender, slightly curved rod, although it may be beaded in appearance. In searching for mycobacteria, examine the smear for 15 minutes before stating that there are no organisms and that the smear is negative. Examine the CSF for at least 30 minutes.

Methylene Blue Stain

Other stains also have a place in ambulatory settings. The methylene blue stain is useful in examining diarrheal stools. Gastroenteritis secondary to viruses, *Vibrio cholerae*, noninvasive *E. coli*, exotoxin from *Staphylococcus aureus*–induced diarrhea (food poisoning), *Clostridium perfringens*, and *Clostridium botulinum* is not usually associated with the presence of fecal leukocytes. In gastroenteritis secondary to *Salmonella*, *Shigella*, invasive *E. coli*, *Campylobacter*, *Giardia lamblia*, and *Entamoeba histolytica*, fecal leukocytes can, however, be seen.[11] The presence or absence of fecal leukocytes and a differential WBC stain can be used to enhance precision in the diagnosis.

The method for stool examination with methylene blue is simple. A wet preparation is made on a glass slide from a small fleck of stool or mucus, two drops of methylene blue are added, a coverslip is placed over the sample, and in 2 minutes the slide is examined—first under a low-power objective to look for WBCs and then under high power to do a differential count.

Many authorities feel that a Gram stain of feces is indicated only if superinfection with *S. aureus* is suspected. In this situation, finding sheets of WBCs and clusters of gram-positive cocci is diagnostic. On the other hand, Quinn et al.[12] found that a Gram stain of rectal exudate is insensitive for the diagnosis of rectal *N. gonorrhoeae*, with up to 50% of culture-positive cases being missed.

AMEBIASIS

In the United States in 1978 it was estimated that 2% to 5% of the population was infected with amebae alone.[13] In more recent times and particularly in the homosexual population, the incidence of *Giardia lamblia* and *Entamoeba histolytica* has been considerably higher. It is therefore extremely important for the primary care provider to identify common parasites under the microscope.

Saline and Iodine Preparation

The use of saline and iodine for evaluation of intestinal parasites is an important diagnostic tool. A wet mount with saline for trophozoites, relatively fragile forms, and an iodine stain for the hardier cysts is accomplished by placing several drops of liquid stool and several drops of these solutions on separate slides and placing a coverslip over each preparation. Nuclear stains such as trichrome stain are important to classify cysts and trophozoites for permanent records but may be too complex for screening in a busy emergency department (ED).

Wet mounts of fungi are useful when evaluating epidermal scales or vaginal discharges, although *Candida* species can easily be seen on Gram stain. *Nocardia* or *Actinomyces* can be seen with the Giemsa stain.

POINTS TO REMEMBER ABOUT STOOL SPECIMENS

Stools containing barium or cathartics and antacids are unsuitable for microscopic examination because these substances may cloud the field. Rectal swabs are usually not sufficient for diagnosis because the sample is too small. Specimens should not be contaminated with urine or water because the fragile trophozoites will be destroyed. Several days must elapse to allow for the passage of these materials before proper stool examination is possible. The specimens must be fresh and warm. At least three fresh specimens are necessary because the parasites may be intermittently excreted in low concentration. Centrifuging loose stool will increase the chance of detecting pathogens.

TIPS FOR A "PERFECT GRAM STAIN"

Because the most common error in Gram stain interpretation is attributable to the staining technique, one safeguard is for physicians to stain their mouth flora on the same slide as the patient's specimen and separate them with a wax line dividing the slide in half. Normal mouth flora includes a number of different gram-positive and gram-negative organisms. If the specimen is overdecolorized, the mouth flora appears to be predominantly gram-negative organisms; if it is underdecolorized, the mouth flora appears to be predominantly gram-positive (see Fig. 6–5). Similarly, if a specimen contains polymorphonuclear leukocytes and the nuclei appear Gram positive, the specimen is underdecolorized.

Trying to salvage a technically inadequate smear by cleaning the oil off with xylol,

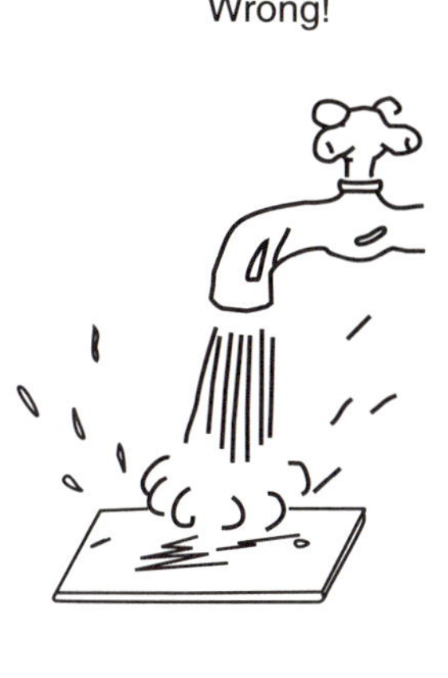

Do not wash the slide under full blast of running water tap!

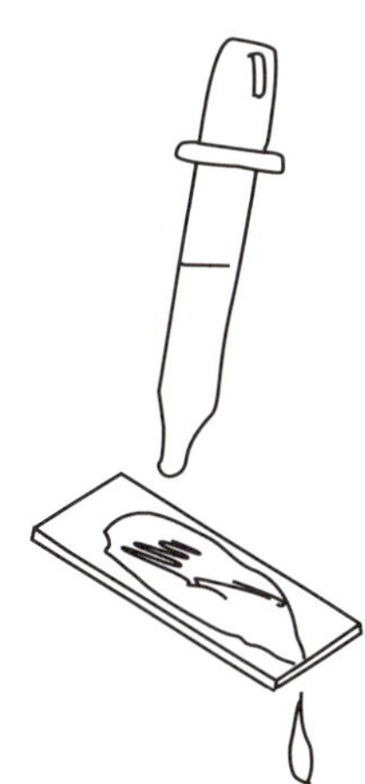

Use a dropper to flood slide gently so that specimen is not washed off.

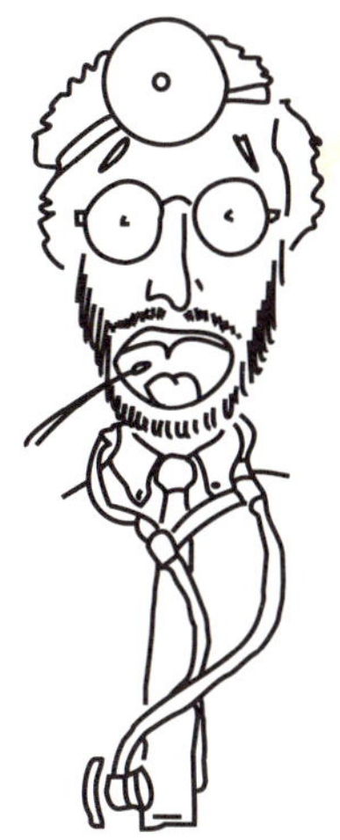

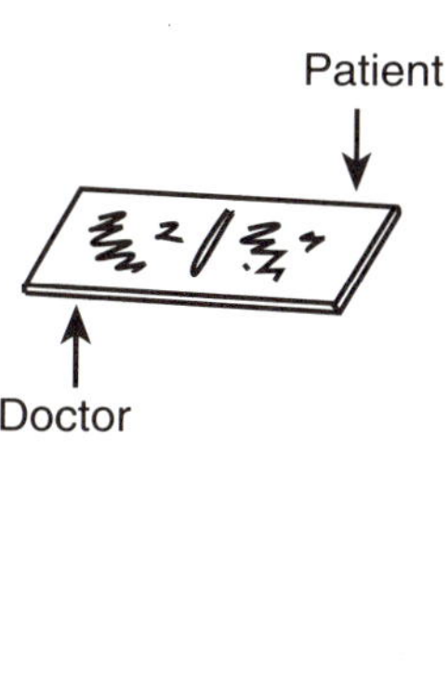

Stain your own mouth flora on the same slide as the patient's specimen—normal mouth flora contains both gram-positive and gram-negative organisms. If the specimen is overdecolorized, the mouth flora will demonstrate predominantly gram-negative organisms; if underdecolorized, the mouth flora will appear to be predominantly gram-positive.

Fig. 6–5. Tips for a perfect Gram stain.

decolorizing, and counterstaining again usually results in further error from poor staining. Starting again from the beginning is recommended. To save time, two slides from the original body material should always be initially prepared. Stain one and save the other .If the first slide does not stain successfully, there is always the other slide with which to work, thus obviating the necessity of obtaining a second specimen. Suspect contamination of the specimen if several types of bacteria are seen unless the provider strongly suspects a polymicrobial infection such as is seen in infected peritoneal aspirates after a ruptured abdominal viscus. Be aware of the varying morphology of a single organism and artifacts such as precipitated reagents or talc crystals from rubber gloves.

The simple technique of performing a Gram stain has changed little in the past hundred years. It remains a rapid, precise means of being cost-effective and intellectually rigorous in the ED while making patients' visits and the ultimate care given more productive.

REFERENCES

1. Provine H, Gardner P: The gram-stained smear and its interpretation, *Hosp Pract* 9:85–91, 1974.
2. Fishbein DB, Daniel B, Palmer DL et al: Bacterial meningitis in the absence of CSF pleocytosis, *Arch Intern Med* 141:1369–1372, 1981.
3. Hirschmann JV: The sputum Gram stain, *J Gen Intern Med* 6:261[B]263, 1991 (editorial).
4. Boerner DF, Zwadyk P: The value of the sputum Gram's stain in community-acquired pneumonia, *JAMA* 247:642–645, 1982.
5. Gleckman R, DeVita J, Hibert D et al: Sputum Gram stain assessment in community acquired bacteremic pneumonia, *J Clin Microbiol* 26:846–849, 1988.
6. Smith B, Vergehese A, Guiterrez C et al: Pulmonary strongyloidiasis diagnosis by sputum Gram stain, *Am J Med* 79:663–666, 1985.
7. Farrington M, French GL: *Legionella pneumophila* seen in Gram stains of respiratory secretions and recovered from conventional blood cultures, *J Infect* 6:123–127, 1983.
8. Olson ML, Shanholtzer CJ, Willard KE, Peterson LR: The slide centrifuge Gram stain as a urine screening method, *Am J Clin Pathol* 96:454–458, 1991.
9. Reik H, Rubin SJ: Evaluation of the buffy coat smear for rapid detection of bacteremia, *JAMA* 245:357–359, 1981.
10. Fisher J, Ganapathy M, Edwards BH, Newman CL: Utility of Grams and Giems stains in the diagnosis of pulmonary tuberculosis, *Am Rev Respir Dis* 141:511–513, 1990.
11. Adler PM: Stool examination: culture versus gram stain, *Ann Emerg Med* 5:337–341, 1986.
12. Quinn T, Corey L et al: The etiology of anorectal infections in homosexual men, *Am J Med* 71:395–403, 1981.
13. Tan J: Common and uncommon parasitic infections in the U.S., *Med Clin North Am* 62:1059–1083, 1978.

Chapter 7

Pregnancy Testing

Stephen Alan Senreich, M.D.

Any female patient capable of menstruating who comes to the emergency department (ED) with almost any complaint, especially an abdominal complaint, must be considered to be potentially pregnant. The following are summaries of four case histories from patients who were seen in various EDs in New York City.

CASE 7–1

A 40-year-old female who had never been pregnant went to the ED because of an inability to void for 24 hours. She had a history of slightly irregular periods and a fibroid uterus. Her last period had been approximately 40 days ago. On examination, she had a large retroflexed fibroid uterus, with the cervix compressing the urethral-vesical junction. She had acute urinary retention. *A hysterectomy was recommended.* She became frightened and left the first hospital and went to a second ED. What additional information is required? What tests can be performed in your ED to reach an appropriate decision for this patient?

CASE 7–2

An 11½-year-old female who had never menstruated went to the ED with her first episode of vaginal bleeding, described by her mother as voluminous, and with severe cramping. She had never had a gynecologic examination, so the gynecologist on call was consulted. What is the diagnosis and how can it be proved?

CASE 7–3

A 26-year-old female with a history of a previous right tubal pregnancy treated by salpingectomy came to the ED with sudden left lower quadrant abdominal pain. She did not remember the exact date of her last period, but she did not think that she was late. Examination revealed a normal-sized uterus and a left cystic adnexal mass. Urinalysis demonstrated 4+ proteinuria. The agglutination-inhibition urine tests for pregnancy were positive. Ultrasound of the pelvis demonstrated a cystic mass in the left adnexa, with no intrauterine pregnancy seen. What is your diagnosis? Are there any other tests that you would recommend in the ED?

CASE 7–4

A 28-year-old female ultrasound technician at the hospital suddenly had right lower quadrant pain. She had a history of occasional missed periods. However, at that time she had been amenorrheic for 2½ months. Two years earlier, she had

had a laparoscopy for similar complaints and had been found to have a functional ovarian cyst. Ultrasound revealed a right cystic adnexal structure consistent with either a corpus luteum or a tubal pregnancy. No intrauterine pregnancy was noted. Her friend, who is a technician in the chemistry laboratory, ran an unspecified type of urine test for pregnancy that she reported as positive. Examination in the ED revealed a normal-sized uterus and left adnexa. The right adnexa contained a slightly tender, perfectly round 3- to 4-cm cystic mobile structure. What would you do?

As will become obvious later, the first two cases represent failure to consider the potential diagnosis of pregnancy. The third and fourth cases represent the appropriate inclusion of pregnancy in the differential diagnosis. But were the patients completely evaluated? Before considering these cases further, it is useful to review how pregnancy may be diagnosed in EDs in the 1990s.

DIAGNOSING PREGNANCY IN THE EMERGENCY DEPARTMENT

The most important factor in diagnosing or ruling out pregnancy or a complication of pregnancy in the differential diagnosis is to *think* of pregnancy as a possibility. The greatest source of error in the diagnosis of pregnancy among emergency department staff is either the failure to think of it or understand how to properly prove or disprove it. *Any woman of menstrual age* (i.e., from approximately 12 to 52 years of age), who comes to the ED has the potential of being pregnant.

The patient's history is rarely totally reliable as a means of excluding pregnancy. Even when the patient states that her last menstrual period was on time or the patient thinks that she is not pregnant or she insists that she could not be pregnant, a recent study demonstrates that there is still at least a 10% chance of pregnancy.[1]

Once pregnancy is considered, it must be confirmed or ruled out. The three absolute signs of pregnancy, i.e., hearing the fetus, seeing the fetus, or feeling the fetus, are not totally applicable in the first trimester. Probable signs of pregnancy such as enlargement of the uterus or softening and cyanosis of the cervix may not be diagnostic.[2]

Ultrasound (also referred to as sonography) has improved our ability to diagnose pregnancy. A transabdominal scan can detect a normal intrauterine pregnancy of 4 weeks or more but is less reliable in detecting early spontaneous abortions or ectopic implantations. Transvaginal ultrasound is now available and is even more sensitive since it detects intrauterine gestations at 3 weeks from conception.[3] However, abnormal pregnancies can still be missed. Over the past several years, ultrasound (abdominal or transvaginal) has become available in EDs, and in some instances, both the obstetric and emergency medicine staffs have been trained and have become proficient in its use. The results are immediate. Ultrasound is certainly reliable if results are positive, i.e., if either an intrauterine or ectopic pregnancy is visible.[4] Sensitivity and reliability have improved, especially with transvaginal ultrasound.[5] However, if the pregnancy is less than 3 weeks' gestation or classic sonographic signs of spontaneous or ectopic abortion are not visible, false-negative results are possible. In the absence of a definitive diagnosis, other means of documenting pregnancy must be used.[6,7] In addition, sonography is relatively expensive (the cost to the patient ranging from $150 to $180).

Until the 1960s, all pregnancy testing was biological in nature. Since 1927 when Aschheim and Zondek found that urine of pregnant women injected into mice resulted in ovarian hyperemia and hemorrhage, many biological tests were used to uncover the presence of gonadotropic activity in pregnant patients.[8] These included the Friedman rabbit test and the Frank-Berman rat ovarian hyperemia test. Each involved killing the animal injected and examining its ovaries. The sensitivity of these methods varied from 1,000 to 6,000 mIU* of human chorionic gonadotropin (hCG) per milliliter.

In 1961, immunologic pregnancy tests became available. A patient's urine containing (an unknown quantity of) hCG would neutralize (a known volume of) anti-hCG antibody so that it could not agglutinate a known quantity of hCG-bound latex particles or red blood cells. This is known as the agglutination-inhibition reaction. Until the late 1980s, this method of testing has been the basis for *all* routine pregnancy testing in hospitals, in laboratories, in physician's offices, and in the home, i.e., the early pregnancy tests.[9] If the test sample would not agglutinate, the patient was considered pregnant. If the sample agglutinated (visible precipitate), there was no hCG in the urine to neutralize antibody and the patient was not considered pregnant.

The sensitivity of the test varied with each manufacturer, from 750 to 3,000 mIU/mL. *Therefore these immunologic tests were not designed to detect normal gestations of less than 4 weeks from conception.* It is extremely important to understand why the sensitivity of these tests was set relatively low (high false-negative rate). Human chorionic gonadotropin is a glycoprotein produced by trophoblastic cells in the placenta and is composed of an α- and β-chain joined covalently to form a quaternary structure.[10] There is a significant cross-reaction between luteinizing hormone (LH) and hCG because both hormones have identical α-chains and similar quaternary structures. Therefore, if the immunologic test sensitivity is too high, false positive tests will result. LH present in the urine can be as high as 300 mIU or more in perimenopausal patients. Since follicle-stimulating hormone (FSH) and thyroid-stimulating hormone (TSH) have a common quaternary structure, they too can lead to false-positive test results if the sensitivity is set too high.

The most significant breakthrough in pregnancy testing occurred during the 1970s with the development of radioreceptor assays for hCG and, more importantly, a radioimmunoassay for the β-subunit of hCG. Although the radioreceptor test "Biocept G" (*not* the β-subunit test) is a rapid blood test for the measurement of biologically active molecule[11] and is sensitive to approximately 200 mIU of hCG per milliliter, it cannot distinguish between hCG and LH. It is therefore susceptible to false-positive results. The tests use the receptor sites of the plasma membranes of bovine corpora lutea, to which the entire hCG molecule binds.

Much more specific and therefore more useful than the radioreceptor test is the radioimmunoassay for the β-chain of the hCG molecule.[10, 12, 13] There are essentially no false-negative results. It can detect as little as 1 to 10 mIU of hCG and can theoretically establish the diagnosis of pregnancy by day 8 after conception, that is, shortly after implantation of the blastocyst. The test is quantitive and is most accurate on serum. At present, the expense of the test and the length of time necessary to perform the assay are its principal problems. Since the radioimmunoassay first became available, these drawbacks have largely been overcome. At present, a good commercial laboratory can perform the test in several hours. The charge to the patient averages $40 to $60.

However, an intriguing problem has resulted from the high degree of sensitivity and specificity of this test for hCG. Although there are no false-positive results *for the detection of hCG,* certain tumors produce ectopic hCG, which can lead to misinterpretation of the test results. Besides gestational trophoblastic tumors, hCG can be secreted by certain gastric and pancreatic adenocarcinomas, hepatomas, and germinal tumors.[14] There are even reports of a small amount of hCG (2 mIU) detected in normal nonpregnant patients.[15, 16] Fortunately, these are unusual situations that should not be a diagnostic problem in treating the average patient in the ED.

*All values refer to the World Health Organization [WHO] First International Preparation [IRP] standard.

Most recently, various serum and urine tests have been developed that use an enzyme-linked immunoabsorbent assay (ELISA) for hCG.[17] Anti–β-hCG monoclonal antibodies bound to a solid support such as latex bind to the unknown amount of hCG in the test sample. Then a second monoclonal anti-α-hCG antibody is added to sandwich the hCG. It is to this second antibody that an enzyme is linked that can be used to produce a colored reaction. Even more recently, the anti–β-monoclonal antibody is linked directly to a colored latex particle instead of an enzyme that will undergo further reactions to produce color. This is an even simpler method known as color immunochromatographic assay (CICA). By using this concept, a variety of qualitative and quantitative tests have been developed that have a sensitivity to 25 to 50 mIU/mL.[18–20] These tests can be run quickly and easily and are relatively inexpensive. *Techniques using this concept are the basis for the newer routine office and home "do-it-yourself" tests.* Although this type of pregnancy evaluation has been vastly improved, there are still some limitations that must be addressed. These will be discussed later under "Pitfalls."

In recent years there has been an explosion of "home" pregnancy tests available to all consumers. The most recent tests use the same ELISA monoclonal antibody technology as discussed above. Articles arguing favorably or unfavorably over the accuracy and interpretation of these home testing kits have been published.[21, 22] The greatest problem with these assays is understanding the limitations of these pregnancy tests. This chapter is written to explain these limitations to professionals. Accuracy is further impaired when these tests are interpreted by an untrained consumer.

The 5-Minute Pregnancy Test

Despite the drawbacks mentioned, the newer immunologic tests on urine have become the standard means of detecting pregnancy in the ED, i.e., those using the ELISA or CICA methods for evaluating the presence of anti–β-subunit hCG monoclonal antibody. They are fast and inexpensive. A package of 30 kits costs the testing facility approximately $85. The charge to the patient averages $15 to $20 in New York.

All tests, regardless of the manufacturer, are performed in similar fashion. Unless the hospital is equipped to perform a serum test for the β-subunit of hCG on demand, it is essential for emergency physicians to be able to do the basic 5-minute qualitative test.

Method

- Obtain a random sample of urine from the patient. If the patient is bleeding vaginally, blood may contaminate the urine and lead to spurious results. In such a patient, a catheterized specimen may be warranted. Also, check for proteinuria. Significant proteinuria can give false-positive results because the protein can inactivate the anti-hCG antibodies.[23]
- There are a variety of rapid enzyme immunoassays for pregnancy testing available today. These assays are all based on the same principles and are performed with similar speed and technique. The companies claim that their tests are sensitive to between 25 and 50 mIU/mL of hCG.
- A sample of urine is added to the test well in the kit. Below the well is an absorbant strip that transfers the specimen through various reactions. The urine will come in contact with anti–β-hCG monoclonal antibodies conjugated to colored particles. If hCG is present in the specimen, it will bind to the antibody-colored conjugate. This congregate moves along the test strip where it is ex-

posed to an anti–α-hCG antibody, which is immobilized in the result window of the test kit. If hCG is present in the urine, a sandwich is created on the test strip, that is, the membrane-fixed anti–α-hCG antibodies, the hCG, and the anti–β-hCG antibodies bound to colored particles. The result is therefore positive if this colored conglomerate is visible in the result window. Depending on the test kit, this could be a colored circle, a colored line, or a colored plus (+). A negative result would occur if there is no hCG-colored conjugate to bind with the membrane-fixed anti–α-hCG antibodies, in which case no visible mark would appear in the result window. The entire reaction takes approximately 5 minutes.

An example of an accurate and easy-to-run CICA test, CARDS ±O·S· HCG-Urine One Step Pregnancy Test from Pacific Biotech, Inc., San Diego, is shown in Figs. 7–1 and 7–2. The test works by the following method:

- Dispense the test sample into the "Add Urine" well. Inside the housing of the test kit below this well is an absorbent pad that transfers the urine to a membrane strip in which the sample moves across the kit while undergoing various reactions.
- As the urine moves through the first zone of the membrane, it comes in contact with anti–β-hCG monoclonal antibodies conjugated to blue latex beads. If there is hCG present in the urine, it will bind and mobilize the antibody–blue latex conjugate.
- This antigen-antibody congregate in the urine continues to move along the test membrane to the second zone, referred to as the "Read Result" window.

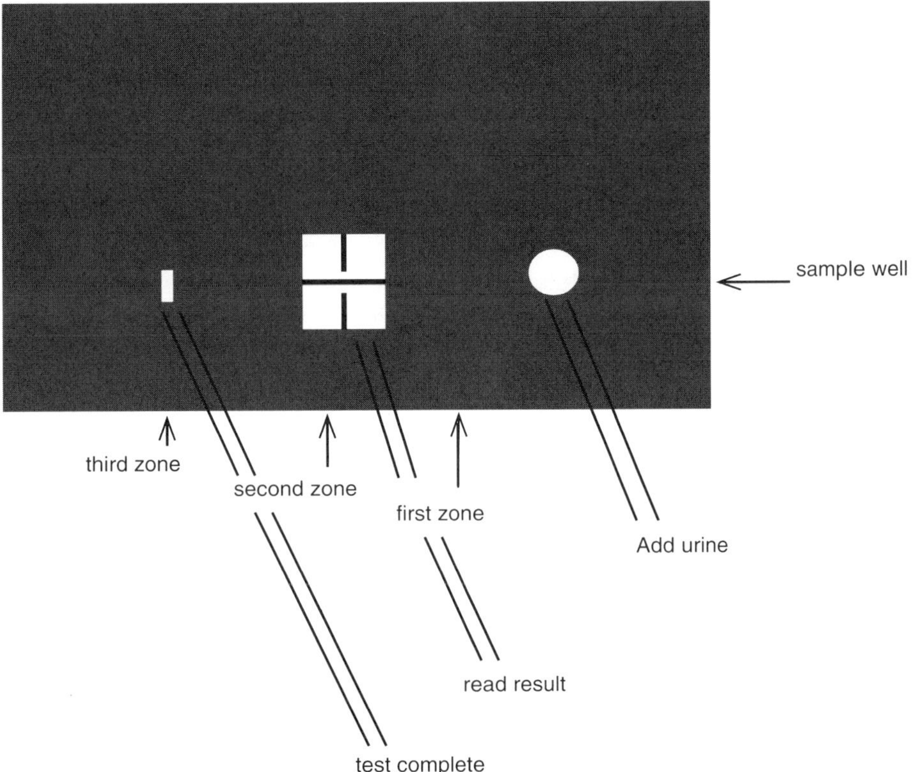

Fig. 7–1. Example of a newer 5-minute monoclonal antibody test for pregnancy. (With permission from Pacific Biotech, Inc.)

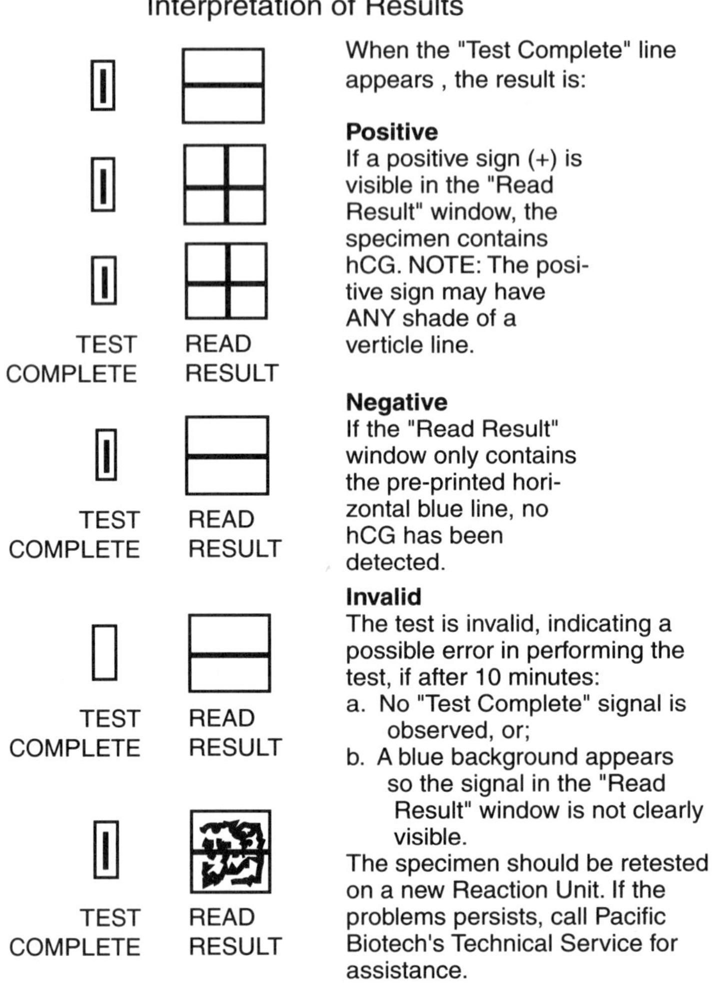

Fig. 7–2. Interpretation of 5-minute pregnancy test results. (With permission from Pacific Biotech, Inc.)

There are two agents immobilized in the second zone: preprinted horizontal blue line is visible that consists of immobilized blue latex beads. The second agent is an anti–α-hCG antibody immobilized on a vertical line. *If hCG is present in the urine,* a "sandwich" is created on this vertical line, i.e., the membrane-fixed anti–α-hCG antibodies, the hCG, and the anti–β-hCG antibodies bound to the blue beads. This vertical line together with the prefixed horizontal line forms a visible positive (+) in the "Read Result" window. *If there is no hCG in the test sample,* there will be no hCG-blue conjugate to bind to the membrane-fixed anti–α-hCG antibodies and only the horizontal blue line will be seen in the "Read Result" window, indicating a negative (−) pregnancy test result.

- The urine continues to move the antibody–blue latex conjugate across the membrane until it makes contact with a binding agent in the "Test Complete" window. Once a blue line is seen in this third zone, the test is considered complete and may be read by the evaluator (Fig. 7–2).

The company claims a detection limit for hCG of 30 mIU/mL.

Pitfalls

Once the test result is available, how reliable is it? What can cause false reactions? As already discussed, the earlier agglutination-inhibition tests of the 1960s through 1980s were specifically designed *not* to be too sensitive to prevent false-positive reactions due to cross-reactivity with LH, FSH, and TSH. Menopause or surgical castration could lead to false-positive results with the older kits because of significant elevation of levels of pituitary gonadotropins. As a result, a pregnancy of less than 4 weeks' gestation may not be producing enough hCG in the urine to give a positive result. *A negative test result therefore did not mean that the patient was not pregnant.* It only meant that she had less than 750 to 2,000 mIU of hCG in the urine.[8] In addition, abnormal pregnancies, which often produce less than normal levels of hCG, may give false-negative results.[24, 25] However, this problem was more serious when attempting to diagnose ectopic pregnancies since up to 50% of such patients did not produce enough hCG in the urine to give a positive result with these older kits.

Now that radioimmunoassay for the β-subunit of hCG in serum has become more rapidly and readily available, this type of problem should theoretically disappear since all pregnancies, normal or otherwise, produce some hCG that should be detected by this test.[26, 27] The opposite problem, false-positive reactions, is possible but, assuming good technique, should be uncommon except in the rare situations where hCG is being produced by the nonpregnancy conditions discussed earlier. As a general rule, a positive result is far more reliable than a negative result.

Sloppy or faulty technique in performance of any of the urine tests by rushed or untrained staff can produce false-positive reactions. Hematuria, vaginal blood contaminating the urine, and proteinuria have already been mentioned as causing false-positive results.[9]

When the older agglutination-inhibition test is used to detect pregnancy, various drugs affecting the central nervous system may cause abnormally high levels of LH and therefore produce a false-positive result.[8] Phenothiazines, "sedative-hypnotic" drugs, antidepressants, anticonvulsants, and methadone are examples. Since many of these patients have amenorrhea and even galactorrhea, one should consider using only the newer assays such as the ELISA or CICA monoclonal antibody assays or the more accurate, albeit more expensive and slower radioimmunoassay for the β-subunit of hCG in a patient with normal pelvic findings (or assume that the patient is pregnant until the radioimmunoassay can be performed).

In the 1990s the only type of rapid urine pregnancy tests that should be used are those employing the monoclonal anti–β-hCG antibodies. These newer test kits, like the one described above, are virtually foolproof. Although false-positive reactions with proteinuria or very turbid urine are still possible, the other conditions that confused earlier types of assays, e.g., those producing high levels of pituitary LH, FSH, or TSH, have been eliminated.[28, 29] This test is specific for the β-chain of hCG. Although the sensitivity of these tests is high (20 to 50 mIU/mL vs. 750 to 1000 mIU/mL with the older tests), there is still the possibility of a false-negative test result. This can occur in very early pregnancy, i.e., less than 2 to 3 weeks from conception, or with early spontaneous abortion or ectopic gestation.

These newer monoclonal antibody immunoassays have an overall false-negative rate of less than 1%.[28] Since 3% of ectopic pregnancies have serum hCG concentrations below 40 mIU/mL, a few will be missed by a urine monoclonal test.[30]

Since the serum quantitative radioimmunoassay for the β-chain of hCG is sensitive to between 1 and 10 mIU/mL, it presently represents the *gold standard* for pregnancy testing (Fig. 7–3).

Fortunately, if a normal or abnormal pregnancy cannot be demonstrated with one

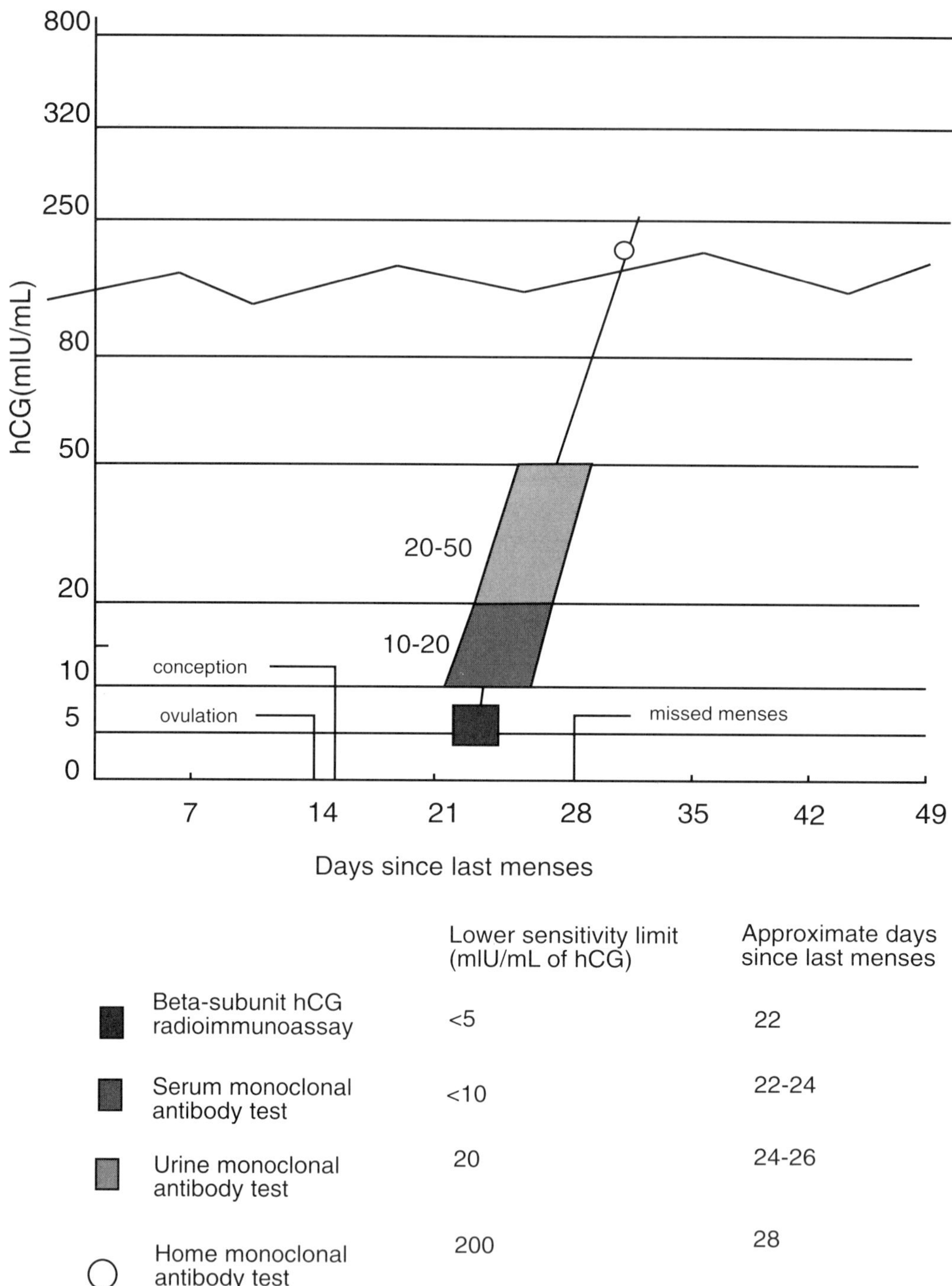

Fig. 7–3. Comparison of sensitivity limits of pregnancy tests. hCG, human chorionic gonadotropin. (With permission from Bluestein D: Postgrad Med 87:58, 1990.)

of the newer tests, that is, hCG levels below 40 mIU/mL, the patient is in no imminent risk, for example, of rupture of an ectopic pregnancy.[28] A patient with such a low level may have pain, but she is rarely debilitated or in immediate danger at that point. Both the physician and patient must be cognizant of all the clinical possibilities and the limitations of the tests. As long as follow-up with serial examinations, quantitative hCG determinations, and ultrasound evaluation is performed, major complications will be avoided.

CLINICAL APPLICATION

Let us now review the four cases presented in the beginning of this chapter.

CASE 7–1 CONTINUED

The first patient was a 40-year-old female with acute urinary retention, possibly 1 to 2 weeks late with her menses, who had a history of fibroids. The initial error at the first ED was that the staff failed to obtain a complete history. The patient had been married for the first time 2 months previously and was trying to become pregnant. This was discovered at the second ED, where the resident did a urine pregnancy test (agglutination-inhibition reaction) that was positive. The pregnant uterus contained multiple fibroids that were stimulated by the estrogens of pregnancy, obstructed the urethra, and caused urinary retention. A Foley catheter attached to a leg bag was left in the bladder. The patient was followed by an obstetrician and a urologist. With continued uterine growth, the uterus became anteroflexed as it filled the pelvis and then no longer compressed the urethra. After 10 days, the patient was able to void spontaneously when the catheter was removed. She was followed with sonography and had elective genetic studies by amniocentesis. She delivered a normal child approximately 30 weeks after her first visit to the ED where the physician recommended a hysterectomy.

CASE 7–2 CONTINUED

The second patient was an 11½-year-old female having her first menstrual bleeding, which was extremely painful and excessive. While waiting for parental consent for pelvic examination, a medical student, practicing how to perform pregnancy tests, used the patient's urine and was surprised when it produced a positive result. The staff correctly suggested that blood contaminating the specimen probably gave a false-positive result. However, the staff was stunned when placental tissue was discovered through a dilated cervix during the girl's pelvic examination; the patient was having a spontaneous abortion. There are two possible explanations. Firstly, this patient may not have told the staff or her family the truth about her menstrual or sexual history. The other possibility is that she conceived before her first menstruation! Although an unusual event, this case reminds the physician that the diagnosis of pregnancy must always be considered and then established or disproved by history and a physical examination and *supplemented* by laboratory tests.

CASE 7–3 CONTINUED

The third patient was a 26-year-old female who had had unilateral pelvic pain, a mass, and a history of tubal pregnancy. The diagnosis of ectopic pregnancy was considered, yet several facts disturbed the staff. The patient was certain that her period was not late. In addition, the patient suggested that she had a history of a left ovarian cyst. Her examination revealed a mobile cystic mass; abdominal ultrasound only corroborated a cystic mass. Finally, the patient had unexplained 4+ proteinuria, which is known to give false-positive pregnancy reactions. Fortunately for the patient, it was daytime and a radioimmunoassay for the β-subunit of hCG could be obtained. The results were available several hours later and were negative. The patient had been admitted for observation while the test results were pending, and the symptoms gradually improved. She had her menses in the hospital and was subsequently followed to see whether the ovarian cyst would totally resolve.

CASE 7–4 CONTINUED

The fourth patient was a 28-year-old ultrasound technician who was unusual in that she had a portfolio of laboratory data, including the results of an abdominal ultrasound examination and a laboratory urine test. Every aspect of her case suggested an ectopic pregnancy; nevertheless, the urine test was repeated by another technician. If positive, the patient would require laparoscopy to corroborate the diagnosis. If negative, serum for radioimmunoassay for the β-subunit of hCG would be obtained to dispel the anxiety of her potential diagnosis. The urine test was negative. A day later the result of radioimmunoassay for the β-chain for hCG returned and was negative. The pain gradually subsided, and the cyst diminished clinically and by ultrasound. She had a period.

The last two cases represent an unusual twist of technology. Because of the time of day and the individual's credentials, a more accurate means of pregnancy detection was used to spare these patients from surgery. If they had gone to a smaller institution at night or on a weekend, the data initially available would have made surgery mandatory.

A SUGGESTED EMERGENCY DEPARTMENT PROTOCOL

When normal, aborting, or ectopic pregnancy is considered in the differential diagnosis of a patient appearing in the ED, the following protocol may be utilized.

1. Test the patient's urine for the β-chain of hCG with one of the newer ELISA or CICA assays. If the test is negative, suspicion for an ectopic pregnancy is low, and the patient does not have severe symptoms, send a serum specimen for a radioimmunoassay test for the β-chain of hCG and ensure appropriate follow-up care. If the patient is moderately or severely symptomatic with pain or vomiting, or if an ectopic pregnancy is suspected, perform or obtain an abdominal pelvic ultrasound examination.
2. If an intrauterine sac with or without an embryo is visible by ultrasonography, ectopic pregnancy is essentially excluded. (However, in this age of technologically assisted pregnancy, a combined intrauterine and ectopic pregnancy occurs in approximately 1 of 7000 pregnancies.) The presence of a pregnancy sac without a visible embryo does not necessarily mean an abnormal gestation. However, such a finding does require careful follow-up care to evaluate fetal development and growth.
3. If an intrauterine pregnancy is not visualized by abdominal ultrasonography, perform or obtain a *transvaginal* ultrasound examination. A gestational sac can be detected at least 1 week earlier when using transvaginal ultrasound than when using abdominal ultrasound.
4. If no gestational sac is visible by transvaginal ultrasound in a patient who also has a negative urine test for hCG, the next step depends on the severity of the patient's symptoms. If symptoms are *mild* and adequate follow-up care can be *ensured*, the patient may be followed carefully as an out-patient. If reliable follow-up care cannot be ensured, or if the patient is potentially too unstable for out-patient management, she may be admitted for observation until the quantitative serum assay for the β-chain of hCG is available, or until symptoms and signs suggest that surgical intervention is indicated. Remember, visualizing an *ectopic* pregnancy by ultrasound can be difficult, with a significant number of false-positive and false-negative results, even by the most experienced examiners.

A positive ELISA urine test for the β-chain of hCG only confirms that there is at least 25 to 50 mIU/mL of hCG present. A pregnancy sac should be visible on transvaginal ultrasound when there is 1000 mIU/mL of hCG. Even a normal pregnancy may not be visualized *below* this level. Therefore, the absence of visual evidence of pregnancy in the patient with a positive *qualitative* test of the urine does not either confirm or exclude a normal or an abnormal pregnancy.

5. Once the quantitative BhCG test result is available, some judgments can be made: If the hCG level is greater than 1000 mIU/mL, the absence of a sac by transvaginal sonography implies an abnormal gestation (spontaneous abortion or ectopic pregnancy), and surgical intervention may be needed (i.e., dilatation and curettage with or without laparoscopy, depending on the symptoms or the endometrial pathology). When the hCG level is less than 1000 mIU/mL, the absence of a sac by transvaginal ultrasonography makes diagnosis more difficult. If symptoms are significant, the patient should be admitted for observation or surgery. If the patient's symptoms are mild, hCG levels may be followed every few days. In a normal pregnancy, hCG levels double every other day; therefore, if levels do not rise, the pregnancy is not normal. When the hCG level rises to above 1000 mIU/mL, transvaginal ultrasound should confirm an intrauterine pregnancy. Absence of an intrauterine sac in the presence of a significant level of hCG requires intervention as above.

6. In the past, culdocentesis was another technique that could be used in the ED to diagnosis or exclude an ectopic pregnancy (especially one that is leaking or clearly ruptured). The presence of free-flowing, nonclotting blood in the pelvis generally indicates a ruptured ectopic pregnancy or ruptured hemorrhagic ovarian cyst. However, culdocentesis is extremely painful and is now rarely indicated—ultrasonography can accurately detect fluid in the pelvis, and the combination of the patient's symptoms and signs (pain, shock) plus the result of the urine hCG, serum hCG, and sonography should make almost all culdocentesis procedures unnecessary for diagnosis.

Since 1982, the serum radioimmunoassay for the β-chain of hCG has been the most accurate means of proving or ruling out pregnancy. American studies have thus far shown essentially no false-negative results in detecting hCG in 100% of ectopic pregnancies.[27] Even if the test were only 98% accurate (as in the enzyme immunoassays), the remaining patients could be followed with serial blood studies and examinations, and thereby the need for surgical procedures would be diminished. However, if a patient's social or educational status is such that she cannot be relied on to return to the hospital when a β-subunit test turns out to be positive, then she must be admitted when ectopic pregnancy is a possibility.

Because the serum radioimmunoassay for the β-subunit of hCG is done more quickly and cheaply without diminishing quality controls, the question of pregnancy in any given patient will essentially be resolved. In the meantime, the newer urine ELISA and CICA immunoassays coupled with a good history, a physical examination, and common sense should suffice for establishing the diagnosis in almost all patients.

REFERENCES

1. Ramoska EA, Sacchetti AD, Nepp M: Reliability of patient history in determining the possibility of pregnancy, *Ann Emerg Med* 18:48–50, 1989.
2. Pritchard JA, MacDonald PC: *Williams obstetrics*, ed 16, New York, 1980, Appleton-Century-Crofts, pp 261–273, 536.
3. Steinkamph MP: Transvaginal sonography, *J Reprod Med* 33:931–938, 1988.
4. Stiller RJ, Haynes de Regt R, Blair E: Transvaginal ultrasonography in patients at risk for ectopic pregnancy, *Am J Obstet Gynecol* 161:930–933, 1989.
5. Kivikoski AI, Martin CM, Smeltzer JS: Transabdominal and transvaginal ultrasonography in the diagnosis of ectopic pregnancy: A comparative study, *Am J Obstet Gynecol* 163:123–128, 1990.

6. Neiger R, Bailey S, Wall AM et al: Diagnosis of ectopic pregnancy using transvaginal ultrasound scanning, *J Reprod Med* 34:52–54, 1989.
7. Timor-Tritsch IE, Yeh MN, Peisner DB et all: The use of transvaginal ultrasonography in the diagnosis of ectopic pregnancy, *Am J Obstet Gynecol* 161:157–161, 1989.
8. Okagaki T: Pregnancy tests. In Gerbie AP, Sciarra JJ, editors: *Gynecology and obstetrics*, vol 2, ed 4, Haggerstown, Md, 1981, Harper & Row, pp 1–9.
9. Derman R, Edelman DA, Berger GS: Current status of immunologic pregnancy tests, *Int J Gynaecol Obstet* 17:190–193, 1979.
10. Batzer FR: Hormonal evaluation of early pregnancy, *Fertil Steril* 34:1–13, 1980.
11. Roy S, Klein TA, Scott JZ et al: Diagnosis of pregnancy with a radioreceptor assay for hCG. *Obstet Gynecol* 50:401–406, 1977.
12. Vaitukaitis JL, Brauntein GD, Ross GT: A radioimmunoassay which specifically measures human chorionic gonadotropin in the presence of human luteinizing hormone, *Am J Obstet Gynecol* 113:751–758, 1972.
13. Goldstein DP, Aono T, Taymor MI et al: Radioimmunoassay of serum chorionic gonadotropic activity in normal pregnancy, *Am J Obstet Gynecol* 102:110–114, 1968.
14. Vaitukaitis JL: Human chorionic gonadotropin—a hormone secreted for many reasons, *N Engl J Med* 301:324–325, 1979.
15. Yoshimoto Y, Wolfsen AR, Hirose F et al: Human chorionic gonadotropin–like material: presence in normal human tissues, *Am J Obstet Gynecol* 134:729–733, 1979.
16. Borkowski A, Muquardt C: Human chorionic gonadotropin in the plasma of normal, nonpregnant subjects, *N Engl J Med* 301:298–302, 1979.
17. Cunningham FG, MacDonald PC, Gant NF: *Williams obstetrics*, ed 18, New York, 1989, Appleton & Lange, pp 14–18.
18. Chatterton RT: Pregnancy tests. In Dilts PV, Sciarra JJ, editors: *Gynecology and obstetrics*, ed 4, Haggerstown, Md, 1991, Harper & Row, pp 1–4.
19. Leach RE, Ory SJ: Modern management of ectopic pregnancy, *J Reprod Med* 34:324–335, 1989.
20. Collins WP: Early pregnancy tests, *Br J Obstet Gynaecol* 97:204–207, 1990.
21. Doshi ML: Accuracy of consumer performed in-home tests for early pregnancy detection, *Am J Public Health* 76:512–514, 1986.
22. Rebar RW, March CM, Resnik R et al: Practical applications of home diagnostic products, *J Reprod Med* 32(suppl):710–717, 1987.
23. Kountz DS, Kolander SA, Rokovsky A: False positive urinary pregnancy test in nephrotic syndrome, *N Engl J Med* 321:1416, 1989.
24. Chartier M, Roger M, Barrat J et al: Measurement of human chorionic gonadotropin (hCG) and β-hCG activities in the late luteal phase: evidence of the occurrence of spontaneous menstrual abortions in infertile women, *Fertil Steril* 31:134–137, 1979.
25. Bloch SK: Occult pregnancy, *Obstet Gynecol* 48:365–368, 1977.
26. Rasor JL, Braunstein GD: A rapid modification of the beta-hCG immunoassay, *Obstet Gynecol* 50:553–558, 1977.
27. Schwartz RO, Di Pietro DL: β-hCG as a diagnostic aid for suspected ectopic pregnancy, *Obstet Gynecol* 56:197–203, 1980.
28. Bluestein D: Should I trust office pregnancy tests, *Postgrad Med* 87:57–68, 1990.
29. Planet G: False positive pregnancy test, *Clin Chem* 36:1522–1523, 1990.
30. Romero R, Kadar N, Copel JA et al: The value of serial human chorionic gonadotropin testing as a diagnostic tool in ectopic pregnancy, *Am J Obstet Gynecol* 155:392–394, 1986.

Chapter 8

Testing for Sexually Transmitted Diseases

Stephen P. Waxman, M.D.

CASE 8–1

A sexually active male complained of a sore throat, arthralgias, and a generalized rash. Two months prior he had had a sore on his penis that resolved without treatment. At that time a friend who was a nurse did a test for syphilis that was negative. With the appearance of the rash, she repeated the same test. It was negative. What are the sources of error in this case?

Comment.—The only specific way of diagnosing syphilis is by identifying *Treponema pallidum* on a darkfield examination of exudate from the lesion. The nontreponemal serologic tests VDRL (Venereal Disease Research Laboratory) and rapid plasmin reagin (RPR) become reactive 1 to 3 weeks after the appearance of the chancre, or about 6 to 8 weeks after exposure. If there is a suspicion of syphilis and the initial test is nonreactive, it may be too early in the course; the test should be repeated at weekly intervals. In this case it is suspected that the patient is in the secondary phase of the infection. Since the serologic tests are virtually 100% sensitive at this stage, the only explanation for a negative result at this time (besides laboratory error) is the prozone phenomenon. The laboratory must be requested to dilute the patient's serum several times before a negative result is accepted. Upon dilution, the RPR became positive. At this stage, without any penile lesions to examine microscopically, correct performance of the serologic test becomes even more important. Of course the fluorescent treponemal antibody absorption (FTA-ABS) and microhemagglutination assay for *T. pallidum* (MHA-TP) would also be positive at this stage without dilution.

Before the current epidemic caused by the human immunodeficiency virus (HIV), most sexually transmitted diseases (STDs) were caused by bacteria and were easily treatable. Management principles included prompt diagnosis, parenteral therapy if compliance was in doubt, screening for multiple and resistant organisms, and contact tracing.

Changing social mores led to an explosion of STDs in the 1970s and 1980s. At the same time, new diagnostic techniques uncovered many other organisms that were sexually transmitted. There are now over 20 organisms that are known to be transmitted sexually (see box). Recent developments in the field include the establishment of a link between genital warts (human papillomavirus) and cancer of the cervix and penis, the discovery that genital ulcers are independent risk factors for the acquisition and transmission of HIV, and insights into the pathogenicity and extensive morbidity of pelvic inflammatory disease.

Sexually Transmitted Pathogens

Bacterial
- *Neisseria gonorrhoeae*
- *Chlamydia trachomatis*
- *Treponema pallidum*
- *Gardnerella vaginalis*
- *Haemophilus ducreyi*
- *Calymmatobacterium granulomatis*
- *Shigella* species
- *Campylobacter* species
- Group B streptococci

Ectoparasitic
- *Phthirus pubis*
- *Sarcoptes scabies*

Mycoplasmal
- *Mycoplasma hominis*
- *Ureaplasma urealyticum*

Protozoal
- *Trichomonas vaginalis*
- *Entamoeba histolytica*
- *Giardia lamblia*
- *Cryptosporidium* species
- *Isospora belli*
- Microsporida organisms

Viral
- Herpes simplex virus
- Hepatitis A, B, and C virus
- Cytomegalovirus
- Human papillomavirus
- Molluscum contagiosum
- Human immunodeficiency virus

Fungal
- *Candida albicans*

With permission from Sargent S: *Postgraduate Med* 91:360, 1992.

There are no cures for the viruses that cause STDs. These are lifelong infections with long latency periods, a high degree of transmissibility, and significant morbidity. In addition, we are now in the middle of a viral epidemic (acquired immunodeficiency syndrome [AIDS]) that has a mortality rate approaching 100%.

These facts make it more important than ever for all health practitioners to include advice about safe sex and barrier forms of contraception during every patient encounter involving an STD.

SYPHILIS

Syphilis is diagnosed by correlating historical, clinical, and serologic data, but darkfield examination of the scrapings of a genital or mucocutaneous lesion is the only way to make an absolute diagnosis. One uses an ordinary compound microscope equipped with a darkfield condenser that prevents direct rays of light from entering the field. Light rays from the periphery reflect off bacteria, treponemes, and other particles on the slide and make them appear brightly highlighted against a black background. Treponemes have a typical corkscrew morphology and demonstrate a characteristic rotating, twisting motion. Because the absence of treponemes on one examination does not exclude the diagnosis of syphilis, multiple darkfield tests are recommended. False-negative results may be due to partial systemic or topical antibiotic therapy or cleansing agents.[1]

Serologic tests for syphilis are categorized according to the test antigen used. The VDRL and the RPR card tests are non–treponeme-specific tests. The test antigen is a cardiolipin-lecithin-cholesterol mixture that combines with reaginic antibodies present in the sera of patients with syphilis. The RPR test is more sensitive than the VDRL test and so will result in a higher titer when compared with that of VDRL. The RPR test is also less specific. Most laboratories will follow a positive RPR with a VDRL test. Results are expressed in terms of tube dilutions, i.e., the number of dilutions required before a test serum turns from positive to negative. The greater the number of dilutions required, the more strongly positive is the test serum. A significant titer change must be a two-tube or greater change. A two-tube or greater decrease in dilutions on serial specimens implies successful therapy. When following a patient over a period of time, the same serologic test (either RPR or the VDRL test) should be used to avoid confusion in comparing titers.[2]

The non–treponeme-specific tests become positive about 2 to 3 weeks after the appearance of a chancre (i.e., 6 weeks after contact). These tests are falsely negative about 25% of the time in the case of primary syphilis. A false-negative result is more likely earlier in the course. In secondary syphilis these tests are 99% sensitive, and a negative result essentially excludes the diagnosis (provided that one has tested for the prozone phenomenon discussed below). In general, after secondary syphilis, the sensitivity of these tests gradually declines to about 75% in late latent and tertiary syphilis. False-negative results are not uncommon in neurosyphilis.[3]

About 1% to 2% of patients with secondary syphilis have a false-negative serologic test result because of the prozone phenomenon. The effect occurs when reaginic antibody is in such abundant supply that the antigen-antibody reaction is overwhelmed and flocculation fails to occur. When the patient's serum is diluted, the test becomes positive.

If the initial test result is negative and secondary syphilis is strongly suspected, the physician should request that the laboratory dilute the serum several times to test for the prozone phenomenon.

It is essential to follow the serologic titers of non–treponeme-specific tests after treating syphilis. The VDRL or RPR titer should decline gradually after treatment and become negative within 1 year of treating primary syphilis and within 2 years of treating secondary syphilis. In general, the longer one has the infection, the longer it takes for the titer to fall and the less likely it is for the patient to become seronegative despite adequate therapy. In late-latent and late syphilis, only 20% to 30% of patients become nonreactive within 5 years of treatment. The remainder are labeled sero-fast, i.e., they retain a positive serologic marker (usually at a low dilution) despite being cured.

Treponeme-specific tests use *T. pallidum* as the test antigen. They are used to confirm the diagnosis of syphilis when the non–treponeme-specific test is positive. If they are negative after a positive non–treponeme-specific test, the physician must conclude that the first test was a biological false positive. The commonly used treponeme-specific tests include the FTA-ABS and the MHA-TP tests.

In the FTA-ABS test, antibodies produced in response to the normal treponemal flora of the patient are absorbed by a charcoal solvent before testing. The treponeme IgG antibodies that remain are specific for *T. pallidum*. When they are added to a suspension of dried *T. pallidum* and fluorescent antihuman globulin, the treponemes will fluoresce under ultraviolet (UV) light.[4] Results are expressed as reactive, nonreactive, or borderline. A borderline test result is nondiagnostic and must be repeated.

The FTA-ABS test becomes positive early in the course of syphilis, about 1 week before the VDRL test, and stays positive indefinitely despite treatment. To accurately assess a patient, the physician must use this test in conjunction with the VDRL and historical and clinical data. In addition, this test has no role in assessing the response to treatment because it remains positive despite adequate therapy. False-negative results approach 20% in primary syphilis, are virtually nonexistent in secondary syphilis, and are present less than 5% of the time in late-latent and late syphilis, i.e., at least 2 years postinfection. False-positive results are seen primarily in the setting of autoimmune or connective tissue diseases such as systemic lupus erythematosus; biological false positives are far rarer with the FTA-ABS test than with the non–treponeme-specific tests.[5]

The MHA-TP test is equivalent to the FTA-ABS test in sensitivity except in cases of primary syphilis, in which case it is less sensitive. Its value is that it is simpler and less costly and can quantify the amount of treponemal antibody. Because the specificity is also in doubt, it should not be used alone as a confirmatory test.

Biological false-positive non–treponeme-specific test results are categorized as acute or chronic depending on the length of time that the test remains positive. If the test is positive for more than 6 months, it is called a chronic false positive; if less than 6 months, it is an acute false positive. Acute false-positive results are associated with acute infections (measles, herpes, mononucleosis, hepatitis), vaccinations, immunizations, and pregnancy. Chronic false positive reactions are associated with autoimmune disorders such as systemic lupus erythematosus, rheumatoid arthritis, scleroderma, and Hashimoto's thyroiditis, as well as drug addiction, chronic hepatitis, and endocarditis. A false-positive test, i.e., a positive non–treponeme-specific test followed by a negative treponeme-specific test (see below), should provoke a thorough investigation for one of these underlying diseases. Most false-positive results occur at low titers (1:2, 1:4). Other treponeme infections such as Lyme disease, yaws, and pinta will also result in positive non–treponeme-specific test results, but these cannot technically be considered biological false positives.[3]

Inasmuch as the treatment for latent syphilis is not necessarily adequate for asymptomatic neurosyphilis, the interpretation of tests in diagnosing neurosyphilis deserves special mention. Neurosyphilis can only be diagnosed by examining the spinal fluid. Recommendations for lumbar puncture in the setting of syphilis are included in the accompanying box. A cell count in excess of 4 leukocytes per cubic milliliter with a total protein content greater than 40 mg/dL indicates possible meningeal involvement. A positive cerebrospinal fluid (CSF) VDRL suggests neurosyphilis but, when considered alone, is not helpful in determining the activity of the disease because the test reaction remains positive for many years, even after successful treatment. Furthermore, the CSF VDRL is an extremely insensitive test with a high degree of false negativity, therefore a negative test result does not rule out neurosyphilis. The CSF FTA-ABS test is not recommended because it is unclear whether a positive result correlates with neurosyphilis. However, a negative test result does provide evidence against neurosyphilis.[6] Only by considering all of the information obtained from the patient interview, the physical examination, the blood serology, the CSF cell count, and CSF protein can the CSF VDRL help to differentiate the stage of the disease process (see Case 8–1).

Syphilis in the setting of HIV disease may result in a more aggressive infection, especially in terms of central nervous system involvement. The serologic response in HIV-infected patients may be unexpectedly high in early syphilis and may be unexpectedly blunted in advanced stages of immunosuppression. Because of this variability, syphilis serology in HIV-infected patients lacks its usual sensitivity. Many investi-

Recommendations for Lumbar Puncture in Patients with Syphilis

Ideal
- All patients with syphilis of 1 year's duration or longer (or latent syphilis of unknown duration)

Definite
- Syphilis of any stage with neurologic signs or symptoms
- Treatment failure in syphilis of any stage
- Syphilis of more than 1 year's duration with a VDRL* or an RPR* titer of 1:32 or greater
- Other evidence of active tertiary syphilis (aortitis, gumma, iritis, etc.)
- Nonpenicillin therapy planned in a patient with syphilis of more than 1 year's duration
- HIV infection in a patient with syphilis of more than 1 year's duration

Controversial
- HIV infection in the presence of syphilis of any stage or duration

With permission from Hansfield H: *Hosp Pract* 15:42, 1991.
**VDRL*, Venereal Disease Research Laboratory; *RPR*, rapid plasma reagin.

gators recommend that any patient who has both HIV infection and syphilis be evaluated for neurosyphilis with a lumbar puncture and that all individuals with dual infections be treated as if they have neurosyphilis.[7] Certainly a lumbar puncture is indicated in any patient who has failed prior therapy or in whom nonpenicillin treatment is planned.

All sexual contacts of individuals infected with syphilis should be evaluated clinically and serologically, and they should be treated prophylactically with antibiotics.

CASE 8–2

A sexually active male had a tender penile ulcer of 1 to 2 weeks' duration. He also complained of tender inguinal adenopathy that started several days before. He had recently been traveling in Southeast Asia on business.

Comment.—The evaluation of a penile ulcer with regional adenopathy begins with a careful interview. A history of vesicles preceding the ulcer or a history of past skin eruptions in the same anatomic area is strongly suggestive of herpes simplex infection. Sexual activity in Southeast Asia, Africa, or the Indian continent increases the risk of chancroid; homosexual contact and contact with prostitutes also increase that risk. A history of a papule or ulcer that healed spontaneously, only to be followed by a tender fluctuant inguinal mass, is suggestive of lymphogranuloma venereum (LGV).

Every penile ulcer should have multiple darkfield microscopic examinations of exudate from the base of the lesion to rule out syphilis. A Gram stain of exudate from the lesion or of an aspirate from regional lymph nodes may reveal the distinctive rods of *Haemophilus ducreyi* (chancroid) or superinfection. A Tzanck preparation may confirm a herpes infection.

In general, the chancre of syphilis is solitary, round, firm, and nontender. Chancroid is usually soft, tender, often irregular, painful, and nonindurated. Herpes simplex, after the vesicle stage, may mimic either. Be mindful that herpes is by far the most common infectious cause of an ulcerated lesion (second only to trauma); syphilis is next. Chancroid, LGV, and granuloma inguinale are far less common. Multiple infections do occur. The darkfield examination of an ulcer was negative, and the patient was treated presumptively for chancroid. Subsequent VDRL tests done weekly for 2 weeks were nonreactive.

CHANCROID

Distinguishing among the statistically minor ulcerating venereal diseases (chancroid, LGV, granuloma inguinale) is often a difficult task for clinicians. Because the laboratory is of limited assistance, a brief description of each infection and some tests that are available may be helpful.

Chancroid is the most common of these minor venereal diseases. Over 20,000 cases were reported between 1986 and 1990 in the United States, with clusters comprising 95% of cases in 5 states (i.e., New York, Texas, California, Florida, and Georgia).[8] The causative organism is *H. ducreyi,* a gram-negative rod. Isolating the organism by culture is possible only on a selective medium and is not performed routinely. Transportation requirements are too rigorous to make this a practical test.

Although chancroid is far less common than herpes or syphilis among the general population, it has exploded as an STD among certain groups, i.e., among inner-city prostitutes and among crack (and other substance) abusers for whom trading sex for drugs is common practice. This is also a group with a high prevalence of HIV infection, and it is postulated that the genital lesion is a prime portal of entry in the transmission of HIV among this group.[9] In Africa where heterosexual spread of HIV is common, acquisition and transmission via a genital ulcer is probably the prime mechanism of spread. Chancroid is the most common cause of genital ulcers in Africa and Southeast Asia.

The infection occurs predominantly in uncircumcised males. The incubation period is from 3 to 5 days. Sites of inoculation are usually the foreskin, the skin under the foreskin, and the coronal sulcus; lesions rarely appear on the shaft of the penis. In women the common sites are the fourchette and the labia. There is often more than one lesion, especially on contiguous skin because of autoinoculation. These are called "kissing lesions."

The lesion of chancroid, in contrast to the firm, round painless chancre of syphilis, is a soft but deep ulcer. It often has irregular contours and erythematous nonindurated margins. It is extremely painful, and there is commonly a gray or yellow exudate covering a red granulating base that bleeds easily with minimal trauma. The lesions are often so painful that the initial complaint may be dysuria, the consequence of urine dripping on the exposed lesions.

Most patients have concurrent genital lesions and unilateral adenopathy. Inflamed regional lymph nodes follow the initial inoculation by about 2 weeks and are usually painful, unilateral, and unilocular, i.e., a single collection of matted fluctuant nodes, or a bubo. The overlying skin may be red and hot.

The laboratory is of limited assistance in making the diagnosis. The organisms are not culturable routinely, and there are no practical serologic tests. To Gram-stain the exudate, the base of the lesion at the periphery should be touched with a cotton swab, which is rolled onto a slide in one direction. This may reveal small gram-negative extracellular organisms that are diagnostic of chanchroid. They form distinctive chains 3 to 20 rods long in a "school-of-fish" pattern. The examiner may also attempt aspirating the bubo (the recommended safe technique is to aspirate with a large-gauge needle through the normal skin adjacent to the bubo) and Gram-stain and culture the pus.

When a venereal disease such as chancroid is suspected, incision and drainage of the fluctuant inguinal mass is contraindicated because this may lead to the formation of chronically draining fistulous tracts.[10] Aspiration of pus from a tense bubo may help avoid spontaneous breakdown of the bubo that could also lead to the formation of draining tracts. As with any genital lesion, chancroid should be considered only after syphilis has been excluded by multiple darkfield examinations and serologic tests.[11]

LYMPHOGRANULOMA VENEREUM

The causative organisms of LGV is *Chlamydia trachomatis*. The species has 15 serotypes, only 3 of which cause LGV. Infections caused by other serotypes include trachoma, inclusion conjunctivitis, and nongonococcal urethritis. This organism is probably responsible for more sexually transmitted infections than any other.

The clinical syndrome has three stages. First, after a 7- to 12-day incubation period, a painless papule appears at the site of the inoculation and heals spontaneously. Over 90% of the time this initial lesion is overlooked by the patient. The second stage occurs 1 to 4 weeks after the primary papule and includes regional adenopathy that is unilateral in two thirds of cases. Unlike chancroid, the adenopathy of LGV usually involves more than one discreet group of nodes or buboes; for example, both the femoral and the inguinal group of nodes will enlarge and, when separated by the inguinal ligament, form the pathognomonic "groove sign." Adenopathy begins as firm, discrete, and tender nodes that gradually coalesce into a matted fluctuant mass.

The third stage, which occurs in only a small percentage of cases, is associated with frank tissue destruction. Deep draining ulcers, fistula formation, and strictures occur most commonly in enteric LGV affecting women and homosexual men as a result of rectal intercourse. These patients may have rectal bleeding, pain, tenesmus, or constipation. Proctoscopy will reveal inflamed, irregular, granulomatous lesions.

The laboratory is of some help in making the diagnosis. Tissue culture is not done routinely; the Frei skin test has been found to be insensitive and is no longer available. Serologic tests for *Chlamydia* antibody include a complement fixation test and a microfluorescence test. The complement fixation test is not specific for LGV; it measures antibody to all chlamydial serotypes without distinction. Because of the widespread prevalence of other chlamydial infections, especially those responsible for nongonococcal urethritis, low titers (less than 1:16) are commonly found in individuals without active infection but with prior exposure. Titers measuring greater than 1:64 may be suggestive of acute LGV in the proper clinical setting, that is, in the presence of inguinal adenopathy or rectal disease suggestive of LGV and in the absence of other chlamydial diseases such as a nonspecific urethritis. Paired sera of acute and convalescent titers that produce a greater than two-tube dilution increase in titer also suggest acute infection.[12] Again, tense buboes should be aspirated through healthy skin to avoid formation of chronically draining fistulous tracts; incision and drainage are contraindicated.

GRANULOMA INGUINALE

Granuloma inguinale is the rarest of the statistically minor venereal diseases; fewer than 100 cases were reported to the Centers for Disease Control (CDC) in 1990.[6] The causative organism is a gram-negative rod, *Calymmatobacterium granulomatis*. After an incubation period that can last up to 3 months, a painless buttonlike papule or subcutaneous nodule forms. This rapidly ulcerates to form a large serpiginous vegetative mass of bright red granulation tissue. Kissing lesions secondary to autoinoculation may result in spread of destructive lesions to the inguinal folds of the lower portion of the abdomen, the thighs, and the perineum. Inguinal adenopathy is rare, although pseudobuboes of granulation tissue may masquerade as adenopathy.

The diagnosis is made on the basis of the distinctive appearance of the lesions, the absence of adenopathy, and the exclusion of other STDs as well as squamous cell carcinoma. No serologic or skin tests are available, and isolating the organism by culture is not practical. A Wright's stain of a biopsy smear may reveal the characteristic

Donovan bodies—clusters of deeply staining rod-shaped organisms within the vacuoles of mononuclear cells.[13]

HERPES SIMPLEX

Herpes simplex virus (HSV) is the most common infectious cause of genital ulcers. The CDC estimates that 700,000 new cases and 20,000,000 episodes of recurrent genital herpes occur yearly. Its significance, however, rests more on a few unique characteristics: (1) there is no cure; (2) there is a high rate of spontaneous recurrence; (3) morbidity includes local symptoms as well as more significant complications such as meningitis, radiculitis, and myelitis; (4) an infected mother presents a risk to the neonate during passage through the birth canal; and (5) there is possible association with carcinomas of the cervix and vulva.

The initial genital lesions appear as a group of thin-walled vesicles on an erythematous base. The vesicles contain clear fluid that is replete with virus. After several days the vesicles are replaced by multiple shallow and painful ulcers that rapidly encrust. Discrete and tender inguinal adenopathy accompanies the lesions. The primary infection lasts 14 to 28 days. Recurrent infections generally heal more quickly and are less symptomatic.

The laboratory is minimally helpful in making the diagnosis. Viral isolation by culture is available. The greatest yield is when the lesions are young. The specimen is obtained by deroofing the vesicle and scraping the base. Papanicolaou smears in women may reveal abnormal cells that can be correlated with herpes, but this is an insensitive and nonspecific test. A Tzanck smear can be prepared in the emergency department by staining scrapings of the base with Wright's stain or methylene blue. Bizarre giant multinucleated cells represent invasion with herpes simplex or varicella virus[14] (see Chapter 15).

Antigen detection tests (direct immunofluorescence and enzyme-linked immunosorbent assay [ELISA or EIA]) are available. Their sensitivity is dependent on the number of cells scraped from the lesion, but when infected cells are present, sensitivities approach 70% to 90%. Newer tests include DNA probe tests that have a sensitivity greater than 90%.

Serologic tests for the diagnosis of herpes simplex (e.g., indirect fluorescent antibody [IFA] or virus neutralization tests) are not very helpful in the acute diagnosis because they do not reliably distinguish between HSV-1 and HSV-2.

By and large, the best "test" for diagnosing herpes is an accurate history and clinical examination. The description of groups of vesicles on a red base that evolve into multiple or coalesced tender shallow ulcers is definitive. The history of similar outbreaks in the past and especially in the same anatomic area is also classic.

For descriptions of STDs that cause genital lesions see Table 8–1.

CASE 8–3

A heterosexual male college student was treated 2 weeks before with intramuscular penicillin. He improved slightly but continued to complain of dysuria and mucoid discharge. His steady girlfriend was also treated for gonorrhea. How do you explain that patient's course?

Comment.—Gonococcal urethritis can be diagnosed by Gram stain. The presence of gram-negative intracellular diplococci of typical morphology is diagnostic. The culture is helpful in diagnosis when the Gram stain is equivocal. The other role for cultures and sensitivity testing is to evaluate for penicillinase-producing *Neisseria gonorrhoeae* (PPNG). The incidence of PPNG is still under 5% in most populations. In

Table 8–1. Sexually Transmitted Diseases Causing Genital Lesions

Disease	Organism	Lesion	Adenopathy	Diagnostic Tests
Chancroid	*Haemophilus ducreyi*	A single, small, circumscribed ulcer; yellow-gray exudate covers a very friable base; painful; kissing lesions secondary to autoinoculation	Tender, unilocular; nodes become matted into a fluctuant mass or bubo; unilateral in ⅔ of cases; erythema of overlying skin	Gram stain of base of lesion or of aspirate from suppurative nodes; gram-negative rods in chains; culture is possible
Lymphogranuloma venereum	*Chlamydia trachomatis*	A single painless papule or ulcer that heals spontaneously; often not present when the patient is seen	Tender, multilocular nodes; often separated by Poupart's ligament, i.e., the "groove sign"; unilateral in ⅔ of cases; erythema of overlying skin	Gram stain is not helpful; acute and convalescent sera for chlamydial group complement fixation titers; culture is not routinely available
Granuloma inguinale	*Calymmatobacterium granulomatis*	Large, spreading irregular ulcers with beefy red, friable base; areas of depigmented scarring and granuloma formation; kissing lesions on contiguous skin	Pseudobuboes, i.e., nodules of infectious tissue—not true adenopathy	Donovan bodies—gram-negative rods within the cytoplasm of macrophages—seen on biopsy or scrapings
Genital herpes	Herpes simplex	Multiple thin-walled vesicles with clear fluid; shallow ulcers with crusting; painful	Tender; discrete; bilateral or unilateral	Tzanck smear with multinucleated giant cells; Papanicolaou smear; acute and convalescent complement fixation titers; culture is possible
Syphilis	*Treponema pallidum*	Solitary, circumscribed, indurated ulcer; painless; not friable; can be multiple	Nontender, discrete, rubbery, firm; bilateral or unilateral; no erythema of overlying skin	Darkfield microscopic examination of exudate; serologic studies (VDRL, RPR, FTA-ABS, MHA-TP)*

*VDRL, Venereal Disease Research Laboratory; *RPR,* rapid plasmin reagin; *FTA-ABS,* fluorescent treponemal antibody absorption; *MHA-TP,* microhemagglutination assay for *Treponema pallidum.*

this case, the presence of PPNG could be the reason for the patient's continuing symptoms. A more likely cause, however, is the presence of a dual infection initially not treated adequately with intramuscular penicillin. *C. trachomatis* is present in 20% to 30% of heterosexual men who are treated for gonorrhea. Chlamydia and other organisms acquired at the time of initial exposure account for 30% to 60% of cases of postgonococcal urethritis that develop in heterosexual men following treatment with intramuscular penicillin. Since chlamydia is an STD, the patient's sexual partner should also be treated for this organism if a nongonococcal infection is documented. The patient had a repeat Gram stain of a urethral swab specimen. More than 10 polymorphonuclear leukocytes per high-power field (PMNs/HPF) but no organisms were found, which suggests a nongonococcal urethritis that was successfully treated with a 1-week course of doxycycline.

URETHRITIS

The urethra is the most common site for STDs in men in the United States. About one third of cases of urethritis are caused by *N. gonorrhoeae* and the remainder by a variety of organisms, including primarily *C. trachomatis*. Complications of local infection in men include epididymitis and prostatitis and in women, cervicitis and pelvic inflammatory disease. The diagnosis and causative organisms are found by epidemiologic, clinical, and laboratory tests.

GONORRHEA

Gonorrhea is a common cause of urethritis in young, inner-city males from low socioeconomic backgrounds, in homosexuals, and among prostitutes and their clients.[15] Clinical signs range from a spontaneous purulent discharge (classic for gonococci) to a mucoid discharge, burning on urination, pruritis around the urethral meatus, or painful ejaculation.

A spontaneous purulent discharge is the hallmark of this infection. When it is present, gonococcus is the causative organism over 90% of the time. On the other hand, a mucoid discharge that must be expressed manually is rarely due to gonorrhea.[16] Only 5% of males with gonococcal urethral infection will be asymptomatic, although a larger percentage of females and even larger percentage of persons with nongenital infection can be asymptomatic carriers with the ability to infect their partners unknowingly.[17]

The laboratory diagnosis of gonococcal urethritis is made by Gram stain and culture of exudate. Specimens are obtained by compressing the urethra proximally and stripping it toward the orifice. A sterile calcium alginate urethral swab is inserted into the urethra no more than 2 cm. The standard cotton swab is inadequate because it cannot be inserted far enough into the urethra to obtain a good specimen. The smear is prepared by rolling the swab onto the slide rather than by rubbing, which may disrupt cell and bacterial morphology. To obtain specimens from the endocervical canal, a cotton-tipped swab is inserted into the canal and moved from side to side while allowing 10 to 30 seconds for absorption of the organisms. The use of lubricants other than possibly warm water should be avoided, and attempts should be made to remove excess cervical mucus with a cotton ball before inserting the swab. Specimens from the anorectal area are best obtained through an anoscope but can be obtained directly by inserting the swab 2 to 3 cm into the canal, moving the swab from side to side, and allowing 10 to 30 seconds to elapse for the absorption of organisms. The use of lubricants should be avoided. Specimens contaminated by stool must be discarded.[18]

The Gram stain typical for gonorrhea shows pairs of gram-negative diplococci (the adjacent sides of each organism in a pair are flattened) that are located within the cytoplasm of PMNs. This "typical" smear, when obtained from the urethra, is confirmed to be gonorrhea by culture in almost 98% of cases. Clearly negative smears (i.e., no organisms seen or organisms that are extracellular and not morphologically like gonococci) are, with an equal level of confidence, not culture-proven gonorrhea. When one sees organisms that appear morphologically like gonococci but are located primarily outside the cells, the urethra must be cultured to make the diagnosis.[10] Gram stains of specimens from the endocervical and anorectal areas are falsely negative greater that 50% of the time, but they are 100% specific, so they are helpful when a typical positive smear is obtained. In these anatomic areas, gonorrhea cannot be excluded by Gram stain; a culture is necessary.[15]

Specimens for culture must be placed on a special medium (modified Thayer Martin agar or New York City agar) that permits only the growth of *Neisseria* organisms. The plate is warmed to room temperature before use, and excess moisture is allowed to evaporate. Agar plates are examined for contamination or drying before use. The specimen is applied in a "Z" pattern and then cross-streaked with a sterile applicator. The plate is placed in the enhanced carbon dioxide environment of a candle jar within 15 to 30 minutes of plating (2 hours is a maximum delay) and incubated at 35° C within 1 to 2 hours. The candle is relit in the jar each time that the jar is opened and allowed to burn at least 45 to 60 seconds to create an adequate carbon dioxide atmosphere.[18] Specimens are incubated for 12 to 24 hours before transportation to the laboratory.

Because of the high incidence of asymptomatic infection at sites other than the urethra and the shifting patterns of antibiotic resistance, specimens for culture should be obtained from all orifices before initiating therapy. Likewise, tests of cure 3 to 5 days after treatment should include all areas from which specimens had previously been cultured and were positive.

As with all venereal diseases, the practitioner must make efforts to diagnose gonococcal infection and treat the patient on the initial visit. Gonococcal infection in the urethra can be diagnosed accurately by a Gram stain of the exudate. As noted above, however, the use of a Gram stain to diagnose infection at other sites is far less accurate. It is not unreasonable, therefore, to treat certain patients presumptively. A homosexual male who practices rectal intercourse regularly with multiple partners and who has lower gastrointestinal symptoms or a female who has intercourse regularly with multiple partners and who has a cervical discharge should be treated for gonorrhea on the first visit even if the Gram stain is not diagnostic for gonococci. The rate of infectivity in these groups is high enough to warrant early therapy. While cultures are pending, other causes should be sought (Case 8–3).

A serologic test for syphilis should be done on all patients as a screen for syphilis and in recognition of the fact that a patient may acquire more than one venereal disease at a time. Only penicillin, second-generation cephalosporins, and some of the new fluroquinones are effective against incubating syphilis. If patients are treated with any other antibiotic, they should return in 3 to 6 weeks for a repeat VDRL test.

NONGONOCOCCAL URETHRITIS

Over half the cases of acute urethritis are caused by nongonococcal organisms. *Chlamydia* types D to K are the organisms responsible 40% to 50% of the time.[19] The

Table 8–2. Clinical Manifestations of Uncomplicated Gonococcal and Chlamydial Infection

Feature	Gonorrhea	Chlamydia
Incubation period	2–10 days	7–20 days
Clinical onset	Sudden	Gradual
Dysuria	Common, sometimes severe	Occasional, usually mild
Urethral or cervical discharge		
Character	Purulent	Mucoid, mucopurulent
Amount	Large	Scant to moderate

With permission from Hansfield HH: *Hosp Pract* 15:43, 1991.

remaining cases are caused by a variety of organisms, including *Ureaplasma urealyticum, Trichomonas,* and herpes simplex. About 20% of cases of nongonococcal urethritis have no known etiology.

C. trichomatis is the most common bacterial cause of STDs. In addition to causing a large percentage of nongonococcal urethritis, it is the most common organism involved in pelvic inflammatory disease, female infertility, and ectopic pregnancy.

Because symptoms of nongonococcal urethritis are milder than those of gonococcal urethritis, patients tend to wait longer before seeking medical help. The discharge of nongonococcal urethritis is not usually purulent or spontaneous and more often is mucoid or mucopurulent in character. It must be expressed manually. A large percentage of infections are asymptomatic.

The diagnosis is made by Gram stain of urethral exudate. The presence of PMNs and the absence of gram-negative intracellular diplococci are suggestive of infection. As noted above, however, only culture can exclude gonorrhea from some areas. In the absence of spontaneous discharge, the penis should be stripped and a urethrogenital swab inserted to obtain a specimen. Greater than 5 PMNs per oil immersion field signifies urethritis. The specimen should be obtained at least 2 hours after urination. In the absence of organisms suggestive of a urinary tract infection, more than 15 to 20 PMNs/HPF (dry) in one or more fields signifies urethritis.[19]

There are several laboratory tests that can help in the diagnosis of *C. trachomatis.* Tissue culture is the most sensitive test but also the most labor-intensive, technically difficult, and expensive. Serologic antibody testing is not helpful because of the ubiquity of the organism in most patients at risk and because it does not distinguish between acute or prior infection. Examination of tissue specimens for antigen by direct fluorescent antibody testing (Micro-Tek), ELISA, or nucleic acid probe is sensitive (>90%) and specific (>97%), especially in symptomatic patients.[20]

Simultaneous infection with gonorrhea and chlamydia is present in up to 35% of men with urethra/gonorrhea.[15] (Table 8–2). All specimens should be cultured for gonorrhea regardless of symptoms. Follow-up tests of cure using the Gram stain on a urethral specimen or by examining the urine for white blood cells are very important, as is a serologic test for syphilis on all patients before therapy. In addition, practitioners must trace, culture, and treat all contacts.

REFERENCES

1. Drisen LM: The diagnosis and treatment of infectious and latent syphilis, *Med Clin North Am* 56:1161–1174, 1972.
2. Felman Y, Nikitas J: Questions physicians ask concerning syphilis serologies, *N Y State J Med* 79:2063–2065, 1979.
3. Lowhagen GB: Syphilis: test procedures and therapeutic strategies, *Semin Dermatol* 9:152-159, 1990.
4. Oates JK: Serologic tests for syphilis and their clinical use, *Br J Hosp Med* 21:612–617, 1979.

5. Felman Y, Nikitas J: Syphilis serology today, *Arch Dermatol* 116:84–89, 1980.
6. Elsner P: Treatment of bacterial sexually transmitted diseases, *Semin Dermatol* 12:342-351, 1993
7. Centers for Disease Control: 1989 sexually transmitted disease guidelines, *MMWR* 38, 1989.
8. Morse SA: Chancroid and *Haemophilus ducreyi, Clin Microbiol Rev* 2:137-157, 1989.
9. Schmid GP: Approach to the patient with genital ulcer disease, *Med Clin North Am* 74:1559-1572, 1990.
10. Felman Y, Nikitas J: Chancroid, *Cutis* 26:464–475, 1980.
11. Hadley AT: Chancroid, *Am Fam Physician* 20:83–86, 1989.
12. Felman Y, Nikitas J: LGV, *Cutis* 25:264–272, 1980.
13. Lynch PJ: Sexually transmitted disease, *Clin Obstet Gynecol* 21:1041–1052, 1978.
14. Curry SS: Cutaneous herpes simplex infection, *Cutis* 26:41–58, 1980.
15. Judson FN: Gonorrhea, *Med Clin North Am* 74:1353-1382, 1990.
16. Jacobs N, Kraus S: Gonococcal and non-gonococcal urethritis in men, *Ann Intern Med* 82:7–12, 1975.
17. Wiesner PJ: Gonorrhea, *Cutis* 27:249–254, 1981.
18. *Criteria and techniques for the diagnosis of gonorrhea,* Atlanta, US Department of Health, Education and Welfare, Centers for Disease Control.
19. Hansfield MM: NGV, *Cutis* 27:208–270, 275–276, 1981.
20. Schacter J: Chlamydial infections, *N Engl J Med* 298:428–435, 490–495, 540–549, 1978.

Chapter 9

Toxicologic Testing

Richard Weisman, Pharm.D.

Mary Ann Howland, Pharm.D.

Karl Verebey, Ph.D.

CASE 9–1

An 18-year-old female came to the emergency department (ED) and stated that 10 hours earlier she had ingested eighteen, 325-mg aspirin tablets. The patient would not provide any additional history other than to complain of nausea. On admission her blood pressure was 96/70 mm Hg, pulse was regular at 88 beats per minute, respirations were 20 breaths per minute, and her oral temperature was 37° C (98.6° F). An intravenous line was placed and blood samples obtained for a complete blood count, electrolytes, glucose, blood urea nitrogen (BUN), a pregnancy test, and a stat salicylate and acetaminophen determination. An arterial blood gas analysis was also obtained.

On examination the patient was awake, alert, and oriented to person, place, and time. The patient appeared somewhat diaphoretic, was well nourished, and appeared to weigh about 50 kg. The remainder of the physical examination was normal except for some diffuse mild abdominal tenderness.

Because the patient refused to drink a slurry of 50 g of activated charcoal and 25 g of sorbitol, she was restrained and a nasogastric tube was placed in her stomach. The activated charcoal and sorbitol were instilled through the nasogastric tube.

The patient also initially refused to provide a urine specimen but 15 minutes later requested to use the bathroom. A bedpan was provided, and a 5-mL aliquot of urine from the bedpan was used to test for the presence of salicylates with a ferric chloride solution. The test was negative.

The stat laboratory reported a salicylate level of 0 mg/dL and an acetaminophen level of 74 μg/mL 10 hours postingestion (the latter value was well above the acetaminophen nomogram level for toxicity). The patient was promptly given oral *N*-acetylcysteine therapy. Subsequent liver function tests and coagulation studies were normal.

CASE 9–2

A 17-year-old female was brought to the ED by her parents 8 hours after an apparent suicide attempt. The patient was awake, alert, and vomiting. When asked what she had taken, she responded "a handful of pills." When the family was questioned about medications available in their home, they responded that the patient's brother was being treated for asthma. Other medications available included aspirin, acetaminophen, and vitamins.

Her blood pressure was 110/70 mm Hg, her pulse was 120 beats per minute, respirations were 24 breaths per minute, and her temperature was 36.9° C. An intravenous line was placed and blood samples obtained for a complete blood count, electrolytes, glucose, BUN, a pregnancy test, and stat theophylline, iron, salicylate, and acetaminophen determinations. An arterial blood gas analysis was also obtained.

On examination the patient was tremulous and agitated and had considerable abdominal pain with protracted vomiting. The patient was obese, weighing approximately 90 kg. The head was atraumatic and normocephalic. Neurologic findings were normal. Her pupils were round, equal (4 mm), and reactive to light. Her chest was clear to auscultation, and heart sounds were normal. The abdomen was distended and tender to palpation in the epigastric area, and bowel sounds were hyperactive. Rectal examination showed good sphincter tone with no masses. Stools were negative for occult blood.

The patient was given 10 mg of metoclopramide intravenously for the vomiting. Sixty grams of activated charcoal and 35 g of sorbitol were administered by mouth. Five minutes later, the patient vomited a large amount of the mixture. Another 5 mg of metoclopramide was administered intravenously.

The laboratory reported that the theophylline level was 52 μg/mL, the salicylate and acetaminophen levels were zero, and the iron level would not be available for several additional hours.

The patient was given repeated 60-g doses of activated charcoal without sorbitol every 2 hours along with additional doses of metoclopramide for vomiting. Repeat theophylline levels at 2, 4, and 6 hours were 61, 50, and 38 μg/mL.

REQUESTING THE RIGHT TESTS

The toxicology laboratory should be used as an adjunct to the diagnostic acumen of the physician. A few specific tests should be ordered after a differential diagnosis has been established. Because of their widespread availability and their potential toxicity, salicylate and acetaminophen determinations should be performed for every adult or adolescent who has attempted suicide. The toxicology laboratory may help in quantitating the extent of toxicity and assessing the adequacy of overdose management in those cases where a clear correlation exists between a level and toxicity.

To use the toxicology laboratory appropriately, one must know which tests to request, when the results are needed, and how soon they can become available. It is also important to determine whether the test should be qualitative or quantitative, when the specimen should be obtained, and what type and quantity of specimen should be sent. Finally, the physician needs to understand the sensitivity and specificity of the analytic methodology that the laboratory will use.

In Case 9–1, the history of salicylate ingestion was entirely incorrect. Because a routine acetaminophen determination was performed, appropriate therapy was initiated to prevent the development of hepatic toxicity and avoid critical complications and a prolonged hospitalization. In Case 9–2, the patient's ingestion was unknown, but the symptoms were consistent with theophylline, aspirin, or iron. Because of the symptoms and the availability of a quantitative assay and antidotal therapy, specific assays were performed.

BEDSIDE DIAGNOSTIC TESTING

There are several diagnostic tests that can be performed at the patient's bedside. In addition to being extremely cost-effective and accurate, they provide the physician with immediate information. These tests include the use of naloxone for opioids, the ferric chloride test for salicylates, the nitroprusside (Acetest) test for ketones, visual inspection of blood for a color change indicative of methemoglobinemia, examination of the urine for oxalate crystals, and abdominal radiography.

Intravenous Naloxone

When administered to patients with central nervous system (CNS) and respiratory depression, naloxone is both diagnostic and specific for reversing the effects of opioids. Patients who respond with an improvement in mental or respiratory status or pupillary dilatation have been exposed to an opioid. Patients who fail to have any response to 10 mg of naloxone do not have an opioid as a major cause of their CNS depression.[1]

Ferric Chloride Test

In Case 9–1, a bedside ferric chloride test was performed to test for the presence of salicylates in the urine. When several drops of 10% ferric chloride solution are added to the urine of a patient who has taken as few as two aspirin tablets several hours earlier, the urine will turn a purple color.[2] If the urine remains a straw color, it is extremely unlikely that the patient has ingested any salicylate and certainly not a toxic quantity. False-positive reactions can be seen in patients who have acetoacetic or phenylpyruvic acid in their urine.

Nitroprusside Tablet Test

Nitroprusside tablets (Acetest tablets) will produce a purple reaction in the presence of a ketone moiety such as that present in acetone or acetoacetic acid. Ingestion of acetone nail polish remover or isopropyl alcohol, which is metabolized to acetone, can be confirmed by the presence of ketones in the urine (or on the breath). This is one of the few clinical conditions where ketones are present in the absence of acid-base disorders. When the presence of ketones is accompanied by a wide–anion gap metabolic acidosis, salicylate poisoning or diabetic, starvation, or alcoholic ketoacidosis[3] is suggested. The combination of a wide–anion gap metabolic acidosis and a positive but weaker than expected nitroprusside tablet test for ketones strongly suggests alcoholic ketoacidosis. Finally, the absence of ketones in the presence of a widened–anion gap metabolic acidosis, is often found with methanol or ethylene glycol ingestions.

Blood Color Test

The color of blood with a methemoglobin concentration of greater than 15% is chocolate brown when compared with the color of normal blood and can help to establish the diagnosis of methemoglobinemia.[4] The most common inducers of methemoglobinemia are oxidants, including nitrites and nitrates, aniline dyes, phenazopyridine (Pyridium), numerous sulfonamides, naphthalene, and many topical anesthetics.[5]

Urinalysis

Calcium oxalate or hippurate crystals in the urine of patients with wide–anion gap metabolic acidosis may help to identify patients who have ingested ethylene glycol.[6] Further inspection of the urine of a patient who is suspected of ingesting ethylene glycol under ultraviolet light (Wood's lamp) may detect the presence of fluorescein or another fluorescent substance.[7] Many antifreeze solutions have a fluorescent substance added to assist mechanics in identifying the source of a leak under a car (i.e., radiator) by the same technique. When antifreeze is the source of an ethylene glycol ingestion, this fluorescent material is usually rapidly eliminated in the urine. Detection of this fluorescence in the urine can help to confirm antifreeze ingestion, but for numerous reasons (such as complete renal shutdown), neither the absence of crystals nor the absence of fluorescence can be used to exclude ingestion of ethylene glycol.

Abdominal Radiography

The finding of radiopaque tablets or substances on an abdominal radiograph or sonogram may be helpful in confirming several ingestions. Substances that are reportedly radiopaque include chlorinated hydrocarbons, chloral hydrate, iron tablets, some of the phenothiazine and cyclic antidepressants, enteric-coated tablets, arsenic, mercury, lead, and some heroin and cocaine drug packages.[8] Diagnostic imaging cannot be used to determine the type of ingestion or definitely determine whether an ingestion actually occurred. An abdominal radiograph may be useful in diagnosing or confirming the presence of condoms, presumably containing drugs such as cocaine or heroin swallowed by "body packers" or "body stuffers." Risk-benefit concerns regarding pregnancy or possible pregnancy in menstruating female patients must be considered (see Chapter 7).

SERVICES OF THE TOXICOLOGY LABORATORY

The toxicology laboratory can be a useful resource for managing poisoned or overdosed patients. Unfortunately, most clinicians have unrealistic expectations of the toxicology laboratory. After ordering a toxicology screen, many physicians have the misconception that if the patient has ingested any of the hundreds of pharmacologic agents available or any of thousands of chemical substances, the toxicology laboratory will be able to establish the diagnosis. Even in the most technologically advanced laboratories it is an unrealistic expectation; the financial, personnel, and time requirements for complete screening are prohibitive.

Before a poisoned patient enters the emergency department, the physician should determine the capabilities of the hospital laboratory, including which tests are performed, when they are performed, and how much time is required for the test to be completed. If all of the essential tests cannot be performed by the hospital laboratory, the physician should inquire about alternative commercial laboratories and their capabilities as well as mechanisms for specimen transport.

AVOIDANCE OF DRUG SCREENS

CASE 9–3

A 4-year-old child was admitted to the hospital because of developmental regression, excessive drooling, irritability, hypotonia, and gastrointestinal disturbances. Over a period of 6 months the child lost the ability to walk, talk, and control his bladder and bowel functions. The child was receiving a Chinese herbal powder, several antibiotics, and allergy medications prescribed by a family physician.

A neurologic evaluation suggested a toxicologic cause for the symptoms and signs. A computed tomographic (CT) scan of the head, a lumbar puncture, and a urine screen for heavy metals were planned. The child's urine was sent for a urine "toxicology screen," which was reported as negative. As a result of the report, heavy metals were excluded by the physician from the differential diagnosis.

The term "toxicology screen" is used by most laboratories to refer to testing for several common drugs of abuse and never for all toxic substances. The tests that were actually performed by the laboratory in Case 9–3 were for amphetamines, barbiturates, opioids, cocaine, and benzodiazepines. The child was discharged without a diagnosis, and the parents continued to administer the Chinese herbal powder.

CASE 9–3 CONTINUED

The child continued to deteriorate and was taken to a second hospital. Here, the Chinese powder (Tse Ku Choy) was found to contain mercurous chloride, and the child's urine was found to contain a toxic amount of mercury. Despite aggressive chelation therapy with dimercaprol, 5 years later the child still had a severe personality disorder, a learning disability, and some coordination difficulties.

Drug "screens" are probably the most frequently ordered toxicology tests. However, interpretation of the data is often meaningless unless one knows how specific and how sensitive the test is for each relevant screened substance as well as whether a substance in question will be included in the analysis. A drug screen may occasionally appear to contradict a clinical diagnosis. For example, a urine drug screen requested on a patient whose history and physical examination suggest a phencyclidine overdose may be reported as negative either because the laboratory does not routinely test for phencyclidine or, if it does test for phencyclidine, the patient may have ingested a congener with insufficient cross-reactivity to produce a positive result. It is important that the physician be as specific as possible about the tests requested and list all possible drugs and medications one can think of that fit the clinical profile as well as provide the laboratory with specific patient information such as mental status, history, and pertinent clinical findings. When the clinical examination strongly suggests a toxicologic cause, the physician should be wary about discarding it solely on the basis of a single negative toxicologic analysis available in the ED.

The physician must pay particular attention to the patient's history and the signs and symptoms. Drugs that should enter into the differential diagnosis of a patient exhibiting agitation, seizures, or CNS excitation include the alcohols, anticholinergic drugs, amphetamines, camphor, carbamazepine, cocaine, cyanide, cyclic antidepressants, isoniazid, lithium, phencyclidine, phenytoin, propoxyphene, salicylates, and theophylline.[9] Rather than order each of these tests, however, the physician should consider the most likely drugs ingested and those for which a laboratory value will alter the course of management.

KNOWING THE LABORATORY'S CAPABILITIES

Notwithstanding the above considerations, many commercial laboratories run panels of similar drugs or several drugs producing similar signs and symptoms that are less expensive than requesting multiple single tests. Health care providers should be familiar with the particular laboratory's routine testing panels, e.g., coma panel, intoxication panel, or drugs-of-abuse panel. For example, many of the drugs that cause CNS depression may be available on a coma panel. Coma panels will usually include ethanol, barbiturates, benzodiazepines, carbamazepine, opioids, phenothiazines, sedative-hypnotics, and cyclic antidepressants. Again, the physician must be aware of which drugs are included and which are not as well as the specificity and sensitivity of the panels.

Patients who have a wide–anion gap metabolic acidosis should have blood tested for ethanol, ethylene glycol, methanol, salicylates, iron, and BUN. Although isoniazid, paraldehyde, cyanide, phenformin, and toluene are also in the differential diagnosis of patients with a wide–anion gap metabolic acidosis, most laboratories do not offer

Table 9–1. Information on Quantitative Tests

Test	Time to Draw Blood Specimen Postingestion*	Time to Repeat	Implications of a Positive Test	Supportive Tests†
Acetaminophen	4 hr	Usually not necessary unless extended release: 8 hr	Use blood level nomogram and *N*-acetylcysteine (Mucomyst) as indicated	LFTs, albumin, PT, PTT
Carboxyhemoglobin	Immediately	1–4 hr	Put patient on 100% oxygen (consider hyperbaric oxygen chamber if very severe)	ECG, ABGs
Digoxin	2–4 hr	2–4 hr	If extreme, consider digoxin antibody fragments (Fab)	ECG, serum potassium
Ethanol	½–1 hr	Usually not necessary	If negative, symptoms are not due to ethanol intoxication; otherwise, positive test is inconclusive (because of possible tolerance)	Serum osmolality—calculated vs. measured
Ethylene glycol	½–1 hr	2 hr and then during dialysis until the level is zero	Use ethanol therapy and hemodialysis	Serum BUN and electrolytes, serum osmolality (calculated vs. measured), ABGs
Heavy metals	1–2 hr	2–4 hr and then during chelation therapy as indicated	Chelation therapy and consider hemodialysis	Measurements of urine volume and concentration of metal

Iron	2–4 hr (liquid iron preparations are absorbed faster than solid ones)	2–4 hr	If serum iron > 500 μg/dL, use deferoxamine.	Deferoxamine challenge test—look for vin rose color of urine
Lithium	½–1 hr	2 hr and then during dialysis until a level of <1 mEq/L	If neurologic symptoms, consider hemodialysis	Renal function tests, ECG
Methanol	½–1 hr	2 hr and then during dialysis until zero	Use ethanol therapy and hemodialysis	Serum BUN and electrolytes, serum osmolality (calculated vs. measured), ABGs
Methemoglobin	1–2 hr	1–2 hr	If patient is symptomatic or level > 30%, use methylene blue	Blood appears chocolate colored to unaided eye
Phenobarbital	1–2 hr	2–4 hr	If CNS depression, consider alkaline diuresis, repeated activated charcoal	
Phenytoin	1–2 hr	2–4 hr	Observe for seizure activity if > 20 μg/mL	
Salicylates	6 hr	2–4 hr	Consider alkaline diuresis if minor toxicity; if severe, consider hemodialysis	Blood gases, serum BUN, electrolytes, ferric chloride test of urine
Theophylline	1 hr—peak level may occur as late as 12 hr after ingesting sustained-release preparation	2–4 hr	Observe for seizure activity if > 20 μg/mL; if severe, consider charcoal hemoperfusion, repeated activated charcoal	ECG, LFTs

*If the time of ingestion is unknown, draw a blood specimen immediately and repeat in 2 to 4 hours.
†*LFTs,* liver function tests; *PT,* prothrombin time; *PTT,* partial thromboplastin time; *ECG,* electrocardiogram; *ABGs,* arterial blood gases; *BUN,* blood urea nitrogen.

these tests with a clinically useful turnaround time. Fortunately, many of these substances have prominent clinical findings that would direct the clinician's thinking toward the correct diagnosis. Most laboratories cannot analyze for ethylene glycol. Thus a physician may ultimately have to presume the presence of ethylene glycol by specifically ruling out other possible causes in conjunction with several bedside diagnostic tests.

Understanding the Time Factor

For toxicologic emergencies, the importance of the laboratory is directly related to the impact that the results will have on patient management. Based on this criterion, critical tests must be available immediately to EDs. After the specimens are obtained, analysis must begin promptly. Immediate testing is often needed for acetaminophen, carboxyhemoglobin, ethylene glycol, arsenic, mercury, lead, iron, lithium, digoxin, methanol, methemoglobin, phenobarbital, salicylates, and theophylline. Rapidly available quantitative results for these substances will significantly improve patient care.

For example, if a young child accidentally ingested a methanol-containing windshield washer antifreeze, having a methanol determination rapidly available will determine the need for ethanol therapy, hemodialysis, and admission or discharge of the patient. These are major high-risk procedures in a child and have the potential for morbidity and mortality, and the availability of such testing will obviate the necessity of basing decisions on the combination of the clinical examination, osmolality, and acid-base analysis.

Qualitative vs. Quantitative Testing

Quantitative laboratory tests generally have longer turnaround times than qualitative analysis. If patient management is not altered by knowledge of a specific blood level of drugs, quantitation may not be necessary. Some of the exposures where qualitative results will suffice include amphetamines, barbiturates, benzodiazepines, cocaine, opioids, and phencyclidine. Exposures that require specific knowledge of a quantitative level include acetaminophen, carboxyhemoglobin, carbamazepine, digoxin, ethanol, ethylene glycol, heavy metals, iron, lithium, methanol, methemoglobin, phenobarbital, phenytoin, salicylates, theophylline, and lidocaine.

The absorption and distribution characteristics of substances should dictate the most meaningful time when specimens for quantitation should be obtained. In overdoses and poisonings, the determination of a peak level may not be possible although that level may have the greatest clinical importance (see Table 9–1). The timing of sample collection may be further complicated by inaccurate or deliberately misleading patient histories or by the ingestion of substances that may delay (gastrointestinal) absorption.[10] It is advisable to repeat quantitative determinations for drugs available in sustained-release formulations or in products capable of forming concretions in the gastrointestinal tract. Repeat quantitative determinations may help to establish whether drug levels are still climbing or decreasing. Gastrointestinal decontamination (emesis, lavage, activated charcoal, cathartics, or whole-bowel irrigation) may be effective in slowing or stopping drug absorption. The slope and direction of a line drawn between two levels can be of prognostic value for patients who have ingested sustained-release products such as theophylline or lithium. Patients with rising levels will require a much higher level of concern than patients whose levels are declining.

Quantitative toxicologic tests are almost always performed on blood samples, with the exception of tests for heavy metals, for which a 24-hour urine collection may be

Table 9–2. Analysis of Common Toxicologic Techniques

Method*	Qualitative or Quantitative	Accuracy	Expense	Specificity	Ease of Performing	Time to Perform
TLC	Qualitative	Least	Least	Least	Least difficult	Slowest
GC	Both	Most	Intermediate	Most	Most difficult	Intermediate
HPLC	Both	Most	Intermediate	Most	Most difficult	Intermediate
RIA	Qualitative	Intermediate	Most	Intermediate	Intermediate	Slowest
EMIT	Qualitative	Intermediate	Most	Intermediate	Least difficult	Fastest
GC/MS	Both	Most	Most	Most	Most difficult	Intermediate

**TLC,* thin-layer chromatography; *GC,* gas chromatography; *HPLC,* high-performance liquid chromatography; *RIA,* radioimmunoassay; *EMIT,* enzyme multiplication immunoassay technique; *MS,* mass spectrometry.

preferred. Most *qualitative* tests can be performed on urine samples. It is advisable to send both blood and urine to the laboratory whenever possible so that the analytic chemist may select the medium that provides the best predictive result. A total of 5 to 10 mL of blood serum (red-topped tube) or plasma (gray-topped [oxalated] tube) and 50 to 100 mL of urine suffice in most cases, depending on the number of tests requested. If the specimens cannot be sent to the laboratory within several hours, they should be refrigerated.

Information for the Laboratory

The specimens should be accompanied by a requisition form describing the patient's clinical symptoms. It should contain the name and the age of the patient; the chart number; the physician's name, telephone number, and address; the estimated time of the ingestion; the time the specimen was taken; the test(s) requested; the medications known to have been taken or administered (at home or in the ED) before the specimen was obtained; and a brief history about the exposure, including vital signs, mental status changes, and specific symptoms.

Table 9–1 provides specific information including timing, interpretation, and therapeutic implications of tests requiring quantitation. When specific questions arise, it is best to consult with a regional poison control center or with the toxicologist at the laboratory where the specimen is analyzed.

Understanding Analytic Techniques

The clinician's understanding of the analytic procedures that will be used by the toxicology laboratory is helpful. Such knowledge allows for an enlightened interpretation of a test's specificity, sensitivity, and time requirements for analysis by the most common laboratory techniques. These data can be found in Table 9–2.

Chromatography is the most frequently used technique in analytic toxicology. It is a separation technique based on the movement of a mobile liquid or gas phase through a solid or liquid stationary phase that interacts with the unknown. The degree of interaction is different for different drugs and molecules, which ultimately results in separation. The greater the affinity between the unknown and the stationary phase, the slower the movement or longer the retention time and vice versa. Thin-layer, gas, and high-performance liquid are all chromatographic techniques.

Thin-layer chromatography (TLC) is the simplest analytic technique; it is commonly used for qualitative screening. A very thin layer of a substance such as silicic acid or aluminum oxide (stationary phase) is applied or glued to glass or plastic plates. A liquid solvent system (mobile phase) is placed in a developing tank. After the test sample to be separated is spotted on the "thin-layer plate," it is placed in the tank for development. As the solvents migrate upward by capillary action, the test specimen begins to move at a rate dependent on its affinity to the developing solvent and the stationary phase. Separation occurs because of the absorption or partition of the test sample molecules as the mobile solvent moves across the stationary sorbent phase. When the solvent front reaches the top, the plate is removed from the tank and then dried, and one of the many developing or detection methods is used to identify the solute. The amount of migration that occurs and the color that develops with the detection method is characteristic for each substance. TLC is rather *specific* because of the migration and color reaction parameters. However, it is not very *sensitive;* thus the method is only effective when a large quantity, at least milligram amounts, of the unknown is present.

Gas chromatography (GC) is considerably more sensitive and can be used quantitatively. The liquid or solid specimen dissolved in an organic solvent is injected into the chromatograph. The specimen is vaporized by heat in the injection port and carried through a column by an inert gas. The column is packed with a stationary phase that interacts with the test sample molecules and changes the rate of its migration as it travels through the column. As the drug reaches the detector, a peak is graphically plotted. The retention time is specific for a particular drug or molecule, and the peak area when compared with a known standard is used to quantitate the drug.

High-performance liquid chromatography (HPLC) is similar in many ways to GC except that it is not restricted to volatile compounds. A high-pressure (1000 to 6000 psi) pump facilitates movement of the specimen through the column at ambient temperatures. HPLC is specific but somewhat less sensitive than GC in most cases.

Radioimmunoassay (RIA) is a sensitive but not very specific technique for drug analysis. Cross-reactivity with closely related substances may occur. For this reason, both RIA and the enzyme multiplication immunoassay technique (EMIT) are used predominantly as screening techniques. A major disadvantage of RIA is that it requires a long preparation time and is too slow in emergency situations. For this reason, the EMIT has become much more popular. No sample preparation is necessary, and the tests takes a few minutes to perform. A major disadvantage to relying on either RIA and EMIT as a screening test is that their analytic capacity is very restricted. For example, if a sample is tested for cocaine and opiates but also contains methamphetamine and amphetamines, RIA and EMIT testing will not alert the chemist to the presence of the amphetamines. In contrast, testing a sample by GC with a nitrogen-phosphorus detector can identify up to 30 to 40 different substances.

Gas chromatography/mass spectrometry (GC/MS) is the ultimate, most sophisticated analytic method for the identification of organic molecules. In the emergency setting it would appear to be most useful in identifying drugs responsible for serious poisonings. GC/MS is capable of positively identifying the specific drug molecules involved. The method is based on separation of the various components of the unknown by GC, with identification of the separated fraction's molecular weight by fragmentation of the drug molecules in a high-energy field. Each different drug molecule breaks in a pattern characteristic for the specific drug. Ratios of the different fragments are characteristic for the specific drug. The method is referred to as "fingerprinting" of molecules.

As impressive as the technology may seem, GC/MS is neither the fastest nor the first-line choice to identify the common drugs or toxins implicated in most poisonings or overdoses. GC/MS is currently used principally in forensic cases where the identity of a drug must be absolute.

In the future when the methodology becomes less expensive and more "user friendly," GC/MS may become part of emergency toxicology's armamentarium.

Atomic absorption spectrophotometry (AAS) is a sophisticated technique for the quantitative identification of heavy metals. The toxicologically important elements determined by AAS are arsenic, mercury, lead, cadmium, barium, manganese, selenium, iron, zinc, chromium, and copper. The method is based on the unique wavelength of light energy emission of single atoms when returning from an excited state to the ground state. Excitation is achieved by energy input using a flame or graphite furnace. The heat is absorbed by the atoms sending their outer electrons to higher orbits. The unique wavelength emission occurs as the electrons return to the stable electron configuration.

Although AAS and other techniques for heavy metal analyses have progressed over the past decade, tests for heavy metals are not routinely offered by hospital laboratories. Emergency physicians and/or administrators should identify regional laboratories offering heavy metal analysis in biological fluids with an acceptable turnaround time. This service should be available when a patient's symptoms are suggestive of poisoning by a heavy metal.

If the laboratory is to be of the greatest possible assistance to the emergency physician, a clinically meaningful relationship must be established based on need and mutual understanding of each other's needs and capabilities.

REFERENCES

1. Moore RA, Rumack BH, Conner CS et al: Naloxone. Underdosage after narcotic poisoning, *Am J Dis Child* 134:156–158, 1980.
2. Weisberg HF: Water and electrolytes. In Dovidsohn I, Wells BB, editors: *Clinical diagnosis by laboratory methods,* Philadelphia, 1962, WB Saunders, p 500.
3. Goldfrank LG, Flomenbaum N, Lewin N et al: Methanol, ethylene glycol and isopropanol. In Goldfrank LG, Flomenbaum N, Lewin N et al, editors: *Goldfrank's toxicologic emergencies,* ed 4, E Norwalk, Conn, 1990, Appleton & Lange, pp 481–498.
4. Kiese M: *Methemoglobinemia: a comprehensive treatise,* West Palm Beach, Fla, 1977, CRC Press.
5. Curry S: Methemoglobinemia, *Ann Emerg Med* 11:214–221, 1982.
6. Terlinsky AS, Grochowski J, Geoly KL et al: Identification of atypical calcium oxylate crystaluria following ethylene glycol ingestion, *Am J Clin Pathol* 76:244–245, 1981.
7. Winter ML, Ellis MD, Snodgras WR: Urine fluorescence using a Wood's lamp to detect the antifreeze additive sodium fluorescein: a qualitative adjunctive test in suspected ethylene glycol ingestions, *Ann Emerg Med* 19:663–667, 1990.
8. Savitt DL, Hawkins HH, Roberts JR: The radiopacity of orally ingested medications, *Ann Emerg Med* 16:331–339, 1981.
9. Messing RO, Closson RG, Simon RP: Drug induced seizures: a 10 year experience, *Neurology* 34:1582–1586, 1984.
10. Nimmo WS: Drugs, diseases and altered gastric emptying, *Clin Pharmacokinet* 1:189–203, 1976.

PART III

An Organ System Approach to Diagnostic Testing

Chapter 10

Pulmonary Testing and Arterial Blood Gas Analysis

Stuart M. Garay, M.D.

The history, physical examination, and chest radiograph are the initial steps in diagnosing most pulmonary disorders. However, arterial blood gas (ABG) analysis, noninvasive oximetric assessment of oxygenation, bedside measurement of minute ventilation, capnographic measurement of end-tidal CO_2, as well as quantitative assessment of airway function have added new dimensions to the emergency physician's ability to diagnose and assess the severity of pulmonary disorders, predict impending respiratory failure, and prescribe proper therapeutic intervention. This discussion of pulmonary diagnostic tests focuses upon the emergency department (ED) and the practical utilization of these tests in that setting.

ARTERIAL BLOOD GAS ANALYSIS

A major breakthrough in the study of the nature of abnormal gas exchange occurred in 1945 when Riley developed the Roughton-Scholander syringe as a tool for measuring the partial pressure of oxygen in small samples of arterial blood. Fifteen years later, the analysis of blood gases remained a measurement used by research fellows. Today, technological advances have made blood gas analysis a routine procedure. The ability to obtain these measurements within minutes permits acute adjustments that are necessary for the care of patients in the ED. The arterial pH, pCO_2, and pO_2 are measured by specifically designed electrodes, whereas the oxygen saturation and bicarbonate concentration are calculated from these data. ABG values reflect both the gas exchange efficiency of the lung and the acid-base status of the patient (the latter is discussed in Chapter 5). Assessment of oxygenation is achieved by determining the arterial pO_2 and the alveolar-arterial O_2 gradient $p(A\text{-}a)O_2$; adequacy of alveolar ventilation is assessed by measuring the arterial pCO_2.

THE TECHNIQUE OF ARTERIAL PUNCTURE

Along with the technological progress mentioned above came the realization that arterial blood can be readily obtained with minimal risk to the patient.[1] The following guidelines should be borne in mind:

1. Superficial arteries are most desirable because they are easily accessible, may be palpated and stabilized between two fingers, and will reveal complications early.

2. Because periarterial hematoma, intraarterial clotting, and arterial vessel spasm may result from an arterial puncture and thereby interrupt blood flow to the tissues supplied by that artery, vessels with collateral blood flow should be used. The use of these vessels is an important protective mechanism if these complications occur. When the radial artery is to be punctured, the Allen test[2] is a simple maneuver that assesses collateral flow through the ulnar artery.

3. For the above reasons, the preferred sites for puncture are the radial and brachial arteries. The femoral artery is least desirable (although it may be used): it is deep under the skin, unnoticed bleeding may occur retroperitoneally, it lies adjacent to the femoral vein, which may be accidentally punctured and thus confuse the blood gas measurements, and it has limited collateral arterial flow.

4. The actual technique requires the use of a 22- to 25-gauge needle. The artery should be palpated from above (middle finger) and below (index finger) while noting the course of the vessel by rolling it under these two fingers; the needle is inserted with the bevel up while feeling the pulse and slowly advancing at an angle (ranging from 45 to 90 degrees above the puncture site) without puncturing the posterior wall of the vessel. After 3 to 5 mL of blood is withdrawn, the needle is quickly withdrawn, pressure is then applied to the site for 5 minutes (longer, if the patient is anticoagulated), and the pulse is checked about 30 minutes later. Newer blood gas analyzers require much less blood, the amount ranging from 0.5 to 1 mL.

- Aseptic technique should be used to prevent infection; cleansing with an alcohol- or povidone-iodine (Betadine)-impregnated pad is usually sufficient.
- Clinicians are divided as to whether a local anesthetic should be administered at the site before arterial puncture. Some observers have documented hyperventilation in patients during the procedure when it is performed without an anesthetic. Others have shown that the hyperventilation is not significant enough to alter blood gas values. Another consideration is that if local anesthetic is not used, the artery may go into spasm when punctured and thus prevent blood sampling. If an anesthetic is used, a small skin wheal is raised with a local anesthetic in a 25-gauge needle.
- Some clinicians advocate skin puncture with the needle alone to allow the needle to be placed parallel to the artery; then the syringe is attached. The technique is accomplished readily with a scalp vein needle ("butterfly"), which allows for the smallest angle between the needle and the artery so that the hole through the arterial wall is oblique and will be sealed off by the circular smooth muscle fibers. There is no evidence to suggest, however, that a larger angle between the needle and the artery leads to more complications. Most physicians puncture the skin with the needle and syringe attached.
- Previously physicians preferred glass syringes because they enable one to differentiate between arterial end venous blood: pulsating arterial blood enters the syringe without the need to pull back upon the plunger whereas venous blood will not. In contrast, a plastic syringe requires manual withdrawal of the plunger. However, during the past five years disposable plastic syringes have been developed that allow pulsating arterial blood to enter the syringe without pulling back on the plunger. Because of the need for sterilization, glass syringes are rarely used in the human immunodeficiency virus (HIV) era. Instead disposable syringes are favored.
- If a heparinized 23-gauge scalp vein needle is used when the artery is punctured, pulsating blood can be seen in the connecting plastic tube. With the needle left in place, blood is aspirated into the attached syringe.

5. Needles should not be capped since percutaneous injuries have most frequently been implicated in the occupational transmission of blood-borne pathogens

such as hepatitis and HIV.[3,4] A study[5] at a university hospital revealed that one third of all needlesticks were related to recapping. Disposable syringes and needles should be placed in puncture-resistant containers for disposal.

6. All samples must be anaerobically drawn into a syringe that has been previously heparinized. Because air bubbles may significantly lower pCO_2 and raise pO_2, the syringe containing the sample should be corked immediately after the arterial blood is drawn. An additional source of error may occur if air is allowed to mix with the sample as it is introduced into the electrode chamber.

7. Too much heparin in a syringe may alter the pH (the pH of sodium heparin is 7)[6]; therefore the syringe must be flushed with sodium heparin (100 units/mL) and then emptied. The dead space of a 5-mL syringe will usually retain about 0.15 mL of heparin, which allows adequate anticoagulation of the blood without affecting the pH.

8. Finally, the clinician must remember that oxygen is consumed and carbon dioxide is produced even after blood is withdrawn into a syringe (in vitro changes: pH = 0.01/10 min, pCO_2 = 1 mm Hg/10 min, and pO_2 = 0.1 vol%/10 min).[7] These changes are temperature dependent. At 20° C, these changes are only 10% of the values at 37° C.[8] Therefore if the blood sample is not immediately analyzed, it should be cooled in ice, which will maintain values up to 1 hour. However, these studies were performed with glass syringes. Recently Liss et al.[9] demonstrated that there is a decline in pO_2 through cooled, plastic syringes and these changes are minimized as the syringes are left at room temperature for 30 minutes or less. Glass syringes should be used and placed in ice if the patient is known to have a severe thrombocytosis, leukocytosis, or a reticulocytosis.

ASSESSMENT OF OXYGENATION: pO_2 AND O_2 SATURATION

The degree of oxygenation of arterial blood is expressed as the partial pressure of oxygen (pO_2) or oxygen saturation (O_2 Sat). These two measurements are related to each other by the sigmoidal oxyhemoglobin dissociation curve. Knowledge of one value enables the clinician to derive the other. Arterial paO_2 values of 40, 50, and 60 mm Hg correspond roughly to O_2 Sat values of 70%, 80%, and 90% (the progression 40 through 90 is easier to remember than the exact O_2 Sat percentages, which are only slightly different). In most clinical situations, after paO_2 is measured, O_2 Sat can be calculated. This is not true, however, for carbon monoxide poisoning. In cases of suspected carbon monoxide poisoning, a co-oximeter (see Oximetry) *must* be used to measure the carbon monoxide concentration (carboxyhemoglobin) and O_2 Sat *directly*. Because paO_2 will not be affected by the carbon monoxide, and O_2 Sat is calculated from the misleadingly normal paO_2, it will also be "normal" and therefore incorrect since the *true* O_2 Sat is very much adversely affected by carbon monoxide poisoning.

Factors that shift the O_2 dissociation curve (such as pH and temperature) must be borne in mind. The blood gas machine analyzes blood at a temperature of 37° C. Various tables, nomograms, and computer programs have been designed to make corrections for temperature discrepancies between the machine and the body.[10] paO_2 and $paCO_2$ change directly with body temperature, but pH varies inversely with temperature. The HCO_3^- and "base excess" that the machine records are not affected by body temperature. The correction factors become clinically significant only at the extremes (temperatures greater than 39° C or less than 35° C).

Disturbances of gas exchange may cause discernible changes in paO_2 and little change in O_2 Sat when the paO_2 is greater than 60 mm Hg because the O_2 dissociation curve is flat in the 60– to 100–mm Hg range. Thus, changes in paO_2 above 60 mm Hg may be of diagnostic value, whereas changes in paO_2 below 60 mm Hg are of critical therapeutic importance. In the latter circumstances, O_2 Sat has decreased to less than 90% and small changes in paO_2 on the steep part of the O_2 dissociation curve (paO_2 less than 60 mm Hg) imply great changes in O_2 Sat.

paO_2 greater than 90 mm Hg on room air is usually considered normal if it is not achieved by hyperventilation. However, arterial oxygen tension is a function of altitude, age, and inspired O_2 concentration. At a given altitude the paO_2 should be multiplied by the fraction local pB/760 (where pB = barometric pressure). The precise reduction in paO_2 with age is somewhat disputed. However, pO_2 values as low as 75 mm Hg may be normal in patients over 70 years of age. Empirically derived formulas for calculating predicted arterial O_2 tension are as follows:

$$paO_2 = 104.2 - 0.27 \times \text{age (seated)}^{11}$$

$$= 103.5 - 0.42 \times \text{age (supine)}^{12}$$

The alveolar gas equation indicates that the fraction of inspired oxygen (FIO_2) is the major determinant of pAO_2 and paO_2. The normal paO_2 for any given FIO_2 is approximately five times the FIO_2 at sea level, assuming that the patient is not hyperventilating and therefore has a normal $paCO_2$.

A discussion of oxygenation must ultimately concern itself with arterial oxygen content inasmuch as this determines the amount of O_2 available to the tissues. Arterial O_2 content is a function of two components. The first component is the oxygen dissolved in the blood plasma (determined by multiplying 0.003 and paO_2); the second component is the O_2 bound to hemoglobin (determined by multiplying 1.34, hemoglobin concentration, and O_2 Sat). Thus, diagnosis of abnormalities in gas exchange requires knowledge of arterial pO_2 and calculation of the alveolar-arterial O_2 gradient (see below); assessment of adequate O_2 in the blood for delivery to tissues requires calculation of the O_2 content (derived from O_2 Sat).

PULSE OXIMETRY

During the past decade, noninvasive measurement of arterial oxygen saturation with pulse oximeters has grown from relative obscurity to an almost indispensable monitoring technique.[13, 14] Oximetry analyzes the percentage of total hemoglobin chemically bound to various substances. Oximeters act as spectrophotometers: they convert light intensity into electric current by determining the intensity of light of specific wavelengths transmitted through a sample of blood. The physics of how a single wavelength of light is absorbed by a substance is described by the Beer-Lambert law: the intensity of light absorbed while passing through a substance is directly proportional to the thickness of the substance. A co-oximeter (not pulse oximeter) measures the concentration of oxyhemoglobin, carboxyhemoglobin, reduced hemoglobin, and methemoglobin by measuring the absorption of light at four different wavelengths, one for each type of hemoglobin. Most co-oximeters are capable of compensating for unmeasured fetal hemoglobin.

Spectrophotometry measures oxygen bound to hemoglobin since the color and optical density of hemoglobin change with the amount of oxygen bound. Oxygenated hemoglobin is bright red, whereas reduced or deoxygenated hemoglobin (deoxyhemoglobin, also referred to as reduced hemoglobin) is dark blue. Each has its own absorption characteristics.

Pulse oximeters combine the principles of spectrophotometry with those of photoplethysmography.[14, 15] Photoplethysmography relies on the finding that when a constant amount of light is transmitted through a pulsatile vascular bed, more light is transmitted through the bed when the arterioles are nearly empty (cardiac diastole) than when the arterioles are full (cardiac systole). Therefore, if a constant light source is transmitted through a blood vessel, the photodetector on the opposite side measures fluxes in intensity with the emptying and filling of the vessel. Since the majority of blood pulsating through vessels is arterial, the pulse oximeter compares absorption during systole and diastole and reflects only arterial blood. Pulse oximeters use only two wavelengths of light, one in the infrared range of 940 nm and one in the red range of 660 nm. Oxyhemoglobin absorbs light in the infrared range, whereas reduced hemoglobin absorbs light in the red range.

The accuracy of most pulse oximeters decreases below O_2 Sat values of 70% to 75%. The accuracy above 70% is $\pm$ 4%, and below 70%, $\pm$ 6%. Pulse oximeters are not routinely calibrated before use. They should be used to monitor *changes* in saturation, and the O_2 Sat reading should never be accepted as an absolute actual saturation. If necessary, a simultaneously drawn ABG sample may be obtained to relate the actual O_2 Sat with the one measured by the pulse oximeter. The difference between the two O_2 Sat measurements can be assessed and the pulse oximeter O_2 Sat used for trend analysis.

Pulse oximetry was first used intraoperatively and postoperatively. Subsequently, pediatric and adult intensive care units began using continuous-pulse oximetry to monitor patients with labile oxygenation as well as during "weaning" trials from mechanical ventilation. When used judiciously, pulse oximetry can be extremely helpful in the ED. Jones et al.[16] used a pulse oximeter in the management of 40 consecutive patients who came to the ED in respiratory distress. Pulse oximetry was useful in assessing overall degree of respiratory distress, titrating the FiO_2 (oxygen concentration) requirement for nonintubated and intubated patients, optimizing positive end-expiratory expiration (PEEP) for patients requiring mechanical ventilation, and serving as an early warning sign for acute respiratory deterioration. The mean duration of usage for the pulse oximeter was 1.8 hours per patient.

It should be emphasized that using pulse oximetry to "spot-check" oxygen saturation may lead to serious errors. Measurements should always be taken in duplicate to demonstrate reproducibility. They should agree within $\pm$2%.[17] In addition, the heart rate displayed on the pulse oximeter should be compared with a palpated or electrocardiographic (ECG) heart rate. Agreement should be within 5 beats per minute to ensure that the pulse oximeter is detecting an appropriate pulse waveform for every heartbeat. A pulse oximeter should not display a saturation reading unless a pulse is recognizable. The American Association for Respiratory Care has published guidelines[17] for the use of pulse oximetry in clinical practice.

Various factors may limit the accuracy of pulse oximetry. *One of the most important limitations of pulse oximetry in the ED is its inability to distinguish carboxyhemoglobin and methemoglobin from oxyhemoglobin.* Carboxyhemoglobin is viewed by the pulse oximeter as if it were predominantly oxyhemoglobin, although some of its absorption is in the reduced hemoglobin range.[18, 19] Thus the pulse oximeter will display a falsely elevated O_2 Sat value by an amount roughly equivalent to the amount of hemoglobin present.[19, 20] The effect of methemoglobin is more complex since methemoglobin absorbs light at both 660 and 940 nm.[17, 21] This results in an "absorbance ratio" of the two wavelengths of approximately 1.0.[14] The pulse oximeter detects this "absorbance ratio" of 1.0, which corresponds to a saturation between 83% and 87%. Thus, in patients with methemoglobinemia, pulse oximetry O_2 Sat is falsely high for O_2 Sat values greater than 85% but falsely low for O_2 Sat values below 85%.[14, 21]

One other major limitation of pulse oximetry involves its use in low-perfusion states.[14, 15] Hypovolemia, hypothermia, hypotension, and vasoconstrictor infusions result in decreased or absent peripheral pulses. Since pulse oximeters must clearly identify an arterial pulse, their performance declines in patients with these conditions. Consequently, pulse oximeters should not be used during cardiac arrests. The earlobe may be a better site for monitoring patients with decreased peripheral perfusion since it is less affected by vasoconstriction than the fingertip.

Other clinical factors may affect the clinical accuracy of pulse oximeters. These include motion; certain vascular dyes such as methylene blue, indigo carmine, and indocyanine green; and certain light sources such as fluorescent, infrared, and xenon lamps. Newer pulse oximeters provide beat-to-beat pulse recognition and synchronization, which decreases the effect of motion. Many radiographic dyes contain methyl blue or green. Thus a significant amount of dye in the blood can be misinterpreted by the pulse oximeter as deoxyhemoglobin and result in a falsely low O_2 Sat value.[22] This effect is usually transient.

Finally, skin and nail pigmentation may affect pulse oximetry readings.[23, 24] Dark skin pigmentation alters the accuracy of pulse oximeters as a function of increased melanin concentration altering light absorption through skin. Inaccurate readings (i.e., 4% variation up or down) are more common in black patients.[24] Furthermore, technical problems (such as an inability to obtain a reading or failure of a warning message indicating poor tissue penetration of a signal) occur more frequently in black patients.[23] Nail polish—especially dark colors such as black, blue, and green—lowers pulse oximetry readings.[25] In contrast, the pulse oximeter is not affected by hyperbilirubinemia.

ALVEOLAR-ARTERIAL OXYGEN GRADIENTS

Assessment of a patient in respiratory failure requires evaluation of both the arterial pO_2 and the arterial pCO_2. Although an arterial pO_2 value of less than 55 mm Hg usually indicates respiratory failure, the etiology remains unknown. Patients may suffer this degree of hypoxemia and have a pCO_2 value of less than 40 mm Hg while hyperventilating (e.g., in cases of adult respiratory distress syndrome [ARDS], acute pulmonary embolism, or acute asthma attack), or they may suffer this degree of hypoxemia and have an increased pCO_2 while hypoventilating (e.g., in cases of drug overdose, neurologic dysfunction, or primary alveolar hypoventilation).

One can differentiate between these two groups of disorders easily in the ED by calculating the "A-a gradient" while the patient is breathing room air. Calculation of the alveolar-arterial oxygen difference $p(A\text{-}a)O_2$ assesses the intrinsic gas exchange properties of the lungs and suggests the cause of a patient's hypoxemia (Table 10–1). An increased A-a gradient implies V/Q, shunt, or diffusion problems. A normal A-a

Table 10–1. Mechanisms of Hypoxemia

Causes of Hypoxemia	pAO_2	paO_2	A-a Gradient (RA)	A-a Gradient on 100% O_2	$paCO_2$	Examples
Decreased F_iO_2	↓	↓	N	N	↓	High altitude
Hypoventilation	↓	↓	N	N	↑	Drug overdose
Diffusion block	N	↓	↑	N	N/↓	Interstitial lung disease, obstructive lung disease
V/Q mismatch (V/Q)	N/↓	↓	↑	N	N/↓/↑	Interstitial lung disease, pulmonary emboli
Right-to-left shunt	↓	↓	↑	↑	N/↓	Intrapulmonary shunt (ARDS), ASD, VSD*

**ARDS*, adult respiratory distress syndrome; *ASD*, atrial septal defect; *VSD*, ventricular septal defect.

gradient implies normal lungs, so an extrapulmonary cause for the patient's hypoxemia should be sought.

When a patient is at sea level and breathing room air ($F_IO_2 = 0.21$), the important mechanisms for arterial hypoxemia include alveolar hypoventilation, V/Q mismatch (low V/Q), and shunt (V/Q = 0). Calculation of the A-a gradient distinguishes these mechanisms: only alveolar hypoventilation is characterized by a normal gradient. Furthermore, the response to 100% O_2 (for a minimum of 20 minutes) distinguishes shunt from V/Q mismatch: in V/Q mismatch, breathing oxygen will normalize the calculated gradient (<100 mm Hg on 100% O_2).

In calculating $p(A\text{-}a)O_2$, the alveolar gas equation (see below) reveals that the alveolar pO_2 (pAO_2) is equal to the partial pressure of the inspired O_2 concentration (P_IO_2) minus $paCO_2$ divided by 0.8 (which is the respiratory exchange ratio in a steady state). $paCO_2$ approximates $paCO_2$ and is substituted for it. Thus,

$$pAO_2 = P_IO_2 - \frac{paCO_2}{R}$$

Because $p_IO_2 = F_IO_2\ (pB - pH_2O)$, these values can be substituted in the equation for p_IO_2:

$$pAO_2 = F_IO_2\ (pB - pH_2O) - \frac{paCO_2}{R}$$

In these equations, *F_IO_2* is the inspired O_2 fraction, *pB* is barometric pressure, and pH_2O is water vapor pressure. On room air, $F_IO_2 = 0.21$, and in a steady state R = 0.8, pB = 760 mm Hg, and $pH_2O = 47$ mm Hg. Therefore,

$$\begin{aligned} pAO_2 &= 0.21(760 - 47) - \frac{paCO_2}{R} \\ &= 150 - 1.25 \times paCO_2 \end{aligned}$$

To summarize,

$$\begin{aligned} p(A\text{-}a)O_2 &= pAO_2 - PaO_2 \\ &= 150 - (1.25 \times paCO_2) - paO_2 \\ &= 150 - 1.25\ (paCO_2 + paO_2) \end{aligned}$$

The normal A-a gradient is 10 to 15 mm Hg. However, because paO_2 varies with age, the A-a gradient normally increases with age.[26] A quick approximation for predicting normal A-a gradients is one third of the patient's age, or 5 + age/4.

The usefulness of calculating the A-a gradient is demonstrated by Cases 10–1 to 10–4.

As noted above, 100% O_2 can be used to differentiate between V/Q and shunt mechanisms causing hypoxemia. If the problem is V/Q mismatch, administration of 100% O_2 will raise paO_2 to about 550 to 575 mm Hg, and the A-a gradient will be reduced to normal (on 100% O_2, the A-a gradient is approximately 100 mm Hg). In the patient described in Case 10–4, the markedly increased A-a gradient suggests that a shunt mechanism is involved.

A shunt may also be referred to as an "intrapulmonary shunt" or "venous admixture" to emphasize that venous blood passes through the pulmonary capillaries without becoming oxygenated. The total, or physiologic, shunt can be determined from the "shunt equation":

$$\frac{Q_S}{Q_T} = \frac{Cco_2 - Cao_2}{Cco_2 - C\bar{v}o_2}$$

where

- Q_S = flow through the shunt
- Q_T = total cardiac output
- Cco_2 = ideal pulmonary capillary O_2 content (determined by assuming pCO_2 = pAO_2)
- Cao_2 = arterial O_2 content
- $C\bar{v}o_2$ = mixed venous O_2 content

When the mixed venous O_2 content is available, the total shunt can be calculated. However, this requires invasive monitoring with a pulmonary artery (Swan-Ganz) catheter.

The numerator of the shunt equation ($Cco_2 - Cao_2$) reflects *pulmonary* pathology, whereas the denominator ($Cco_2 - C\bar{v}o_2$) reflects *nonpulmonary* pathology. Therefore hypoxemia secondary to pulmonary disease results in an increased shunt fraction, Q_S/Q_T, whereas hypoxemia secondary to nonpulmonary disease affects the shunt fraction to a lesser degree. The shunt equation also suggests that a decreased $C\bar{v}o_2$ may result in a reduced Cao_2. Finally, the greater the shunt fraction, Q_S/Q_T, the less likely spontaneous ventilation can be sustained.

As noted above, a true determination of Q_S/Q_T can only be achieved by invasive monitoring. Alternatively, the shunt can be found by using one of several published nomograms.[27,28] Calculation of $p(A\text{-}a)O_2$ has been used to assess the severity of the shunt fraction. The major limitation of the $(A\text{-}a)O_2$ gradient in this setting is its variability with changes in the FiO_2; patients with severe respiratory failure require FiO_2 values greater than 0.21. It is difficult to compare various $(A\text{-}a)O_2$ gradients calculated from different FiO_2 values. If a patient's cardiac output is normal (the difference in $(a\text{-}v)O_2$ is 5 mL per 100 mL of blood), the $p(A\text{-}a)O_2$ value can be used to estimate the shunt fraction: each 20–mm Hg increment in $p(A\text{-}a)O_2$ corresponds to a 1% shunt. This is only valid when paO_2 is greater than 150 mm Hg. Recently two other calculations have been proposed: paO_2/FiO_2 and paO_2/pAO_2. The problem with paO_2/FiO_2 is that it is also dependent on FiO_2 as well as $paCO_2$. paO_2/pAO_2 is not affected by FiO_2 and $paCO_2$. The ratio is normally greater than 0.7 in healthy individuals regardless of FiO_2.[29]

ASSESSMENT OF ADEQUATE VENTILATION: pCO_2

$paCO_2$ values normally range between 37 and 43 mm Hg. The partial pressure of arterial CO_2 measures the adequacy of the lung to remove CO_2 from the blood entering the lung. In contrast to paO_2, altitudes below 8000 ft and age have minimal effect on this value. $paCO_2$ can be used as an accurate estimate of alveolar ventilation because CO_2 rapidly equilibrates between alveolar gas and pulmonary capillary blood (in contrast to the different values for arterial and alveolar oxygen). If CO_2 production is held constant, arterial pCO_2 is inversely related to alveolar ventilation:

$$paCO_2 = \frac{1}{VA}$$

where VA is alveolar ventilation.

Thus an increased $paCO_2$ value indicates alveolar hypoventilation; conversely, a reduced $paCO_2$ value indicates alveolar hyperventilation. When the $paCO_2$ value is abnormal, one must determine whether this condition is a primary ventilatory abnormality (intrinsic or extrinsic to the lung) or whether the value merely represents compensation for a primary metabolic disturbance in an attempt to achieve acid-base balance. $paCO_2$ values are determined in part by acid-base homeostasis because the $paCO_2$ value is directly proportional to the H_2CO_3 concentration, which is the body's primary buffer system.

Measurements of minute ventilation (VE) at the bedside are usually a non–steady-state estimate, but they can be very helpful in identifying the mechanism of arterial hypercapnia. Portable, relatively accurate, inexpensive flowmeters that measure individual tidal breaths and summate to VE are now available (e.g., Wright, Boehringer, or Drager respirometers). Minute ventilation is the product of tidal volume and respiratory rate. During each tidal breath, some of the air reaches the alveoli and participates in gas exchange (alveolar ventilation, VA), whereas some air remains in the conducting airways (dead space ventilation, VDS). Thus, over a 60-second interval, VE is the sum of VA and VDS (VE = VA + VDS). Minute ventilation ranges from 5 to 8 L/min, whereas VA is roughly two thirds of VE.[30] If hypercapnia develops in a patient, VA must be reduced. A mathematical solution of the equation governing VE reveals that VA = VE − VDS. Thus when hypercapnia results in a reduced VA, the mechanism must be either a reduced VE or an increased VDS.

When a patient comes to the ED with an increased $paCO_2$ and a reduced VE, the mechanism for hypercapnia is alveolar hypoventilation (when VE is reduced, VA must be reduced). As $paCO_2$ increases, pAO_2 decreases because

$$pAO_2 = 150 - \frac{paCO_2}{R}$$

(see the alveolar gas equation above).

If the A-a gradient remains normal, this decrease in PAO_2 must produce arterial hypoxemia. Diseases that should be considered are those that result in a decreased ventilatory drive (e.g., sedative drugs, anesthesia, head injuries, and medullary infarct) or decreased chest bellows output (e.g., neuromuscular disease and thoracic cage abnormalities).

If arterial hypercapnia is present and measured VE is increased, then diseases such as recurrent pulmonary emboli that result in increased dead space (anatomic and physiologic) are responsible for the patient's hypercapnia. In this instance, the increased VE is not adequate to compensate for the increased VDS. Ventilation of nonperfused areas results in increased VDS. Alveolar ventilation (VA) is decreased, and hypercapnia results. VDS may also be increased because of increased airway resistance (as in the case of asthma or bronchitis) or increased lung compliance (as in the case of emphysema). The local alterations in resistance and compliance produce underventilation of local lung units and so increase regional arterial pCO_2 values. When lung disease is extensive, compensation by hyperventilating normal lung units cannot prevent systemic arterial hypercapnia.

Arterial hypocapnia indicates the presence of hyperventilation, which can also be verified by measuring VE. The causes for a reduced $paCO_2$ value include pulmonary (interstitial, airways, or vascular processes) and nonpulmonary (anxiety, drugs, meningitis, fever, or pain) causes.

CAPNOGRAPHIC ANALYSIS OF EXHALED CO_2

As discussed above, carbon dioxide is metabolically produced in body tissues and is ultimately exhaled. The capnograph records the exhalation of CO_2. The capnogram is the displayed waveform of CO_2 exhalation. Originally a research tool, technological advances have brought this type of monitoring to the bedside and the ED.[31, 32] Fig. 10–1 displays a normal capnogram. There are two recording speeds at which capnograms may be visualized. Fast-speed capnograms provide breath-by-breath analysis of the waveform.

Slow-speed capnograms provide trend analysis of the end-tidal pCO_2 ($pETCO_2$) over time. Normal fast-speed capnograms have a characteristic waveform analyzing different parts of the respiratory cycle. During inspiration, the pCO_2 is normal. At the start of exhalation (point A, phase I) the pCO_2 is zero and represents the conducting airways (anatomic dead space), which contain little if any CO_2. The graph rises sharply (segment AB, phase II) as alveolar gas mixes with dead space gas. Near the end of exhalation, the CO_2 rise is minimal and the graph plateaus as the alveolar gas is exhaled (segment BC, phase III). The pCO_2 at the end of the alveolar plateau is called the end-tidal pCO_2 ($pETCO_2$). The end-tidal pCO_2 represents the highest concentration of CO_2 at the end of exhalation and is assumed to represent alveolar gas. Normal $pETCO_2$ ranges between 4.5% and 5.5%. As inspiration begins, pCO_2 rapidly declines. Measurement of end-tidal pCO_2 provides a noninvasive estimate of $paCO_2$. It is usually 4 to 6 mm Hg below $paCO_2$.

End-tidal pCO_2 represents $paCO_2$ and is the net flux of CO_2 into and out of the alveolus. CO_2 entry into the alveolus is determined by CO_2 production (vCO_2) as well as venous blood flow, i.e., perfusion (Q). Clearance of alveolar CO_2 is a function of alveolar ventilation (V_A). Thus $paCO_2$ or $pETCO_2$ is directly proportional to varying V/Q relationships. Normal V/Q relationships result in $pETCO_2$ approximating $paCO_2$. If ventilation is reduced (low V/Q), $pETCO_2$ rises toward mixed venous pCO_2 ($p\bar{v}CO_2$). If ventilation increases or perfusion decreases (increased dead space), $pETCO_2$ approaches inspired pCO_2, which is usually zero. Various clinical situations may affect $pETCO_2$. Conditions that increase CO_2 production such as fever, seizures, and sepsis increase end-tidal pCO_2. A reduction in alveolar ventilation regardless of etiology (chronic ob-

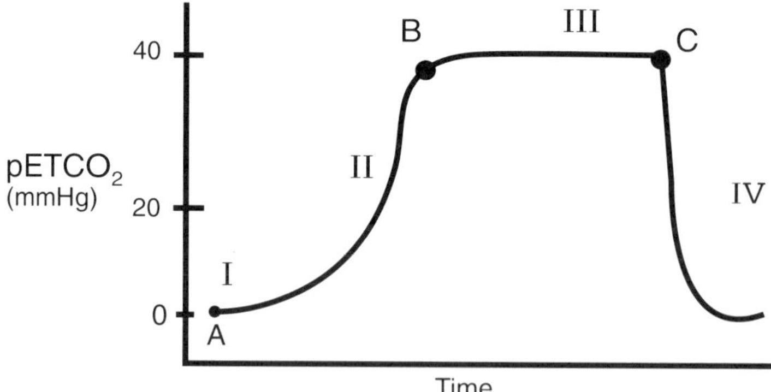

Fig. 10–1. A normal capnogram depicting a single respiratory cycle. Point *A*, phase I—start of exhalation; segment *AB*, phase II—alveolar gas mixes with dead space gas, increasing the alveolar gas concentration; segment *BC*, phase III—end of exhalation marks the plateau phase or "pure" alveolar gas.

structive pulmonary disease [COPD], hypoventilation, central nervous system [CNS] depression, or neuromuscular disease) will increase $pETCO_2$. Equipment malfunction such as a leak in the ventilator circuit will result in an increased $pETCO_2$. Alternatively, conditions that reduce CO_2 production and/or reduce delivery of CO_2 to the lungs such as hypothermia, cardiac arrest, pulmonary embolism, hypotension, and hemorrhage will decrease $pETCO_2$. Hyperventilation will lower end-tidal CO_2. A reduced $pETCO_2$ may be secondary to such equipment malfunction as endotracheal cuff leak or disconnected ventilator or esophageal intubation. It should be noted that compensatory changes may occur and preclude the "predicted" end-tidal pCO_2 response.

When $paCO_2$ is measured, an arterial–end-tidal pCO_2 gradient can be calculated ($paCO_2 - pETCO_2$). This gradient is usually less than 5 mm Hg. In conditions that result in high V/Q (increased dead space), $pETCO_2$ is considerably less than $paCO_2$, which results in an increased gradient (see below). Other causes of an increased $paCO_2 - pETCO_2$ gradient include cardiac arrest as well as positive-pressure ventilation (especially when PEEP is used). Thus this gradient lacks specificity.

Two techniques are used for CO_2 monitoring: infrared absorption spectrophotometry and mass spectroscopy.[31, 32] This discussion will focus on the former since the latter is considerably more complex, more expensive, and less available to the ED.

The ability of infrared analyzers to measure CO_2 is based on their capability of absorbing infrared radiation of a particular wavelength. An infrared light beam is directed to a sample of exhaled gas of unknown CO_2 concentration. Within the sample, CO_2 molecules absorb some of the infrared energy. A photodetector compares the relative amount of light absorbed with that of a reference containing a comparison gas free of CO_2. The difference represents the CO_2 concentration. The respiratory rate may be determined by counting the number of CO_2 pulses over a time period.

Capnometers are classified according to their gas sampling technique as either mainstream or sidestream. The former connects directly to an endotracheal tube, thereby avoiding response time delays. However, mainstream capnometers are bulky, require sterilization, need heating to prevent condensation and secretions from interfering with their sensor windows, and do not function if CO_2 is present in the inspired gas. Sidestream analyzers can be used in both intubated and nonintubated patients, are lighter, and lack mechanical dead space. The major disadvantages of sidestream analyzers is the slow response time to CO_2 changes since gas must travel from the sample size to the analyzer. In addition, condensation and secretions may also accumulate in the tubing, and prevent accurate pCO_2 measurements.

Various animal models of cardiac arrest have demonstrated that $pETCO_2$ is useful for evaluating the effectiveness of cardiopulmonary resuscitation (CPR).[33–35] As previously discussed, $pETCO_2$ is determined by V/Q relationships. Thus, changes in perfusion (Q) are reflected by $pETCO_2$. During cardiac arrest, dead space is markedly increased since ventilation continues without perfusion (i.e., high V/Q); $pETCO_2$ declines to zero. As CPR restores part of this circulation, $pETCO_2$ increases and may approach levels as high as 15 to 20 mm Hg. When circulation is restored to normal, $pETCO_2$ returns to normal. $pETCO_2$ correlates with cardiac output during CPR.[36, 37] Sanders et al.[38] found that the $pETCO_2$ level obtained during CPR identified patients more likely to be resuscitated. Patients who survived resuscitation had a $pETCO_2$ of 15 ± 4 mm Hg during resuscitation as compared with those who did not survive who had a $pETCO_2$ level of 7 ± 5 mm Hg.[38] Callahan and Barton[39, 40] subsequently demonstrated that an initial $pETCO_2$ determination during CPR correctly predicted 71% of the patients who would be successfully resuscitated with a 98% specificity.

Measurement of $pETCO_2$ may be helpful in two other situations in the ED: esophageal intubation and diagnosis of pulmonary emboli. Accidental intubation of the esophagus can occur during attempted endotracheal intubation, especially during an acute cardiopulmonary arrest. Monitoring end-tidal pCO_2 may help detect esophageal intubation; failure of $pETCO_2$ to rise to normal or a significant decrease after several breadths suggests this problem.[41] Although significant levels of CO_2 can be present in the esophagus and stomach following the ingestion of carbonated beverages, CO_2 is usually rapidly cleared after 10 to 15 seconds of esophageal or gastric ventilation.[42] Monitoring of $pETCO_2$ to detect esophageal intubation during a cardiac arrest may be limited since $pETCO_2$ may be very low during an arrest because of poor pulmonary perfusion (Q). Sayah et al., however, have recently demonstrated in a dog model of cardiac arrest that esophageal intubation may be detected by monitoring end-tidal pCO_2 in this situation.[41]

Measurement of $pETCO_2$ as well as the $paCO_2 - pETCO_2$ gradient has been advocated as a noninvasive means for diagnosing acute pulmonary embolism.[43, 44] A normal gradient is less than 7 mm Hg. An increased $paCO_2 - pETCO_2$ gradient has been correlated with an increased VDS/VT, i.e., as a measure of increased dead space ventilation, which is observed in patients with acute pulmonary emboli. Unfortunately, this measurement is more sensitive than specific. Chopin et al.[45] compared capnography with angiography in 44 patients with COPD and documented pulmonary emboli. Although 100% sensitive, an increased gradient was only 65% specific with a false positive rate of 35%.

ASSESSMENT OF ACUTE AIRWAY DYSFUNCTION IN THE EMERGENCY DEPARTMENT

In recent years it has become apparent that the severity of an asthmatic attack cannot always be evaluated by the history and physical examination alone. Although sternocleidomastoid retraction[46] and pulsus paradoxus[47] have been correlated with expiratory flow rates (the former corresponding to a forced expiratory volume in 1 second [FEV_1] of less than 1 L, the latter corresponding to an FEV_1 of less than 1.25 L), these findings are not always reliable.[48, 49] More objective criteria are therefore needed to assess the severity of asthmatic exacerbations. Generally, serial ABG values are needed to assess the degree of hypoxemia and hypercapnia only in patients with severe exacerbations. During an acute exacerbation of asthma, the typical ABG analysis reveals mild to moderate hypoxemia, hypocapnia, and (therefore) a widened alveolar-arterial O_2 gradient (see the section on $p(A\text{-}a)O_2$). Significant hypoxemia (pO_2 less than 60 mm Hg) usually does not occur unless the FEV_1 is less than 1 L, and hypercapnia usually does not occur until the FEV_1 is less than 0.5 L.[50] Because there are exceptions to these correlations, however, ABG analysis should be performed whenever the patient's clinical situation suggests the need.

Although blood gas analysis helps assess severe exacerbations, it is less helpful in assessing mild to moderate attacks. It is often difficult to decide prospectively which patient has a severe enough exacerbation to warrant a blood gas determination. In 1990, the National Heart, Lung and Blood Institute[51] convened a National Asthma Education Program (NAEP) workshop to present a comprehensive approach for diagnosing and treating asthma. In its recommendations, it stressed that all patients should acquire their own peak flowmeters in an effort to more objectively monitor the severity of their symptoms. During the last 10 years, measurement of expiratory flow rates—FEV_1 and the peak expiratory flow rate (PEFR)—by using portable spirometers or peak flowmeters has helped in the ED assessment and management of acute asthmatic attacks. The NAEP Expert Panel Report[51] categorized the severity of asthma according to measured flow rates. These measurements have been used for deciding therapeutic options (such as adding corticosteroids), as well as for determining the need for hospitalization. Acute asthmatic attacks have been categorized into three stages of severity based on the FEV_1 and PEFR measurements (see Table 10–2).[52] Further-

Table 10–2. Severity of Asthma

	Stage	FEV_1 (L)	PEFR (L/min)	pCO_2 (mm Hg)
Mild	1	2	200	—
Moderate	2	1–2	80–200	—
Severe	3	1	<80	—
	3A	0.75–1.0	60–80	35
	3B	0.75	60	35–45
	3C	Unable to perform	—	>45

more, variations of these measurements are now used for admission and discharge criteria.

Measurements of Expiratory Flow Rates

The most sensitive measurement of airflow is obtained by a pneumotachograph and is usually available only in research laboratories. A simpler clinical approach at the bedside uses a peak flowmeter. The PEFR is defined as the maximal flow that can be sustained for 10 ms during a forced expiration starting from total lung capacity. Normal PEFR ranges from 400 L/min to 800 L/min but is markedly dependent on age, body size, and sex[53, 54] (Table 10–3). When compared with FEV_1, PEFR is more variable and more effort dependent. Patient motivation and cooperation are essential to ensure that a decreased flow rate is not effort related. The mean or best of three determinations (usually after one or two practice attempts) correlates well with the FEV_1.[53–56]

The patient is asked to take a deep breath (inspiration), insert the mouthpiece, and finally, blow into the meter as hard as possible. It is *not* necessary to empty the lungs as is done in a timed vital capacity maneuver. Thus the advantage of measuring PEFR rather than FEV_1 is that it is easier to perform, it is less tiring, and it is less likely to promote dynamic compression of the airways, which may result in a cough and increased obstruction.

Portable peak flowmeters are used frequently in the ED; almost always only the mouthpiece is changed between patients. Shapiro et al.[57] have found that greater than 200 uses lead to deterioration in the accuracy of some peak flowmeters (mini-Wright) but not others (the Assess). Although no known transmission of any disease has been documented, it is probably wise to change the entire flowmeter frequently (not just the disposable mouthpieces). Ideally, a new peak flowmeter should be used for each patient and then given to the patient for home monitoring.

As of mid-1993 there were at least eight different peak flowmeters in widespread clinical use: Wright, mini-Wright, Assess, Personal Best, Vitalograph, Ferraris (also called the Wright Pocket Peak Flow Meter), Spira, and Astech. They appear to be comparable and differ mainly in size and cost. Certain technical differences will be dis-

Table 10–3. Predicted Peak Expiratory Flow Rates

	55 in		60 in		65 in		70 in		75 in		80 in	
Age (yr)	M	F	M	F	M	F	M	F	M	F	M	F
20	—	390	550	420	600	460	650	500	700	530	740	—
30	—	380	530	450	580	450	620	480	660	520	710	—
40	—	370	500	400	550	440	600	470	640	500	680	—
50	—	360	480	490	530	420	570	460	610	490	650	—
60	—	350	460	380	500	410	540	450	580	475	620	—

Modified with permission from Leiner GC, Abramowitz S, Small MJ et al: *Am Rev Respir Dis* 88:644, 1963.

cussed below. Methods are now available for reproducing expiratory flow patterns from computer-driven syringe pumps with a high degree of accuracy. The American Thoracic Society (ATS) has introduced a standard computerized forced expiratory maneuver. Miller et al.[58] demonstrated that several peak flowmeters (mini-Wright, Ferraris, and Vitalograph meters) give reproducible results. However, they were not accurate over the entire range with a significant nonlinearity: overreading by 40 to 80 L/min was found in the midflow range from 300 to 500 L/min, whereas underreading by 30 to 80 L/min was found in the high range above 500 L/min. Similar overestimating of flow rates in the midflow range has been found by Gardner et al.,[59] who studied the three flowmeters cited above as well as the Assess, Spira, and Wright peak flowmeters.

The Wright peak flowmeter has been used since 1959.[60] A circular device about 12.7 cm in diameter and 3.6 cm deep, the meter has a radial inlet nozzle for a disposable mouthpiece. It weighs about 900 g and costs about $450. The meter consists of a rotating vane that drives a clockwork mechanism. Initially closed by the vane, the orifice area is variable. During expiration, the vane is deflected through an angle, which is a function of the rate of flow of air, and the deflection is recorded on the dial in liters per minute. The instrument is calibrated by comparison with a pneumatachograph. The Wright peak flowmeter usually reads lower than the highest value. Because it is bulky and expensive, its use has declined in recent years.

The mini-Wright peak flowmeter, introduced in 1977, is lighter than the standard Wright peak flowmeter and less expensive and is made of plastic rather than metal.[61] It is 15 cm (15 × 18 × 5.3 cm) and consists of a spring piston that slides freely on a rod within the body of the instrument. The piston drives an independent sliding indicator along a slot marked with a scale graduated from 60 to 800 L/min. The indicator records the maximum movement of the piston and remains in that position until manually returned to zero by the operator. The meter should be held horizontally with the air vents uncovered.

Tested by several groups, the mini-Wright peak flowmeter appears to be as accurate as the standard Wright peak flowmeter; values obtained correlate well to flow rates measured by the more sensitive pneumotachograph.[62, 63] However, the meter does have several minor limitations. There appears to be about a 5% intra-instrument variation. In addition, wide fluctuations may occasionally occur and are due to sliding of the plastic indicators independent of engagement of the spring-loaded piston system. This problem may be due to sticking of the membrane caused by mucus and dirt. Subsequent release of the membrane can cause erroneously high readings.[64] Thus peak flowmeters—like spirometers—need periodic calibration.[65, 66] Appropriate cleaning appears to eliminate this problem (detailed instructions are given by the manufacturer). Despite these drawbacks, the cost (about $20 to $30), the ease of handling, the relative accuracy, and the reproducibility make this a valuable tool in the ED.

Several newer peak flowmeters have been designed and tested. One of the meters, the Assess by Healthscan, which has been available for approximately 10 years, has been shown to be extremely accurate, even more so than the mini-Wright peak flowmeter.[67] The increased accuracy may be due to the fact that the Healthscan peak flowmeter operates as a rotameter with airflow directed through a precisely drilled orifice. Two scales are provided together with a removable end piece so that flow ranging from 80 to 520 L/min can be determined. In contrast, the mini-Wright peak flowmeter design uses a single expanding spring to measure flow. Variability of the length-tension relationship for any particular spring will alter the accuracy and reproducibility of the instrument. This peak flowmeter has been economically priced ($18 to $25). The Vitalograph, Ferraris-Wright Pocket Peak Flow Meter, and Astech are the most recent peak flowmeters to became available, and all appear to have a similar degree of accuracy and cost, although clinical experience with these meters is relatively short.[68]

The Wright Pocket Peak Flow Meter uses a flexible vane of tempered steel, fixed at one end, that bends in relation to the patient's exhaled flow rates to move a sliding scale indicator. This vane mechanism avoids the traditional piston and spring design (as do the Assess and Personal Best peak flowmeters), which leads to less wear and fatigue of the meter over time.

FEV_1 Measurements

A simple spirometer measures volume changes during a forced expiration. By measuring the volume expired per unit time the physician can obtain useful information about the presence and degree of airway obstruction. Originally introduced by Tiffeneau and Gaensler 40 years ago, the timed vital capacity in 1 second (FEV_1) has been the standard approach for evaluating airway function, i.e., documenting airway obstruction. Although more recent analysis of maximum expiratory flow rates (the flow-volume loop) has become routine in the pulmonary function laboratory, this more sophisticated test is neither routinely available nor usually necessary in emergency situations. The development of inexpensive, portable spirometers brought these instruments and the FEV_1 measurements to the ED. The plethora of machines that have been introduced during the past decade has required the ATS to provide strict guidelines to manufacturers.[69] Only spirometers conforming to these guidelines should be used.

In performing the timed vital capacity maneuver, patient motivation and cooperation are important. The patient should wear a nose clip, although this may be unrealistic for an acute asthmatic who is dyspneic. Patients are told to take a maximum inspiration, to place their mouth over the mouthpiece leading to the spirometer, and while keeping their lips tightly closed, to blow out as hard and as fast as they can. The procedure should be repeated once or twice to ensure reproducibility (although ATS guidelines suggest that three to seven attempts may be necessary to ensure reproducibility). Volume is recorded by the spirometer at body temperature and ambient pressure, saturated (BTPS). A 1-second time line marks off the desired volume. The observed total volume expired and the volume expired in 1 second are compared with a height- and age-related predicted nomogram. Most modern spirometers are computerized and offer a choice of different predicted values, depending on the patient population.[70] Because flow rates are a function of lung volume, all FEV_1 measurements must be related to the observed total volume expired (i.e., the forced vital capacity [FVC]), which differentiates a reduced FEV_1 in obstructive airways dysfunction from restrictive interstitial, chest wall, or neuromuscular processes. The FEV_1 is recorded as a percentage of FVC (the total volume expired during the maneuver). Values less than 70% to 75% are usually abnormal.

During an asthmatic attack there is a greater proportionate change in flows at small lung volumes than at large volumes. Since the FEV_1 is relatively insensitive to minor changes in flow at low lung volumes, it reflects maximal flow over a wide range of vital capacity and may therefore be more accurate than measurements of peak flow. A reduced peak flow rate may be due to airflow limitation but can also be seen in patients with expiratory muscle weakness and restrictive lung disease. These other conditions are usually apparent. The potential for discrepancy between the FEV_1 and peak flow is probably greatest in patients in the middle of the range of flow rates, with overreading of the PEFR with respect to the FEV_1 in those patients with intermediate and poor function. The major limitation in obtaining FEV_1 measurements in acute asthmatic patients is that the forced expiratory maneuver requires total exhalation of air, which may paradoxically increase air trapping, and create greater discomfort and dysfunction.

ASSESSMENT

Banner et al.[71] suggested that patients require hospitalization if their PEFR value is less than 16% of that predicted and if it remains less than 60 L/min or if there is less than a 16% improvement in the PEFR after a 0.3-mL subcutaneous injection of epinephrine. Nowak et al.[72] demonstrated that patients with an initial FEV_1 value of less than 1 L or a PEFR value of less than 100 L/min usually require hospitalization: if such patients are discharged, they usually relapse. In addition, most patients who have an FEV_1 value less than 1.6 L or a PEFR value less than 250 L/min after treatment have a similar poor outcome.[72, 73] Patients whose FEV_1 values improve by at least 0.4 L or whose PEFR values improve by 100 L/min after bronchodilator treatment can usually be discharged.[72, 73] It appears that the degree of improvement is as important as—if not more important than—the absolute values for flow rates. Thus an increase of 400 mL in a patient with an FEV_1 value of 1 L may be better evidence of improvement than an increase of 200 mL in a patient with an FEV_1 value of 2 L. It should be stressed that some patients require admission despite improved performance on these tests, so these criteria cannot be considered absolute. In addition, at extreme heights (men whose height is greater than 185 cm or less than 155 cm and women whose height is greater than 175 cm or less than 150 cm), the percentage predicted may be more accurate than absolute values for admission or discharge criteria. Thus it is most prudent to require an FEV_1 increment of at least 0.4 L after bronchodilators *as well as* an FEV_1 value greater than 1.5 L (or 40% of predicted) *or* an increase in PEFR by 100 L/min *as well as* a PEFR value greater than 250 L/min (or 40% of predicted).[74] In addition, it should be noted that spirometry and peak flow readings may sometimes underestimate the degree of physiologic recovery. This situation occurs in the case of patients with low FEV_1 values and significant hyperinflation (increased residual volume and total lung capacity). Initial recovery in these patients results in a reduction in residual volume and total lung capacity (decreased airway trapping and hyperinflation). Subsequently, such patients demonstrate improvement in flow rates.

CASE 10–1

A 25-year-old man comes to the ED because of an acute exacerbation of his asthma. An arterial blood gas determination reveals the following values: pH = 7.48, pCO_2 = 28 mm Hg, pO_2 = 75 mm Hg, and HCO_3^- = 23 mEq/L.

Comment.—The A-a gradient calculation is as follows:

$$pAO_2 = FIO_2\,(pB - pH_2O) - \frac{pCO_2}{R}$$

$$= 0.21(760 - 47) - \frac{28}{R}$$

$$= 0.21(713) - 1.25\,(28) = 150 - 35 = 115$$

Therefore,

$$\text{A-a gradient} = 115 - 75 = 40$$

The calculation reveals an abnormally increased gradient, indicating intrinsic lung pathology. Thus, even though this patient had an O_2 Sat of 90% and a mild reduction in pO_2, his gas exchange, revealed by the increased A-a gradient, is markedly abnormal. This condition is typical of an acute asthmatic attack in which bronchospasm and mucous plugging result in V/Q mismatch.

CASE 10–2

A "double overdose" brings two 30-year-old patients to the ED. Both have ingested substantial amounts of barbiturates and diazepam. Blood gases drawn on room air revealed these values: patient 1: pH = 7.18, pCO_2 = 70 mm Hg, pO_2 = 50 mm Hg, and HCO_3^- = 24 mEq/L; patient 2: pH = 7.31, pCO_2 = 50 mm Hg, pO_2 = 50 mm Hg, and HCO_3^- = 25 mEq/L.

Comment.—The A-a gradient calculation for patient 1 is as follows:

$$pAO_2 = FIO_2\,(pB - pH_2O) - \frac{pCO_2}{R}$$

$$= 0.21(760 - 47) - \frac{70}{0.8} = 150 - 88 = 62$$

Therefore,

$$\text{A-a} = 62 - 50 = 12$$

The calculation reveals a normal gradient, indicating that the cause for hypoxemia and hypoventilation is *extrinsic* to the lung itself.

The A-a gradient calculation for patient 2 is as follows:

$$pAO_2 = 0.21(760 - 47) - \frac{50}{0.8} = 150 - 63 = 87$$

Therefore,

$$\text{A-a} = 87 - 50 = 37\text{, an abnormally increased gradient}$$

Thus one can be reasonably confident that patient 1 sustained hypoventilation because of the effect of the ingested drugs on the brain stem. Temporary mechanical ventilation restored this patient's gas exchange. Patient 2, on the other hand, had an increased A-a gradient, indicating a lung problem in addition to any central cause for hypoventilation. The chest radiograph revealed that this patient's overdose was complicated by aspiration pneumonitis and that the patient required treatment with antibiotics in addition to mechanical ventilation.

CASE 10–3

A confused 53-year-old woman is brought by ambulance to the ED. Her husband states that she has a chronic cough and dyspnea on exertion. One week ago, an upper respiratory tract infection (URI) developed. One hour ago, she was oriented and responsive. Blood gas analysis revealed the following values: pH = 7.10, pCO_2 = 95 mm Hg, and pO_2 = 105 mm Hg.

Comment.—The A-a gradient calculation is as follows:

$$pAO_2 = F_IO_2\ (pB - pH_2O) - \frac{pCO_2}{R}$$

$$= 0.21(760 - 47) - 1.25(95) = 31$$

Therefore,

$$A\text{-}a = 31 - 105 = -69$$

The negative A-a gradient is impossible. The above calculation *assumed* an inspired O_2 of 21% (room air). However, this result should be a clue that the patient received oxygen on her way to the ED, which resulted in hypercapnia and disorientation.

CASE 10–4

A 44-year-old tachypneic man arrives in the ED. The chest radiograph reveals that he has a bilateral lower lobe pneumonia. On room air, ABG analysis revealed these values: pH = 7.48, pO_2 = 44 mm Hg, pCO_2 = 29 mm Hg, and HCO_3^- = 24 mEq/L. On 100% oxygen, the ABG determination revealed these values: pH = 7.43, pO_2 = 110 mm Hg, pCO_2 = 30 mm Hg, and HCO_3 = 24 mEq/L.

Comment.—The A-a gradient calculation of the ABG values based on room air is as follows:

$$pAO_2 = F_IO_2\left(pB - \frac{pH_2O}{R}\right) - pCO_2$$

$$= 0.21(760 - 47) - \frac{30}{0.8} = 150 - 1.25(30) = 112$$

Therefore,

$$A\text{-}a = 112 - 44 = 68$$

The calculation based on 100% O_2 is as follows:

$$pAO_2 = 1.0(760 - 47) - \frac{pCO_2}{1^*}$$

$$= 713 - 30 = 683$$

Therefore,

$$A\text{-}a = 683 - 110 = 573$$

The markedly increased $(A\text{-}a)O_2$ gradient suggests that a shunt mechanism is involved.

*NOTE: When the patient is breathing 100% O_2, R is approximately 1 rather than 0.8.

REFERENCES

1. Petty TL, Bigelow DB, Levine BE: The simplicity and safety of arterial puncture, *JAMA* 195:693–695, 1966.
2. Greenhow DE: Incorrect performance of Allen's test—ulnar artery flow erroneously presumed inadequate, *Anesthesiology* 37:356–357, 1972.
3. Centers for Disease Control: Guidelines for prevention of transmission of human immunodeficiency virus and hepatitis B virus to health care and public safety workers. *MWR* 38(suppl 2):95–110, 1989.
4. Henderson DK, Fahey BJ, Willy M et al: Risk for occupational transmission of human immunodeficiency virus type 1 (HIV-1) associated with clinical exposures, *Ann Intern Med* 113:740–746, 1990.
5. Jagger J, Hunt FH, Brand-Elnaggar J, Pearson RD: Rates of needlestick injury caused by various devices in a university hospital, *N Engl J Med* 319:284–288, 1988.
6. Yoshimura H: Effects of anticoagulants on the pH of the blood, *J Biochem (Tokyo)* 22:279–296, 1935.
7. Kelman GR, Nunn JF: Nomograms for correction of blood po_2, pco_2, pH and base excess for time and temperature, *J Appl Physiol* 21:1484–1490, 1966.
8. Foster JM, Terry ML: Studies on the energy metabolism of human leukocytes: I. Oxidative phosphorylation by human leukocyte mitochondria, *Blood* 30:168–175, 1967.
9. Liss HP, Payne CP Jr: Stability of blood gases in ice and at room temperature, *Chest* 103:1120–1122, 1993.
10. Andritsch RF, Muravchick S, Gold MI: Temperature correction of arterial blood gas parameters, *Anesthesiology* 55:311–315, 1981.
11. Raine JM, Bishop JM: A-a difference in O_2 tension and physiologic dead space in a normal man, *J Appl Physiol* 18:284–288, 1983.
12. Sorbini CA, Grassi V, Solinas E, Muisan G: Arterial oxygen tension in relation to age in healthy subjects, *Respiration* 25:3–13, 1968.
13. Severinghaus JW, Honda Y: History of blood gas analysis. VII. Pulse oximetry, *J Clin Monit* 3:135–138, 1987.
14. Welsh JP, DeCesare R, Hess D: Pulse oximetry: instrumentation and clinical applications, *Respir Care* 35:584–601, 1990.
15. Tremper KK, Barker SJ: Pulse oximetry, *Anesthesiology* 70:98–108, 1985.
16. Jones L, Heiselman D, Cannon L et al: Continuous emergency department monitoring of arterial saturation in adult patients with respiratory distress, *Ann Emerg Med* 17:463–468, 1988.
17. Shrake K, Blonshine S, Brown R, et al: AARC Clinical Practical Guidelines: pulse oximetry, *Respir Care* 36:1406–1409, 1991.
18. Eisenkraft JB: Carbon monoxide and pulse oximetry, *Anesthesiology* 68:300, 1988.
19. Barker SJ, Tremper KK: The effects of carbon monoxide inhalation on pulse oximeter signal detection, *Anesthesiology* 67:599–603, 1987.
20. Raemer DB, Elliott WR, Topulos GP, Philip JH: The theoretical effect of carboxyhemoglobin on the pulse oximeter, *J Clin Monit* 5:246–249, 1989.
21. Watch MF, Connor MT, Hing AV: Pulse oximetry in methemoglobinemia, *Am J Dis Child* 143:845–847, 1989.
22. Scheller MS, Unger RJ, Kenler MJ: Effects of intravenously administered dyes on pulse oximetry readings, *Anesthesiology* 65:550–552, 1986.
23. Jubran A, Tobin MJ: Reliability of pulse oximetry in titrating supplemental oxygen therapy in ventilator-dependent patients, *Chest* 97:1420–1425, 1990.
24. Ries AL, Prewitt LM, Johnson JJ: Skin color and ear oximetry, *Chest* 96:287–290, 1989.
25. Cote CJ, Goldstein EA, Fuschsman WH, Hoaglin DC: The effect of nail polish on pulse oximetry, *Anesth Analg* 67:683–686, 1989.
26. Mellengaard K: The alveolar-arterial oxygen difference: its size and components in normal man, *Acta Physiol Scand* 67:10–26, 1966.
27. Benatar SR, Hewlett AM, Nunn JF: The use of iso-shunt lines for control of oxygen therapy, *Br J Anaesth* 45:711–718, 1973.
28. Shapiro AR, Peters PM: A nomogram for planning respiratory therapy, *Chest* 72:197–200, 1977.

29. Hess D, Maxwell C: Which is the best index of oxygenation—$p(A\text{-}a)O_2$, $paCO_2/P_{AO_2}$ or $paCO_2/F_{IO_2}$, *Respir Care* 30:961–963, 1985.
30. Nunn JF: *Applied respiratory physiology,* ed 2, London, 1977, Butterworth, pp 178–212.
31. Hess D: Capnometry and capnography: technical aspects, physiologic aspects, and clinical applications, *Respir Care* 35:557–576, 1990.
32. Gravenstein JS, Paulus DA, Hayes TJ: *Capnography in clinical practice,* Boston, 1989, Butterworths.
33. Weil MH, Bisera J, Trevino RP et al: Cardiac output and end-tidal carbon dioxide, *Crit Care Med* 13:907–909, 1985.
34. Sanders AB, Atlas, M, Ewy GA et al: Expired pCO_2 as an index of coronary perfusion pressure, *Am J Emerg Med* 3:147–149, 1985.
35. Gudipati C, Weil MH, Bisera J et al: *Circulation* Expired carbon dioxide: a noninvasive monitor of cardiopulmonary resuscitation, 77:234–239, 1988.
36. Falk JL, Rackow EC, Weil MH: End-tidal carbon dioxide concentration during cardiopulmonary resuscitation, *N Engl J Med* 318:607–611, 1988.
37. Garnett AR, Ornato JP, Gonzalez ER et al: End-tidal carbon dioxide monitoring during cardiopulmonary resuscitation, *JAMA* 257:512–515, 1987.
38. Sanders AB, Kern KB, Otto CW et al: End-tidal carbon dioxide concentration during cardiopulmonary resuscitation. A prognostic indicator for survival, *JAMA* 262:1347–1351, 1989.
39. Callahan M, Barton C: Prediction of cardiopulmonary resuscitation from end-tidal carbon dioxide concentration, *Crit Care Med* 18:358-362, 1990.
40. Barton C, Callahan M: Lack of correlation between end-tidal carbon dioxide concentrations and $paCO_2$ in cardiac arrest, *Crit Care Med* 19:108–110, 1991.
41. Sayah AJ, Peacock WF, Overton DT: End-tidal CO_2 measurement in the detection of esophageal intubation during cardiac arrest, *Ann Emerg Med* 19:857–860 1990.
42. Garnett AR, Gervin CA, Gasvin AS: Capnographic waveforms in esophageal intubation: effect of carbonated beverages, *Ann Emerg Med* 18:387–390, 1989.
43. Hatle L, Rokseth R: The arterial–to–end-expiratory carbon dioxide tension gradient in acute pulmonary embolism and other cardiopulmonary diseases, *Chest* 66:352–357, 1974.
44. Eriksson L, Wollmer P, Olsson CG et al: Diagnosis of pulmonary embolism based upon alveolar dead space analysis, *Chest* 96:357–362, 1989.
45. Chopin C, Fesard P, Mangalaboyi J et al: Use of capnography in diagnosis of pulmonary embolism during acute respiratory failure of chronic obstructive pulmonary disease, *Crit Care Med* 18:353–357, 1990.
46. McFadden ER, Kiser R, deGroot WJ: Acute bronchial asthma: relations between clinical and physiologic manifestations, *N Engl J Med* 288:221–225, 1973.
47. Rebuck AS, Read J: Assessment and management of severe asthma, *Am J Med* 51:788–798, 1971.
48. Kelsen SG, Ketsen DP, Fleegler BF et al: Emergency room assessment and treatment of patients with acute asthma, *Am J Med* 64:622–628, 1978.
49. Shim C, Williams MH: Pulsus paradoxus in asthma, *Lancet* 1:530–531, 1978.
50. McFadden ER, Lyons HA: Arterial blood gas tensions in asthma, *N Engl J Med* 278:1027–2119, 1968.
51. National Heart, Lung and Blood Institute: *Guidelines for diagnosis and management of asthma,* Pub No 91–3042, NIH, Bethesda, Md, 1991, National Institutes of Health.
52. Snider GL: Staging therapeutic schedules to clinical severity in status asthmaticus. In Weissled EB, ed: *Status asthmaticus,* Baltimore, 1978, University Park Press, pp 152–153.
53. Leiner GC, Abramovitz S, Small MJ et al: Expiratory peak flow rate, *Am Rev Respir Dis* 88:644–651, 1963.
54. Gregg I, Nunn AJ: Peak expiratory flow in normal subjects, *BMJ* 3:282–284, 1973.
55. Rosenblatt G, Alkalay I, McGann et al: The correlation of peak flow rate with maximal expiratory flow rate, one-second forced expiratory volume and maximal breathing capacity, *Am Rev Respir Dis* 87:589–591, 1963.
56. Ritchie B: A comparison of forced expiratory volume and peak flow in clinical practice, *Lancet* 2:271–273, 1962.
57. Shapiro SM, Hendler JM, Ogirala RG et al: An evaluation of the accuracy of Assess and mini-Wright peak flow meters, *Chest* 99:358–362, 1991.

58. Miller MR, Dickinson SA, Hitchings DJ: The accuracy of portable peak flow meters, *Thorax* 47:904–909, 1992.
59. Gardner RM, Grapo RO, Jackson BR et al: Evaluation of accuracy and reproducibility of peak flow meters at 1,400 m, *Chest* 101:948–952, 1992.
60. Wright BM, McKerrow CB: Maximum forced expiratory flow rate as a measure of ventilatory capacity, *BMJ* 2:1041–1047, 1959.
61. Wright BM: A miniature Wright peak-flow meter, *BMJ* 2:1627–1628, 1978.
62. Perks WH, Tams IP, Thompson DA et al: An evaluation of the mini-Wright peak flow meter, *Thorax* 34:79–81, 1979.
63. Levin E, Gold MI: The mini-Wright expiratory peak flow meter, *Can Anaesth Soc J* 28:285–287, 1981.
64. Brown LA, Sly RM: Comparison of mini-Wright and standard Wright peak flow meters, *Ann Allergy* 45:72–74, 1980.
65. Morrill CG, Dickey DW, Weiser PC et al: Calibration and stability of standard and mini-Wright peak flow meters, *Ann Allergy* 46:70–73, 1981.
66. Fisher J, Shaw A: Calibration of same Wright peak flow meters, *Br J Anaesth* 52:46–464, 1980.
67. Eichenhorn MS, Beauchamp RK, Harper PA, Ward JC: An assessment of three portable peak flow meters, *Chest* 82:306–309, 1982.
68. Nolan KM, Dornelly SM, Hughhes DT, Stronin L: Evaluation of the Ferraris pocket peak flow meter for the measurement of peak expiratory flow rate (PEFR) and forced expiratory volume in the first second (FEV_1). *Respir Med* 86:525–526, 1992.
69. Cherniack RM, Chatburn R, Gardner RM et al: *Statement on technical standards for peak flow meters,* Pub No 92–2113a, Bethesda, Md, 1992, National Institutes of Health.
70. Moris JF: Spirometry in the evaluation of pulmonary function, *West J Med* 125:110–111, 1976.
71. Banner AS, Shah RS, Addington WN: Rapid prediction of need for hospitalization in acute asthma, *JAMA* 235:1337–1338, 1976.
72. Nowak SG, Gordon KR, Wroblewski DA, et al: Spirometric evaluation of acute bronchial asthma, *JACEP* 8:9–12, 1979.
73. Nowak RM, Pensler MI, Sarker DD et al: Comparison of peak expiratory flow and FEV_1: admission criteria for acute bronchial asthma, *Ann Emerg Med* 11:64–69, 1982.
74. Wyner P, Myers R, Feldman M, Garay S: Spirometric assessment in acute asthma: a prospective study, *Chest* 82:245, 1982.

Chapter 11

Cardiologic Evaluation

Richard I. Levin, M.D.
Itzhak Kronzon, M.D.

CASE 11–1: HEMODYNAMIC COMPROMISE IN AN ELDERLY MAN

A 73-year-old man was brought to the emergency department (ED) with complaints of chest discomfort and dyspnea. He had been hospitalized for an acute, inferior wall myocardial infarction several weeks before. During that admission he had received thrombolysis, had made an uneventful recovery, and was discharged in an asymptomatic state. Physical examination revealed an anxious, elderly man who was dyspneic and diaphoretic. The pulse was 110 per minute and regular, and his blood pressure was 80/50. No paradoxical pulse was noted. There were no additional physical findings of note. The electrocardiogram (ECG) showed Q waves in leads II, III, and aV_F and was unchanged from his previous admission. A portable chest film revealed apparent cardiomegaly that was not appreciated during his recent hospitalization.

In the presence of an enlarged cardiac silhouette and in the absence of a paradoxical pulse, the physicians considered occult infarct extension or expansion with resultant cardiogenic shock to be a leading diagnostic possibility. Pericardial effusion with "early tamponade" was also considered. The patient received intravenous fluids and inotropic support, and an emergency echocardiogram was requested. A large, intrapericardial echo-free space was clearly visualized (Fig. 11–1), indicative of a probable large pericardial effusion. The addition of Doppler color-coded flow imaging demonstrated a high-velocity jet flowing from the left ventricle into the echo-free space in systole and from the echo-free space back into the left ventricle in diastole (Fig. 11–2). This condition, a small rupture of the free wall of the heart with blood flow into the pericardial sac, defines a pseudoaneurysm and is a surgical emergency. The patient was taken to the operating room, the diagnosis confirmed, the pseudoaneurysm resected, and the myocardial perforation sutured.

This case illustrates the two main themes of this chapter: the key to a diagnosis is almost always embedded in the history, but our extraordinary technology aids immeasurably in extracting it. When primary reliance is placed on technology, however, *instead* of on our clinical skills, the resultant waste of time and resources may be detrimental (or even fatal) to the patient. Moreover, recent evidence suggests that our reliance on technology may have diminished our clinical skills,[1] a concern particularly relevant to the ED where rapid cardiologic treatment requires that initial decisions be based solely on the history.

This chapter describes cardiologic diagnostic tests and techniques useful in the ED setting. In the description of each, we have tried to indicate the circumstances in which the test should be used. Some of the tests can be performed by all physicians,

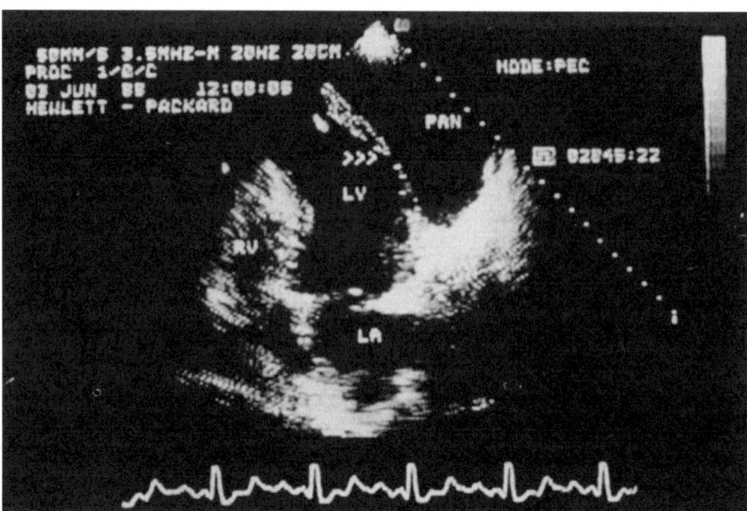

Fig. 11–1. Two-dimensional apical view showing the left ventricle *(LV)* and the large adjacent pseudoaneurysm *(PAN)*. A defect is seen in the lateral left ventricular wall *(arrows)*. *LA*, left atrium; *RV*, right ventricle.

and some require the help of a cardiologist. This review of a very large area of knowledge is necessarily limited, and the reader is referred to several excellent and comprehensive texts for additional information.[2–6]

THE ELECTROCARDIOGRAM

Diagnosis of Ischemic Heart Disease

The ECG remains a standard of care in the evaluation of a patient with chest pain. It should be done as soon as the patient reaches the examining area and while the initial history is being obtained. The standard 12-lead ECG should then be supplemented with continuous ECG monitoring. Despite its "premier status," however, the ECG's diagnostic accuracy for both ischemia and infarction is only fair.[7,8] For example, an ECG obtained while a patient is experiencing chest pain *in unstable angina* has a sensitivity of only 35% and a specificity of 68% for ischemia.[9,10] Sensitivity of the ECG for the diagnosis of acute myocardial infarction ranges from 51% to 80%, and the specificity ranges from 64% to 99% depending on the characteristics of the group studied.[11–13] The extraction of otherwise "invisible" information from the scalar ECG by computerized discriminant analysis may improve the accuracy only slightly[14]; even more sophisticated techniques such as body-surface potential mapping may improve the accuracy close to 100%, but these techniques are currently too impractical for use in the ED. The impact of these data is clear: although the ECG may establish or suggest the diagnosis of acute myocardial infarction, it cannot be used to rule out the diagnosis in the ED. The history prevails again.

The changes in the ECG that may occur during myocardial ischemia and infarctions are listed in Table 11–1 along with some conditions other than ischemia that can induce the same changes. All of the morphologic changes listed here occur in the portion of the tracing occurring after depolarization of the ventricles, i.e., the ST segment and T wave. The ST segment is inscribed during ventricular contraction, during which the state of polarization is unchanging. Therefore the change in amplitude is 0, and the segment is inscribed along the isoelectric line (TP or PR segments). Empirical observations have demonstrated that the ST segment is indeed isoelectric in

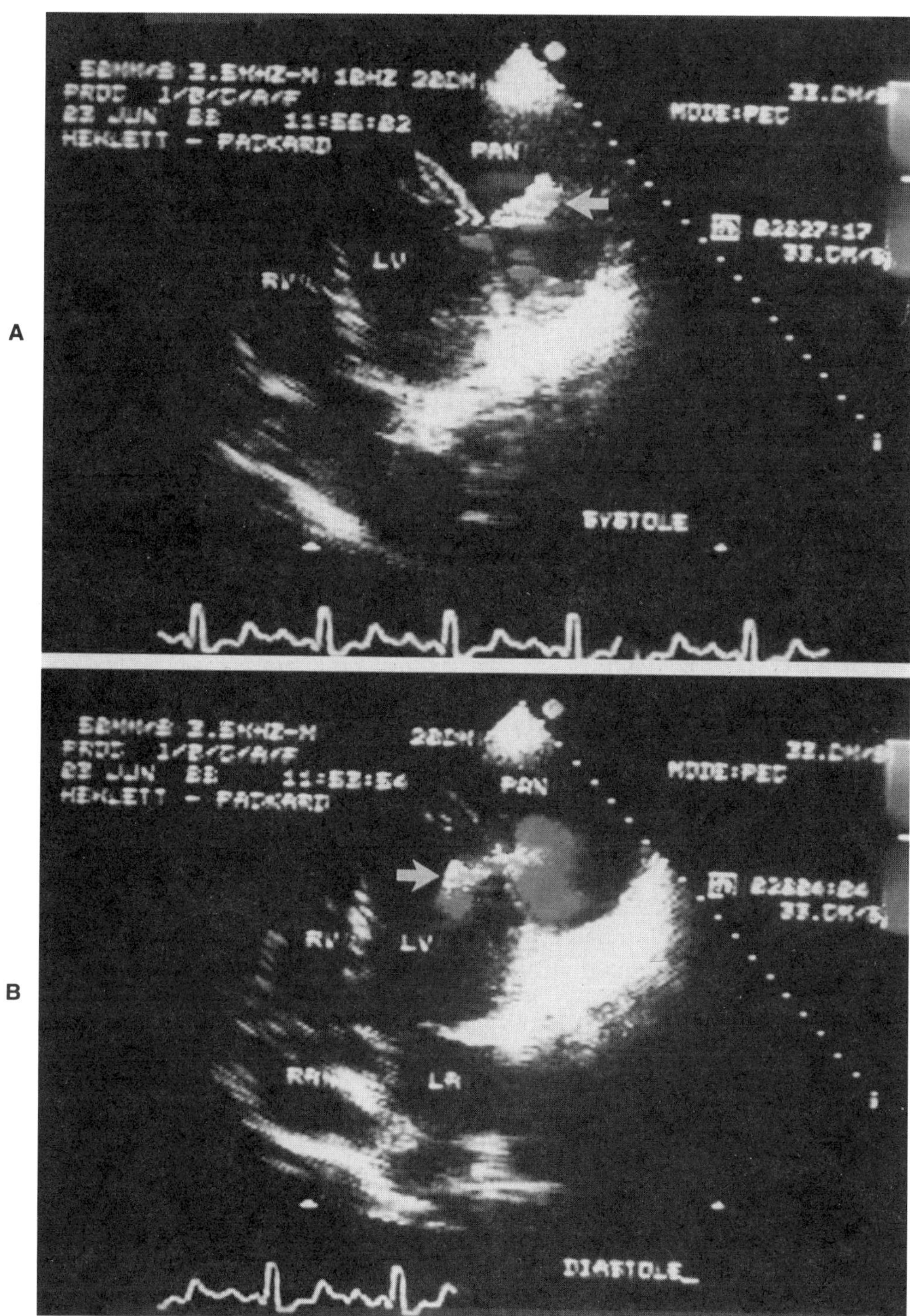

Fig. 11–2. A, Doppler showing a jet of flow into the pseudoaneurysm in systole *(arrows). LV,* left ventricle; *PAN,* pseudoaneurysm; *RV,* right ventricle. **B,** Doppler showing a jet of flow back into the left ventricle from the pseudoaneurysm in diastole *(arrow). LA,* left atrium; *LV,* left ventricle; *RA,* right atrium.

Table 11–1. Electrocardiographic Changes in Myocardial Ischemia

Change	Significance in Ischemia	Differential
Tall T waves	"Hyperacute" change of early MI*	Normal variant, hyperkalemia, intracranial hemorrhage
Inverted T waves	Non–Q-wave MI	Normal variant, Stokes-Adams, posttachycardias, intracranial disease (hemorrhage), pericarditis, mitral valve prolapse, others
ST depression	Myocardial ischemia, non–Q-wave MI	Digitalis effect, acute cor pulmonale
ST elevation	Myocardial ischemia, early infarction	Normal variant, MI, pericarditis, ventricular hypertrophy, others
Nonspecific ST and T changes	Possible ischemia	Normal variant, many others

*MI, myocardial infarction.

the limb leads in approximately 75% of adults; however, in the precordial leads, some ST elevation is present in over 90% of normal individuals.[15] This is one of the causes of the weak diagnostic efficiency of the ECG for myocardial infarction.

Notwithstanding the above statistics, the most widely recognized ECG change due to myocardial ischemia is deviation of the ST segment. This deviation of ischemia is due to complex electrical events, including abnormal resting membrane potential, abnormal depolarization, and repolarization.[16] These changes in turn result in both a "diastolic current" and a "systolic current" that cause a displacement of the ST segment from the isoelectric line.[16] Although it was once thought that classic angina induced *only* ST depression and variant angina induced *only* ST elevation, it is now recognized that depression and elevation can be seen in both and that the type of deviation may vary in the same individual over time.[17] This new understanding of ST deviation is important because ST elevation is also one of the early signs of myocardial infarction. The question then becomes, "does ST elevation represent ischemia or infarction?" If a patient coming to the ED demonstrated ST elevation that disappeared promptly with the relief of pain after nitroglycerin or a calcium channel blocker is administered and no other ECG changes are present, it is very likely that an anginal episode rather than infarction had taken place.

ECG changes present in acute myocardial infarction include alterations of the ST segment, T wave, and QRS complex as well. The sequence of ECG changes that can be seen is shown in Fig. 11–3. It should be noted that there is marked variability in both the time course and the magnitude of these evolutionary changes. Because the average patient with myocardial infarction does not arrive in the ED until 2 hours after the onset of chest pain, the hyperacute T waves, which tend to be transient, may not be seen.[18] Although ST elevation may be seen in a wider area than that in which Q waves develop, the amplitude of the elevation may vary from almost nothing to 10 mm (1.0 mV) or more. The period of time required for the development of the Q wave is also extremely variable (hours to days), but in general, the Q wave begins to develop while the ST segment is still elevated. The Q wave develops because no electrical potential is generated by the dead or dying myocardial cells in the infarct zone. The ECG looks through this electrical "hole" in the myocardium to electrical potential generated by the opposite side of the heart, which is moving in a direction away from the exploring electrode instead of toward it, hence a negative rather than positive deflection.

This same process can result in the loss of R-wave voltage as well. However, there are many causes of small R waves, and therefore the new Q wave remains the single most important ECG sign of myocardial infarction.[19, 20] Even so, Q waves can be due

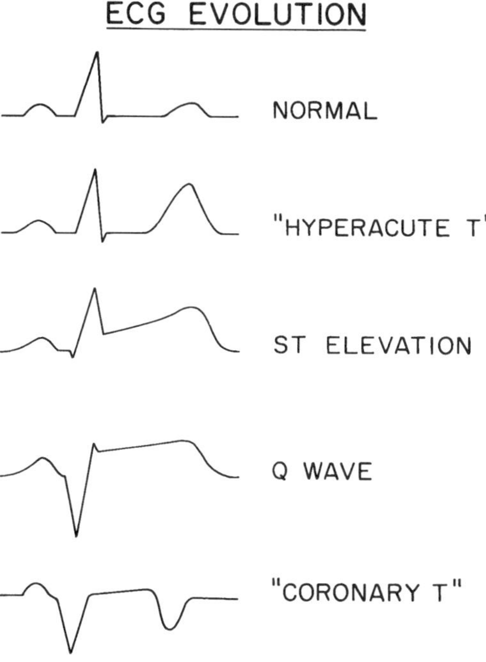

Fig. 11–3. Evolutionary changes in the electrocardiogram in myocardial infarction. The temporal sequence is portrayed from top to bottom. The development of each component is quite variable, and complete evolution may take several days.

to other causes such as cardiac position in the chest, ventricular hypertrophy or strain, idiopathic hypertrophic subaortic stenosis, and conduction abnormalities including the Wolff-Parkinson-White (WPW) syndrome.[21] Therefore, as noted above, the specificity of ECG changes in acute myocardial infarction is much less than 100%.

These issues regarding the ECG have enormous clinical significance. Despite the many causes of ST deviation, including normal variance, the *only* criteria required for administration of a thrombolytic agent in the huge, multicenter trials that have proved the efficacy of thrombolytic drugs were chest pain and ST deviation.[22–30] Nevertheless, in current practice, the physician's time would be better spent relying more on the history to administer definitive therapy than debating the significance of "minor" ECG changes.

There are other modern approaches to the diagnosis of myocardial infarction in the ED that use computerized, statistical analysis.[31–34] Both Pozen and colleagues[32] and Goldman et al.[33] found that the use of an empirically derived logistic function significantly improved the diagnosis of myocardial infarction. Of the nine independent variables described by Pozen et al.,[32] four were ECG related although the most significant factor was historical (i.e., a history of previous myocardial infarction). Such techniques have now been validated in prospective, multicenter studies[35] but have not been widely adopted. Since the methods have been shown to be both diagnostically efficient and cost-effective and computers are ubiquitous, it is not clear why.

Diagnosis of Dysrhythmias and Conduction Blocks

A thorough review of the abnormalities of electrical impulse formation and conduction that can affect the heart is beyond the scope of this chapter. Interested read-ers are referred to the many excellent general cardiology texts or volumes specifically dealing with ECG analysis or dysrhythmias.[36–38] The purpose of this section is therefore to offer a standard approach to the diagnosis of dysrhythmias and to note some of the common problems encountered in the ED.

The threshold for obtaining an ECG should be quite low. Patients who have a history of altered mental status, syncope, chest discomfort, dyspnea, fatigue, and a previous history of cardiac problems and those found to have bradycardia (pulse rate less than 60), tachycardia (pulse rate over 100), or an irregular pulse should have an ECG performed. When a dysrhythmia is in the differential diagnosis, the physician should be present when the ECG is taken so that a variety of diagnostic/therapeutic maneuvers may be instituted while the patient is initially connected to the electrode leads. ECG analysis is a difficult science. It must be approached logically, with attention to each detail of the cardiac cycle in sequence rather than by *gestalt.* A simplified approach to dysrhythmia recognition is demonstrated in Fig. 11–4. This approach is an example of the logical dissection of the information on the ECG to yield specific conclusions about the status of the sinus node, atrioventricular (AV) conduction, and ventricular conduction. It is presented merely as one of many possible systems and is not all-inclusive. Similarly, physicians should recognize their limitations as electrocardiographers and be prepared to consult with available experts when necessary.

Tachycardias

The common tachycardias and some of their distinguishing characteristics are listed in Table 11–2. Sinus tachycardia is seen frequently in the ED and occurs in an extremely wide variety of circumstances, including approximately one third of patients with acute myocardial infarction. There is no specific treatment for sinus tachycardia because its presence generally indicates an appropriate physiologic response to stress. The ventricular rates of all the supraventricular dysrhythmias may overlap, and so, especially at more rapid rates, the type of dysrhythmia may not be distinguishable by standard ECG analysis alone. Although the sawtooth pattern of the baseline in atrial flutter and the irregularly irregular ventricular response in atrial fibrillation are helpful signs, they are not always present.

In dealing with tachycardias, diagnosis and therapy may overlap. In the presence

Table 11–2. Tachydysrhythmias

Tachycardia	Rate	Features
Sinus tachycardia	100–160[a]	A response to stress
PAT, PSVT[b]	140–220[c]	Abnormal P wave, isoelectric PP Regular rhythm Block with digitalis
Atrial flutter	250–350[c]	Undulating "sawtooth" baseline[d] Variable block
Atrial fibrillation	100–180[e]	No P waves, irregularly irregular
Junctional tachycardia	140–220	P wave may be hidden by QRS or T
Ventricular tachycardia	140–200[f]	Regular, AV[b] dissociation Fusion beats, bizarre QRS

[a]Rates up to 200 can be seen in young individuals.
[b]*PAT,* paroxysmal atrial tachycardia; *PSVT,* paroxysmal supraventricular tachycardia; *AV,* atrioventricular.
[c]This is the atrial rate; the ventricular rate depends on whether a block is present.
[d]The sawtooth pattern is seen generally in the inferior leads (II, III, aV_F) and may not be seen at all in other leads.
[e]This refers to the ventricular rate; the atrial rate, if measurable at all, is 400 to 800.
[f]Rates as slow as 100 and as rapid as 280 have been recorded.

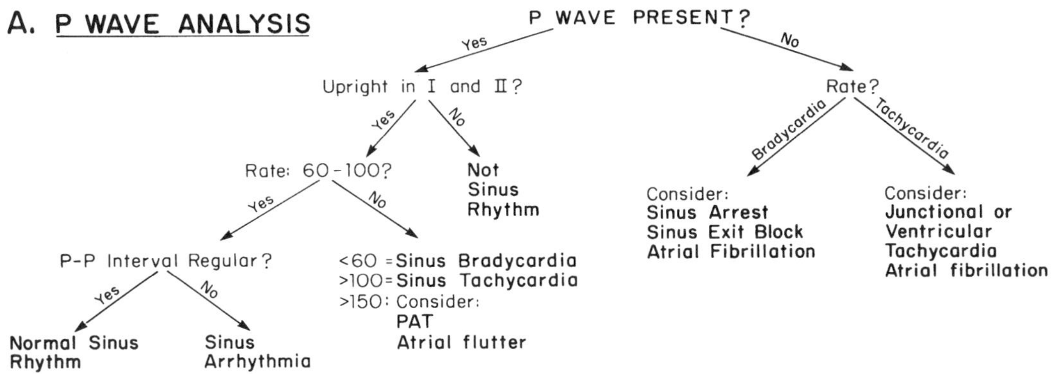

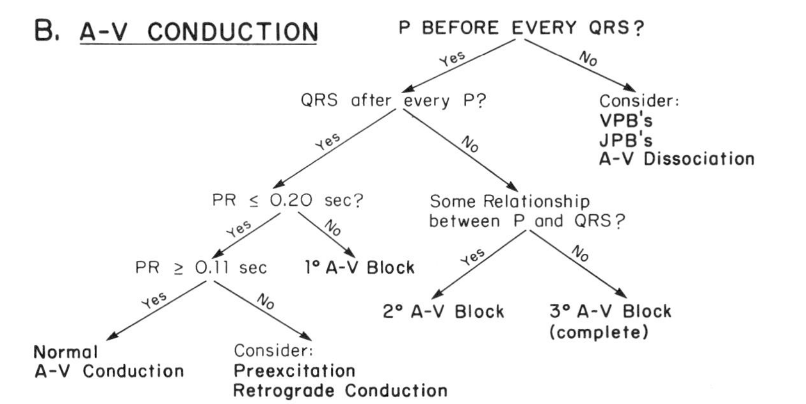

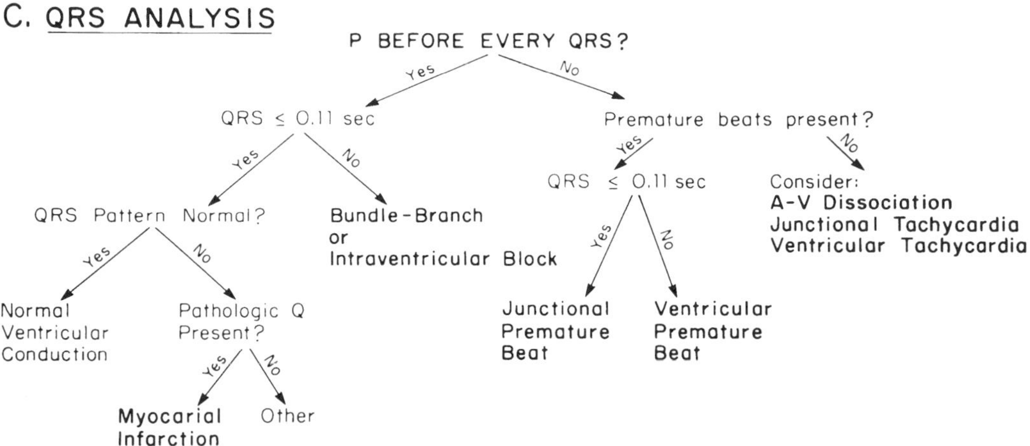

Fig. 11–4. Flow chart for electrocardiographic analysis. Use of these three decision trees allows categorization of the major dysrhythmias. It is neither complete nor applicable in all circumstances. For example, when severe tachycardia is present, it may be impossible to locate P waves even though they are present. *PAT,* paroxysmal atrial tachycardia; *VPB,* ventricular premature beat; *JPB,* junctional premature beat; *A-V,* atrioventricular.

Table 11–3. Response to Vagal Stimulation During Tachycardia

	Response			
Tachycardia	Termination	Transient Slowing	Ventricular Slowing/Increased Block	No Response
Sinus*		+	+/–	
PAT, PSVT†	+		+/–	+
Atrial flutter			+	
Atrial fibrillation				+
Ventricular tachycardia‡				+

*The general response is for transient slowing of the sinus rate while the maneuver is applied; rarely an atrioventricular block is induced and leads to a slower ventricular rate. This latter response is also transient.
†*PAT,* paroxysmal atrial tachycardia; *PSVT,* paroxysmal supraventricular tachycardia.
‡Rare instances of cessation of ventricular tachycardia by vagal maneuvers have been reported. (With permission from Waxman MB et al: Phenylephrine (Neo-Synephrine) terminated ventricular tachycardia, *Circulation* 50:656–664, 1974.)

of myocardial ischemia or infarction and a tachycardia that originates from other than the sinus node, rapid termination is in order. Although many physicians refrain from its use, the quickest and most certain method for termination of many continuous, nonsinus tachycardias is electrical cardioversion.[39] Intravenous injection of adenosine is over 90% effective in terminating paroxysmal supraventricular tachycardia (PSVT)[40–42] and has replaced calcium antagonists or digoxin as the drug of choice for PSVT in the opinion of many experts.

Since both the sinus and AV nodes are richly supplied by the vagus nerve, maneuvers that increase vagal tone will alter tachycardias whose mechanisms involve either of these tissues. Vagal maneuvers may be useful in less urgent circumstances. Table 11–3 presents the expected response of the common tachycardias to vagal maneuvers. As noted, these maneuvers may be therapeutic[43] as well as diagnostic[44] and result in termination of the majority of episodes of PSVT.

Maneuvers that increase vagal tone and can be used in the ED include the Valsalva maneuver, Müller's maneuver (sucking hard on the thumb placed in the mouth), carotid sinus pressure, gagging, the diving reflex (facial immersion in cold water),[45] and the administration of either edrophonium chloride (Tensilon) or metaraminol bitartrate (Aramine). We would recommend that nondrug interventions be attempted first, alone and in combination; if these are unsuccessful, edrophonium or metaraminol can then be used alone and in combination with the physical maneuvers. When multiple approaches including facial immersion are used, these techniques convert perhaps 90% of episodes of PSVT.[43] Many clinicians are unfamiliar with cold water facial immersion, but the technique is quite simple, easily administered, and highly effective. With the patient sitting upright on a stretcher, in bed, or on a chair, an adjustable table is wheeled to rest above the patient's lap. A large bowl is filled with ice-cold water (containing some ice if the patient can tolerate it) and placed in front of the patient. Then the patient is asked to take in a deep breath as though he were about to dive into a pool of water and immerse his face for 30 to 45 seconds. Monitoring is continued throughout the procedure.

Cessation of the tachycardia is characteristically preceded by a slight slowing of the rate, which may not be perceptible on cursory examination of the ECG, and may be followed by a period of asystole or ventricular premature beats (or both) or a short run of ventricular tachycardia.[43, 46, 47] If these maneuvers do not terminate the tachycardia, another ECG response may be noted: as detailed in Table 11–3, transient, progressive slowing of both sinus and ventricular activity with a slow acceleration after release of the vagal maneuver establishes that the tachycardia is sinus in origin. In the case of atrial flutter, vagal maneuvers may increase the AV block that is present. If the ECG has been confusing because of the superimposition of QRS and T waves on

Table 11–4. Bradydysrhythmias

Bradycardia	Rate	Features
Sinus bradycardia*	<60	P:QRS is 1:1
Junctional escape†	35–60	RR constant
Idioventricular†	20–50	QRS is a "ventricular" type; RR is generally constant

*Sinus bradycardia is common during sleep and a variety of other conditions that require no therapy.
†The presence of either of these rhythms indicates the failure of higher pacemakers to fire or to conduct adequately. The junctional beat generally has a normal-appearing QRS, but the QRS of idioventricular rhythm resembles a ventricular premature beat.

the P wave, one can then observe the unobscured flutter waves and make the diagnosis. Thus, vagal maneuvers may be extremely useful diagnostically and therapeutically when treating tachycardias.

Bradycardias

Bradycardias are seen less commonly in a general ED than tachycardias, but they may be equally serious and symptomatic. Several common bradycardias are listed in Table 11–4. Sinus bradycardia is common in athletes and others during sleep. In the elderly, rates above 50 generally need not be treated; however, rates below 50, especially in the setting of ongoing myocardial ischemia, may require treatment.[39] Any condition associated with increased vagal tone may transiently induce sufficient sinus slowing, or AV block, so that one of two escape rhythms, junctional or idioventricular, will occur. In the setting of an acute viral illness with nausea and emesis, the bradycardia will disappear as the acute illness subsides. However, patients who have primary complaints of syncope, presyncope, or fatigue and who demonstrate junctional or idioventricular rhythms may have serious cardiac disease and may require temporary or permanent pacemakers as part of their therapy.

Table 11–5. Atrioventricular Block

Degree	Characteristics
1st	PR > 0.20 sec P:QRS is 1:1
2nd Mobitz type I (Wenckebach phenomenon)	PR lengthens and RR shortens* until P is blocked P:QRS > 1:1 (3:2, 4:3, etc.)
Mobitz type II	PR not variable Intermittent blocking of the P wave P:QRS > 1:1 (2:1, etc.)
3rd (complete)	Ventricles are *completely* independent of the atria† P:QRS depends on independent rates of atria and ventricles

*Generally there is progressive lengthening of the PR interval before the dropped beat, but such absolute order need not be seen.
†In general, the atrial rate will be faster than the ventricular rate. If the ventricular rate is faster, atrioventricular dissociation may be present without complete heart block also being present.

Atrioventricular Block

AV block need not result in bradycardia or symptoms but may require therapy if symptomatic or if the block occurs during myocardial infarction—a condition that has been reported to occur in up to 20% of cases.[48] The classification of AV block is shown in Table 11–5. The circumstance in which these blocks are seen determines the therapy. Furthermore, the rhythms may be quite confusing; expert opinion may be needed.

Intraventricular Block

The final category of block is intraventricular. This category includes left and right bundle-branch block, left anterior and posterior hemiblocks, and combinations of these, as well as diffuse intraventricular blocks distal to the bundle branches. It is beyond the scope of this review to discuss these blocks and their implications, so the reader is again referred to standard texts.[36–38]

Wolf-Parkinson-White Syndrome and J Wave

Two additional ECG findings require some discussion. The first is the WPW syndrome, an interesting condition in which an abnormal electrical pathway exists between the atria and the ventricles that allows the AV node and its timing functions to be bypassed. The bypass tract allows an abnormal excitation of ventricular muscle to occur earlier than would occur if the signal traveled the normal route through the AV node and specialized conduction system. This "preexcitation" results in distinctive ECG findings that are shown diagrammatically in Fig. 11–5. Because the extra pathway bypasses the physiologic delay of the AV node, the PR interval becomes shortened. Further, because the ventricular muscle is stimulated abnormally by the early signal, the first portion of the QRS complex is slurred as the signal spreads slowly through muscle rather than rapidly by way of the His-Purkinje system; the result is a delta wave (see Fig. 11–5). In turn, the abnormal ventricular depolarization results in abnormal repolarization as reflected in ST-segment and T-wave abnormalities.

The importance of recognizing this anomaly is the understanding that extremely rapid tachycardias may occur and that their therapy may be difficult. In particular, atrial fibrillation can be life-threatening because the bypass tract may allow the ventricular rate to rise to intolerable levels and result in acute cardiac failure or ventricular fibrillation.[49] Digitalis, which for many physicians is the drug of choice for slowing the ventricular response in atrial fibrillation, may paradoxially *speed* the rate of ventricular firing in WPW syndrome and thus result in ventricular fibrillation.[50, 51] Cardioversion, the group 1 antidysrhythmics, β-blockers, and amiodarone may be help-

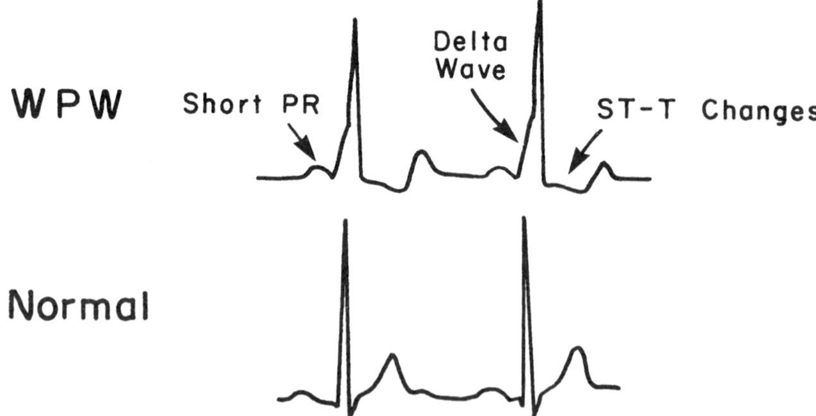

Fig. 11–5. Electrocardiographic findings in Wolff-Parkinson-White syndrome *(WPW)*. An aberrant conduction pathway between the atria and ventricles results in "preexcitation" of the ventricular muscle, which causes (1) a shortening of the PR interval; (2) an abnormal, slow, initial wave of ventricular depolarization, the delta wave; and (3) secondary ST and T-wave changes.

ful in the ED,[52–56] but surgical or radio-frequency ablation of the bypass tract may be required for long-term management.[57–59]

The second ECG manifestation particularly relevant to the ED is the J wave, which is a broad wave that occurs between the QRS complex and ST segment in patients with hypothermia and body temperatures below approximately 25° C.[60] This morphologic change can be confused with bundle-branch or intraventricular block, but it disappears completely on rewarming.

BLOOD STUDIES

Analysis of the components of blood is not a "cardiovascular" test, but a determination of the levels of certain enzymes and elements may be critical to complete evaluation of a cardiac patient.

Serum Enzymes and Isoenzymes in Myocardial Ischemia and Infarction

There are three criteria that generally allow the unequivocal diagnosis of acute myocardial infarction to be made: chest pain, a positive ECG, and elevated cardiac enzyme levels. The last may be the most sensitive antemortem test available. The release of enzymes from the myocardium appears to be a specific marker of cell death, and only the most sensitive tests for these proteins become positive in unstable angina or in prolonged, transmural ischemia.[61–63] Therefore, their presence in elevated concentrations in the blood indicates death of myocardium. Furthermore, each enzyme, on the basis of molecular weight and other characteristics, has unique times of first appearance, peak activity, and duration of release. Thus by making serial measurements from the time of admission through the fourth day of hospitalization, the clinician can map the pattern of release and the absolute level of the enzyme as further validations of the hypothesis that an infarction has occurred.

Many enzymes show elevated activity in the serum after myocardial infarction,[64] but three have become the standards for the diagnosis. Creatine kinase (CK) is the first to be elevated in the serum at 2 to 3 hours after the onset of chest pain. It reaches a peak at approximately 24 hours and returns to normal in 3 to 5 days.[65] Because the MB isoenzyme of CK is found in highest concentration in the heart,[66] elevation of CK-MB levels is the most accurate test for myocardial damage.[12, 13, 61, 66–68] Aspartate aminotransferase (AST, [serum glutamic-oxaloacetic transaminase—SGOT]) is the second enzyme whose levels become elevated 6 to 12 hours after infarction. It peaks at 18 to 36 hours and returns to normal in 3 to 5 days. Lactate dehydrogenase (LDH) activity rises above normal in 12 to 48 hours, reaches a peak in 2 to 6 days, and returns to normal after 1 to 2 weeks. There are five isoenzymes of LDH. The heart contains primarily LDH_1; however, red blood cells are also rich in this isoenzyme, and so caution must be exercised in order to prevent hemolysis during venipuncture and a consequent false positive assay. Normally, LDH_2 has greater activity in the serum than LDH_1. The ratio reverses, however, in myocardial infarction; therefore, an $LDH_1:LDH_2$ ratio greater than 1 (an "LDH flip") is highly suggestive of infarction.[69] From a practical and cost-efficient perspective, measuring CK-MB levels alone at admission and 12 to 24 hours later supplemented by LDH measurements for admissions greater than 12 hours after onset provides all the diagnostic efficiency necessary.[70]

Recently, the field of enzyme analysis has advanced on several fronts, which makes the tests more important and useful in the ED. All of the enzymes require at least 2 hours to become elevated in the serum after the onset of chest pain during myocardial infarction. Since this is approximately the time that it usually takes a patient with an acute infarction to arrive in the ED, a sensitive test should allow a definitive diag-

Table 11–6. Effect of Electrolyte Abnormalities on the Electrocardiogram

Electrolyte	ECG Findings
Hyperkalemia	Tall peaked T waves QRS widens ST elevation
Hypokalemia	Small T wave; prominent U wave QRS may widen (rare) ST depression
Hypercalcemia	Shortening of the QT_c*
Hypocalcemia	Prolongation of the QT_c
Hypernatremia	No changes noted
Hyponatremia	No changes noted

*QT_c, QT interval corrected for the heart rate.

nosis very quickly. The assays for the key enzymes were previously assays of catalytic activity. Rapid assays for the actual concentration or mass of CK-MB are now available, and they are equal to if not more accurate than the traditional activity assays and should allow a definitive diagnosis in the ED.[67, 71, 72] An extremely sensitive enzyme-linked immunosorbent assay (ELISA) for the sarcomeric component troponin T has recently been reported to have a diagnostic efficiency for infarction greater than CK-MB with an appearance time at least as rapid.[63] Unfortunately, it may be positive in "unstable angina" as well. The implication is interesting and has long been suspected by many: the syndrome of unstable angina includes death of myocardium, and therefore the syndrome could be classified as a miniinfarction. As such extremely sensitive assays become available, the current classification of ischemia and infarction will necessarily change.

Electrolyte Abnormalities

Electrolyte imbalance can cause a variety of abnormal states that might result in an ED visit by the patient. Because the generation of the ECG tracing is dependent on normal electrolyte concentrations, alterations from normal will result in specific ECG changes (Table 11–6). The most striking changes occur in the case of hyperkalemia. Above 5.5 mEq/L, the T wave becomes tall; above 6.5 mEq/L, the QRS complex begins to widen.[73] The QRS complex may become so wide that only a continuous sine wave pattern appears. In the case of severe hyperkalemia, an AV block of any variety may occur. Ventricular standstill, tachycardia, or fibrillation may be the cause of death. The other electrolyte imbalances do not present as striking morphologic changes in the ECG and may also be less dangerous. A variety of dysrhythmias may be seen in the case of hypokalemia, including paroxysmal atrial tachycardia (PAT), AV block, and ventricular ectopy; however, these are much more likely to occur when digitalis is present than when hypokalemia exists by itself.

Hematocrit

An occasionally overlooked cause for tachycardia or worsening angina is anemia. A patient, especially if elderly, who has nonspecific complaints or complaints of worsening angina or congestive heart failure and an unexplained tachycardia should have a hematocrit determination. We have seen many examples in which pallor was not recognized, the hematocrit was not obtained, and the results were disastrous.

CHEST RADIOGRAPHY

In Chapters 18 and 19, Drs. Rosen et al. discuss the indications for and the selection of appropriate views for chest radiography in the ED, and we will not discuss this important topic further. We wish to merely emphasize that the chest x-ray film is most helpful in cardiovascular diagnosis when the physician is attempting to determine the cause of acute dyspnea. The differentiation of chronic obstructive pulmonary disease from congestive heart failure or pericardial disease can be difficult to make on the basis of historical and physical diagnostic criteria alone. Fortunately, the radiographic patterns in these diseases are quite different.

HEMODYNAMIC MEASUREMENT WITH THE PULMONARY ARTERY CATHETER

Cardiac catheterization has belonged to the armamentarium of clinical cardiology since Dr. Forssman's experiments on himself in 1929. The experience that has accumulated during the ensuing years has enabled cardiologists to measure intracardiac pressures, transvalvular gradients, intracardiac blood flow, and a variety of other indices of cardiac function. With the addition of angiography, it has become possible to accurately diagnose a wide range of congenital and acquired heart disease.

Cardiac catheterization requires trained and skilled personnel and expensive and complicated equipment, however. In the late 1960s, Swan, Ganz, and Forrester[74] of Cedars-Sinai Hospital in California introduced a soft balloon-tipped catheter that could be inserted through a peripheral vein and advanced to the right atrium. When the balloon is inflated in the right atrium, the catheter becomes flow directed and can easily be manipulated into the pulmonary artery and to a pulmonary "wedge" position. Because the pressure at the catheter tip can be measured continuously during its positioning, the catheter can be monitored and manipulated without the aid of fluoroscopy. Once in place, the balloon is usually deflated and its tip left in the pulmonary artery for continuous hemodynamic monitoring.

In the case of an acutely ill patient who comes to the ED, pulmonary artery (Swan-Ganz) catheterization can be used for diagnosis, determination of prognosis, and hemodynamic monitoring to evaluate the patient's cardiovascular status and response to therapy.

Diagnosis

Diagnosis of cardiovascular catastrophes may be extremely difficult. Common, easily obtained physical findings may sometimes be nonspecific, even misleading. For example, a hypotensive patient with myocardial infarction and findings of bibasalar rales may be hypovolemic. These findings of pulmonary congestion, which may be confirmed by chest radiographs, may lag behind an improving hemodynamic status that can change rapidly. Hemodynamic measurements in this example would clearly demonstrate the actual state of hydration.

The state of hydration (preload) is reflected in the measurement of left ventricular filling pressure or left ventricular end-diastolic pressure (LVEDP), which is done indirectly by recording the "pulmonary artery wedge" (PAW) pressure. In the absence of mitral valve obstruction, PAW pressure equals diastolic left atrial pressure, which in turn approximately equals diastolic left ventricular pressure. Table 11–7 lists normal measurements that can be obtained by the pulmonary artery (Swan-Ganz) catheter; Fig. 11–6 depicts the normal pressure patterns.

Pulmonary artery (Swan-Ganz) catheterization is performed by inserting the catheter percutaneously and advancing it from the right atrium across the tricuspid valve

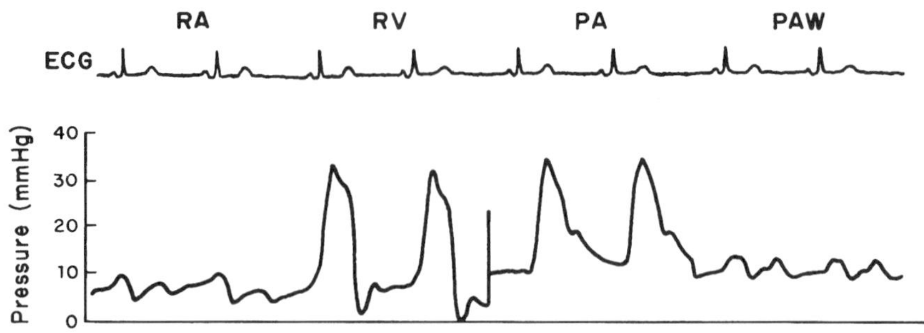

Fig. 11–6. Pressure curves obtained with the pulmonary artery catheter. The pulmonary artery wedge *(PAW)* pressure is generally an excellent reflection of the left ventricular end-diastolic pressure *(LVEDP)*, even in the presence of severe elevations of the pulmonary vascular resistance. *ECG*, electrocardiogram; *RA*, right atrium; *RV*, right ventricle; *PA*, pulmonary artery.

to the right ventricle and then to the pulmonary artery and into the wedge position. Modifications of the catheter, including the addition of a second lumen, an oximetry probe, and a pacing wire allow, respectively, a determination of cardiac output by thermodilution, the status of oxygen delivery to the tissues, and emergency pacing as well.

To determine cardiac output by thermodilution, a chilled solution (usually saline) is rapidly injected into the right atrium and temperature change is determined by a small temperature transducer located at the catheter tip, which changes its electrical resistance as a function of the change in temperature. The chilled solution becomes thoroughly mixed with the blood by the time it reaches the pulmonary artery. The extent of the mixing determines the increase in temperature of the injectate and depends on the volume of blood "added" to the iced saline. The higher the cardiac output, the closer the mixture's temperature to blood temperature. The determination of output can be repeated frequently within short periods of time; it is reproducible and reliable and compares favorably with other more elaborate techniques. Currently available equipment permits the results to be digitally displayed within seconds after injection.

The cardiac index, stroke volume, stroke volume index, and systemic vascular resistance can then be calculated easily according to the following formulas:

$$\text{Cardiac index} = \frac{\text{Cardiac output}}{\text{Body surface area}}$$

$$\text{Stroke volume} = \frac{\text{Cardiac output}}{\text{Heart rate}}$$

$$\text{Stroke volume index} = \frac{\text{Cardiac index}}{\text{Heart rate}}$$

$$\text{Systemic vascular resistance} = \frac{\text{Mean arterial pressure} - \text{Right atrial pressure}}{\text{Cardiac output}}$$

Although right-sided pressures most often reflect left-sided pressure and although elevation of left ventricular diastolic pressure and left atrial pressure frequently causes elevation of pulmonary artery and right ventricular systolic pressure, it is not uncommon that a cardiopulmonary, hemodynamic catastrophe may selectively "attack" one side of the heart. Hemodynamic measurements can clearly distinguish between situations that mainly affect the left ventricle, the right ventricle, or both. In addition, the

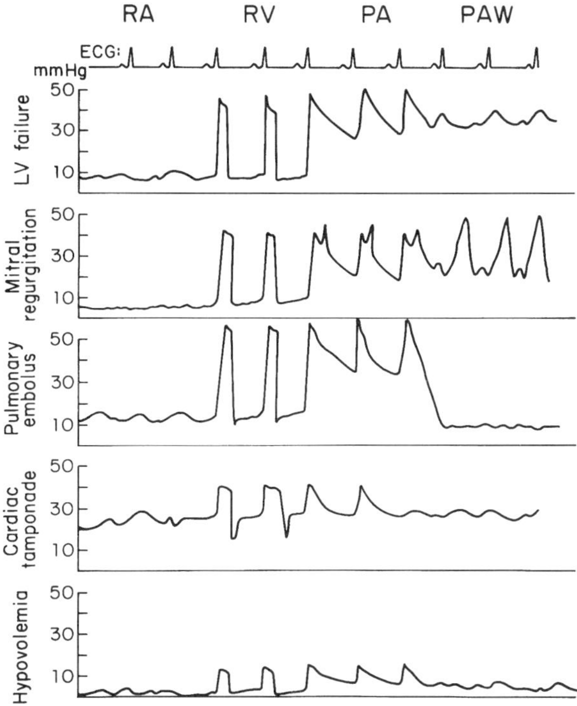

Fig. 11–7. Abnormal pressure curves obtained with the pulmonary artery catheter. Abbreviations are as in Fig. 11–6; *LV*, left ventricle.

diagnosis of such complications of myocardial infarction as mitral regurgitation or ventricular septal defect can be made easily.

The pressure patterns seen in a variety of pathologic states are displayed in Fig. 11–7. The first panel demonstrates the findings in the case of left ventricular failure. This pattern is seen most frequently in cases due to coronary artery disease and less frequently in those due to cardiomyopathy, infiltrative left ventricular disease, and myocarditis; it is usually associated with an elevated LVEDP and therefore an elevated PAW pressure. In the case of mitral regurgitation (Fig. 11–7), there is a marked elevation of left atrial pressure during systole, which gives a characteristically tall CV wave. In contrast, patients who have primarily a right ventricular disorder show isolated elevated right ventricular pressures. The right atrial pressure is accordingly also elevated. The most common cause for right ventricular failure is left ventricular failure.

Table 11–7. Normal Hemodynamic Measurements

Site	Pressure (mm Hg)			
Right atrium	a = 2–7	c = 1–6	v = 2–8	Mean = 0–6
Right ventricle	15–25/0–6			
Pulmonary artery	15–25/4–13			Mean = 9–20
Pulmonary artery wedge	a = 4–16		v = 5–20	Mean = 4–13
Cardiac index = 2.5–3.5 L/min/m²				
Pulmonary vascular resistance = 0.5–2.0 clinical units				
Systemic resistance* = 11–22 clinical units				

*Arterial pressure recording is required. The systemic resistance is calculated as

$$\text{Systemic resistance} = \frac{\text{Mean arterial pressure} - \text{Mean right atrial pressure}}{\text{Cardiac output}}.$$

a, c, v = refer to waves visualized in a continuous recording of pressure versus time in the identified chamber

Table 11–8. Differential Diagnosis of Cardiac Catastrophes by Pulmonary Artery (Swan-Ganz) Catheterization

	Pressures (mm Hg)*			
Condition	RA	RV	PA	PAW
Normal	Mean, 0–6	15–25/0–6	15–25/4–13	Mean, 4–13
Left ventricular failure‡	↑ or →‡	↑/↑ or ↑	↑/↑	↑ ↑
Right ventricular failure (pulmonary disease)	↑ ↑	↑ ↑/↑ ↑	↑ ↑/↑ ↑	→
Right ventricular infarction	↑ ↑	↑ or →/↑ ↑	↑ or →/→	→
Cardiac tamponade§	↑ ↑	↑ or →/↑ ↑	↑ or →/↑	↑ ↑
Hypovolemia	↓	↓	↓	↓

**RA,* right atrium; *RV,* right ventricle; *PA,* pulmonary artery; *PAW,* pulmonary artery wedge.
‡↑, elevated; ↑ ↑, markedly elevated; ↓, decreased; →, unchanged.
†Prominent "CV" wave in mitral regurgitation.
§In cardiac tamponade, all diastolic pressures are equal and elevated (PAW = diastolic pulmonary artery = right ventricular diastolic pressure = right atrial pressure).

In patients with lung disease or pulmonary obstruction to blood flow (e.g., cor pulmonale or acute pulmonary embolus), however, the pulmonary artery pressure is elevated, whereas the left atrial pressure (pulmonary artery *wedge* pressure) may still be within normal limits. (Fig. 11–7 demonstrates these discordant effects of a pulmonary embolus.)

The hemodynamics of right ventricular infarction have been understood only during the last decade. This disorder, usually associated with acute inferior wall infarction, may manifest itself with distended neck veins and a shock-like syndrome. Right heart catheterization shows elevated right ventricular diastolic pressure, frequently with normal or low PAW pressure. This condition of right ventricular pump failure due to infarction should be treated by volume replacement; when diagnosed and properly treated, it carries a much better prognosis than shock due to left ventricular pump failure.

In the case of cardiac tamponade, when the entire heart is encased and compressed by pericardial fluid under high pressure, all diastolic pressures are high and equal to the intracardiac diastolic pressure. Right-sided catheterization therefore shows an elevated PAW pressure that equals (or is within 5 mm Hg of) the elevated right atrial pressure. Both ventricular diastolic pressures are elevated and have the characteristic shape of a dip and a plateau (Fig. 11–7). In the case of hypovolemia, on the other hand, all diastolic pressures are low. Thus the differential diagnosis of a patient with clinical signs of diminished cardiac output or congestive heart failure (with or without severe hypotension) can be clearly distinguished by right heart catheterization. Some relatively common cardiopulmonary catastrophes that can be diagnosed with the Swan-Ganz catheter are summarized in Table 11–8.

Prognosis

The determination of cardiac output is an extremely important and reliable factor in the prognostic evaluation of patients with acute cardiac disorders. When the cardiac index is above 2 L/min/m^2, the probability of survival is quite high. However, when this value falls below 1.5 L/min/m^2, survival probability drops below 30%. Very low cardiac indices (1 L/min/m^2 or less) are associated with death within a short period. Decreased cardiac output is a much more sensitive indicator for determining the prognosis than are other parameters frequently used such as blood pressure, heart rate, physical findings of rales over the lungs, and other indications of heart failure. Even when other clinical findings are lacking, a diminished cardiac output due to any cause may lead to an ominous outcome and require aggressive therapy.

Indications for Pulmonary Artery (Swan-Ganz) Catheterization

Complications of a myocardial infarction*
- Hypotension
- Congestive heart failure (pulmonary edema or right ventricular infarction)
- Signs of low cardiac output
- New murmur
- Mitral regurgitation
- Ventricular septal defect

Cardiac tamponade
Hypovolemia
Pulmonary embolization with complications (hypotension, congestive heart failure)
Adult respiratory distress syndrome (ARDS)
Gram-negative sepsis
Drug intoxication
Acute renal failure

*Each of these items may be an indication even in the absence of infarction.

Evaluation of Therapy

In the past, therapy was mainly given to correct abnormal physical findings. Thus vasopressors were prescribed for hypotensive patients and digitalis and diuretics for patients with findings of congestive heart failure. Modern management of a patient with acute, severe, hemodynamic abnormalities requires accurate knowledge of all hemodynamic parameters, including ventricular preload (filling pressure or LVEDP) and afterload, as well as frequent determination of cardiac output. Attempts should be made to keep the LVEDP near the optimum (approximately 18 mm Hg) and the cardiac index as close to normal as possible. Improvement in cardiac index can often be obtained by the use of vasodilators, which decrease peripheral vascular resistance, the major determinant of left ventricular afterload. Hypovolemia requires volume replacement. The accurate fine-tuning of preload and afterload by using pulmonary artery (Swan-Ganz) catheterization in conjunction with medications, solutions, and mechanical devices to obtain the best cardiac output in an acutely ill patient is the hallmark of state-of-the-art therapy. (See the accompanying box for a list of indications for the use of hemodynamic monitoring and Table 11–9 for a selection of diagnostic tests for cardiac emergencies.)

As a final comment on the pulmonary artery catheter, it should be noted that there is substantial controversy about the use of this technique.[75–79] Although its effectiveness in several small well-defined groups of patients is clear,[75–77] its effectiveness in reducing mortality in the general population of the critically ill has never been determined prospectively or adequately[77–79]; at least one regulatory agency has called for severe restrictions on its use.[79] The pulmonary artery catheter allows the physician to "see" the hemodynamic problem quantitatively, but such quantification may not help the patient. Its current widespread use cannot be condemned, but it will likely be limited and focused in the future.

ECHOCARDIOGRAPHY

The most prominent technological cardiovascular achievement during the last two decades has been the creation of noninvasive methods for obtaining accurate infor-

Table 11–9. Selection of Diagnostic Tests for Cardiac Emergencies*

	Test†							
	ECG		PA Cath		TTE		TEE	
Condition	Sens	Spec	Sens	Spec	Sens	Spec	Sens	Spec
Myocardial infarction	+++	++	0	0	+++	+	+++	+
Mitral regurgitation	0	0	++	+	+++	+++¶§	++++	++++
Aortic insufficiency	0	0	+	0	+++	+++¶§	++++	++++
VSD	++	0	++++	+++	++++	+++¶	+++	+++
Tamponade	+	0	+++	+++	++++	++¶	+++	++
Dissection	0	0	0	0	++	++	++++	++++¶
Pulmonary embolus¶‖	+	+	++	+	+	+	++	++
Prosthetic dysfunction	0	0	+	+	++	++¶§	+++	+++

*Shown is the relative usefulness in the ED of each test for *diagnosing* the condition listed.
†*ECG,* electrocardiogram; *PA Cath,* pulmonary artery catheterization; *TTE,* transthoracic echocardiogram; *TEE,* transesophageal echocardiogram; *Sens,* sensitivity; *Spec,* specificity; *VSD,* ventricular septal defect.
¶Indicates the test of choice.
§TTE should be used first, and if the diagnosis is not clear, then TEE should be performed.
‖All of the tests listed here are ancillary to the performance of arterial blood gas analysis, ventilation-perfusion scanning, and arteriography.

mation about cardiac anatomy and function.[80] The one method among these techniques most readily available to the ED is echocardiography, where its application, as demonstrated by Case 11–1, can be lifesaving.

Echocardiography is now widely used in emergency cardiology. This test, noninvasive and harmless, can provide rapid bedside evaluation of cardiac anatomy, physiology, and pathology. With a transducer placed on the chest wall, high-frequency (2 to 5 mHz) sound waves that are reflected from cardiac interfaces can provide superb two-dimensional multiplanar tomographic imaging of all cardiac structures. Within a short period of time (usually 10 to 20 minutes) information can be obtained about the size of each cardiac chamber, the thickness and motion of each wall, the anatomy (or pathoanatomy) of each valve, and the condition of the proximal part of the great vessels as well as the pericardium and its contents.

Most commercial diagnostic systems now also have the capability for Doppler echocardiography. There are several Doppler modalities; each of them measures and displays flow velocity. *Pulsed Doppler* can evaluate flow velocity at any given point within the heart. Although it has excellent depth resolution, i.e., it describes blood flow velocity patterns at a particular spot and a particular depth, it cannot measure high flow velocity such as that across a markedly stenosed aortic valve. In contrast, *continuous-wave Doppler* can measure high flow velocity and provide flow information along the entire path of the interrogating beam, but it lacks depth resolution. Finally, *color Doppler* provides instantaneous *imaging* of blood flow velocity in the entire imaging field. In most commercial units, blood flowing toward the transducer appears red whereas blood flowing away from the transducer appears blue. Turbulent flow such as that seen across a stenosed or regurgitant valve has a mosaic pattern. In most units, the higher the velocity, the brighter the color. The color-coded image of blood flow velocities is displayed simultaneously with the two-dimensional echocardiographic structural image. These images can be evaluated directly on the diagnostic unit screen and can be recorded on videotape for further evaluation and analysis.

Transesophageal echocardiography (TEE) is the newest addition to the technology.[81] An echocardiographic probe is mounted on a gastroscope and is inserted through the mouth and placed in the esophagus, just behind the heart. The juxtaposition of the esophagus and the heart provides a superb window for evaluation of the heart, especially its posterior aspect. This image is not masked or shadowed by struc-

Indications for Transesophageal Echocardiography in the Emergency Department

Suspicion of aortic dissection.

Suspicion of prosthetic valve dysfunction in patients with acute congestive heart failure.

When a cardiac source of embolization is suspected and the diagnosis cannot be established by transthoracic echocardiography.

Patients with acute cardiac symptoms when echocardiography is essential for the diagnosis (transesophageal echocardiography may be indicated if the transthoracic echocardiogram is not of diagnostic quality)

tures that interfere with the path of the ultrasound beam such as bone or lung, and the higher frequencies available (5 to 7.5 mHz) provide higher-resolution images. This test is "semiinvasive" and should be used only when indicated as discussed in the accompanying box.

Evaluation of Patients with Chest Pain

Although the history, physical examination, and ECG are frequently sufficient to establish the cause of chest pain, as described earlier in this chapter they may be completely inconclusive. Evaluation of the heart by echocardiography can confirm the clinical diagnosis and can clarify the nature of the pain when the clinical approach alone cannot.

Ischemic Heart Disease

One of the first manifestations of myocardial ischemia is an abnormality of motion of the affected wall.[82] An ischemic wall fails to thicken normally during systole and later fails to move normally. The pattern of contraction may be diminished *(hypokinetic)*, absent *(akinetic)*, or bulging *(dyskinetic)*. In the temporal sequence of abnormalities associated with myocardial ischemia, wall motion abnormalities precede both ECG changes and pain. The echocardiographic demonstration of abnormal wall motion is especially helpful in patients with possible ischemic chest pain and abnormal ECG tracings that prevent the diagnosis of ischemia (e.g., left ventricular hypertrophy). In contrast, patients who have normal wall motion during chest pain are very unlikely to be suffering from myocardial ischemia.[83] Finally, the extent and degree of wall motion abnormality are valuable in determining the prognosis of patients with myocardial ischemia and myocardial infarction.

Acute Pericarditis

Echocardiography can demonstrate with high diagnostic efficiency an echo-free space around the heart, which is pathognomonic of pericardial effusion[84] (Fig. 11–8). In addition, the echocardiographic examination can demonstrate the quantity of the effusion and its hemodynamic sequelae, such as impending or extant cardiac tamponade.[85] Echodense signals from within the effusion suggest the presence of fibrin or pus, whereas echolucent signals suggest simple transudates.[86] The thickness of the pericardium can also be evaluated.

Aortic Dissection

The diagnosis of aortic dissection is always a challenge in the ED. Confirmation previously required expensive, cumbersome, and potentially dangerous technologies such as computed tomographic (CT) scanning, magnetic resonance imaging (MRI), or

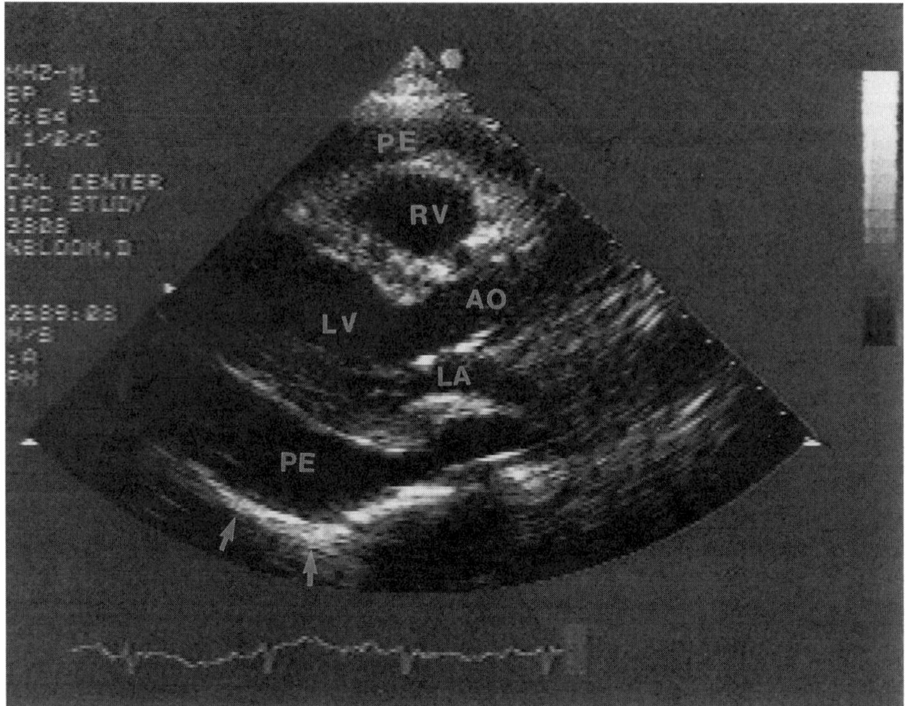

Fig. 11–8. Two-dimensional long-axis view from a patient with pericarditis. Moderately large pericardial effusion *(PE)* is noted behind as well as in front of the heart. The bright pericardial echoes are marked by arrows. *RV,* right ventricle; *AO,* aorta; *LV,* left ventricle; *LA,* left atrium.

angiography. Echocardiography is now the test of choice. Routine transthoracic echocardiograms may show dissections of the aortic root, but viewing of the aortic arch and the descending aorta is difficult and of low sensitivity. TEE, on the other hand is extremely sensitive and specific in this diagnosis.[87] It can clearly demonstrate the intimal flap, the intimal tear, and with color Doppler, blood flow within the true and false lumen (Fig. 11–9). Color Doppler can also demonstrate associated aortic insufficiency when present. Although MRI rivals TEE in diagnostic efficiency, TEE is considered the technique of choice for the diagnosis of dissection because it can be performed at the bedside.

Pulmonary Embolism

The pain of a large pulmonary embolus may be indistinguishable from that of myocardial ischemia. TEE can demonstrate clots within the main pulmonary artery or its main branches (Fig. 11–10) and changes secondary to the embolus such as acute right ventricular dilatation, and evidence of acute pulmonary hypertension (using Doppler echocardiography) may also be demonstrated.[88, 89] Occasionally echocardiography can actually reveal blood clots traveling through the right heart chambers. In the setting of severe hemodynamic compromise, specific thrombolytic therapy may be initiated on the basis of TEE demonstration of clots within the pulmonary artery.

Evaluation of Acute Congestive Heart Failure

Shortness of breath is a common ED finding that may be due to myriad diseases and may indicate a life-threatening condition. The differential diagnosis includes left-sided valvular dysfunction and left ventricular dysfunction, and the echocardiogram

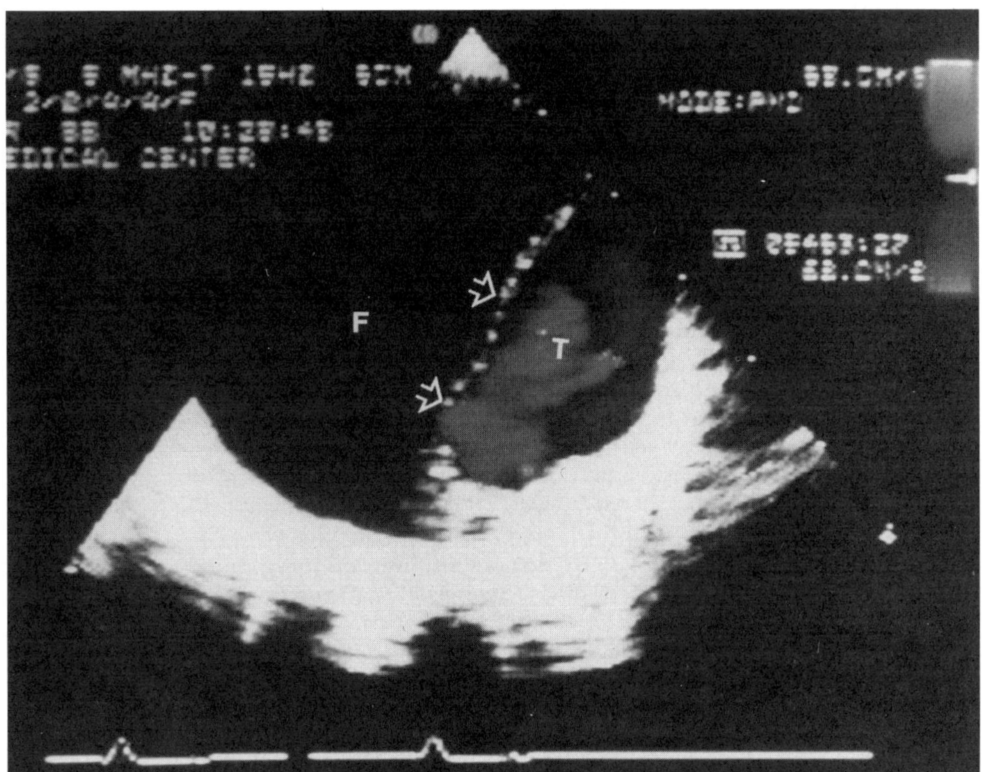

Fig. 11–9. Transesophageal echocardiogram in aortic dissection. The intimal flap *(arrows)* separates the true lumen *(T)* from the false lumen *(F)*.

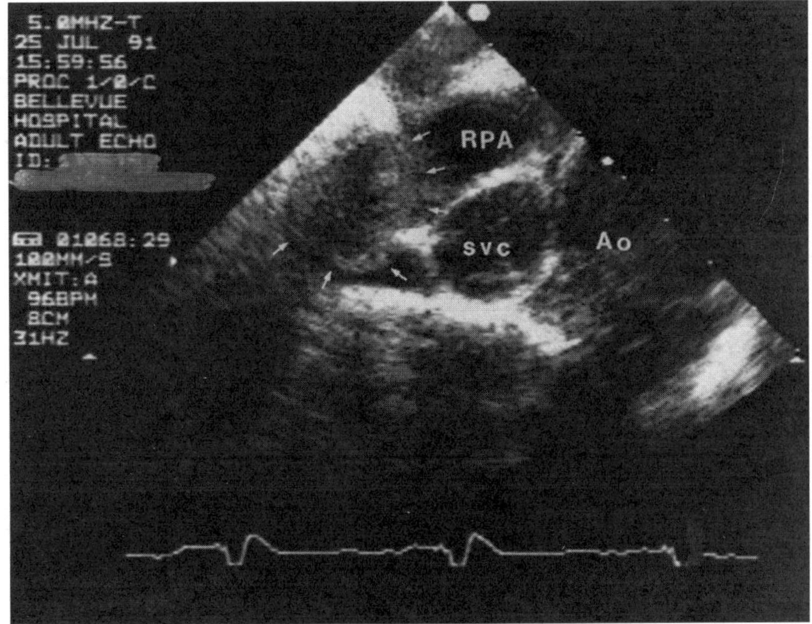

Fig. 11–10. Transesophageal echocardiogram in pulmonary embolus. The embolus lodged in the right pulmonary artery is outlined by arrows. *RPA,* right pulmonary artery; *SVC,* superior vena cava; *Ao,* aorta.

offers remarkable discriminating ability between these two. A brief case history may be illustrative.

CASE 11–2: ACUTE BREATHLESSNESS IN AN ELDERLY WOMAN

A 62-year-old female was told of a heart murmur in childhood but was asymptomatic until a few weeks before when she noted some shortness of breath on exertion. She was examined by her physician who found mild congestive heart failure and prescribed salt restriction, digoxin, 0.25 mg daily, and furosemide, 40 mg daily. The patient's symptoms then increased, and she was rushed to the ED with severe shortness of breath. On admission, she was markedly dyspneic. The pulse was 130 per minute and regular, and the blood pressure was 110/80 mm Hg. Auscultation of the lungs revealed rales bilaterally well up both posterior lung fields. There was a loud systolic murmur audible along the left sternal border. The murmur was also audible at the apex but did not radiate to the carotids. ECG revealed sinus tachycardia and left ventricular hypertrophy. Portable chest radiography suggested pulmonary venous congestion and mild interstitial edema. The cardiac silhouette was only mildly enlarged, with a configuration suggestive of left ventricular dilatation.

The patient was treated with oxygen and intravenous furosemide, 40 mg. Thirty minutes later, the shortness of breath increased markedly and frank pulmonary edema developed. An additional 40 mg of furosemide and 3 mg of morphine sulfate were administered, and an infusion of nitroprusside was begun. Pulmonary edema persisted in spite of rotating tourniquets, and ultimately a phlebotomy of 400 mL was performed. An echocardiogram was then recorded (Fig. 11–11). This study revealed a normal-sized left ventricle. There was marked asymmetrical left ventricular hypertrophy with a septal thickness of 22 mm and a posterior wall thickness of 13 mm. The left ventricular cavity was small and the wall motion markedly

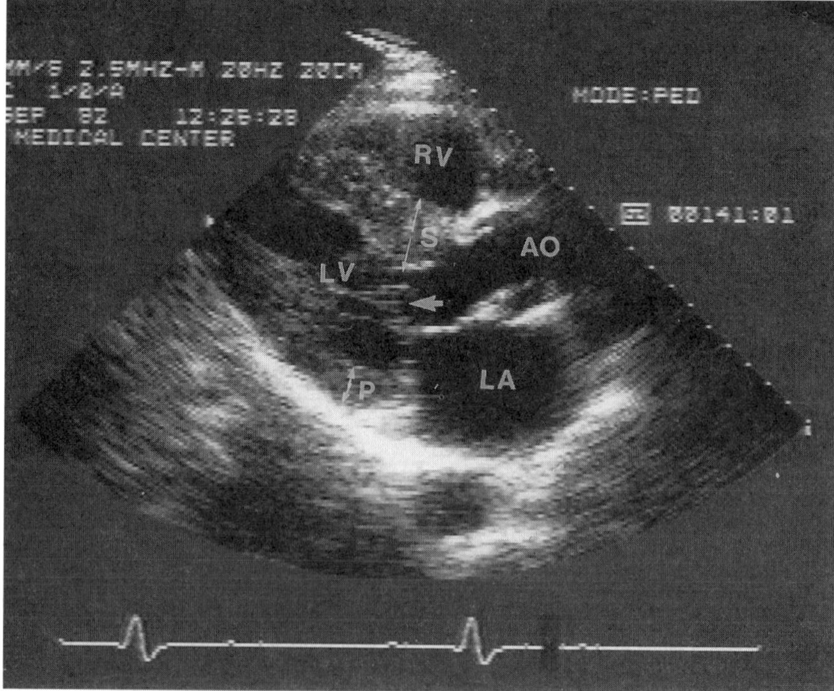

Fig. 11–11. Two-dimensional echocardiogram (systolic frame) in hypertrophic cardiomyopathy. Note that the hypertrophic septum *(S)* is much thicker than the posterior wall *(P)*. Abnormal systolic anterior motion of the anterior mitral leaflet obstructs the left ventricular *(LV)* outflow tract *(arrow)*. *RV,* right ventricle; *AO,* aorta; *LA,* left atrium.

hyperkinetic with cavity obliteration. The mitral valve opened normally in diastole, but there was abnormal systolic anterior motion of the anterior mitral leaflet that achieved coaptation with the septum throughout most of systole. Doppler echocardiography showed evidence of severe left ventricular outflow tract obstruction as well as evidence of severe mitral regurgitation. The echocardiographic and clinical diagnosis was idiopathic hypertrophic subaortic stenosis with secondary, severe mitral regurgitation.

Obviously, the problem with this patient was not left ventricular systolic dysfunction. The left ventricle was hyperkinetic, and the cavity size was small. A relatively narrow left ventricular outflow tract, when associated with higher than normal blood flow velocity in this region, causes systolic anterior motion of the anterior mitral leaflet by the venturi effect. This results in left ventricular outflow tract obstruction and, because of failure of the mitral leaflets to coapt fully in systole, mitral regurgitation. Mitral regurgitation in turn leads to diminished afterload and therefore even more vigorous left ventricular contraction that results in higher flow velocity across the left ventricular outflow tract, more systolic anterior motion of the anterior mitral leaflet, more obstruction, and more mitral regurgitation. This cycle continues and is accelerated by any therapeutic maneuvers that either increase left ventricular contractility or diminish left ventricular size. Inotropic agents, diuretics, vasodilators, or maneuvers that cause hypovolemia (such as phlebotomy or rotating tourniquets) are in fact contraindicated in this condition. Echocardiography revealed the true nature of the underlying pathology of this patient with congestive heart failure and resulted in an immediate change in therapy to β- and calcium blockade to decrease contractility and thereby diminish left ventricular outflow tract obstruction.

This case is an uncommon but dramatic example of how echocardiography can be essential in correctly identifying the cause of acute shortness of breath. We will now consider the more common cardiac causes of acute shortness of breath that may be diagnosed in the ED with echocardiography.

Mitral Stenosis

Mitral stenosis may induce acute and sometimes unexpected pulmonary edema. Characteristic auscultatory findings may be absent or difficult to hear because of the noise created by labored respiration or pulmonary edema. The ECG may show nonspecific changes and may not be contributory. Echocardiography is diagnostic (Fig. 11–12). It shows the narrow mitral orifice, the area of which can actually be planimetered in a diastolic frame in the short-axis view. The fused commissures are seen. The anterior mitral leaflet bows as it reaches its maximal opening, and the smaller posterior leaflet that is attached to the anterior leaflet by the fused commissures has abnormal anterior motion during valve opening.[90, 91]

Doppler echocardiography demonstrates increased flow velocity across a narrow mitral orifice.[92] Measurement of flow velocity across the valve provides the transmitral gradient as calculated by the simplified Bernoulli formula $\Delta P = 4V^2$, where ΔP is the pressure gradient between the left atrium and the left ventricle (in mm Hg) and V is the flow velocity across the valve (in m/sec). The pressure gradient across the stenosed mitral valve decays slowly. Obviously, the narrower the mitral orifice, the longer it will take to equalize the pressures of the left atrium and the left ventricle. This rate of pressure gradient decay is therefore inversely related to the mitral valve area, and the mitral valve area can thus be calculated from the Doppler spectral signal.[93] Therefore, in a patient with acute shortness of breath, echocardiography not only diagnoses mitral stenosis with practically 100% accuracy but also quantifies the magnitude of the mitral valve gradient and the mitral valve area and demonstrates associated lesions such as left atrial dilatation, left atrial clots, or mitral regurgitation.

A

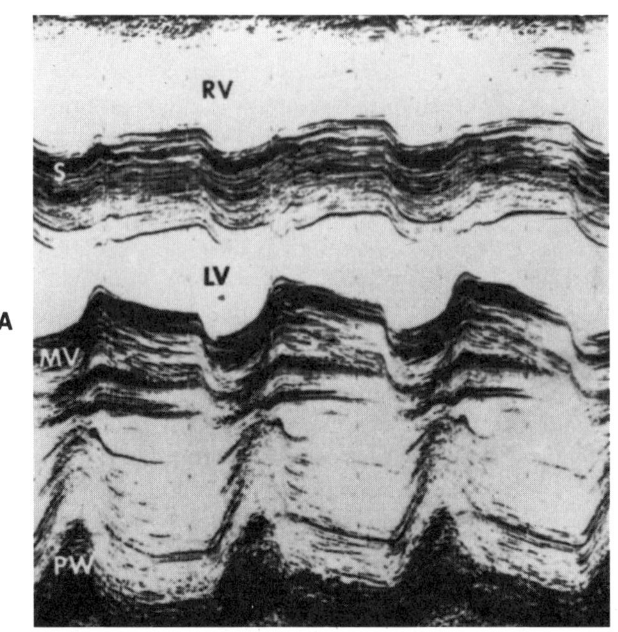

B

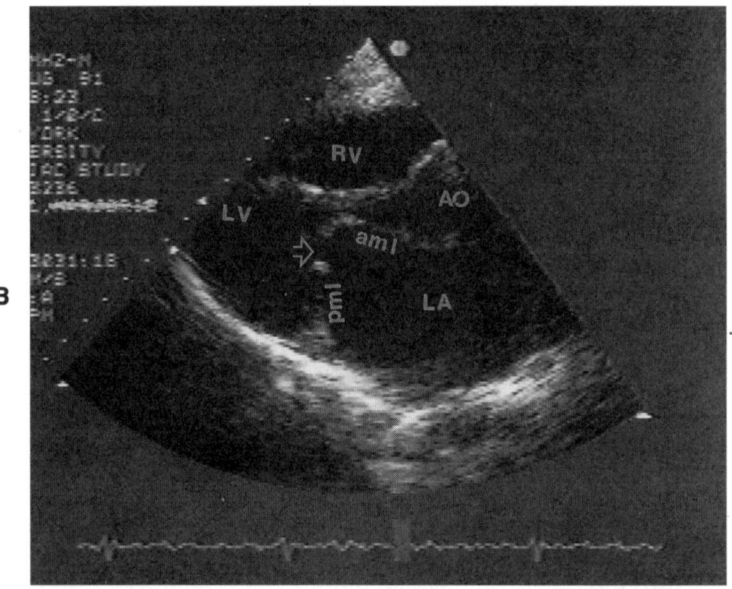

C

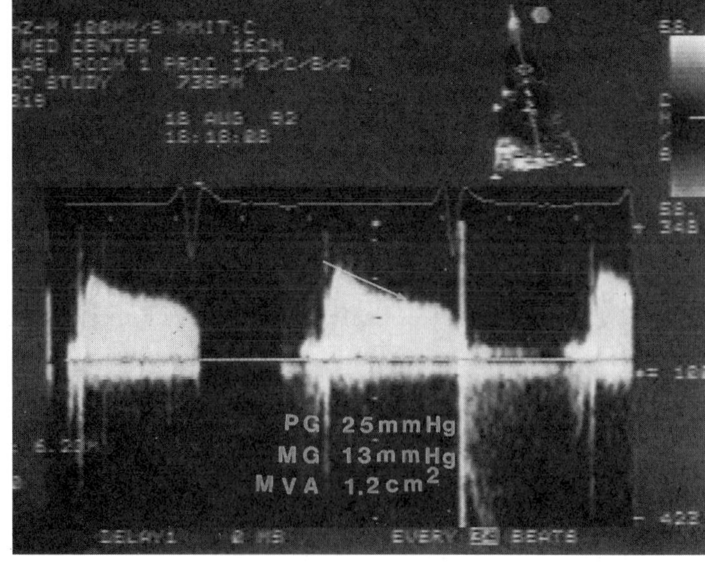

Mitral Regurgitation

Acute mitral regurgitation is usually the result of valve destruction that may be secondary to valvular perforation, chordal rupture, or papillary muscle disruption. Whereas the first two are usually secondary to endocarditis or trauma, papillary muscle disruption is usually secondary to papillary muscle infarction. In fact, this is the one example in which a very small myocardial infarction, *sometimes less than 1% of the myocardium,* may create acute, life-threatening mitral regurgitation. Since the left atrium is not prepared and therefore not preconditioned for the sudden, huge volume of blood transmitted across the destroyed mitral valve with each systole, there is a marked elevation of left atrial pressure that decreases the systolic gradient between the left ventricle and the left atrium. Because of this diminished gradient, the characteristic mitral regurgitation murmur may be absent or faint. When present, the murmur is frequently masked by noises created by labored respiration and pulmonary edema.

Echocardiography is extremely useful in this situation (Fig. 11–13). It can precisely show mitral valve pathology including vegetations, perforations, flail leaflet, or ruptured papillary muscle.[94–96] Doppler echocardiography also clearly demonstrates the regurgitant jet and can be used to quantify the severity of regurgitation. Usually the wider the jet and the larger the jet area, the more severe the mitral regurgitation.[97] Associated lesions such as left ventricular dilatation and left atrial dilatation (less impressive in acute than in chronic mitral regurgitation) can also be evaluated. In selected cases, TEE may be required to better evaluate the details of the mitral valve and better demonstrate the jet of mitral regurgitation.

Aortic Regurgitation

Aortic regurgitation may also be responsible for acute congestive heart failure. Most commonly, chronic aortic regurgitation leads to left ventricular dysfunction and symptoms that may range from mild shortness of breath to frank pulmonary edema. Occasionally, these symptoms may start suddenly because of acute aortic regurgitation. The causes include destruction of the aortic valve by bacterial endocarditis, blunt or penetrating trauma, aortic dissection, or spontaneous rupture of a defective valve, most frequently due to myxomatous degeneration.

In each case, the diagnosis of acute aortic regurgitation may not be apparent since the auscultatory findings as well as the peripheral signs of aortic insufficiency may be absent or difficult to detect. This is because the markedly elevated left ventricular diastolic pressure may decrease the diastolic pressure gradient between the aorta and the left ventricle and thus the intensity of the murmur may be diminished or completely inaudible. High left ventricular diastolic pressure may abolish the low diastolic pressure in the aorta as well and thus diminish the characteristic wide pulse pressure of aortic insufficiency.

Echocardiography may delineate the abnormality that led to aortic insufficiency. It can easily evaluate the aortic root and diagnose aortic valve vegetation and pro-

---

Fig. 11–12. Echocardiography in mitral stenosis. **A,** M-mode echocardiography shows a thickened mitral valve *(MV)* diminished EF slope, and abnormal diastolic anterior motion of the posterior mitral leaflet. *RV,* right ventricle; *S,* septum; *LV,* left ventricle; *PW,* posterior wall. **B,** Two-dimensional echocardiography (diastolic frame) reveals characteristic "bowing" of the anterior mitral leaflet *(aml).* The posterior leaflet *(pml)* is pushed forward because of function of the commisures. The mitral orifice is small *(arrow).* The left atrium *(LA)* is dilated. *AO,* aorta. **C,** Doppler echocardiography allows the calculation of the peak *(PG)* and mean *(MG)* gradients across the stenotic mitral valve. The rate of pressure gradient equalization is reduced *(arrow).* The mitral valve area *(MVA)* was calculated from the "pressure half time" (the time required for the LA-LV pressure gradient to reach its half maximal value).

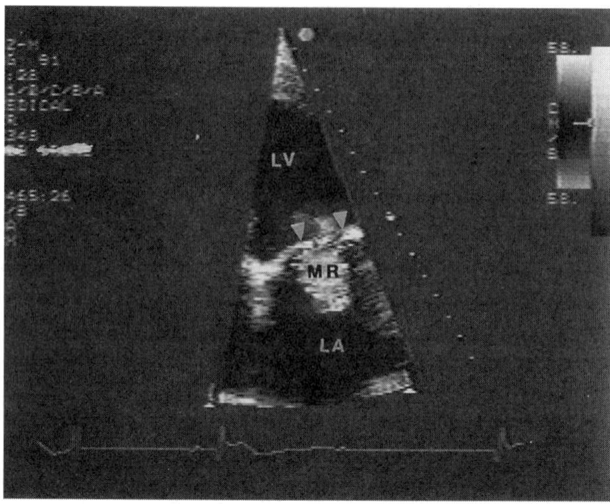

Fig. 11–13. Apical two-dimensional echocardiogram (systolic frame) in mitral regurgitation. The mitral valve *(arrows)* is thickened. The left atrium *(LA)* is dilated. A jet of mitral regurgitation *(MR)* is clearly depicted. *LV,* left ventricle.

lapsed or flail aortic cusps.[98] As described earlier, dissection of the ascending aorta is frequently identified by regular transthoracic echocardiography, whereas the degree of extension to the aortic arch and descending thoracic aorta can be better evaluated by TEE. The degree of aortic regurgitation can be readily assessed by the Doppler technique,[99] and the size and function of the left ventricle can be evaluated (Fig. 11–14). Clinical decisions about the mode of therapy can be based on the results of the echocardiographic examination.[100] Although many patients will require an emergency operation, others may be treated medically.

Acute Prosthetic Valve Dysfunction

Acute prosthetic valve dysfunction is becoming a more common reason for sudden acute congestive heart failure. Bioprostheses are prone to calcification and gradual stenosis that frequently occur within a decade after valve replacement. Bioprosthesis leaflet rupture is also a complication that is not uncommon; it may lead to acute valvular insufficiency with a syndrome very similar to acute mitral or acute aortic insufficiency. Endocarditis is a common complication that may lead to destruction of valvular and perivalvular tissue; in turn, these may lead to acute valvular regurgitation and severe congestive heart failure. Mechanical valves may break or disintegrate. Moving disks or balls may stick because of thrombosis or panus formation in an open position or in an almost closed position and lead to severe, sometimes acute valvular regurgitation or stenosis. In both cases, severe, acute congestive heart failure may be the initial clinical finding. Endocarditis and paravalvular abscesses with fistula formation may frequently lead to further valve destruction, dehiscence, and perivalvular leak.

Although routine, transthoracic echocardiography may frequently demonstrate the pathology that caused prosthetic valve dysfunction and Doppler echocardiography can demonstrate both valvular stenosis and regurgitation,[101] we emphasize that TEE is superior to transthoracic echocardiography in the evaluation of most forms of mitral prosthetic dysfunction.[102] In these cases, the metallic part of the prosthetic material shadows the posteriorly located left atrium, and thus structures and blood flows behind the valve cannot be evaluated with an echo beam originating on the anterior surface of the chest. Important findings such as clots or vegetations and also the jet of mitral regurgitation may not be depicted. TEE, on the other hand, is performed

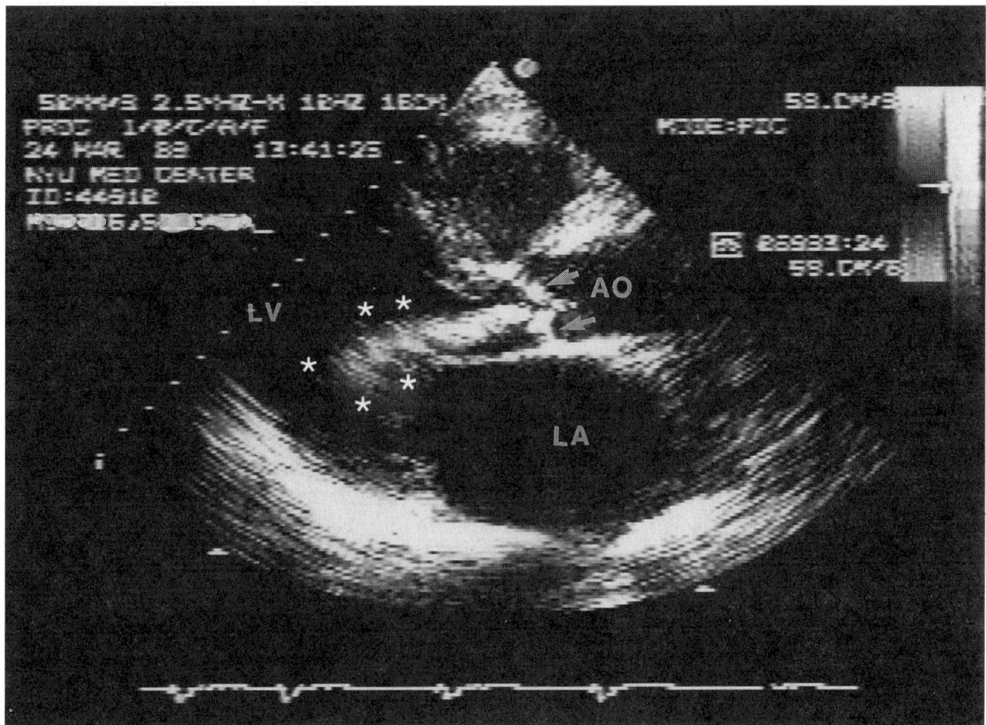

Fig. 11–14. Two-dimensional echocardiogram (diastolic frame) in aortic regurgitation. The aortic valve *(arrows)* is thickened. The left ventricle *(LV)* and left atrium *(LA)* are dilated. The jet of blood extending to the left from the aortic valve is identified here by the asterisks and was clearly demonstrated by the technique of color Doppler echocardiography. *AO,* aorta.

with the transducer in the esophagus, behind the heart. The left atrium and the posterior aspect of the mitral valve are therefore unmasked, and the pathology and abnormal flow behind the valve can easily be demonstrated (Fig. 11–15). Therefore TEE is indicated in patients with symptomatic prosthetic valve dysfunction. An absence of prosthetic mitral regurgitation on transthoracic echocardiography does *not* rule out severe, acute mitral regurgitation.

Systolic Left Ventricular Dysfunction

Left ventricular dysfunction is probably the most common reason for acute congestive heart failure. As noted, echocardiography can promptly and rapidly evaluate the size of the chambers and their wall motion. Parameters of left ventricular function such as global left ventricular ejection fraction, stroke volume, and left ventricular output can be easily calculated. Segmental wall motion can be analyzed, and areas of hypokinesis, akinesis, or dyskinesis due to any cause can be rapidly identified. These parameters of left ventricular function have not only diagnostic value but also significant prognostic value. Obviously, the lower the ejection fraction, the worse the prognosis. Ejection fractions below 30% (regardless of the cause) indicate high short-term mortality, whereas an ejection fraction of more than 50% usually indicates an excellent prognosis.[103]

Diastolic Left Ventricular Dysfunction

Up to 40% of patients with congestive heart failure have normal left ventricular systolic function.[104] In many of these patients there is nothing wrong with myocardial contractility; in fact, many of them have compensatory hyperkinesis with a high ejection fraction. Instead, they suffer from poor left ventricular distensibility (low com-

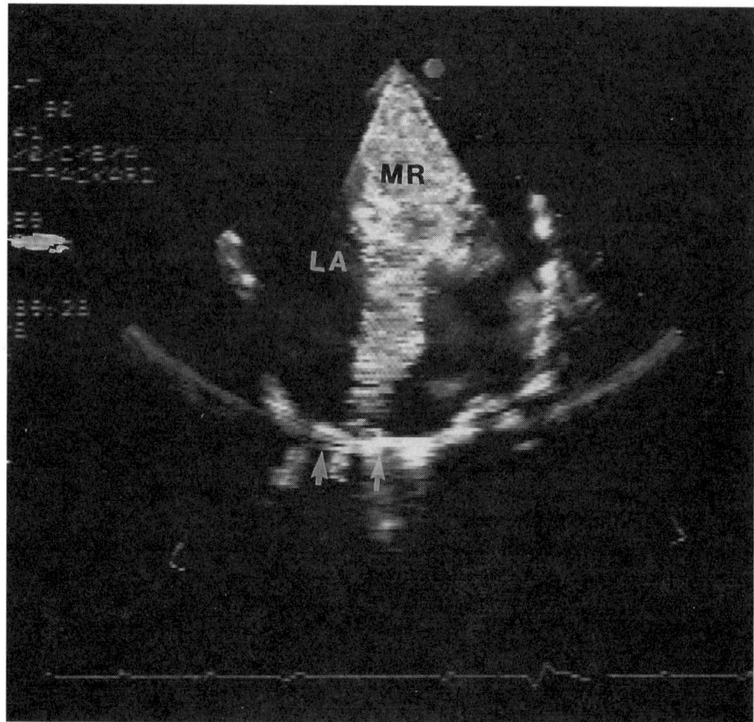

Fig. 11–15. Transesophageal echocardiogram (systolic frame). A prosthetic, mechanical valve is noted in the mitral position *(arrows).* A jet of mitral regurgitation *(MR)* is clearly noted. This jet was not seen on the transthoracic echocardiogram because of "shadowing" by the metallic prosthetic valve. *LA,* left atrium.

pliance). The high diastolic left ventricular pressure leads to elevated left atrial pressure and pulmonary venous hypertension, which may lead to severe symptoms of congestive heart failure. Echocardiography in these patients demonstrates normal systolic function and discloses the cause for diastolic dysfunction such as severe left ventricular hypertrophy (symmetrical, as seen in hypertensive left ventricular disease, or asymmetrical, as seen in patients with hypertrophic cardiomyopathy). Doppler echocardiography may be of further assistance by showing an abnormal left ventricular filling pattern.[105] A combination of systolic and diastolic dysfunction is frequently present in patients with ischemic, infarcted, hypertrophic, or infiltrated myocardium. This combination will also be easily identified by echocardiography.

Evaluation of a Patient with Hypotension

Symptomatic hypotension is a life-threatening condition that requires immediate diagnosis and treatment. Diagnostic techniques require a determination of blood volume, filling pressure, left ventricular function, and peripheral vascular resistance. Pulmonary artery catheterization, as discussed above, can provide most of the information required for immediate management of the patient. However, as noted, the technique is invasive and not without risks and may not alter the outcome. A good echocardiographic examination can provide much of the required information and may, in many cases, replace or at least supplement the invasive procedure. Below we describe characteristic echocardiographic findings that are associated with cardiac conditions inducing hypotension.

Acute Hypovolemia

Left ventricular chamber size is typically smaller than normal, and wall motion is well preserved and usually hyperkinetic with cavity obliteration. There is no other evidence of cardiac pathology. Often, minor degrees of tricuspid regurgitation (present in many normal adults) permit the measurement of pulmonary artery systolic pressure that is lower than normal.[106]

Acute Profound Left Ventricular Dysfunction

This is usually secondary to massive myocardial damage, the most common reason being acute, extensive myocardial infarction. However, myocarditis, cardiac contusion, and toxic and radiation damage are also in the differential diagnosis. Symptoms of congestive left heart failure frequently coexist. As mentioned before, left ventricular segmental wall motion as well as global wall motion can be easily analyzed by echocardiography. The pulmonary artery pressure, assessed noninvasively by Doppler, is elevated. Standard parameters including left ventricular diastolic and systolic dimension, the percentage of circumferential fiber shortening, ejection fraction, stroke volume, and cardiac output can be calculated. Prognosis can be assessed and the response to various modes of therapy monitored by echocardiography.

Acute Cardiac Rupture

Types of cardiac rupture include papillary muscle rupture inducing acute mitral regurgitation, septal rupture causing an acute left-to-right shunt, and rupture of the free wall of the heart causing cardiac tamponade. The most common cause for these conditions is myocardial infarction. Blunt or sharp cardiac trauma is another obvious cause. Cardiac tamponade associated with rupture of the free wall of the heart usually has an extremely rapid course (frequently seconds) ending in sudden death. For this reason the physician is more likely to see other forms of cardiac tamponade, which will be discussed in more detail below. In acute papillary muscle rupture, echocardiography will show a flail mitral leaflet with attached ruptured muscle and severe mitral regurgitation. Rupture of the left ventricle, as described in Case 11–1, is easy to diagnose by echocardiography. The site of the rupture can be identified, usually in an infarcted area that is characterized by hypokinesis or akinesis and an absence of systolic thickening. A high-velocity blood flow jet can be easily identified by Doppler echocardiography across the newly created defect.[107] The left ventricle and left atrium may be dilated, and signs of pulmonary hypertension can be demonstrated.

Cardiac Tamponade

Echocardiography is the technique of choice for demonstration of pericardial effusion and is specifically helpful in the diagnosis of cardiac tamponade. An echo-free space separating the pericardium from the epicardium is diagnostic of pericardial effusion. The volume of pericardial effusion is directly related to the size of this echo-free space. An echo-free space may or may not be associated with cardiac tamponade.

Signs of cardiac tamponade include respiratory variations in chamber size.[108] This is the echocardiographic equivalent of paradoxical pulse. With inspiration, the left ventricular dimension decreases and the right ventricular dimension increases. During expiration, there is expansion of the left ventricle and diminishing right ventricular diameter. Doppler echocardiography can show respiratory variations in intracavitary flow velocities.[109] With inspiration, left-sided transvalvular flow velocities (i.e., flow velocity across the mitral and aortic valve) diminish, whereas right-sided transvalvular flows increase in velocity. These findings are characteristic of other conditions such as chronic obstructive pulmonary disease or pulmonary embolization that may produce a paradoxical pulse; the findings are not associated with cardiac tamponade and are therefore considered nonspecific. However, when seen together with a large pericardial effusion, they are suggestive of cardiac tamponade.

More specific for cardiac tamponade is the finding of diastolic chamber collapse.[85, 110] Frequently the intrapericardial pressure exceeds that of the right-sided chambers during diastole and therefore produces diastolic collapse of these chambers. This finding is sensitive and confirms the clinical observation of cardiac tamponade in symptomatic patients.

Echocardiography can also serve as a guide for needle pericardiocentesis.[111] The site of puncture as well as pericardial fluid evacuation can be monitored. When medical therapy is offered for pericardial effusion, repeat echocardiography can document the change in pericardial effusion size and the nature of its hemodynamic effects.

Pulmonary Embolus

Pulmonary embolus may be a cause for sudden hypotension. In patients hypotensive because of a pulmonary embolus, the left ventricle is frequently small and hyperkinetic whereas the right-sided chambers are dilated. As mentioned before, a thrombus can occasionally be seen in the right heart chambers and TEE can reveal a thrombus lodging in the main pulmonary artery or the main branches.[88] Doppler echocardiography can frequently demonstrate evidence of severe, acute pulmonary hypertension.[89] Findings consistent with paradoxical pulse may be present in the absence of pericardial effusion.[112]

Evaluation of a Patient with Syncope

Although the differential diagnosis of syncope is extensive and many causes are not cardiac in nature, echocardiography may be quite helpful in evaluating cardiac causes. Obviously, when the culprit is a dysrhythmia, ECG monitoring will be superior to echocardiography. Echocardiography may nevertheless infrequently reveal the underlying pathology that might have led to the dysrhythmia. Cardiac conditions that are frequently associated with syncope are discussed below.

Aortic Stenosis

The aortic valve is clearly visualized by transthoracic echocardiography (Fig. 11–16). In adults, severe aortic stenosis is always associated with aortic calcification noted by echocardiography and is frequently associated with left ventricular hypertrophy. Doppler echocardiography is now capable of accurately evaluating the transaortic valve gradient and allows the aortic valve area to be calculated.[113, 114] Severe aortic stenosis is defined as an aortic valve area of 0.8 cm^2 or less. With normal cardiac output, the pressure gradient across a severely stenosed aortic valve is usually 50 mm Hg or more. However, severe stenosis with low cardiac output may be present with much smaller gradients. In these cases, the characteristic murmur may also be soft.

Idiopathic Hypertrophic Subaortic Stenosis

This was the cause of the patient's symptoms in Case 11–2. The condition is associated with left ventricular outflow obstruction and high flow velocity demonstrated in the subvalvular region where the anterior mitral leaflet coapts with the septum during systole. Characteristic echocardiographic findings are (1) asymmetrical septal hypertrophy; (2) abnormal systolic anterior motion of the anterior mitral leaflet, and (3) high flow velocity (as evidence for a high gradient) that reaches its peak in late systole.[115, 116]

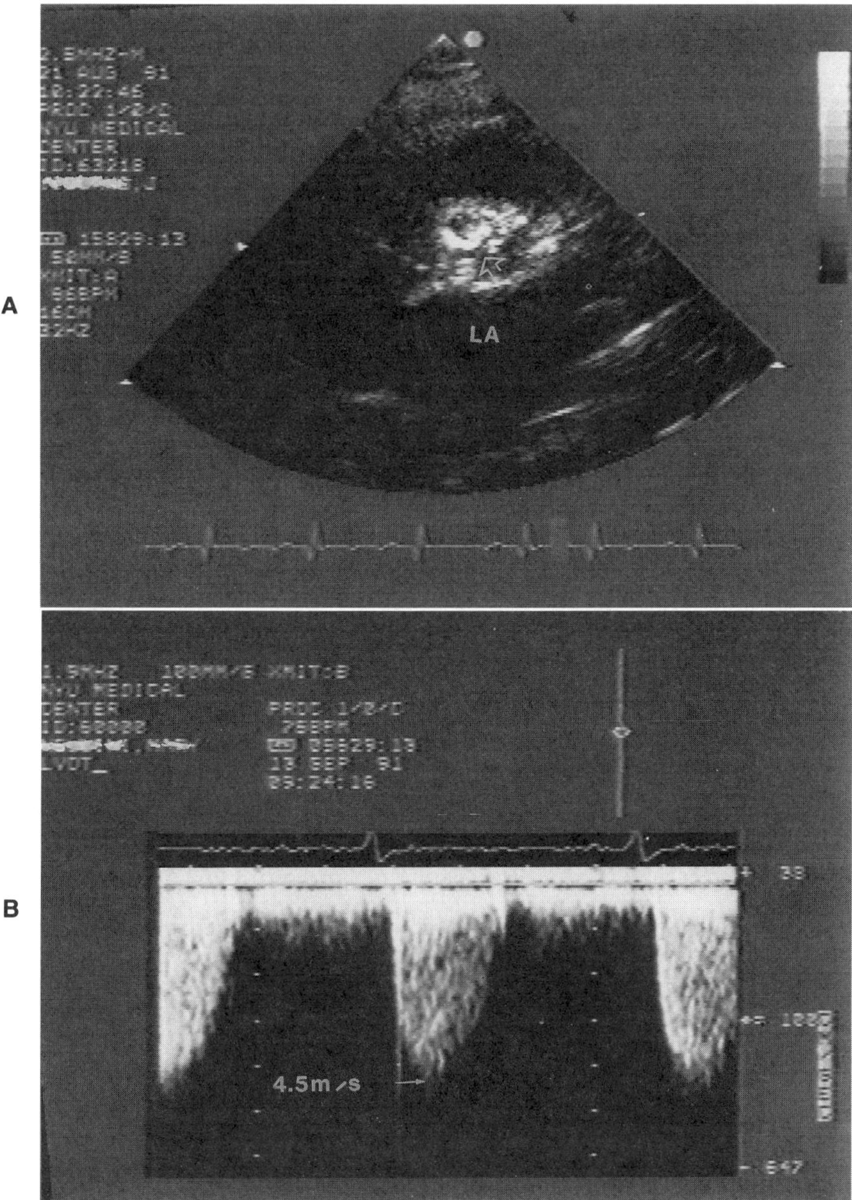

Fig. 11–16. Echocardiography in aortic stenosis. **A,** Short-axis two-dimensional echocardiogram (systolic frame). The thickened and calcified aortic valve *(arrow)* has limited opening during systole. *LA,* left atrium. **B,** Continuous-wave Doppler shows high flow velocity across the stenosed aortic valve during systole. By using the modified Bernoulli equation, the peak gradient across the value is $\Delta P = 4V^2 = 4(4.5)^2 = 84$ mm Hg (*ΔP,* pressure; *V,* velocity).

Left Atrial Myxoma

Left atrial myxoma is a rare cause of sudden syncope. A change in body position may result in a change in the location of the neoplastic mass, which may move into the mitral orifice and obstruct it. The result may be sudden syncope. More commonly, the symptoms are those of congestive heart failure and shortness of breath or those of systemic illness with fever and night sweats. Occasionally the first symptoms may be those of tumor embolism to the brain or to a peripheral organ. The echocardio-

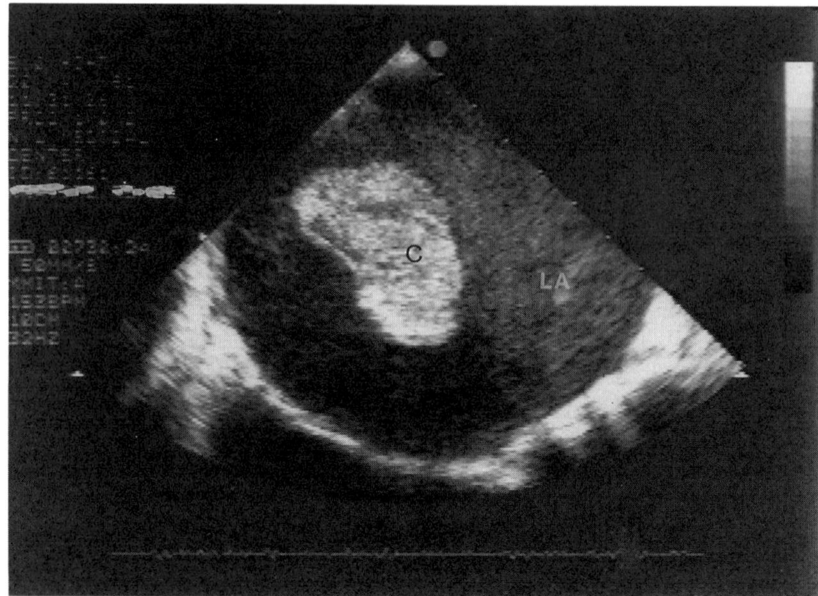

Fig. 11–17. Transesophageal echocardiography. A large clot *(C)* is noted within the dilated left atrium *(LA)*.

gram of an atrial tumor is always diagnostic.[117] It is usually connected to the interatrial septum and frequently moves in diastole toward the mitral orifice and in systole back into the left atrial cavity.[118] Other intracardiac tumors may cause various symptoms depending on their location. They can also be identified by echocardiography.

Evaluation of Patients with Stroke, Transient Ischemic Attacks, and Peripheral Embolization

A cardiac source of embolization should be considered in every patient who has focal neurologic signs or evidence of acute arterial occlusion. The major source for cardiac embolization is intracardiac clots (especially in patients with stagnation of blood in dilated chambers). These clots form because of left atrial dilatation secondary to mitral stenosis, left ventricular dilatation with wall motion abnormalities such as those seen in patients with prior infarction, left ventricular aneurysm, and diffuse left ventricular wall motion abnormalities due to cardiomyopathy, etc. In all of these conditions, echocardiography can identify the underlying disease and very often demonstrate the clot. Left atrial clots are frequently found in the left atrial appendage, which is not well seen on transthoracic echocardiography, so TEE is a better test for identifying clots in the left atrium and left atrial appendage[119] (Fig. 11–17). Not infrequently, TEE demonstrates spontaneous, smokelike, swirling echocardiographic contrast[120] (Fig. 11–18). This finding is the echocardiographic equivalent of stagnation of blood and is often a precursor of clot formation. In fact, the finding of this "smoke" is currently considered an indication for anticoagulation therapy since it is associated with embolic episodes.

Intracardiac Tumors

The most common tumor, as noted above, is left atrial myxoma. However, many other tumors, benign as well as malignant, may also be seen first as embolic disorders.

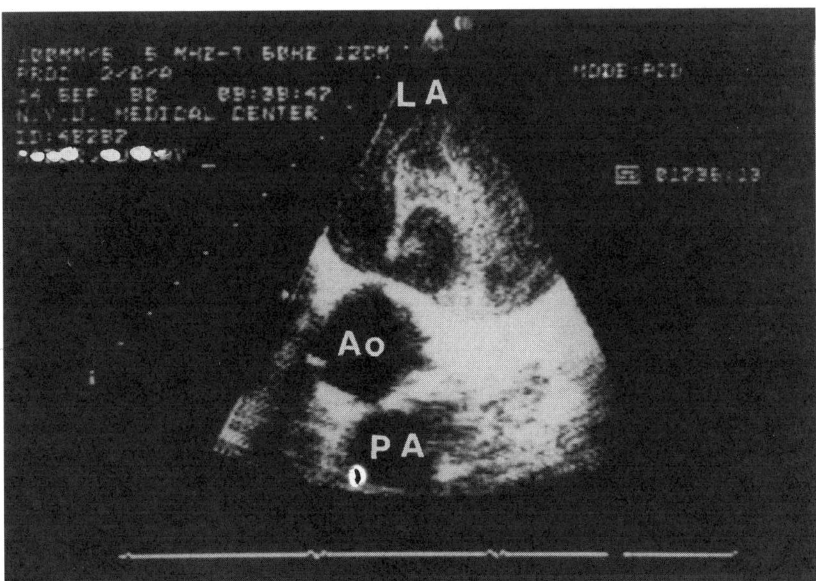

Fig. 11–18. Transesophageal echocardiography. Swirling, spontaneous echoes are present within the left atrium *(LA)* of this patient with mitral stenosis. This spontaneous "smoke" is frequently seen in patients with stagnation of blood and is considered a precursor of clot formation. *Ao,* aorta; *PA,* pulmonary artery.

Valvular Vegetations

Echocardiography clearly identifies valvular vegetations in patients with endocarditis.[95, 121] It is important not only to diagnose endocarditis but also to image it. Embolic complications are quite common in acute and subacute bacterial endocarditis, and the risk for embolization can be predicted by analyzing the echocardiographic data. Larger vegetations have a higher incidence of embolization. Mobile vegetations embolize more frequently than sessile vegetations, and fresh vegetations (characterized by decreased brightness) pose a higher risk for embolization than older ones.[122] Echocardiography can also identify complications of endocarditis such as valvular disruption and regurgitation, myocardial abscesses,[123] and fistulous communication between chambers.[124] The echocardiographic findings can accurately predict the prognosis of the patient and may be used to determine whether medical or surgical therapy is appropriate (Fig. 11–19).

Aortic Atheromas

Recently TEE has helped to identify a new clinical syndrome and demonstrate its importance. Protruding mobile atheromas in the aortic arch that are only visible by TEE may detach spontaneously or during cardiac catheterization and embolize to the brain or to the periphery[125, 126] (Fig. 11–20).

Other Conditions

Echocardiography identifies valvular conditions known to be associated with embolic events.[127, 128] Those conditions include mitral valve prolapse, valvular calcification, mitral annular calcification, mitral valve strands, and noninfected valve thrombi associated with lupus erythematosus or anticardiolipin antibody syndromes. Finally, echocardiography can identify cardiac structural abnormalities that are known to be associated with embolic events. These include atrial septal defect and patent foramen ovale, which may be responsible for paradoxical emboli. Atrial septal aneurysm, a clinical entity only recently diagnosed by echocardiography (better seen by TEE than

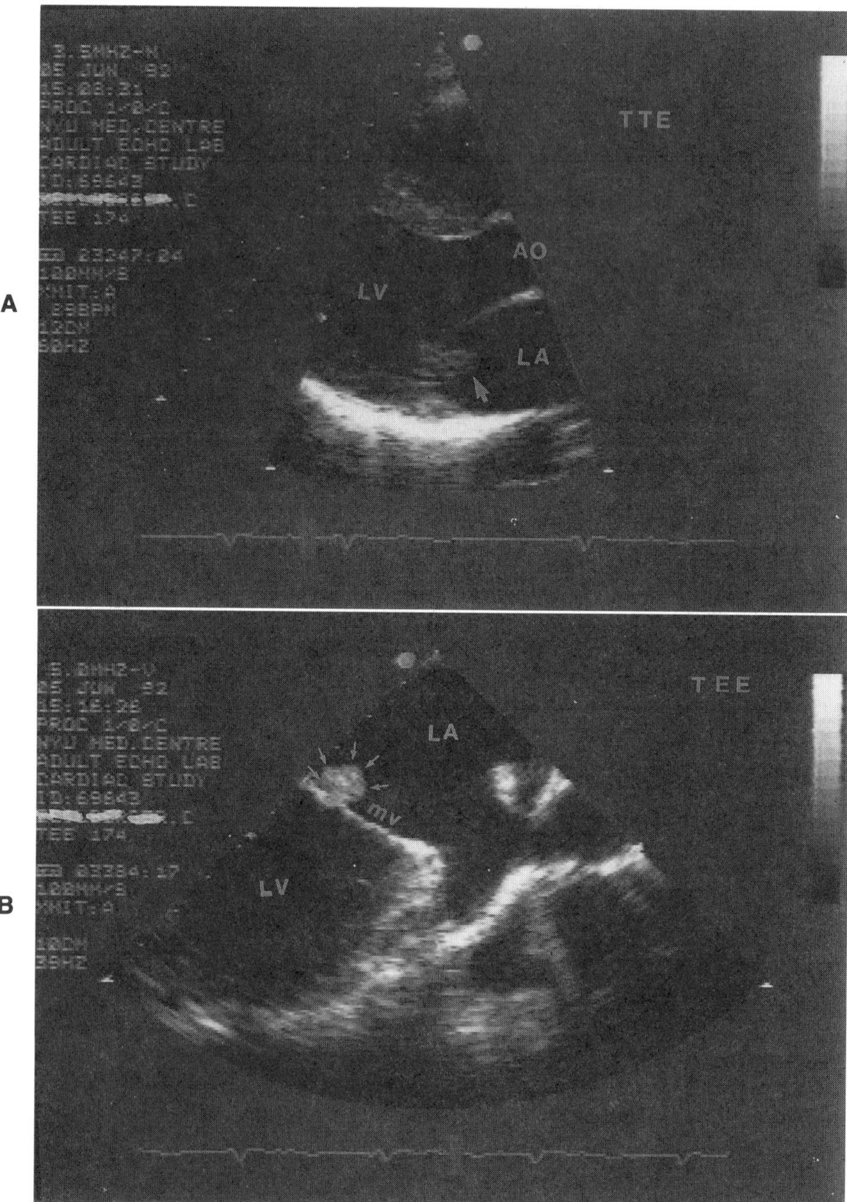

Fig. 11–19. Echocardiography in bacterial endocarditis. **A,** Vegetation *(arrow)* is noted on the left atrial *(LA)* side of the mitral valve. *TTE,* transthoracic echocardiogram; *AO,* aorta; *LV,* left ventricle. **B,** Same patient, transesophageal echocardiogram *(TEE)*—the vegetation is better delineated (*MV,* mitral valve).

by transthoracic echocardiography), is a congenital disorder that is also associated with embolic disorders. It is quite possible that stagnation of blood within this aneurysm may lead to platelet aggregation and, rarely, even to clot formation. Atrial septal aneurysm is frequently associated with a patent foramen ovale, which may be an additional risk factor.

CONCLUSION

In this chapter we have discussed the roles of various cardiovascular diagnostic tests in the ED. The indications for these studies vary, and their availability is not uni-

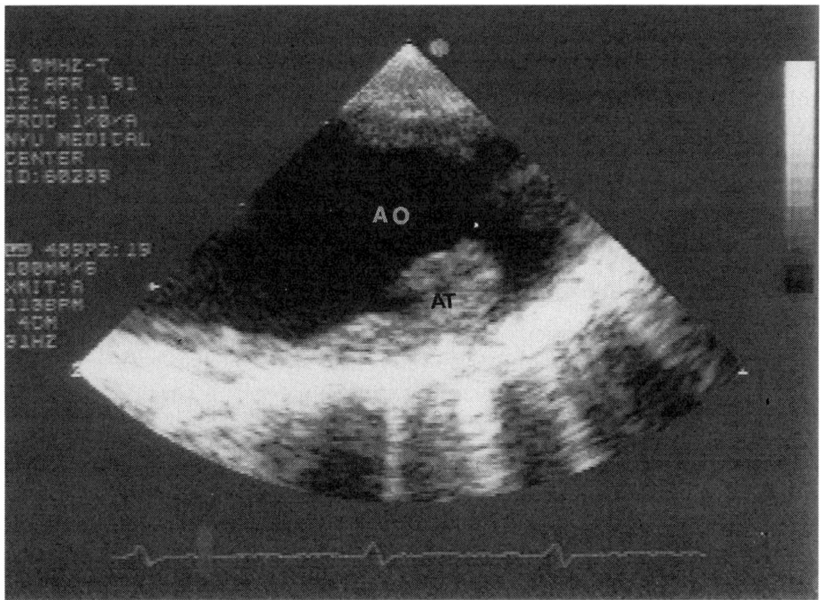

Fig. 11–20. Protruding, mobile atheroma *(AT)* in the aortic arch of a patient with recurrent embolic stroke. *AO,* aorta.

versal. Table 11–9 on page 186 lists suggestions for the selection of tests that will offer the greatest help in the diagnosis of selected cardiac emergencies. However, we would like to conclude as we began: the most important cardiovascular examination is the history. When sufficient attention is paid to the history, appropriate testing provides confirmation of a clinical hypothesis. Testing alone cannot be a substitute for the physician's skill in formulating that hypothesis.

REFERENCES

1. Goldman L, Sayson R, Robbins S: The value of autopsy in three medical eras, *N Engl J Med* 308:1000–1005, 1983.
2. Goldberger E, Wheat MW: *Treatment of cardiac emergencies,* St Louis, 1977, Mosby Inc.
3. Mason, DT, ed: *Cardiac emergencies,* Baltimore, 1978, Williams & Wilkins.
4. Chung EK, ed: *Cardiac emergency care,* Philadelphia, 1980, Lea & Febiger.
5. Eliot RS, Saenz A, Forker AD, eds: *Cardiac emergencies,* Mount Kisco, NY, 1982, Futura Publishing.
6. Sheinman MM, ed: *Symposium on cardiac emergencies,* Philadelphia, 1979, WB Saunders.
7. Gorlin R: *Coronary artery disease,* Philadelphia, 1976, WB Saunders.
8. Cohn PF: Evaluation of anginal syndromes using standard clinical procedures. In Cohn PF, editor: *Diagnosis and therapy of coronary artery disease,* Boston, 1979, Little, Brown.
9. Gregoire J, Theroux P: Detection and assessment of unstable angina using myocardial perfusion imaging: comparison between technetium-99m sestamibi SPECT and 12-lead electrocardiogram, *Am J Cardiol* 66:42–46, 1990.
10. Bilodeau L, Theroux P, Gregoire J et al: Technetium-99m sestamibi tomography in patients with spontaneous chest pain: correlations with clinical, electrocardiographic and angiographic findings, *J Am Coll Cardiol* 18:1684–1691, 1991.
11. Justis DL, Hession WT: Accuracy of 22-lead ECG analysis for diagnosis of acute myocardial infarction and coronary artery disease in the emergency department: a comparison with 12-lead ECG, *Ann Emerg Med* 21:1–9, 1992.
12. Herlitz J, Hjalmarson A, Waldenstrom J: The diagnostic value of different enzymes and standard ECG in acute myocardial infarction, *Scand J Clin Lab Invest* 45:413–420, 1985.

13. Turi ZG, Rutherford JD, Roberts R et al: Electrocardiographic, enzymatic and scintigraphic criteria of acute myocardial infarction as determined from study of 726 patients (a MILIS study), *Am J Cardiol* 55:1463–1468, 1985.
14. Kornreich F, Selvester RH, Montague TJ et al: Discriminant analysis of the standard 12-lead ECG for diagnosing non–Q wave myocardial infarction, *J Electrocardiol* 24(suppl):163–172, 1992.
15. Hiss RG, Lamb LE, Allen MF: Electrocardiographic findings in 67,375 asymptomatic patients, *Am J Cardiol* 6:200–231, 1960.
16. Horan LG, Flowers NC: Electrocardiography and vectorcardiography. In Braunwald E, editor: *Heart disease: a textbook of cardiovascular medicine*, Philadelphia, 1980, WB Saunders, pp 231–252.
17. Chiercha A, Brunelli C, Simonetti I: Sequence of events in angina at rest: primary reduction in coronary flow, *Circulation* 61:759–768, 1980.
18. Dressler W, Roesler H: High T waves in the earliest stage of infarction, *Am Heart J* 34:627–645, 1947.
19. Horan LG, Flowers NC, Johnson JC: Significance of the diagnostic Q wave in myocardial infarction, *Circulation* 43:428–436, 1971.
20. Helfant R: Q waves in coronary heart disease: newer understanding of their clinical implications, *Am J Cardiol* 38:662–664, 1976.
21. Goldberger AL: Recognition of ECG pseudo-infarct patterns, *Mod Concepts Cardiovasc Dis* 49:13–18, 1980.
22. Gruppo Italiano per lo Studio della Streptochinasi nell'infarto miocardico (GISSI): Effectiveness of intravenous thrombolytic treatment in acute myocardial infarction, *Lancet* i:397–402, 1986.
23. Gruppo Italiano per lo Studio della Streptochinasi nell'infarto miocardico (GISSI): Long-term effects of intravenous thrombolysis in acute myocardial infarction: final report of the GISSI study, *Lancet* 2:871–874, 1987.
24. ASSET Study Group: Trial of tissue plasminogen activator for mortality reduction in acute myocardial infarction, *Lancet* 2:525–530, 1988.
25. ISIS-2 Collaborative Group: Randomised trial of intravenous streptokinase, oral aspirin, both, or neither among 17,187 cases of suspected acute myocardial infarction, *Lancet* 2:349–360, 1988.
26. AIMS Trial Study Group: Long-term effects of intravenous anistreplase in acute myocardial infarction: final report of the AIMS study, *Lancet* i:427–431, 1990.
27. The International Study Group: In-hospital mortality and clinical course of 20,891 patients with suspected acute myocardial infarction randomised between alteplase and streptokinase with or without heparin, *Lancet* i:71–75, 1990.
28. Gruppo Italiano per lo Studio della Streptochinasi nell'infarto miocardico (GISSI): GISSI-2: a factorial randomised trial of alteplase versus streptokinase and heparin versus no heparin among 12,490 patients with acute myocardial infarction, *Lancet* i:65–71, 1990.
29. de Bono DP, Simoons ML, Tijssen J et al: Effect of early intravenous heparin on coronary patency, infarct size, and bleeding complications after alteplase thrombolysis: results of a randomised double blind European Cooperative Study Group trial, *Br Heart J* 67:122–128, 1992.
30. ISIS-3 (Third International Study of Infarct Survival) Collaborative Group: ISIS-3: a randomised trial of streptokinase vs tissue plasminogen activator vs anistreplase and of aspirin plus heparin vs aspirin alone among 41,299 cases of suspected acute myocardial infarction, *Lancet* ii:753–770, 1992.
31. Diamond GA, Forrester JR, Hirsch M: Application of conditional probability analysis to the clinical diagnosis of coronary artery disease, *J Clin Invest* 65:1210–1221, 1980.
32. Pozen MW, D'Agostine RB, Mitchell JB et al: The usefulness of a predictive instrument to reduce inappropriate admissions to the coronary care unit, *Ann Intern Med* 92:238–242, 1980.
33. Goldman L, Weinberg M, Weisberg M: A computer-derived protocol to aid in the diagnosis of emergency room patients with acute chest pain, *N Engl J Med* 307:588–596, 1982.
34. Lee TH, Juarez G, Cook EF et al: Ruling out acute myocardial infarction. A prospective multicentral validation of a 12-hour strategy for patients at low risk, *N Engl J Med* 324:1239–1246, 1991.

35. Goldman L, Cook EF, Brand DA et al: A computer protocol to predict myocardial infarction in emergency department patients with chest pain, *N Engl J Med* 318:797–803, 1988.
36. Hurst JW, Schlant RC: *The heart, arteries and veins,* ed 7, New York, 1990, McGraw-Hill.
37. Chung EK: *Principles of cardiac arrhythmias,* ed 3, Baltimore, 1983, Williams & Wilkins.
38. Braunwald E: *Heart disease: a textbook of cardiovascular medicine,* ed 4, Philadelphia, 1992, WB Saunders.
39. American Heart Association: *Textbook of advanced cardiac life support,* Dallas, 1987, The Association.
40. DiMarco JP, Sellers TD, Berne RM et al: Adenosine: electrophysiologic effects and therapeutic use for terminating paroxysmal supraventricular tachycardia, *Circulation* 68:1254–1263, 1983.
41. DiMarco JP, Miles W, Akhtar M et al: Adenosine for paroxysmal supraventricular tachycardia: dose ranging and comparison with verapamil. Assessment in placebo-controlled, multicenter trials. The adenosine for PSVT Study Group, *Ann Intern Med* 113:104–110, 1990.
42. Cairns CB, Niemann JT: Intravenous adenosine in the emergency department management of paroxysmal supraventricular tachycardia, *Ann Emerg Med* 20:717–721, 1991.
43. Wald RW, Sharma AD et al: Vagal techniques for termination of paroxysmal supraventricular tachycardia, *Am J Cardiol* 46:655–664, 1980.
44. Puech P, Grolleau R, Figac E: The diagnosis of supraventricular arrhythmias and the differentiation between supraventricular tachycardias with aberrant conduction and ventricular tachycardias. In Sandoe E, Flensted-Jensen E, Olesen KH, editors: *Symposium on cardiac arrhythmias,* Sodertalje, Sweden, 1971, AB Astra, pp 199–222.
45. Wildenthal K, Atkins JM: Use of the "diving reflex" for the treatment of paroxysmal supraventricular tachycardia, *Am Heart J* 98:536–537, 1979.
46. Hellerstein HK, Levine B, Feil H: Electrocardiographic changes following carotid sinus stimulation in paroxysmal supraventricular tachycardia, *J Lab Clin Med* 38:820–821, 1951.
47. Klein HO, Hoffman BF: Cessation of paroxysmal supraventricular tachycardias by parasympathomimetic interventions, *Ann Intern Med* 81:48–50, 1974.
48. Rotman M, Wagner GS, Wallace AG: Bradyarrhythmias in acute myocardial infarction, *Circulation* 45:703–722, 1972.
49. Gallagher JJ, Pritchett ELC, Sealy WC et al: The preexcitation syndromes, *Prog Cardiovasc Dis* 20:285–327, 1978.
50. Wellens HJJ, Durrer D: Effect of digitalis on atrioventricular conduction and circus-movement tachycardias in patients with Wolff-Parkinson-White syndrome, *Circulation* 47:1229–1233, 1973.
51. Sellers T, Bashore TM, Gallagher JJ: Digitalis in the preexcitation syndrome. Analysis during atrial fibrillation, *Circulation* 56:260–267, 1977.
52. Rosenbaum MB, Chiale PA, Ryba D: Control of tachyarrhythmias associated with Wolff-Parkinson-White syndrome by amiodarone hydrochloride, *Am J Cardiol* 34:215–223, 1974.
53. Markel ML, Prystowsky EN, Heger JJ et al: Encainide for treatment of supraventricular tachycardia associated with the Wolff-Parkinson-White syndrome, *Am J Cardiol* 58:41–48, 1986.
54. Kreeger RW, Hammill SC: New antiarrhythmic drugs: tocainide, mexiletine, flecainide, encainide, and amiodarone, *Mayo Clin Proc* 62:1033–1050, 1987.
55. Miles WM, Zipes DP, Rinkenberger RL et al: Encainide for treatment of atrioventricular reciprocating tachycardia in the Wolff-Parkinson-White syndrome, *Am J Cardiol* 62:20–25, 1988.
56. Bolognesi R: The pharmacologic treatment of atrial fibrillation, *Cardiovasc Drugs Ther* 5:617–628, 1991.
57. Jackman WM, Wang XZ, Friday KJ et al: Catheter ablation of accessory atrioventricular pathways (Wolff-Parkinson-White syndrome) by radiofrequency current, *N Engl J Med* 324:1605–1611, 1991.
58. Schluter M, Geiger M, Siebels J et al: Catheter ablation using radiofrequency to cure symptomatic patients with tachyarrhythmias related to an accessory atrioventricular pathway, *Circulation* 84:1644–1661, 1991.
59. Calkins H, Langberg J, Sousa J et al: Radiofrequency catheter ablation of accessory atrio-

ventricular connections in 250 patients. Abbreviated therapeutic approach to Wolff-Parkinson-White syndrome, *Circulation* 85:1337–1346, 1992.
60. Trevino A, Razi B, Beller B: The characteristic electrocardiogram of accidental hypothermia, *Arch Intern Med* 127:470–473, 1971.
61. Roberts R: Diagnostic assessment of myocardial infarction based on lactate dehydrogenase and creatine kinase isoenzymes, H & L, *J Crit Care* 10:486–506, 1981.
62. Klein MS, Ludbrook PA, Mimbs JW: Perioperative mortality in patients with unstable angina selected by exclusion of myocardial infarction, *J Thorac Cardiovasc Surg* 73:253–257, 1977.
63. Katus HA, Remppis A, Neumann EJ et al: Diagnostic efficiency of troponin T measurements in acute myocardial infarction, *Circulation* 83:902–912, 1991.
64. West M, Eshchar J, Zimmerman HJ: Serum enzymology in the diagnosis of myocardial infarction and related cardiovascular conditions, *Med Clin North Am* 50:171–191, 1966.
65. Sobel BE, Shell WE: Serum enzyme determinations in the diagnosis and assessment of myocardial infarction, *Circulation* 45:471–482, 1972.
66. Roberts R, Gowda KS, Ludbrook PA: Specificity of elevated serum MB creatine phosphokinase activity in the diagnosis of acute myocardial infarction, *Am J Cardiol* 36:433–437, 1975.
67. Marin MM, Teichman SL: Use of rapid serial sampling of creatine kinase MB for very early detection of myocardial infarction in patients with acute chest pain, *Am Heart J* 123:354–361, 1992.
68. Gama R, Swain DG, Nightingale PG et al: The effective use of cardiac enzymes and electrocardiograms in the diagnosis of acute myocardial infarction in the elderly, *Postgrad Med J* 66:375–377, 1990.
69. Rapaport E: Serum enzymes and isoenzymes in the diagnosis of acute myocardial infarction, *Mod Concepts Cardiovasc Dis* 46:47, 1977.
70. Lee TH, Goldman L: Serum enzyme assays in the diagnosis of acute myocardial infarction. Recommendations based on a quantitative analysis, *Ann Intern Med* 105:221–233, 1986.
71. Green GB, Hansen KN, Chan DW et al: The potential utility of a rapid CK-MB assay in evaluating emergency department patients with possible myocardial infarction, *Ann Emerg Med* 20:954–960, 1991.
72. Mair J, Artner-Dworzak E, Dienstl A et al: Early detection of acute myocardial infarction by measurement of concentration of creatine kinase-MB, *Am J Cardiol* 68:1545–1550, 1991.
73. Surawicz B: Relationship between electrocardiogram and electrolytes, *Am Heart J* 73:814–834, 1967.
74. Swan HJC, Ganz W, Forrester J: Catheterization of the heart on man with use of a flow-directed balloon-tipped catheter, *N Engl J Med* 283:447–451, 1970.
75. Hines RL: Pulmonary artery catheters: what's the controversy? *J Cardiovasc Surg* 5(suppl):237–239, 1990.
76. Matthay MA, Chatterjee K: Bedside catheterization of the pulmonary artery: risks compared with benefits, *Ann Intern Med* 109:826–834, 1988.
77. Robin ED: The cult of the Swan-Ganz catheter: overuse and abuse of pulmonary flow catheters, *Ann Intern Med* 103:445–449, 1985.
78. Saarela E, Kari A, Nikki P et al: Current practice regarding invasive monitoring in intensive care units in Finland. A nationwide study of the uses of arterial, pulmonary artery and central venous catheters and their effect on outcome, *Intensive Care Med* 17:264–271, 1991.
79. Technology Subcommittee of the Working Group on Critical Care Ontario Ministry of Health: Hemodynamic monitoring: a technology assessment, *Can Med Assoc J* 145:114–121, 1991.
80. Feigenbaum H: *Echocardiography*, ed 4, Philadelphia, 1986, Lea & Febiger.
81. Seward JB, Khanderia BK, Oh JK et al: Transesophageal echocardiography: technique, anatomic correlations, implementation, and clinical applications, *Mayo Clin Proc* 63:649–680, 1988.
82. Horowitz RS, Morganroth HJ, Parrotto G et al: Immediate diagnosis of acute myocardial infarction by two dimensional echocardiography, *Circulation* 65:323–328, 1982.

83. Pandian NG, Kerber RE: Two dimensional echocardiography in experimental coronary stenosis, *Circulation* 66:597, 1982.
84. Feigenbaum H, Waldhausen JA, Hyde LP: Ultrasonic diagnosis of pericardial effusion, *JAMA* 191:107–109, 1965.
85. Kronzon I, Cohen ML, Winer HE: Diastolic atrial compression: a sensitive sign of cardiac tamponade, *J Am Coll Cardiol* 2:770–774, 1983.
86. Martin RP, Bowden R, Filly K et al: Intrapericardial abnormalities in patients with pericardial effusion: findings by two dimensional echocardiography, *Circulation* 61:568–572, 1980.
87. Ezbel R, Engberding R, Daniel WG et al: Echocardiography in the diagnosis of aortic dissection, *Lancet* 1:457–461, 1989.
88. Klein AL, Stewart WC, Cosgrove DM et al: Visualization of acute pulmonary emboli by transesophageal echocardiography, *J Am Soc Echocardiogr* 3:412–415, 1990.
89. Kasppar W, Meinertz T, Kersting F et al: Echocardiography in assessing acute pulmonary hypertension due to pulmonary embolism, *Am J Cardiol* 45:567–569, 1980.
90. Nichol PM, Gilbert BW, Kisslo JA: Two dimensional echocardiographic assessment of mitral stenosis, *Circulation* 55:120–125, 1977.
91. Wann LS, Weyman AE, Feigenbaum H et al: Determination of mitral valve area by cross sectional echocardiography, *Ann Intern Med* 88:337–340, 1978.
92. Hatle L, Angelsen B: *Doppler ultrasound in cardiology*, Philadelphia, 1985, Lea & Febiger.
93. Hatle L, Angelsen B, Tromsdal A: Noninvasive assessment of atrioventricular pressure half time by Doppler ultrasound, *Circulation* 60:1096–1104, 1979.
94. Cziner DG, Rosenzweig BP, Katz ES et al: Transesophageal vs transthoracic echocardiography for diagnosis of mitral valve perforation, *Am J Cardiol* 69:1495–1497, 1991.
95. Martin RP, Meltzer RS, Chia K et al: Clinical utility of two dimensional echocardiography in infective endocarditis, *Am J Cardiol* 46:379–385, 1980.
96. Himmelman RB, Kusumoto F, Oken K et al: The flail mitral valve: echocardiographic findings by precardial and transesophageal imaging and Doppler color flow mapping, *J Am Coll Cardiol* 17:272, 1991.
97. Nanda NC, Cooper JW, Philpot EF et al: Evaluation of valvular regurgitation by color Doppler, *J Am Soc Echocardiogr* 12:56–62, 1989.
98. Grayburn PA, Smith MD, Handshoe R et al: Detection of aortic insufficiency by standard echocardiography, pulsed Doppler echocardiography and auscultation, *Ann Intern Med* 104:599, 1986.
99. Perry GJ, Helmcke F, Nanda NC et al: Evaluation of aortic insufficiency by Doppler color flow mapping, *J Am Coll Cardiol* 9:952, 1987.
100. Slater J, Gindea AJ, Freedberg RS et al: A comparison of cardiac catheterization and Doppler echocardiography in the decision to operate in aortic and mitral valve disease, *J Am Coll Cardiol* 17:1026–1036, 1991.
101. Daniel LB, Grigg LE, Weisel RD et al: Comparison of transthoracic and transesophageal assessment of prosthetic valve dysfunction, *Echocardiography* 7:83–95, 1990.
102. Nellesen U, Schnittger I, Appleton CP et al: Transesophageal two-dimensional echocardiography and color Doppler flow velocity mapping in the evaluation of cardiac valve prostheses, *Circulation* 78:848–855, 1988.
103. Gradman A, Deedwania P, Cody R et al: Predictors of total mortality and sudden death in mild to moderate heart failure, *J Am Coll Cardiol* 14:564, 1989.
104. Nishimura RA, Housmans PR, Hatle LK et al: Assessment of diastolic function of the heart. Part I: physiologic and pathophysiologic features, *Mayo Clin Proc* 64:71, 1989.
105. Nishimura J, Hatle LK, Abel MD et al: Assessment of diastolic function of the heart: background and current application of Doppler echocardiography. Part II: Clinical studies, *Mayo Clin Proc* 64:181, 1989.
106. Yock PG, Popp RL: Non-invasive estimation of right ventricular systolic pressure by Doppler ultrasound in patients with tricuspid regurgitation, *Circulation* 70:657, 1984.
107. Helmcke F, DeSouza A, Nanda NC et al: Two dimensional and color Doppler assessment of ventricular septal defect, *Am J Cardiol* 63:1112, 1989.
108. Kronzon I, Cohen ML, Winer HE: Contribution of echocardiography to the understanding of the pathophysiology of cardiac tamponade, *J Am Coll Cardiol* 1:1180–1983, 1983.
109. Leeman DE, Levine MJ, Come PC: Doppler echocardiography in cardiac tamponade: ex-

aggerated respiratory variation in transvalvular blood flow velocity integrals, *J Am Coll Cardiol* 11:572, 1988.

110. Schiller NB, Botvinick EH: Right ventricular compression as a sign of cardiac tamponade, *Circulation* 56:774, 1977.
111. Callahan JA, Seward JB, Nishimure RA et al: Two dimensional echocardiographically graded pericardiocentesis: experience in 117 consecutive patients, *Am J Cardiol* 55:476, 1985.
112. Kronzon I, Weiss E, Winer HE et al: Echocardiographic observations of paradoxical pulse without pericardial disease, *Chest* 48:474–479, 1980.
113. Currie PJ, Seward JB, Reeder GS et al: Continuous wave Doppler echocardiographic assessment of severity of calcific aortic stenosis: a simultaneous Doppler-catheter correlative study in 100 adult patients, *Circulation* 54:396, 1985.
114. Zoghbi WA, Farmer KL, Soto JG et al: Accurate non-invasive quantification of stenotic aortic valve area by Doppler echocardiography, *Circulation* 73:452, 1986.
115. Henry WL, Clark CE, Epstein SE: Asymmetric septal hypertrophy (ASH). Echocardiographic identification of the pathognomonic anatomic abnormality of IHSS, *Circulation* 47:225, 1973.
116. Sasson Z, Yock PG, Hatle LK et al: Doppler echocardiographic determination of the pressure gradient in hypertrophic cardiomyopathy, *J Am Coll Cardiol* 11:752, 1988.
117. Mugge A, Daniel WG, Haverdich A et al: Diagnosis of noninfective cardiac mass lesions by two dimensional echocardiography. Comparison of transthoracic and transesophageal approach, *Circulation* 83:70–78, 1991.
118. Freedberg RS, Kronzon I, Remancik WM et al: The contribution of magnetic resonance imaging to the evaluation of intracardiac tumors diagnosed by echocardiography, *Circulation* 77:96–103, 1988.
119. Aschenberg W, Schluter M, Kremer P et al: Transesophageal two dimensional echocardiography for the detection of left atrial appendage thrombus, *J Am Coll Cardiol* 7:163–166, 1986.
120. Daniel WG, Mellesen U, Schroeder E et al: Left atrial spontaneous echo contrast in mitral valve disease: an indicator for an increased thrombotic risk, *J Am Coll Cardiol* 11:1204–1211, 1988.
121. Daniel WG, Schroeder E, Mugge A et al: Transesophageal echocardiography in infective endocarditis, *Am J Card Imaging* 2:78–85, 1988.
122. Sanfillipo AJ, Picard MA, Newell JB et al: Echocardiographic assessment of patients with infectious endocarditis: prediction of risk for complications, *J Am Coll Cardiol* 18:1191–1200, 1991.
123. Daniel WG, Mugge A, Martin RP et al: Improvement in the diagnosis of abscesses associated with endocarditis by transesophageal echocardiography, *N Engl J Med* 324:795–800, 1991.
124. Trehan N, Goldfarb A, Gindea AJ et al: Echocardiographic diagnosis of atrioventricular septal perforation caused by an aortic valve vegetation, *J Am Soc Echocardiogr* 1:150–151, 1988.
125. Tunick PA, Kronzon I: Protruding atherosclerotic plaque in the aortic arch of patients with systemic embolization: a new finding seen by transesophageal echocardiography, *Am Heart J* 120:658–660, 1990.
126. Tunick PA, Perez JL, Kronzon I: The association between protruding atheromas in the thoracic aorta and systemic embolization: a new finding seen by transesophageal echocardiography, *Ann Intern Med* 115:423–427, 1991.
127. Brenner B, Blumenfeld Z, Markiewitz W et al: Cardiac involvement in patients with primary antiphospholipid syndrome, *J Am Coll Cardiol* 18:931–936, 1991.
128. Lee RJ, Bartzokis T, Yeoh TK et al: Enhanced detection of intracardiac sources of cerebral emboli by transesophageal echocardiography, *Stroke* 22:734–739, 1991.

Chapter 12

Hematologic Evaluation

Daniel Brookoff, M.D., Ph.D.

EVALUATION OF BLOOD CELLS

In the first modern textbook on the subject, Downey called hematology "the study of the blood and all the organs through which it flows." Diseases of nearly every organ system produce hematologic changes that can be assessed with simple laboratory tests. While primary hematologic diseases are relatively rare, hematologic manifestations of other diseases occur frequently. Examination of the blood is performed in all patients with major illness because of the importance of determining the presence of anemia or leukocytosis. Evaluation of platelet counts and coagulation factors is important in patients with unexplained bleeding and in those expected to undergo a hemostatic stress such as surgery.

Erythrocytes

Physiology and Pathology

Erythrocytes, the major cellular components of blood, mediate oxygen transport from the lungs to the tissues. In order to perform this function they are densely packed with the oxygen-carrying protein hemoglobin. Hemoglobin is unique not only for its ability to carry and unload oxygen but also for its fluidity. If red cells contained a similar protein such as myoglobin at the same concentration, they would have the flow characteristics of bricks. The erythrocyte membrane is also a specialized structure with an underlying layer of the protein spectrin, which maintains the erythrocyte's disk shape and gives it the distensibility to ensure smooth flow through narrow capillaries. Erythrocytes survive for only 120 days in the circulation, and the continuous processes of erythrocyte production and destruction lend themselves to laboratory evaluation.

Most of the laboratory tests of erythrocytes requested by emergency physicians are concerned with the detection and evaluation of anemia. The causes of anemia can be broadly categorized into two groups: defects in production or accelerated destruction of erythrocytes. Another useful way to categorize anemias is by the size of the circulating erythrocytes: microcytic, normocytic, or macrocytic (see accompanying box). These classifications have a physiologic basis in the development of erythrocytes from nucleated precursors in the bone marrow.

Classification of Common Anemias by Red Cell Size

Microcytic (MCV* < $80\mu m^3$)
- Iron deficiency anemia
- Thalassemia
- Immune hemolytic anemia
- Microangiopathic anemia

Normocytic (MCV, $80-100\mu m^3$)
- Hemorrhage
- Chronic disease
- Bone marrow failure or infiltration (e.g., by tumor)
- Lead poisoning

Macrocytic anemia (MCV > $100\mu m^3$)
- Vitamin B_{12} deficiency
- Folate deficiency
- Chemotherapy (e.g., with methotrexate)
- Hypothyroidism
- Severe liver disease

*MCV, mean corpuscular volume

DETERMINANTS OF RED CELL SIZE

During their development in the marrow, the increasing concentration of hemoglobin in the cytoplasm of nucleated erythroblasts feeds back upon the nucleus and controls nuclear development and cellular division. When a critical concentration of hemoglobin is reached, DNA synthesis halts, no more divisions take place, and the nucleus is extruded. With each division, the ultimate size of the daughter cells decrease. If heme synthesis is impaired (e.g., due to iron deficiency) or globin synthesis is disrupted (e.g., thalassemia), then the buildup in cytoplasmic hemoglobin will be slowed and the erythroblast will undergo excess divisions resulting in small erythrocytes (microcytosis). When DNA synthesis is impaired (e.g., vitamin B_{12} or folate deficiency or antimetabolite chemotherapy), nuclear development is slowed and will be arrested before the usual number of cell divisions can take place. The resultant erythrocytes will be macrocytes. In some instances, metabolic abnormalities can impair both hemoglobin formation and nuclear development (e.g., lead poisoning), and the resultant cells are of normal size (normocytic anemia).

Different modes of cell destruction can also influence cell size (e.g., many types of intravascular hemolysis cause loss of membrane and microcytosis). Severe liver disease can result in the circulation of abnormal lipids that are incorporated into the red cell membrane and cause macrocytosis. Cell loss due to extravascular hemolysis or acute hemorrhage usually results in normocytic anemia.

Hemoglobin

The World Health Organization defines anemia by quantifying hemoglobin. For males, anemia is defined as a hemoglobin concentration of less than 13 g/dL; for menstruating females, less than 12 g/dL; and for pregnant females, less than 11 g/dL. The most accurate determinations result from using venous blood samples. Fingerstick samples can give falsely low values.[1] Capillary blood from a cold extremity is especially likely to produce a low hemoglobin reading.[2] At least 5 mL of blood should be collected in a test tube containing ethylenediaminetetraacetic acid (EDTA), which is provided in a lavender-topped tube. Samples will remain stable at room temperature for up to 12 hours.

In the laboratory, erythrocytes are lysed by using a measured volume of saponin. Potassium cyanide and potassium ferricyanide are added to convert hemoglobin to cyanomethemoglobin, the concentration of which is then measured by absorption at 540 nm in a photometer.[3] Falsely high values may result from increased plasma turbidity due to abnormal plasma proteins, hyperlipidemia, or very high white cell counts (greater than 50,000).

Hematocrit

The hematocrit is the proportion of the blood volume occupied by erythrocytes. It was originally ascertained by packing the red cells with a centrifuge and determining the ratio of packed cell volume to the total volume of the entire sample. With current cell counters, the hematocrit is a calculated value derived from the total erythrocyte count and the mean corpuscular volume (MCV).

Erythrocyte Indices

Most emergency departments (EDs) use laboratories with automated cell counters. The cell counter works by forcing a metered volume of a suspension of blood cells through a small orifice and calculating the cell count by measuring the electrical impedance or the scatter of light transmitted across the opening of the aperture.[4] In addition to cell counts, automated counters determine red cell indices, including the MCV (normal range, 80 to 100 μm^3), which is the factor by which one can discriminate among microcytic, normocytic, and macrocytic anemias.[5] By dividing the hemoglobin by the erythrocyte count, the cell counters also calculate mean corpuscular hemoglobin (MCH; normal value, 26 to 34 pg). This value will be low in thalassemia and can be high in disorders such as immune hemolytic anemia where the cells lose relatively more membrane than hemoglobin. Dividing hemoglobin by hematocrit yields the MCH concentration (normal range, 31 to 36 g/dL of red cells). This value is classically low in iron deficiency anemias and can also be low in thalassemia. Automated cell counters will also calculate a measure of red cell size distribution known as the red cell distribution width (RDW). This is a measure of anisocytosis, and the normal range is a value less than 14 μm. The RDW is increased in hemolytic anemias, folic acid and vitamin B_{12} deficiency, patients receiving chemotherapy, and alcoholics. An RDW of more than 20 μm is usually an indicator of thalassemia.[6]

Blood Films

Microscopic examination of blood yields information on red cell size, shape, and variation. In some instances, cell shape can be an important indicator of the diagnosis (e.g., schizocytes in microangiopathic anemias, spherocytes in immune hemolytic anemia, teardrop cells in myelophthisic disorders or sickled cells). Hemoglobin concentration can be estimated by evaluating the cells for hypochromia or signs of hemoglobinopathy (e.g., target cells). Examining blood films for erythrocyte inclusions can make the diagnosis of parasitemia.

Although blood smears are usually made on slides, better morphology can be obtained by using coverslips. A small drop of anticoagulated blood is placed in the center of a coverslip, and another coverslip is placed to contact the drop. The coverslips are quickly pulled away from each other and allowed to completely air-dry. The coverslips can be stained with Wright's stain, which is allowed to set for 3 minutes. Buffer is then added to the stain on the coverslip until a green surface sheen appears. After

3 minutes, the coverslip is rinsed off in distilled water and allowed to dry. It is then placed on a slide and examined. Red cells should be of uniform size (roughly 80% of the diameter of a small lymphocyte) should contain a central pallor that spans a third to half the diameter and should have no cellular inclusions.

Reticulocyte Counts

The most useful measure of erythrocyte production in emergency practice is the reticulocyte count. Reticulocytes are immature forms of erythrocytes that circulate for 1 to 2 days before maturing into erythrocytes. Reticulocytes do not have a biconcave shape and thus no central pallor on a blood film. Reticulocytes can also be distinguished from erythrocytes on a blood film by their basophilic cytoplasm. Reticulocytes have a higher mean cell volume than erthrocytes. Because of this, blood with a high proportion of reticulocytes may have a macrocytic MCV (but will have a low RDW). Much of the process of reticulocyte maturation takes place in the spleen, where portions of the cell membrane and cytoplasm are removed in a process called "splenic conditioning." Asplenic patients cannot "condition" their reticulocytes and thus will appear to have macrocytosis.

In the laboratory test for reticulocytes, ribosomal RNA is precipitated and stained with a supravital dye such as new methylene blue or cresyl violet. The blood is then microscopically examined and the number of erythrocytes containing stained precipitate counted and expressed as a percentage of the total number of red cells examined.[7] The normal range for reticulocytes is between 1% and 2%. In cases of anemia with inadequate red cell production, the reticulocyte count may appear increased because of the dearth of mature erythrocytes. A *corrected reticulocyte count* (the reticulocyte index) can be obtained by using the following simple formula:

$$\text{Reticulocyte count (\%)} \times \text{Patient's hematocrit/Normal hematocrit.}$$

A "normal" reticulocyte count (usually 1% to 2%) is *not* normal in the face of anemia and instead indicates inadequate erythrocyte production.

TESTS OF ERYTHROCYTE DESTRUCTION

Certain syndromes involving accelerated erythrocyte destruction are associated with other abnormal laboratory values. For example, blood loss due to upper gastrointestinal hemorrhage is associated with elevations in blood urea nitrogen levels. Intravascular hemolysis will often cause rises in the serum level of bilirubin, lactate dehydrogenase, and aspartate aminotransferase (AST) (serum glutamic-oxaloacetic transaminase [SGOT]). Brisk hemolysis typically causes *hemosiderinuria* (stainable iron in the urine), and *hemoglobinuria* can be an important sign of overwhelming hemolysis (e.g., major transfusion reaction).

Sickle Cell Preparation

Patients with sickle cell disease will usually have some sickle cells on a regular blood smear. The proportion of sickled cells is not related to the severity of crisis or hemolysis. If the diagnosis of sickle cell disease is in doubt, a sickle cell preparation can be ordered. In this test red cells are exposed to a solution of sodium metabisulfite, a reducing agent that induces the polymerization of sickle hemoglobin (HbS). The cells are then examined microscopically. This test cannot be used to distinguish between sickle cell disease (HbSS) and sickle cell trait (HbSA).

CASE 12–1

A 50-year-old man came to the ED with complaints of transient left-sided weakness. On examination, he was neurologically intact but noted to have a ruddy complexion. His hemoglobin was 21 g/dL and his oxygen saturation was normal.

Comment.—This patient has polycythemia vera due to clonal overproduction of erythrocytes, which is considered by many to be a preleukemic state. Hemoglobin levels over 18 g/dL lead to severely increased blood viscosity and increased risk of stroke. This patient requires emergent phlebotomy to reduce his hemoglobin level below 17 g/dL.

CASE 12–2

Three days after starting treatment for an infection with sulfamethoxazole, a 10-year-old male began to complain of severe abdominal and back pain. His mother brought him to the ED 3 days later when she noted that his urine had turned dark. Laboratory tests in the ED were remarkable for a hemoglobin of 8 g/dL, a hematocrit of 22, a reticulocyte count of 25%, and an MCV of 100 μm^3. Heinz bodies (red cell inclusions made up of precipitated hemoglobin) were noted on the smear.

Comment.—This boy has glucose-6-phosphate dehydrogenase (G6PD) deficiency, a condition that leads to self-limited hemolysis after exposure to certain drugs (see box on the next page).[8] Patients usually do well after discontinuation of the offending drug.[8] His corrected reticulocyte count of 13% was appropriately high for his degree of anemia.

CASE 12–3

A 16-year-old male with sickle cell disease came to the ED because of worsening weakness and progressive dyspnea following a viral syndrome. At that time his weakness was severe, and he had dyspnea on mild exertion. His hemoglobin was 4 g/dL (he told the physician that his hemoglobin usually runs between 8 and 10). His reticulocyte count was 0.2% and the smear was positive for occasional sickle cells.

Comments.—This patient is having an aplastic crisis. In this case it was due to infection with parvovirus, which commonly infects children and teenagers and destroys cycling erythroblasts. Since most normal erythroblasts are dormant, most people experience only a mild transient anemia with this infection. In patients whose erythrocyte production is maximal (e.g., sickle cell disease, severe thalassemia) the virus can destroy all the differentiated erythroid elements in the marrow. Since up to 2 weeks is required to replenish the erythroid cell lines from stem cells, a severe but self-limited nonregenerative anemia results. Patients with such aplastic crises are usually admitted for supportive care until the aplasia resolves. In patients with sickle cell disease, aplastic crises are not necessarily associated with vasoocclusive crises and are rarely seen beyond the age of 20 years.

LEUKOCYTE COUNTS AND DIFFERENTIALS

White blood cell counts and differential counts are among the most common laboratory tests requested by emergency physicians. They are usually requested to help evaluate a patient for bacterial infection. Either an elevated neutrophil count or an increase in the proportion of immature neutrophils is an important sign of bacterial infection. However, as the box on page 215 demonstrates, there are many noninfec-

Common Causes of Hemolytic Anemia

- Microangiopathies
  - Disseminated intravascular coagulation
  - Thrombotic thrombocytopenic purpura
  - Artificial heart valve
  - *Shigella*
  - Aortic stenosis
  - Polyarteritis nodosa
  - Acute glomerulonephritis
- IgM mediated (cold agglutinin positive)
  - Epstein-Barr virus
  - Cytomegalovirus
  - Chronic lymphocytic leukemia
  - Lymphomas
  - Lupus
  - Varicella
  - Measles
- IgG mediated (warm agglutinin positive)
  - Idiopathic
  - Chronic lymphocytic leukemia
  - Lupus
  - Non-Hodgkin lymphoma
- Drug induced
  - Procaine
  - Triamterene
  - Quinidine
  - α-Methyldopa
  - Penicillin in high doses
  - Rifampin
  - Isoniazid (INH)
  - Thiazides
  - Ibuprofen
- Metabolic
  - Sickle cell disease
  - Hereditary spherocytosis
  - Paroxysmal nocturnal hemoglobinuria
  - Drugs that commonly cause hemolysis in glucose-6-phosphate dehydrogenase (G6PD) deficiency
    - Sulfamethoxazole
    - Nitrofurantoin
    - Primaquine
    - Sulfacetamide
    - Nalidixic acid
- Environmental causes
  - Heat stroke
  - Severe burns
  - Insect venom
- Other causes
  - Arsine gas
  - Copper sulfate
  - Chlorates
  - Ulcerative colitis
  - Malaria
  - Babesiosis

Modified from Beutler E: Hemolytic anemia. In Williams W et al, editors: *Hematology,* New York, 1983, McGraw-Hill.

Noninfectious Causes of Neutrophilia

Drugs and medications
- Epinephrine
- Lithium
- Cocaine
- Corticosteroids

Cigarette smoking
Recent surgery
Malignancy
Hemolytic anemia (e.g., sickle cell disease)
Seizures (can increase leukocyte counts to over 30,000/mm^3[3,31])
Hemorrhage
Inflammatory disease
Burns and trauma (can increase leukocyte counts threefold[32])
Exercise (short sprints can increase counts to over 35,000/mm^3[3,33])
Diabetic ketoacidosis
Uremia
Eclampsia
Pregnancy

tious causes of neutrophilia, which is defined as an elevation in the absolute neutrophil count (usually ranging from 1800 to 7700/mm^3) by two standard deviations above the mean. Other instances where the white blood cell counts are of clinical significance in emergency practice include the evaluation of neutropenia in patients who have undergone cancer treatment and in the assessment of a patient for hematologic malignancy.

To obtain a leukocyte count, blood collected in EDTA is suspended in a saponin solution that lyses erythrocytes. Counts made "by hand" with a hemacytometer are not precise and have more than 20% variance.[9] Results from automated cell counters are more consistent. In these machines, a fixed volume of cells suspended in saponin flows through an aperture, and the count is determined by measuring electrical impedance or light scatter.

Differential cell counts are currently performed by microscopically examining the stained blood smear. The proportion of different cell types are recorded, as are the number of immature circulating forms (e.g., stabs, bands). The presence of precursor cells that are normally restricted to the marrow (e.g., blasts, nucleated erythroid cells) are also noted. An excess of immature cells (termed a "shift to the left" because of the position of the keys for counting immature cells on the cell counter) is a ratio of immature to mature granulocytes of greater than 10%. The differential count is time-consuming and imprecise and is being replaced by automatic counters that use light scatter or microfluorimetry to distinguish different types of cells. The different types of cells are often expressed as a percentage of the total count (Table 12–1).[10] Since percentages carry a greater variance than absolute counts, many laboratories also report absolute counts for the various cell types (Table 12–2).[11–13]

Normal values for leukocyte counts vary among different populations: children have higher leukocyte counts than adults, and leukocytes peak soon after birth with an average count of 22,000.[14] Children between the ages of 6 months and 4 years usually have a higher proportion of lymphocytes than granulocytes. Leukocyte counts are also normally elevated in pregnancy with increased neutrophils, monocytes, and eosinophils.[15] Leukocyte counts in black patients average 1000 to 1200/mm^3 lower than those in white patients.[16]

Table 12–1. Average Differential Counts

Cell	Count (%)
Segmented neutrophils	58.9 ± 0.3
Band forms	0.2
Lymphocytes	35.9 ± 0.4
Monocytes	2.9 ± 0.2
Eosinophils	2.0 ± 0.2
Basophils	0.1

Data from National Health and Nutrition Survey: *Vital Health Stat* 220:1–2, 1982.

Table 12–2. Normal Ranges of Absolute Leukocyte Counts (cells/mm^3)

Cell	All Subjects[12]	Males[13]	Females[13]
Neutrophils	1,830–7,250	1,539–5,641	1,861–6,821
Lymphocytes	1,500–4,000	1,168–3,262	1,149–3,664
Eosinophils	0–700	30–592	20–582
Monocytes	200–950	217–849	225–836
Basophils	0–150	0–136	0–138
Total	4,300–10,000	3,480–9,200	3,800–10,100

Stained blood smears can also be used to examine the morphology of individual granulocytes for features related to the presence of infection. These include toxic granulations, Döhle bodies, and vacuolization. Of the three, only neutrophil vacuolization appears to be reasonably specific for bacterial infection.[17]

Interpreting Leukocyte Counts and Differentials

The utility of a laboratory test is measured by whether an abnormal reading represents disease. In light of the variability of white cell counts and differentials[18] and physiologic variance,[19] moderate variations from normal values are often not clinically significant. In other words, it is usually fruitless to pursue an abnormal leukocyte count unless some specific disease process is suspected [20] (see Chapters 1 and 25). Extreme values are often associated with disease, but even when there is neutrophilia, neither the actual leukocyte count nor the differential can distinguish between bacterial and viral infection [21] in all instances. On the other hand, a differential count is often not necessary to confirm the presence of infection when leukocytosis is documented by the cell count. The management of most cases of acute bacterial infection will not be influenced by the differential count.[20]

The Leukocyte Count as a Screening Test

There is no evidence to support the use of leukocyte counts as a "screening" test for a patient who is not suspected of having an infection, having neutropenia, or having a hematologic malignancy.[11] Even the rare occurrence of making an early diagnosis of leukemia in an asymptomatic patient is of questionable clinical utility.[21] The differential count is even less reliable than the leukocyte count as a screening tool. Fifty percent of healthy patients have abnormal differential counts.[22] Although the actual cost of performing a white cell count and differential is relatively inexpensive, the real costs are not limited to the actual cost of the test but also include the physician's response to an abnormal result,[23] including repeat and "follow-up" tests. The use of the leukocyte differential as a routine admission test has also come into question. Again, differential counts can be valuable to support the diagnosis of infection or neutropenia, but in other patients admitted to the hospital abnormal leukocyte differentials are rarely of clinical value.[24]

Leukocyte and Differential Counts in Infection

Many infections cause neutrophilia. Most patients with bacterial sepsis have elevated leukocyte counts, but up to 10% of patients whose blood cultures are positive for bacteria have normal leukocyte and differential counts.[25] In many cases of sepsis, either the leukocyte count or the differential may be abnormal, but not both. In one study of children with documented bacterial infections, 25% had abnormalities in only one of the two tests.[26]

The leukocyte count takes on added significance in neonates suspected of infection because these patients often cannot generate fevers in the first 2 weeks of life. In obtaining a blood specimen for a leukocyte count it is important to remember that the leukocyte count of capillary blood can be significantly higher than that of venous blood, which in turn can be significantly higher than that of arterial blood. It is also important to take into account the fact that vigorous crying can, by itself, cause a marked elevation of the leukocyte count. With neonates as with other patients, the laboratory results must be correlated with the overall clinical evaluation in order to be meaningful.[27]

The Leukocyte Count in Diagnosing Appendicitis

Although the leukocyte count and differential are always used in evaluating a patient with abdominal pain who is suspected of having appendicitis, these tests by themselves cannot serve as the basis for the decision on whether to surgically intervene.[28] More than 15% of adult patients with appendicitis will not have a leukocyte count greater than 9000, which is the number frequently included as the minimum "required" to consider the diagnosis of appendicitis.[29] The differential count by itself is even less sensitive for the diagnosis of appendicitis,[30] but it does appear to increase the sensitivity of the leukocyte count in these cases. In one large series, 21% of patients with appendicitis had normal leukocyte counts, but only 4% had both a normal count and a normal differential.[31]

EVALUATION OF NEUTROPENIA

Leukocyte counts are vital in evaluating febrile patients who are receiving cancer chemotherapy. A neutrophil count of less than 1000/mm^3 in a febrile patient receiving chemotherapy should prompt quick treatment for bacterial sepsis. Cancer patients with neutropenic sepsis usually die within 48 hours of the onset of fever.[32] If the white count is greater than 4500/mm^3, a differential count is not necessary.[33] Other causes of neutropenia are listed in the box on the next page and except for the infectious causes, aplasia, and chemotherapy-induced neutropenia, they are not usually predictors of overwhelming sepsis.

CASE 12–4

A 48-year-old man came to the ED with a complaint of painful swelling of his left calf. He had diffuse massive adenopathy, splenomegaly, and a large mass in the left politeal space. Hemoglobin, hematocrit, and platelet counts were all within normal limits. The leukocyte count was 89,000/mm^3, and the differential showed 98% lymphocytes.

Causes of Neutropenia

Chemotherapy
Sepsis
Specific bacterial infections
- *Salmonella typhi*
- *Brucella abortus*
- *Salmonella paratyphi*
- *Pasteurella tularensis*

Protozoal infection
Rickettsial infection
Viral infection
Radiation
Chemicals
- Lead
- Ethanol
- Benzene

Hypersplenism
Myelodysplastic syndromes and aplastic anemia
Drugs (dose related)
- Antihistamine
- Carbamazepine
- Chloramphenicol
- Colchicine
- Imipramine
- Isoniazid
- Penicillamine
- Phenothiazine
- Propylthiouracil (PTU)
- Rifampin

Drugs (hypersensitivity)
- Ampicillin
- Chloramphenicol
- Nonsteroidal antiinflammatory drugs (NSAIDS)
- Penicillin
- Procainamide
- Quinidine
- Sulfonilamides

Comment.—This patient has chronic lymphocytic leukemia. Leukostasis is not a problem in this disease if the lymphocyte count is below 1 million. On the other hand, leukostasis is seen in myeloid leukemias at counts above 100,000/mm^3. In this case venogram demonstrated a deep venous thrombosis secondary to occlusion of the patient's popliteal vein by enlarged lymph nodes. His adenopathy soon regressed with oral prednisone and chlorambucil.

CASE 12–5

A 32-year-old women with a 5-day history of fatigue and myalgias began medicating herself with a family member's trimethoprim-sulfamethoxazole. She came to the ED with continued myalgias, a temperature of 99.1° F, and nonfocal examination findings. Her hemoglobin was 11.5, the platelet count was 230,000, and the leukocyte count was 2900 with 50% neutrophils.

Comment.—This patient had a hypersensitivity reaction to sulfamethoxazole. Use of the drug was discontinued, and her leukocyte count returned to normal in 4 days.

EVALUATION OF HEMOSTASIS

Platelets

Physiology and Pathology

The formation of a platelet plug at the site of vessel injury is critical for effective hemostasis. The platelet plug is responsible for immediate hemostasis, and patients with platelet defects will suffer from excessive bleeding immediately following an injury, phlebotomy, or operative procedures. Epistaxis, gastrointestinal bleeding, or menorrhagia may also be signs of platelet disorders.

In order to maintain hemostasis, functioning platelets must be present in adequate concentrations, usually 150,000 to 400,000/mm^3 of blood. Thrombocytopenia, defined as a platelet count below 100,000/mm^3, is the most common cause of defective platelet plug formation.[37] The risk of bleeding when thrombocytopenia is present is inversely related to the platelet count. Patients with counts below 50,000/mm^3 are at risk for severe bleeding from trauma, and counts below 20,000/mm^3 pose a significant risk for spontaneous intracerebral hemorrhage.[38]

Thrombocytopenia can be manifested by petechiae, mucosal bleeding or, if platelet counts are very low, purpura or deep tissue bleeding. Petechiae, nonblanching reddish macules, are a manifestation of pinpoint dermal hemorrhages. They can often be found in the oral mucosa or at sites of skin compression, such as areas underlying elastic bands, belts, blood pressure cuffs, or tourniquets (hence the name "tourniquet sign"). Thrombocytopenia can be caused by the underproduction or accelerated destruction of platelets, which normally have a circulating half-life of 4 days.

Abnormalities of platelet production may be due to marrow hypoplasia caused by cytotoxic drugs, radiation, or idiopathic hypoplastic syndromes. Marrow infiltration by cancer cells or fibrosis can also result in decreased platelet production. Several noncytotoxic drugs can cause selective impairment of platelet production, the most common of which are thiazides, sulfonamides, gold, and trimethoprim-sulfamethoxazole.[39] Other causes of platelet production abnormalities include viral infection (e.g., rubella), heatstroke, vitamin B_{12} deficiency, folic acid deficiency, and profound iron deficiency. Another substance that commonly causes underproduction of platelets is ethanol, and chronic alcoholics will often have platelet counts in the 50,000 to 80,000/mm^3 range.

Accelerated destruction of platelets and removal of platelets from the circulation are common causes of thrombocytopenia. Platelets may be destroyed by immune mechanisms,[40] as is the case in idiopathic thrombocytopenic purpura, lupus, lymphoma, or certain cases of hemolytic anemia (Evan's syndrome). Thrombocytopenia due to heparin, gold, quinidine, and quinine is the result of drug-induced antibody formation, and antibodies may also play a role in thrombocytopenic syndromes associated with phenytoin, diazepam, thiazides, acetaminophen, and sulfisoxazole.[41] Platelets can also be destroyed by nonimmunologic mechanisms in cases of disseminated intravascular coagulopathy (DIC), thrombotic thrombocytopenic purpura, preeclampsia, and gram-negative septicemia. Hypersplenism can result in platelet sequestration, which can reduce the number of circulating platelets by up to 80%. Common causes of hypersplenism are cirrhosis, congestive heart failure, portal vein obstruction, tuberculosis, and other granulomatous diseases and connective tissue disorders.[42] Another form of thrombocytopenia frequently seen in the ED is due to washout from massive transfusion of stored blood or packed red cells. A common rule in the management of severe hemorrhage is that a patient who is transfused with more than 10 units of packed cells or blood will require platelet transfusions (usually 8 to 10 units of properly stored platelets) to maintain hemostasis. When a large blood loss is anticipated from surgery or trauma, platelet washout can be avoided by transfusing 4 units of platelets after every 4 units of blood or packed cells.[39]

Thrombocythemia, that is, *excessive* concentrations of platelets, can be as serious a problem as thrombocytopenia. Platelet dysfunction can be detected at counts greater than 1,000,000/mm^3 and generally becomes clinically significant at counts above 2,000,000/mm^3, for which emergency treatment is required. Counts this high are usually due to a myeloproliferative disorder, *essential thrombocythemia,* although they can be associated with a variety of cancers.[43]

There are three separate platelet functions necessary for the formation of a competent platelet plug: adhesion, aggregation, and secretion.[44] The platelet plug begins to form when there is disruption of the endothelial lining of a blood vessel and exposure to the bloodstream of components of the subendothelium such as collagen and elements of the basement membrane. Contact with these substances causes platelets to adhere to the injured area and undergo activation, a process that involves a change in shape and release of secretory granules containing adenosine diphosphate (ADP), serotonin, fibrinogen, and various enzymes. A plasma protein, von Willebrand factor, is necessary for platelet adhesion, and deficiency of this factor results in a hemorrhagic disease, von Willebrand syndrome.[45] Since this disease is almost always congenital, patients coming to the ED with von Willebrand syndrome almost always relate a history of a bleeding disorder (e.g., with dental extraction).

Once platelets adhere to the subendothelium and become activated, they release mediators that initiate a second process called aggregation whereby additional platelets are recruited into the plug. Platelet aggregation is dependent on the presence of fibrinogen, and patients with afibrinogenemia will have prolonged bleeding times. Aggregated platelets next progress to the secretion phase. In this phase contractile proteins mediate the large-scale release of secretory granules that cause vasoconstriction and recruit even more platelets into the plug. Secretion is largely dependent on prostaglandins generated by enzymes on the platelet membrane. Aspirin irreversibly acetylates and inactivates membrane cyclooxygenases and causes defects in platelet function by inhibiting secretion. The effect of aspirin is usually dose related, but in patients with subclinical platelet disorders, one aspirin can cause profound platelet dysfunction for up to a week. Since the effect of aspirin is irreversible, aspirin-poisoned platelets must be replaced by new platelets before the defect can be corrected.[46]

Nonsteroidal antiinflammatory drugs such as ibuprofen and indomethacin cause reversible enzyme inhibition and therefore usually do not prolong the bleeding time. Other drugs that can interfere with platelet function include carbenicillin and penicillin—usually when used in large parenteral doses for prolonged periods.[47] Platelet dysfunction has also reportedly been associated with antihistamines and antipsychotic medications. Uremia, chronic liver disease, and macroglobulinemia are also associated with severe platelet dysfunction. In these diseases the platelet dysfunction is probably due to serum-borne factors that interfere with activation and aggregation since the platelets in these patients function normally in vitro.

LABORATORY TESTS OF PLATELET FUNCTION

The Platelet Count

Thrombocytopenia is the most common cause of serious bleeding. The most important initial test of clinical importance is the platelet count. Blood for platelet counting should be collected in EDTA (lavender-topped tube). If the blood is kept unagitated at room temperature, a reliable platelet count can be obtained from the specimen for up to 18 hours. The platelet concentration can be quickly estimated by examination of a properly prepared Wright-stained smear. A normal platelet concentration corresponds to the presence of 8 to 12 platelets per high-power field or, alternatively, 1 platelet per 20 erythrocytes (providing, of course, that the erythrocyte concentration is near normal). Precise platelet counts can be obtained by lysing erythrocytes with ammonium oxalate and then using a hemocytometer or an electronic cell counter that counts the cells by using electrical impedance or laser light scatter. In this instance, although the machines are much quicker than hemocytometers, they are less precise and result in broader normal ranges. The machines are also unreliable when the platelet count is less than 50,000/mm^3 or when the white blood cell count is greater than 100,000/mm^3. In these instances, the platelet count should be confirmed by using a hemocytometer.[39] Occasionally, a patient will have a low platelet count due to laboratory artifact. Termed pseudothrombocytopenia, this occurrence is due to an IgM antibody that, in the presence of EDTA, causes platelet agglutination.[48] This antibody is of no clinical import, but it will result in artificially low counts. The blood smears of patients with pseudothrombocytopenia will show clumped platelets. If the blood is recollected in citrate or heparin, it will usually yield a normal platelet count.

Bleeding Time

The bleeding time is an overall screening test for platelet function. It is also one of the most overused and misunderstood tests in hematology. It should only be used if there is a reason to suspect a platelet disorder, such as a recent history of aspirin use in a preoperative patient, a history suggestive of von Willebrand disease, or a history of an intercurrent disease that can interfere with platelet function. The bleeding time test can also be used to evaluate the effects of platelet transfusion in certain limited cases. Bleeding time tests are not part of the routine preoperative workup and can result in considerable cost and inconvenience if used correctly because of the large proportion of false positive results.[49]

In the template bleeding time test (Ivy)[50] a 10-mm-long incision, 1 mm deep, is made midway down the volar surface of the arm. A blood pressure cuff on the upper part of the arm is kept inflated to 40 mm Hg. A stopwatch is started as the incision is made, and blood is blotted away with filter paper every 30 seconds. When blood no longer stains the paper, the test is finished. Usually two cuts are made, and if the bleeding times are within 3 minutes of each other, the average bleeding time is reported. In many institutions a spring-loaded device (Mielke) has replaced the blade and template. With platelet counts above 100,000/mm^3 the average bleeding time is 4.5 minutes; a normal bleeding time is 10 minutes or less. Some hematologists feel that it is not useful to obtain bleeding time tests in patients with platelet counts of less than 100,000/mm^3. Other hematologists use a formula that takes into account the decrease in platelet concentration:

$$\text{Bleeding time (minutes)} = 30 - (\text{Platelet count}/4000).$$

A bleeding time of over 10 minutes with a platelet count of over 100,000/mm^3 establishes the diagnosis of platelet dysfunction. If an inflated blood pressure cuff cannot be used or is contraindicated (e.g., bilateral arm casts, wounds, rash), the Duke bleeding time test can be performed. The Duke test is similar to the Ivy method but does not use a cuff. It is less precise than the two types of Ivy bleeding time tests and has a normal range of 1 to 3.5 minutes.

Platelet Aggregometry

For patients who have a normal platelet count but an abnormally prolonged bleeding time, the specific platelet defect can be defined by platelet aggregometry.[51] An aggregometer records the transmission of light through a suspension of platelets. The platelets are collected in citrate (blue-topped tube) and exposed to various substances that should induce aggregation such as ADP, epinephrine, collagen, or ristocetin. When the platelets aggregate, light is transmitted through the suspension more readily. This test can differentiate among acquired platelet abnormalities (such as aspirin use or myeloproliferative syndromes), hereditary disorders (e.g., von Willebrand disease), and serum or collagen abnormalities unrelated to the quantity or quality characteristics of platelets that may result in a prolonged bleeding time (e.g., Ehlers-Danlos syndrome, Marfan syndrome, uremia, amyloidosis, and scurvy).[52]

COAGULATION AND FIBRINOLYSIS

Physiology

In addition to activating platelets, injuries to blood vessels activate the coagulation system, which will normally result in the formation of a fibrin clot.[53] The fibrin clot is responsible for prolonged hemostasis. Disorders of the coagulation system usually manifest themselves in delayed hemorrhage following injury or in deep tissue bleeding (e.g., hemarthrosis). The precursor to fibrin, fibrinogen circulates as a large, multichained protein. Interaction with thrombin results in the cleavage of these chains into fibrin monomers and fibrinopeptides A and B (also called fibrin split products). The fibrin monomers then polymerize to form the clot and bind more fibrinogen in the process. Factor XIII, which is made both in the liver and by platelets, cross-links the fibrin polymers and binds the ends to fibronectin, a component of basement membranes. Factor XIII strengthens and stabilizes the clot and promotes wound healing.

The coagulation cascades are series of chemical reactions that result in the activation of thrombin.[54] When a blood vessel is injured, damaged cells release tissue thromboplastin, which activates factor VII and sets off the "extrinsic pathway" of coagulation (Fig. 12–1). The exposure of subendothelial collagen to the plasma activates factor XII, which sets off the "intrinsic pathway" (see Fig. 12–1). Knowing about these separate cascades is essential to understanding and interpreting coagulation tests. In vivo, the two systems probably interact and are interdependent[55] (e.g., factor VII can directly activate factor IX). The two most commonly used tests of the coagulation system, the prothrombin time (PT) and the partial thromboplastin time (PTT), are tests of the extrinsic and intrinsic pathways, respectively. Unfortunately, they are very sensitive to factors that may be clinically insignificant[56] (see below).

Just as the coagulation system exists to establish fibrin clots, the fibrinolytic system exists to remove fibrin and reestablish flow in thrombosed vessels. With the increasing use of fibrinolytic drugs, understanding and monitoring of the fibrinolytic system are becoming increasingly important in the ED as well as in special care units.[57] Plasmin, a serine protease like many of the coagulation factors, is the main agent of fibrinolysis and cleaves fibrin in both its monomer and polymer form. Plasmin can also cleave factors V and VIII and lead to a coagulopathy. Plasmin can become activated from its inactive form (plasminogen) through the action of the coagulation factors that initiate the intrinsic pathway of coagulation. Other activators of plasminogen can be found in injured tissues, notably endothelial cells (tissue plasminogen activator), and in minute amounts in normal urine (urokinase). Streptokinase is a nonenzymatic protein derived from bacteria that is used therapeutically to enhance fibrinolysis. Streptokinase binds to molecules of plasmin or plasminogen and turns them into potent plasminogen activators.[58] The use of fibrinolytic agents is steadily increasing. They are currently indicated for (some cases of) acute myocardial infarction, deep venous thrombosis, pulmonary embolism, retinal artery occlusion, peripheral arterial occlusion, vertebrobasilar stroke, and occluded indwelling vascular catheters.[59]

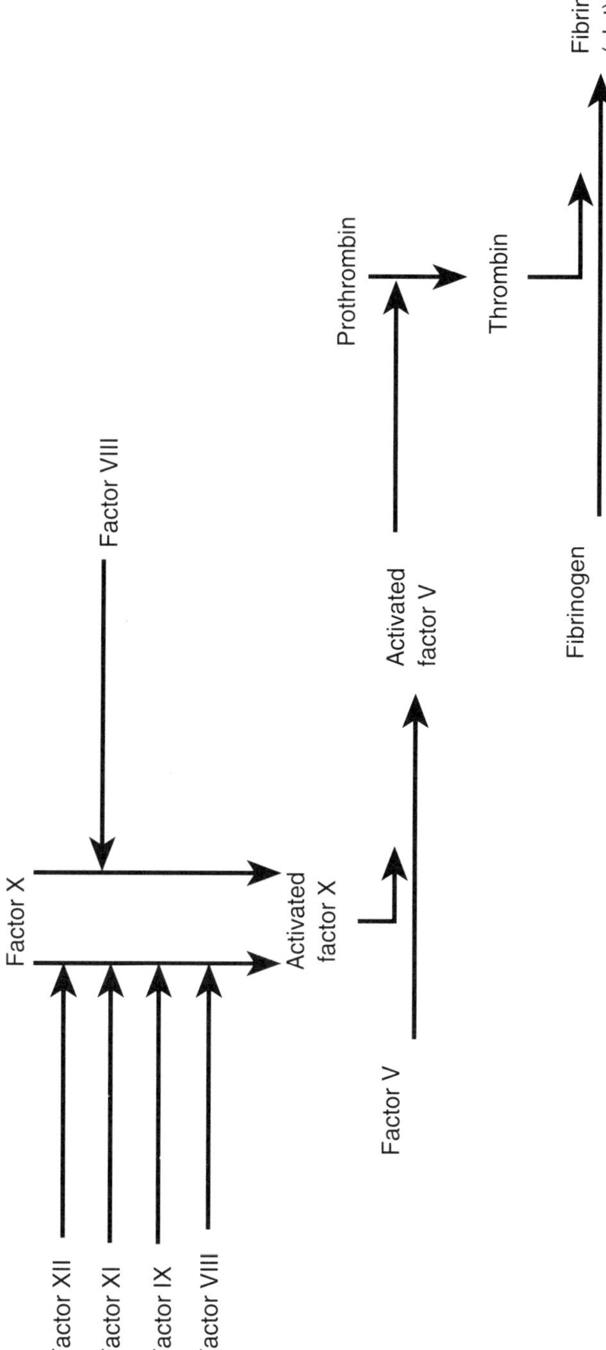

Fig. 12–1. Schematic representation of coagulation cascade.

Tests of Coagulation

Since calcium is required for most of the coagulation reactions, blood for most coagulation studies is collected in tubes with chelators such as citrate (blue-topped tube) to effectively remove the calcium.

Prothrombin Time

In 1832 de Blainville discovered the extrinsic pathway of coagulation when he injected suspensions of brain tissue into various animals and found that they all died immediately: their blood vessels were filled with clotted blood. In 1935 Quick invented the PT test (also called the Quick test) by adding tissue thromboplastin and calcium to citrated plasma and measuring the time to clot formation. The normal ranges of the PT vary among laboratories and are usually between 10 and 13 seconds. The PT is used to measure activity of the vitamin K–dependent factors (factors II (thrombin), VII, IX, and X).

The PT is particularly sensitive to the level of factor VII, a short-lived factor ($t_{1/2}$= 6 hours) that itself may not be clinically important but serves as a useful measure of the liver's ability to synthesize protein or, alternatively, of the degree of vitamin K depletion resulting from the use of the anticoagulant coumarin.[60] Since the goal of coumarin therapy is to cause anticoagulation by reducing the concentration of factors II and X, the PT may reach "therapeutic" levels a day or two before the patient is adequately anticoagulated. Conversely, when treating vitamin K deficiency, the PT may show a rapid return to normal (usually within 6 hours of an injection of phytonadione [Aquamephyton]) despite a persistent coagulopathy.

As noted, in addition to serving as an assessment of coumarin therapy and/or vitamin K deficiency, the PT serves as a rapid but crude test of the liver's ability to synthesize protein. In general, the PT does not become prolonged until the levels of vitamin K–dependent factors are less than 40% of normal. In cases of acute hepatitis, a PT of 1½ times normal can be an indicator of fulminant hepatic necrosis.[61] Other factors that can prolong the PT are low levels of fibrinogen or dysfibrinogenemia, the presence of fibrin split products, and blood specimens left in unstoppered tubes or collected in the wrong anticoagulant (e.g., EDTA). Clinically important factor deficiencies involving components of the extrinsic pathway are very rare. The PT is not a useful preoperative test in a patient who does not have a history of coumarin use, liver disease, or malnutrition.

International Normalized Ratio

Many centers are now using International Normalized Ratios (INRs) to monitor warfarin therapy. The INR is calculated by the following formula:

$$\text{INR} = (\text{observed prothrombin ratio})^{\text{ISI}}$$

where ISI is the index of sensitivity for the thromboplastin reagent used for the test. Because different thromboplastins used in the United States have a wide range of ISIs, recommendations for the intensity of warfarin therapy are given in terms of INR. In general, patients on warfarin should be kept at an INR between 2.0 and 3.0 for all indications (including recurrent systemic embolism) except mechanical prosthetic heart valves, for which an INR of 2.5 to 3.5 is recommended.[62]

The Activated Partial Thromboplastin Time

Ellagic acid, a substance found in the bezoar stones of goats and llamas, has been used as a medicine since the fifteenth century. The stones were said to stop bleeding when placed on wounds, and the high demand for these stones in Europe in the sixteenth and seventeenth centuries helped finance many of the expeditions to the New World, where bezoar stones were harvested from Peruvian llamas.[56] These days ellagic acid is used in the activated partial thromboplastin time (aPTT) test as a surface activator of the intrinsic pathway of coagulation. Other substances that can be used as surface activators include kaolin or silica. In the original version of the test (the PTT), the glass sides of the test tube were used to initiate surface activation. Today, nearly all laboratories use an activator and may use the term PTT to mean aPTT.

The aPTT test also requires the addition of calcium and phospholipid to citrated plasma. In vivo, the platelet membrane rather than phospholipid is the site of many of the reactions of the intrinsic system as well as a source of some of the factors in the pathway (V and VIII). Because of this, severe thrombocytopenia can also cause a functional coagulopathy. Since the phospholipid used will potentiate the intrinsic pathway but will not activate factor VII, it is considered only a "partial" thromboplastin, hence the name of the test. The normal ranges for the PTT are between 25 and 42 seconds.[39] Prolongation of the PTT implies either a deficiency of any of the coagulation factors other than VII or XIII or the presence of a circulating anticoagulant. Mixing studies (see below) can differentiate between the two.

Deficiencies of factors that determine the PTT may have little clinical significance (e.g., XII [Hageman factor], prekallikrein [Fletcher factor], and high–molecular-weight kininogen [Fitzgerald factor]). A deficiency of other factors has potential clinical significance (e.g., factor XI, deficiency of which produces various bleeding risks, notably worse with urologic surgery). Finally, some deficiencies have great significance (factors VIII and IX, the hemophilic factors).

If an abnormally prolonged PTT persists after mixing equal volumes of normal and patient plasmas, this is presumptive evidence for a circulating inhibitor. The most common anticoagulant detected by the PTT is heparin, which works by deactivating factors II and X. Other anticoagulants include circulating antibodies to the coagulation factors, which are rare but can pose serious bleeding problems, and an antibody to phospholipid called the *lupus anticoagulant.*[63] The lupus anticoagulant, which is rarely associated with lupus despite its name, does not act as an anticoagulant in vivo. Rather, it has some association with thrombosis and causes increased risk of fetal wastage, deep venous thrombosis, and cerebral thromboembolism. This property is probably due to its ability to cause intravascular aggregation of platelets. The PTT is useful in the workup of abnormal bleeding, the monitoring or detection of heparin, and the preoperative evaluation of a patient requiring major surgery (see box on page 226).[64]

ASSAYS FOR FIBRINOGEN AND FIBRIN DEGRADATION PRODUCTS

In the assay for fibrinogen, thrombin is added to plasma and the amount of clottable fibrinogen determined either by solubilizing it in urea and measuring its spectrophotometer absorbence or by measuring the clotting time and comparing it with a standard curve.[65] The normal range for fibrinogen is between 180 and 400 mg/dL. This level may increase twofold to fourfold in acute inflammation (fibrinogen is the acute-phase reactant responsible for an increased erythrocyte sedimentation rate). A low fibrinogen level can be found in DIC, severe liver disease, or hypofibrinogenemia. Since the fibrinogen assays are not as sensitive to fibrin degradation products (FDPs) or the presence of heparin as are the PT and PTT (see box on page 227), they are useful as monitors of therapy in DIC. For example, heparin therapy can be adjusted to obtain the clinically desirable fibrinogen level of greater than 100 mg/dL.

There are currently several tests of FDPs, and they vary in their specificity. Al-

Preoperative Hemostatic Evaluation

All patients should complete the following screening questionnaire:

1. Have you ever bled for a long time or developed a swollen tongue or mouth after cutting or biting your tongue, cheek, or lip?
2. Do you develop bruises larger than a silver dollar without being able to remember when or how you injured yourself?
3. Have you ever had prolonged bleeding after a tooth extraction? Has the bleeding ever started up again the day after the extraction?
4. What operations have you had, including minor procedures? Have you ever had abnormal bleeding or bruising after surgery?
5. Have you been under the care of a doctor in the past 5 years? If so, for what?
6. What medications—including aspirin or any other remedies for headache, colds, menstrual cramps, arthritis, or other pains—have you taken in the last 10 days?
7. Has any blood relative had a problem with unusual bleeding or bruising after surgery? Were blood transfusions required to control this bleeding?

Answers to this questionnaire help place the patient at one of four levels:

Level 1: The screening history is negative and the surgery planned is minor. No screening tests are recommended.

Level 2: The screening history is negative and surgery is major (e.g., bowel resection). A PTT* and platelet count are recommended.

Level 3: The screening history suggests the possibility of defective hemostasis and/or the patient is facing a very high-risk procedure (e.g., cardiac bypass, surgery of the central nervous system, or major urologic surgery). A PT*, PTT, platelet count, and bleeding time test are recommended.

Level 4: The screening history is highly suggestive of a bleeding disorder. A PT, PTT, platelet count, and bleeding time are recommended. If the results of these tests are normal, consider platelet aggregation tests (for von Willebrand's disease), assays for factors VIII and IX (for mild hemophilia the PTT can be normal even if one of these factors is at 20% of normal level), or a thrombin time to detect dysfibrinogenemia.

Adapted with permission from Rappaport SI: *Blood* 61:229–231, 1983. **PTT*, partial thromboplastin time; *PT*, prothrombin time.

though most normal plasma will contain some FDPs, the level is usually elevated in liver disease (since the liver clears these fibrinopeptides from the bloodstream) and in DIC.

Thrombin Time

This test is used to monitor the effect of systemic fibrinolytic therapy. A low concentration of thrombin is added to plasma and the clotting time determined. The normal range is 18 to 20 seconds. Besides fibrinolytic therapy, other causes of a prolonged thrombin time include hypofibrinogenemia, dysfibrinoginemia, the presence of heparin, uremia, hyperbilirubinemia, and a high concentration of FDPs. The thrombin time is usually measured every 4 hours during systemic fibrinolytic therapy.[66] In some centers, baseline fibrinogen levels, PT, and aPTT are obtained and may be used as secondary monitors.

Differential Diagnosis of Prolonged Prothrombin Time and Partial Thromboplastin Time

- Isolated prolonged PT
  - Vitamin K deficiency
  - Coumarin effect
  - Isolated factor VII deficiency
  - Liver disease
- Isolated prolonged PTT
  - Lupus anticoagulant
  - Heparin
  - Disseminated intravascular coagulation
  - Hemophilia A or B, antibody to factors VIII or IX
- Prolonged PT and PTT
  - Severe vitamin K deficiency
  - Disseminated intravascular coagulation
  - Heparin
  - Severe liver disease
  - Antibody to or deficiency of factors X, V, or II
  - Lupus inhibitor
  - Amyloidosis

CASE 12–6

A 15-year-old male with a history of hemophilia A was brought to the ED because of pain in his left quadriceps area. There was no antecedent history of trauma. Physical examination revealed mild swelling without ecchymosis. The PTT was 75.

Comment.—Muscle hematomas in hemophiliacs can occur spontaneously or following minor trauma. Deep muscle hematomas involving the quadriceps or iliopsoas muscles can lead to serious complications. Initially these hematomas can be seen with little or no swelling or ecchymoses. Factor VIII levels should be kept at 50% to 70% of normal levels to control the bleeding from a deep muscle hematoma. This patient should have a factor VIII level determination. The dose of clotting units needed for replacement is calculated by the following formula:

$$\text{Weight (kg)} \times \text{plasma volume (40 mL/kg)} \times \text{\% of factor VIII needed.}$$

If this boy weighs 40 kg, his dose would be $40 \times 40 \times 0.70 = 1120$ clotting units. There are several ways to replace this factor. One unit of plasma contains 200 to 250 clotting units, cryoprecipitate contains 100 clotting units, and lyophilized factors generally contain 500 units per bottle. This patient would have to receive treatment every 12 hours to keep factor VIII levels above 50% until the hematoma has resolved.

CASE 12–7

A 53-year-old male came to the ED because of bladder outlet obstruction and was admitted to the urology service. He had undergone coronary artery bypass surgery 2 years before, and at that time he was told that he had some type of blood abnormality. Nevertheless, the surgery was performed without bleeding complications. He had also had prior dental extractions without incident. Screening laboratory tests showed a PT of 12 seconds and an aPTT of 82 seconds. He was taking several cardiac medicines.

Comment.—Upon further testing a significant factor XI deficiency was identified. Deficiency of this factor has a variable effect on the duration of bleeding. Patients with factor XI deficiency can go through life without bleeding problems until they encounter a major hemostatic stress. One such stress is urologic surgery where hemostasis can be particularly problematic because urokinase literally bathes the tissues of the urinary tract. Mixing studies demonstrated that the bleeding problem was the result of a factor deficiency, and the patient's factor XI level was increased with fresh frozen plasma. The differential diagnosis for an increased aPTT included lupus anticoagulant (which would not be clinically significant), other factor deficiency, a factor inhibitor, or heparin therapy. All abnormal aPTTs deserve a timely and complete workup.

REFERENCES

1. Nelson DA, Morris MW: Basic methodology. In Henry JB, editor: *Clinical diagnosis and management by laboratory methods,* Philadelphia, 1984, WB Saunders.
2. Gaillard HM, Hamilton GC: Hemoglobin, hematocrit and other erythrocyte parameters, *Emerg Clin North Am* 4:15–40, 1986.
3. International Committee for Standardization in Hematology: Proposal for standardization of hemoglobinometry, *Blood* 26:104–110, 1965.
4. Saunders AM, Scott F: Hematologic automation by use of continuous flow systems, *J Histochem Cytochem* 22:707–714, 1974.
5. Seward SJ, Safran C, Morton K, Robinson SH: Does mean corpuscular volume help physicians evaluate anemia? *J Gen Intern Med* 5:187–191, 1990.
6. Bessman JD: Improved classification of anemias by MCV and RDW, *Am J Clin Pathol* 80:322–331, 1983.
7. Mial JB: *Laboratory medicine,* St Louis, 1972, Mosby Inc.
8. Beutler E: Hemolytic anemia. In Williams W, Beutler E, Erslev AJ, Lichtman MA, editors: Hematology, New York, 1983, McGraw-Hill.
9. Wintrobe MM: *Clinical hematology,* Philadelphia, 1981, Lea & Febiger.
10. National Health and Nutrition Survey: *Vital Health Stat* 220:1–2, 1982.
11. Shapiro MF, Greenfield S: Complete blood counts and leukocyte differential counts, *Ann Intern Med* 106:65–74, 1987.
12. Orfanakis NG, Ostlund RE, Bishop CR: Normal blood leukocyte concentrations, *Am J Clin Pathol* 53:647–653, 1970.
13. Bain BJ, England JM: Normal hematological values—sex differences in leukocyte counts, *BMJ* 1:306–309, 1975.
14. Albritton EC: *Standard values in blood,* Philadelphia, 1952, WB Saunders.
15. Pitkin RM, Witte DL: Platelet and leukocyte counts in pregnancy, *JAMA* 242:2696–2672, 1979.
16. Korpman RA, Bull B: Whither the WBC differential? *Blood Cells* 6:421–429, 1980.
17. Zieve P, Spriggs D, Wisch JS, Kufe DW: Vacuolization of the neutrophil, *Arch Intern Med* 118:356–357, 1966.
18. Koepke JA, Dotson MA, Shifman MA: A critical evaluation of differential leukocyte counting, *Blood* 11:1753–1786, 1985.
19. Bull B, Korpman RA: Characterization of the white blood cell differential count, *Blood Cells* 6:411–419, 1980.
20. Young GP: CBC or not CBC, that is the question, *Ann Emerg Med* 15:367–371, 1986.
21. Griffin JD, Mercado T, Austin M, Schumacher HR: Treatment of preleukemic syndromes, *J Clin Oncol* 3:982–991, 1985.
22. Wesson SK, McClain MP, Crowson TW, Benson ES: Differential counts and overuse of the laboratory, *Lancet* 1:552–558, 1980.
23. Badgett RG, Hansen CJ, Rogers CS: Clinical usage of the leukocyte count in emergency department decision making, *J Gen Intern Med* 5:198–202, 1990.
24. Connelly DD, Read R, Goebel SL et al: The use of the differential leukocyte count for inpatient casefinding, *Hum Pathol* 13:294–300, 1982.

25. Weitzman M: Diagnostic utility of white blood cell and differential counts, *Am J Dis Child* 129:1183–1189, 1975.
26. Rasmussen NH, Rasmussen LN: Predictive value of peripheral white blood cell counts to bacterial infection in children, *Acta Paediatr Scand* 71:775–778, 1982.
27. Crain EF, Shelov SP: Febrile infants, predictors of bacteremia, *J Pediatr* 101:686–689, 1982.
28. Hubbel DS, Barton WK, Solomon OD: Leukocytosis in appendicitis in older persons, *JAMA* 175:139–141, 1961.
29. Miskowiak N, Burcharth F: White cell count in acute appendicitis, *Dan Med Bull* 29:210–211, 1982.
30. Lee PW: The leukocyte count in acute appendicitis, *Br J Surg* 60:618–624, 1973.
31. Sasso D et al: Leukocyte and neutrophil counts in acute appendicitis, *Am J Surg* 120:563–566, 1970.
32. Ketchel SJ, Rodriguez V: Acute infections in cancer patients, *Semin Oncol* 5:167–178, 1978.
33. Benson AS, Bennett JS, McDonough M, Turnbull J: Correlations between leukocyte counts and abnormal granulocyte counts in patients receiving chemotherapy, *Cancer* 56:1350–1355, 1985.
34. Prokesch RC, Rimbaud D: Cerebrospinal fluid after seizures, *South Med J* 76:322–327, 1983.
35. Kirov SM et al: Intraoperative and postoperative changes in white blood cell count, *N Z J Surg* 49:738–742, 1979.
36. Moorthy AV, Zimmerman SN: Human leukocyte response after an endurance race, *Eur J Appl Physiol* 38:271–276, 1978.
37. Day HJ, Rao AK: Evaluation of platelet function, *Semin Hematol* 23:89–101, 1986.
38. Slichter SJ, Harken LA: Thrombocytopenia: mechanisms and management of defects in platelet production, *Clin Hematol* 7:523–541, 1978.
39. Thompson AR, Harker LA: *Manual of hemostasis and thrombosis*, Philadelphia, 1983, FA Davis.
40. Karpatkin S: Autoimmune thrombocytopenic purpura, *N Engl J Med* 304:1135–1143, 1981.
41. Moss RA: Drug-induced immune thrombocytopenia, *Am J Hematol* 9:439–457, 1980.
42. Harker LA: Platelet survival time, *Prog Hemost Thromb* 4:321–337, 1978.
43. Murphy S: Thrombocytosis and thrombocythemia, *Clin Hematol* 12:89–106, 1983.
44. Shattil SJ, Bennett JS: Platelets and their membranes in hemostasis: physiology and pathophysiology, *Ann Intern Med* 94:108–118, 1980.
45. Bloom AL: The von Willebrand syndrome, *Semin Hematol* 17:215–243, 1980.
46. Packham MA, Mustard JF: Pharmacology of platelet-affecting drugs, *Circulation* 62:26–47, 1980.
47. Shattil SJ, Hirsh J, Marder VJ, Salzman EW, eds: Carbenicillin and penicillin G inhibit platelet function in vitro by impairing the interaction of agonists with the platelet surface, *J Clin Invest* 65:329–337, 1980.
48. Van Vliet HH, Kappeis-Klunne MC, Abel J: Pseudothrombocytopenia: a cold auto-antibody against platelet glycoprotein GP II^b. *Br J Haematol* 82:501–511, 1986.
49. Lind SE: Prolonged bleeding time, *Am J Med* 77:305–310, 1984.
50. Mielke CH: The standardized normal Ivy bleeding time and its prolongation by aspirin, *Blood* 34:204–212, 1969.
51. Chanoff D, Feinman RD, Detwiler TC: Interrelation of platelet aggregation and secretion, *J Clin Invest* 60:866–873, 1977.
52. Malpass TW, Harker LA: Acquired disorders of platelet function, *Semin Hematol* 17:242–263, 1980.
53. Robert HR, Lozier VN: New perspectives on the coagulation cascade, *Hosp Pract* pp. 97–112, 1992.
54. Lammle B, Griffin JH: Formation of the fibrin clot, *Clin Hematol* 14:281–331, 1985.
55. Furie B, Furie BC: Molecular and cellular biology of blood coagulation, *N Engl J Med* 336:800–805, 1992.
56. Wintrobe MM: *Blood, pure and eloquent*, New York, 1980, McGraw-Hill.
57. Marder VJ: Fibrinolytic therapy. In Colman RW et al, editors: *Hemostasis and thrombosis—basic principles and practice*, Philadelphia, 1987, JB Lippincott.
58. Sharma GV: Thrombolytic therapy, *N Engl J Med* 306:1268–1279, 1982.

59. Collen D, Veistreate M: Thrombolytic therapy in the eighties, *Blood* 67:1529–1540, 1986.
60. Erban SB, Kinnar JL, Schwartz SJ: Routine use of the prothrombin and partial thromboplastin times, *JAMA* 262:2428–2432, 1989.
61. Gregory SA, McKenna R, Sassetti RJ, Knospe WH: Hematologic emergencies, *Med Clin North Am* 70:1129–1149, 1986.
62. Hirsh J, Dalen JE, Deykin D, Poller L: Oral anticoagulants: mechanism of action, clinical effectiveness, and optimal therapeutic range, *Chest* 102:312S-326S, 1992.
63. Schleider MA, Nachman R, Jaffe E: A clinical study of the lupus anticoagulant, *Blood* 48:499–509, 1976.
64. Rappaport SI: Preoperative hemostatic evaluation, *Blood* 61:229–231, 1983.
65. Exner T: Evaluation of currently available methods for plasma fibrinogen, *Am J Clin Pathol* 71:521–537, 1979.
66. Bell WR, Meek AG: Guidelines for the use of thrombolytic agents, *N Engl J Med* 301:1266–1272, 1979.

Chapter 13

Endocrinologic Tests and Evaluation of Endocrine Function

Samuel Engel

Harry Shamoon

True endocrine emergencies are uncommon. However, because of the systemic nature of many endocrinologic and metabolic disturbances, endocrinologic disorders enter into the differential diagnosis of a wide variety of clinical situations. Although hormonal assay results are ordinarily not available on a "stat" basis, some functional assessments of endocrine gland function are available in the emergency department (ED) (e.g., urine-specific gravity as an index of antidiuretic hormone (ADH) secretion, serum ketones as an index of insulin secretion). Finally, although in most cases results of endocrine tests done in the ED will not be available before the patient leaves the ED, obtaining the appropriate serum or urine samples before instituting therapy may be necessary to establish the diagnosis.

In this chapter the types of testing available in the ED as well as the tests that should be performed for subsequent consideration will be reviewed. Most dynamic assessments of endocrine gland function, however, are not intended for ED settings and should be carried out only under controlled settings (e.g., insulin tolerance tests, dexamethasone suppression tests), often under the supervision of an endocrinologist.

DISORDERS OF GLUCOSE METABOLISM

CASE 13–1

A 23-year-old male with insulin-dependent diabetes mellitus was brought to the ED by his roommate. He had not eaten all day and was in a lethargic, confused state. After intravenous access was established and a sample of blood obtained, the patient was given 25 g of glucose intravenously for presumptive hypoglycemia. He appeared somewhat more responsive within 3 to 5 minutes; bedside analysis of the patient's blood specimen revealed a blood glucose level of 800 mg/dL and positive serum ketones. Therapy for diabetic ketoacidosis was then initiated.

Comment.—Therapy for presumed hypoglycemia should not be withheld pending laboratory confirmation of the diagnosis. Nevertheless, rapid determination of blood glucose values can allow for early adjustment of therapy, if so indicated.

The most common classes of endocrinologic disorders seen in the ED are those related to disorders of glucose metabolism. Patients with a known history of diabetes

Table 13–1. Glucose Oxidase Reagent Strips

Product	Range of Blood Glucose (mg/dL)	Maximum Time for Test
Chemstrip bG (meter)	20–500	2 min
Chemstrip bG (visual)	20–800	3 min
Glucostix (meter)	40–399	50 sec
Glucostix (visual)	20–800	2 min
Glucofilm (meter/visual)	20–500	1 min
One Touch (meter)	0–600	45 sec

and symptoms of worsening diabetic control usually pose no diagnostic problem. Diabetics with altered states of consciousness who are unable to provide the historical clues necessary for diagnosis and undiagnosed diabetics are most in need of rapid evaluation and treatment.

The development of glucose oxidase–impregnated test strips that can be accurately read has made assessment of blood glucose a rapid bedside test.[1] The various available strips use the ability of the enzyme glucose oxidase to generate hydrogen peroxide from glucose; the hydrogen peroxide then oxidizes the color indicators to different degrees to allow a semiquantitative estimate to be made by visual comparison with standards on the bottle or vial label. Reflectance meters can be used in conjunction with all of the commercially available strips. These meters provide a quantitative measure of the degree of oxidation of the color indicators and therefore a more precise measurement of the blood glucose.

Chemstrip bG (Table 13–1) uses two different reagent zones with different color indicators; each goes through a series of color changes dependent on the blood glucose concentration, and values from 20 to 800 mg/dL can be estimated relatively accurately. The test is performed by spreading a drop of whole blood on the strip; after 60 seconds, the blood is wiped off with dry cotton, and the strip is allowed to develop for another 60 seconds before comparing it with the 2-minute reference chart. If the blood glucose concentration appears to be equal to 240 mg/dL, 60 more seconds are allowed for further development and the strip is then compared with the 3-minute reference chart. Chemstrip bG strips can also be inserted into the Accuchek series of reflectance meters for quantitative measurements.

Table 13–2. Reflectance Meters

Product Name	Manufacturer	Strip Used
Accuchek II	Bio Dynamics	Chemstrip bG
Accuchek III	Bio Dynamics	Chemstrip bG
Glucometer II	Ames	Glucostix
Glucometer III	Ames	Glucofilm
One Touch	Life Scan	One Touch strips
One Touch II	Life Scan	One Touch strips

Glucostix and Glucofilm, which are used with the Glucometer II and III meters, respectively, can also provide a visual estimate of the blood glucose level. In addition, several reagent strips are available (e.g., One Touch) that do not require precise timing or wiping of the specimen (Table 13–2).

It should be noted that reflectance meter accuracy may be limited at very low (<40 gm/dL) or very high (>400 mg/dL) glucose levels. This does not usually limit the clinical utility of the information. A second potential source of error may arise in hypotensive patients: artifactually lower glucose readings from *fingerstick* samples have been shown to occur. When a patient is hypotensive, accurate readings with a reagent strip may be obtained with whole blood from a vein. Finally, faulty technique, especially under adverse conditions in the ED, may significantly affect results. For example, failure to allow alcohol on the skin to dry and allowing it to wet the reagent strip pad or touching the pad to the skin instead of the blood droplet may artificially lower the values.

The treatment of uncontrolled diabetes mellitus differs depending on the presence or absence of *ketoacidosis.* The presence of ketone bodies can be assessed by the nitroprusside reagent, which forms a purple color in the presence of acetoacetate and, to a somewhat lesser extent, acetone. However, β-hydroxybutyrate, the predominant circulating ketone body, does not react with nitroprusside. Nitroprusside reagent is available in tablet form (Acetest) or in strip form (Ketostix or Chemstrip uK). To assess the presence of ketonuria, the strips are covered with a film of urine as per the manufacturer's instructions; then the degree of color change is compared with a reference chart. Ketonuria is often present in the absence of ketonemia because of the rapid renal clearance of ketone bodies. Thus, when ketonuria is demonstrated, the nitroprusside test should then be used to test the *blood* qualitatively and, in some circumstances, semiquantitatively for the presence of ketone bodies. Acetest tablets can be used for assessment of ket*onemia* as well as ket*onuria* as follows: the tablet is placed on a clean surface, preferably a piece of white filter paper, and crushed and one drop of the serum or plasma placed on the crushed tablet. After 2 minutes, the color of the tablet is compared with the reference chart. (When testing urine, comparison to the reference chart should be made at 30 seconds). The clinician can make a semiquantitative assessment of the degree of ketonemia by making serial dilutions of the plasma with normal saline and noting the dilution at which the nitroprusside reaction becomes negative.

The use of serial ketone measurements over time (not serial dilutions) to follow the course of ketoacidosis is potentially misleading because the ratio of (the unmeasured) β-hydroxybutyrate to (the measured) acetoacetate may be as high as 30:1. As the ketoacidosis resolves, the redox state of the cell is altered, i.e., the ratio of intracellular reduced nicotinamide-adenine dinucleotide (NADH)/NAD falls and more β-hydroxybutyrate is converted to acetoacetate, which results in a more strongly positive nitroprusside test as the patient's clinical state improves.[2] In most cases, after the initial determinations it is sufficient to simply test for the presence of ketone bodies in undiluted plasma or serum (until negative).

In patients with uncontrolled diabetes, an arterial blood gas (ABG) analysis should be obtained initially to assess the presence and severity of (metabolic) acidosis, as well as the adequacy of respiratory compensatory mechanisms (hyperventilation resulting in hypocapnea and a compensatory respiratory alkalosis). Subsequently the patient's course can be followed with venous pH measurements inasmuch as venous pH is only approximately 0.04 pH units below the arterial pH and is more easily obtained. Serum *electrolytes* must be obtained frequently and particular attention paid to the serum potassium concentration. In the presence of severe diabetic ketoacidosis, the serum potassium level may be elevated, normal, or slightly depressed, all in the face of severe total-body potassium depletion. With correction of the acidosis, the *serum* potassium value can fall rapidly and dramatically, which in turn can cause or contribute to dangerous dysrhythmias; potassium supplementation should be prompt and should in fact begin before the onset of frank hypokalemia, but not while the patient is hyperkalemic.

The blood urea nitrogen and serum creatinine concentrations should also be obtained as an index of renal function and as a guide to the degree of volume depletion. In the presence of significant impairment of renal function, potassium supplementation should, of course, be undertaken even more cautiously.

Serum sodium values may be artifactually low in the face of marked hyperglycemia. Glucose, acting as an osmotic load, draws free water into the intravascular compartment, which results in dilutional hyponatremia but without an effective change in osmolality. A rough guide for correction of the effects of hyperglycemia on the serum sodium concentration is that for each 100 mg/dL of glucose above 100 mg/dL, the serum sodium value should fall by 1.6 mEq/L.

CASE 13–2

A 37-year-old male was brought into the ED by his wife, a physician, because of the onset of stupor. His past medical history was noteworthy only for a prior episode of coma 6 months previously, from which he recovered without any permanent neurologic deficit. Evaluation at that time had been unrevealing. The physical examination was remarkable for a pulse rate of 130, a blood pressure of 120/70 mm Hg, a respiratory rate of 16, a temperature of 95° F, and diaphoretic skin; neurologic examination revealed an obtunded male responsive only to extreme noxious stimuli. His blood glucose level by glucose oxidase strip determination was 20 mg/dL. After additional blood was obtained, the patient was given 25 g of glucose intravenously and recovered normal neurologic function. Because of the unexplained hypoglycemia, a specimen of the patient's pretreatment blood was analyzed for the presence of insulin and C-peptide. Although high levels of insulin were present, C-peptide was not. The patient's wife was indicted for attempted murder.

Comment.—In cases of unexplained hypoglycemia it is critical to obtain samples of blood at the time of hypoglycemia for subsequent evaluation of the cause of the low blood glucose level.

Insulin is synthesized in the pancreas in a precursor form, proinsulin.[3] The proinsulin molecule is cleaved within the β-cell to equimolar amounts of insulin and an inactive fragment C-peptide; both are then secreted into the circulation. Excessive secretion of endogenous insulin (e.g., in the case of patients with insulin-producing tumors) should consequently result in high circulating levels of insulin as well as C-peptide. Overtreatment with oral hypoglycemic agents, which stimulate endogenous insulin secretion, results in a similar pattern. Commercially available insulin is purified by chromatographic methods and contains essentially no measurable C-peptide. Thus the presence in a patient's blood of high levels of insulin along with the simultaneous absence of C-peptide is diagnostic of exogenous insulin administration. Conversely, the absence of elevated insulin immunoreactivity rules out the diagnosis of insulin-mediated hypoglycemia.

Non-insulin–mediated hypoglycemia may have a variety of causes (see the accompanying box). Hypoadrenalism (cortisol deficiency) or hypopituitarism (combined cortisol and growth hormone deficiency) may cause hypoglycemia as a result of impair-

Causes of Non–Insulin-Mediated Hypoglycemia

- Adrenocortical insufficiency
- Growth hormone deficiency
- Inborn errors of glucose production
  - Errors of glycogen storage
  - Errors of gluconeogenesis
- Drug-induced impairment of gluconeogenesis
  - Ethanol
  - Salicylates
- Extrapancreatic neoplasms

ment of the counterregulatory mechanisms that maintain hepatic production of glucose. In fact, a diabetic with a recent increase in the frequency of hypoglycemia and no other obvious cause should be evaluated for adrenal and pituitary insufficiency. Drugs such as salicylates or alcohol can interfere with hepatic glucose production and should be considered in the differential diagnosis. When hypoglycemia results from salicylate toxicity or methanol or ethylene glycol poisoning, the anion gap may be elevated. Critical to all of these diagnoses is the demonstration of inappropriate (or appropriate) plasma insulin levels *at the time* of hypoglycemia. Thus the laboratory should be instructed to save the pretreatment sample (of the serum or plasma) and to freeze it for subsequent analysis if the situation warrants (Fig. 13-1).

DISORDERS OF THE THYROID GLAND

CASE 13–3

A 26-year-old intensive care unit (ICU) nurse came to the ED with complaints of nervousness and palpitations. She had noted several months of heat intolerance,

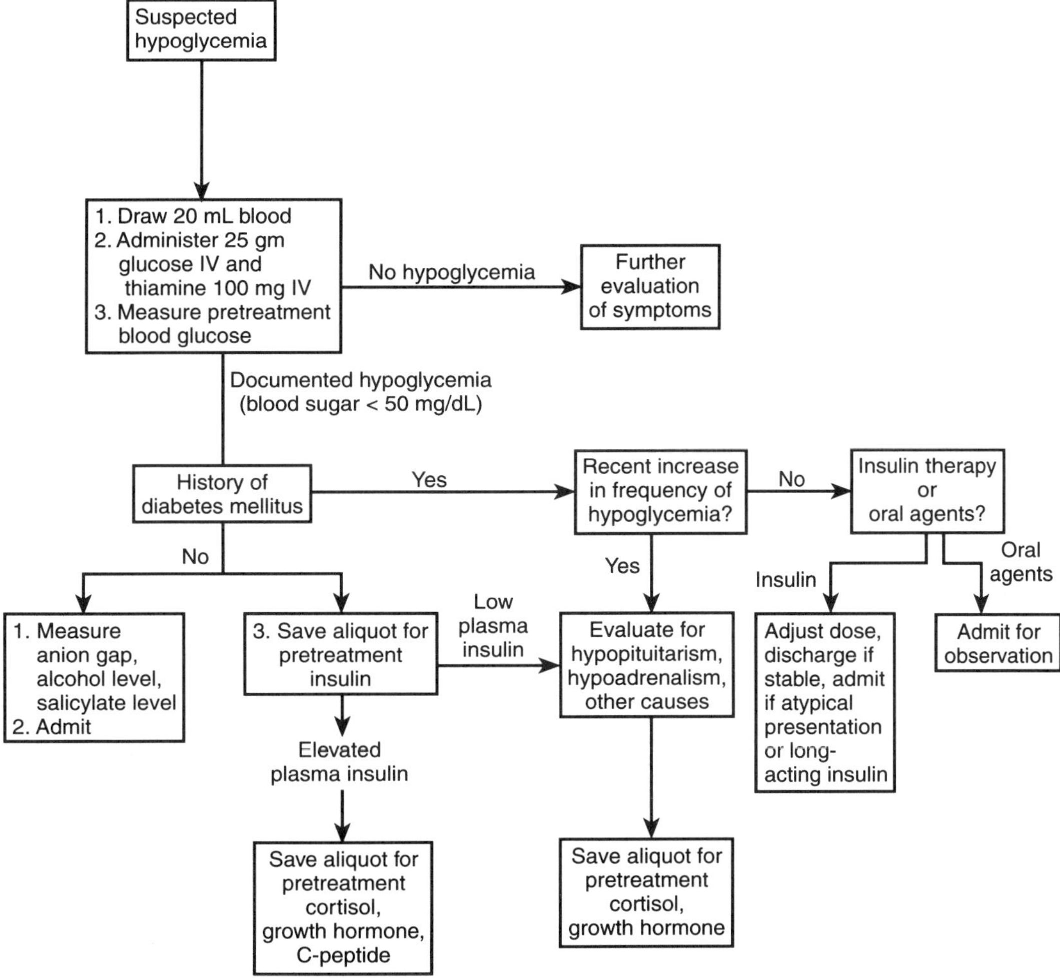

Fig. 13–1. Treatment algorithm for suspected hypoglycemia.

hyperdefecation, and irregular menses. She had lost 30 lb during the same period because, she stated, she had been dieting. Physical examination was noteworthy for a pulse of 130/min, moist smooth skin, lid lag and stare, but no proptosis, no goiter, and no hyperactive reflexes. Thyroid function tests done by the employee's health service 1 week earlier disclosed the following values: thyroxine (T_4), 18 μg/dL (normal is 4 to 11); triiodothyronine (T_3) uptake, resin (T_3RU), 45% (normal, 25% to 35%); and total T_3, 340 ng/dL (normal 80 to 180). She was referred for a radioactive iodine uptake (RAIU) test, which showed less than 1% uptake at 24 hours. When confronted with this information, she admitted to taking exogenous thyroid hormone in an attempt to lose weight.

Comment.—The absence of a goiter in a patient with clinical and chemical evidence of hyperthyroidism suggests that the thyrotoxicosis is not caused by *thyroidal* overproduction of thyroid hormones. The demonstration of low RAIU in the neck confirms that the thyroid is not the site of excessive hormone synthesis.

Results of thyroid function testing are generally unavailable in an ED; therefore *definitive* therapy for suspected hyperthyroidism must often be delayed until the biochemical diagnosis is established. The most useful and widely available screening test for hyperthyroidism is the radioimmunoassay for total T_4 concentration. A highly sensitive thyroid-stimulating hormone (TSH) assay (to show suppressed levels) may also be obtained. The total T_4 combined with an index of the thyroid hormone binding capacity such as the T_3 RU test can be used to calculate a free T_4 index. The free T_4 index takes into account any perturbations in thyroid hormone binding proteins (e.g., the rise in T_4 binding globulin seen in women receiving estrogen therapy) that would affect the total T_4 level but not the amount of free T_4.[4]

Almost all hyperthyroid patients have elevated free T_4 indices. Rarely a patient may have "T_3-thyrotoxicosis," a situation wherein the T_4 level is within the normal range but the total T_3 level is elevated. This may occur in early hyperthyroidism or in relatively iodine-deficient hyperthyroid states. Thus measurement of the serum T_3 by radioimmunoassay should probably be included in an evaluation of a patient with suspected hyperthyroidism. The serum T_3 test is also useful in the recognition of a less common entity, *hereditary dysalbuminemia.*[5] In this syndrome patients have an abnormal protein that binds T_4 but not T_3. The increased pool of protein-bound T_4 results in an increase in the total T_4 level but no change in the actual concentration of free unbound hormone. Inasmuch as this abnormal protein does not bind T_3, it has no effect on T_3 RU; thus the free T_4 index, which is derived from the total T_4 and the T_3 RU, is elevated despite a normal concentration of free unbound hormone. Since the total T_3 levels are unaffected, measurement of T_3 levels will alert the physician to the possibility of the presence of this syndrome. Even more rarely, thyroxine binding prealbumin (TBPA) may excessively bind T_4 and present the same difficulty in diagnosis.

RAIU measurement at 24 hours provides information regarding the functional status of the thyroid, i.e., the ability of the thyroid to concentrate an administered dose of radioactive iodine and incorporate it into hormones. Uptake is determined by simply counting the number of β-emissions over time and calculating the percentage of the administered dose of radioactivity that is localized to the thyroid.

The administration of exogenous thyroid hormone, by suppressing the pituitary-thyroid axis, will result in a low RAIU. Subacute thyroiditis, an inflammatory process of the thyroid gland that can result in dysfunction of thyroid tissue and release of stored hormone into the circulation, can give a similar picture of hyperthyroxinemia and a depressed RAIU. A low RAIU due to thyroiditis is usually distinguished from exogenous thyroid hormone administration by the presence of a tender thyroid and by the relatively acute onset and short duration of hyperthyroid symptoms. Occasionally, subacute thyroiditis can be painless.[6] In this situation an elevation of the erythrocyte sedimentation rate (ESR) or other acute-phase reactants may be useful in diagnosis. Antithyroid antibodies may be present in the patient's serum, but the antibody titers are not as elevated as those in Hashimoto's thyroiditis. One final note should be remembered about measuring RAIU: the thiourea class of drugs (propylthiouracil, methimazole) blocks thyroidal uptake of iodine. Thus, if possible, patients should have their RAIU measured before being treated with these agents.

Thyroid scanning provides information regarding the structure of the thyroid, i.e., the pattern of the distribution of radioactivity throughout the neck. Thyroid scans are therefore also useful to evaluate the functional status of structural lesions, e.g., masses. Thyroid nodules that function as well as the adjacent normal thyroid tissue are usually benign. Thyroid nodules that do not concentrate iodine (i.e., "cold" nodules) have a 20% incidence of malignancy.

Ultrasonography can be useful in the evaluation of a thyroid nodule. If a nonfunctioning nodule is demonstrated to be cystic, further evaluation is generally unnecessary. Physical examination is notoriously unreliable for distinguishing solid thyroid nodules from cystic lesions, so ultrasonography is favored by some authors as an essential part of the workup of a thyroid mass. However, ultrasonography is frequently bypassed in evaluation of "cold" nodules, with the diagnostic evaluation proceeding directly to fine-needle aspiration for cytology.

Patients may come to the ED with a recently discovered and occasionally painful thyroid nodule. Rarely, hemorrhage into a thyroid cyst or nodule may require decompression for symptomatic relief. This procedure should be performed by physicians experienced in the technique of fine-needle aspiration of the thyroid. In most cases, referral for outpatient evaluation is sufficient.[7]

Suspected *hypothyroidism* is best evaluated by measurements of the total T_4 levels and the T_3 RU. It is also important to measure the serum TSH level. In patients with primary thyroidal failure, or primary hypothyroidism, the pituitary secretion of TSH *increases* as a result of the absence of the normal negative feedback by thyroid hormone. An elevated TSH concentration thus serves as confirmatory evidence of primary hypothyroidism, the most common cause of thyroidal failure. A "normal" TSH value in the face of a low T_4 level, however, is suggestive of secondary hypothyroidism, that is, inadequate thyroidal stimulation because of insufficient secretion of TSH by the pituitary. In this setting, other pituitary functions would also be expected to be abnormally low, and further evaluation is needed. Indeed, if secondary hypothyroidism is suspected, therapy with thyroid hormone should be withheld because administration of thyroid hormone to a patient with coincident secondary hypoadrenalism could precipitate acute adrenal insufficiency. In addition, patients with suspected hypothyroidism should not be treated with sedative-hypnotics because they are particularly sensitive to central nervous system (CNS) depressant effects.

Measurement of total T_3 levels is generally not of value in the patients suspected of having hypothyroidism. T_3 levels tend to fall rather late in the course of hypothyroidism. Furthermore, T_3 concentrations may be deceptively low in a euthyroid individual who has the "low-T_3 syndrome" because of starvation, illness, or the use of various drugs. Thus, the serum T_3 concentration is not predictive of hypothyroidism.

In summary, for patients suspected of having hyperthyroidism, serum should be obtained for the total T_4 level, T_3 RU, and the total T_3 level. The patient should be referred for a 24-hour RAIU, especially if no goiter is palpable. For patients with suspected hypothyroidism, the T_4 level, T_3 RU, and TSH level should be measured. Patients with a solitary thyroid nodule should be referred for RAIU and scan. Ultrasonography is useful for evaluating a thyroid nodule that has undergone a rapid change in size or a unilaterally enlarged, tender thyroid.

DISORDERS OF THE ADRENAL GLAND

CASE 13–4

A 43-year-old female came to the ED with complaints of abdominal pain and nausea. During the preceding 2 days a low-grade fever and a nonproductive cough had developed. On the day of admission she had a temperature of 103° F and complained of nausea, vomiting, and sharp periumbilical pain. Physical examination revealed a pulse rate of 140/min, a blood pressure of 80/40 mm Hg, a respiratory rate of 18, a temperature of 39.5° C, hyperpigmented skin, hypoactive bowel sounds, and mild diffuse abdominal tenderness without rebound tenderness. Laboratory tests disclosed the following values: white blood cell (WBC) count, 19,300/mm^3 with 60% neutrophils, 20% lymphocytes, 3% monocytes, and 17% eosinophils; Na, 134 mEq/L; K, 6.2 mEq/L; Cl, 94 mEq/L; HCO_3^-, 15 mEq/L. A chest radiograph revealed a lingular infiltrate. She was treated for septic shock with broad-spectrum antibiotics and large doses of steroids, and her blood pressure rose to 100/70 mm Hg. Cultures of blood drawn in the ED remained negative. Forty-eight hours later, upon discontinuance of the high-dose corticosteroids, she again became hypotensive. At that point she was evaluated for and found to have adrenal insufficiency. She was treated successfully with steroid replacement.

Comment.—In the face of hypotension of unclear etiology, low sodium, high potassium, and eosinophilia, the physician must have a high index of suspicion for adrenal insufficiency.

Adrenal insufficiency, although uncommon, must be considered in a wide variety of clinical circumstances. The serum electrolytes often give an important clue to this diagnosis. Hyponatremia caused by deficiencies of both cortisol and aldosterone is most commonly seen. Cortisol deficiency impairs the ability to excrete a free water load, which results in a dilutional hyponatremia; aldosterone deficiency results in an inability to conserve sodium at the collecting tubule. This deficiency may result in hyponatremia if hypotonic fluids are ingested.

Hyperkalemia occurs secondary to aldosterone deficiency and is aggravated by diminished distal delivery of sodium from intravascular volume depletion. Metabolic acidosis may also play a role. Inasmuch as cortisol deficiency by itself usually does not result in hyperkalemia, patients with secondary adrenal insufficiency (due to pituitary dysfunction or withdrawal of glucocorticoid therapy) may simply have a modest dilutional hyponatremia and no hyperkalemia. Another useful clue to the presence of glucocorticoid deficiency due to primary *or* secondary adrenal insufficiency is the presence of an absolute eosinophilia.

Once adrenal insufficiency is considered on clinical grounds, several diagnostic and therapeutic steps should be undertaken immediately: an intravenous infusion of adrenocorticotropic hormone (ACTH) should be begun. Different authors have proposed different methods of performing the ACTH infusion test.[8] A simple method is to obtain a plasma specimen for cortisol levels, inject 250 μg of synthetic ACTH (Cortrosyn) as a bolus, and then obtain additional plasma cortisol levels 30 and 60 minutes after administration. The results of this test will enable the physician to subsequently determine the need for glucocorticoid therapy (Table 13–3). An alternative method of performing an ACTH test is to obtain a baseline cortisol level, add the ACTH to the intravenous fluids, and then infuse it over the course of 2 to 6 hours, with additional measurements of the plasma cortisol level at the conclusion of the infusion.

A hypotensive, volume-depleted patient with an intact adrenal gland will normally have increased aldosterone secretion. Pharmacologic doses of ACTH can induce a further rise in aldosterone levels. Thus obtaining aldosterone levels before and during the ACTH infusion test may also be useful in differentiating between primary and secondary adrenal insufficiency.

Simultaneously with these diagnostic steps, therapy should be undertaken. Dexa-

Table 13–3. Expected Responses to Adrenocorticotropic Hormone Infusion

Condition	Response
Normal adrenal function	Doubling of initial plasma cortisol *or* Attaining plasma cortisol levels of >20 μg/dL
Primary adrenal insufficiency	No increase in plasma cortisol
Secondary adrenal insufficiency	No increase in plasma cortisol unless prolonged (48 hr) infusion is performed

methasone, a potent glucocorticoid that does not interfere with the radioimmunoassay for cortisol, can be given without affecting the results of the ACTH infusion test. Volume replacement with isotonic fluids is essential and is effective even in the absence of mineralocorticoid replacement. Of course, other specific abnormalities such as hyperkalemia or hypoglycemia should be treated independent of the cause of adrenal insufficiency.

The possibility of hypercortisolism is often raised in the ED setting, e.g., in a hypertensive diabetic patient with hypokalemia and mild hypernatremia; however, the diagnostic workup can only be carried out under prolonged, stress-free conditions, i.e., after admission to the hospital. The overnight dexamethasone suppression test has gained popularity as an easily performed screening test for Cushing's syndrome.[9] The clinician performs the test by administering 1 mg of dexamethasone at 11 P.M. and then obtaining a serum cortisol level the following morning at 8 A.M. The expected suppression of ACTH and cortisol secretion does not occur in patients with any cause of Cushing's syndrome. There is, however, a substantial (~20%) incidence of false-positives, i.e., normal individuals who fail to suppress cortisol production. False-positive test results are seen most frequently in stressed, hospitalized, or obese patients and in those with psychiatric illness. A normal response eliminates any need for further testing, but a positive result will identify a large "false-positive" group of normal individuals in addition to a small "true-positive" group of patients with hypercortisolism. There is universal agreement, however, that *random* serum cortisol determinations are of little value in establishing the diagnosis of hypercortisolism inasmuch as the range seen in Cushing's syndrome may not differ from the range of random serum cortisol values seen in the normal population.

In summary, in the case of patients with suspected hypoadrenalism, serum electrolytes and a complete blood count (CBC) with a differential WBC count should be obtained. In addition, an ACTH infusion test should be performed and the patient simultaneously treated for presumed adrenal insufficiency with dexamethasone and volume replacement. Patients with suspected hypercortisolism may have an overnight dexamethasone suppression test performed, but the high incidence of false-positive results often necessitates a more formal, prolonged evaluation.

DISORDERS OF THE PITUITARY

CASE 13–5

A 35-year-old female was brought to the ED because her husband could not awaken her in the morning. She had had no medical illnesses, recent complaints, or medications. She had no history of substance abuse. She was gravida 3, para 3 and had been amenorrheic since her last pregnancy 10 years before admission. Examination revealed an obtunded female with no focal neurologic findings, a blood pressure of 90/60 mm Hg, a pulse of 112/min and regular, a respiratory rate of 16, and a temperature of 36.4° C rectally. After receiving intravenous naloxone (2 mg), dextrose (50 g), and thiamine (100 mg), she became arousable and was lucid within 10 minutes. Her laboratory data disclosed a glucose level of 26 mg/dL before treatment. Additional testing eventually revealed no evidence of exogenous insulin, and a head computed tomographic (CT) scan soon after admission revealed an empty sella turcica. After recovery, the patient related a history of severe postpartum blood loss 10 years earlier requiring transfusion.

Comment.—The clinical picture suggests that the patient had had pituitary necrosis (Sheehan's syndrome) 10 years before her admission. Together with a history of amenorrhea suggesting gonadotropin loss, the hypoglycemia may reflect ACTH, growth hormone, or combined deficiencies. Hypothyroidism may or may not accompany the other trophic hormone deficiencies. In this case, ACTH deficiency should be *assumed* and an infusion of dexamethasone administered. This can be given concurrently with an ACTH test as described previously.

Evaluation of the anterior pituitary for hypofunction depends largely on evaluation of the other endocrine glands that it controls. If hypopituitarism is suspected, a formal evaluation of total pituitary function should be undertaken (usually in an inpatient setting).

Patients with diabetes insipidus may come to the ED in a confused, disoriented state. ADH deficiency can result in severe hypernatremia and hyperosmolality. In addition to serum electrolyte studies, a urine sample should be obtained to document the inappropriately low urine osmolality or specific gravity. Measurements of ADH levels are not widely available and are not necessary to make the diagnosis of diabetes insipidus. More important may be testing for medications that cause central diabetes insipidus (ethanol, α-adrenergic agents, phenytoin) and nephrogenic diabetes insipidus (lithium, democlocycline). Hypercalcemia and hypokalemia also cause nephrogenic diabetes insipidus.

HYPOCALCEMIA AND HYPERCALCEMIA

CASE 13–6

A 42-year-old male with chronic alcoholism was brought to the ED by the police after having suffered a grand mal seizure in the street. He remained obtunded. When obtaining his vital signs, the nurse noted the development of carpal spasm while the sphygmomanometer was on the patient's arm. An electrocardiogram (ECG) revealed a QT interval of 0.42 seconds (normal is between 0.3 and 0.4 seconds for a rate over 60/min and less than 100/min). The patient was treated for presumptive hypocalcemia. During the course of the next 2 hours he continued to have generalized seizures. The pretreatment serum calcium level was 6.4 mg/dL; the posttreatment level was unchanged. A serum magnesium level was then obtained, and the patient was treated with intramuscular magnesium sulfate with subsequent resolution of the signs and symptoms of hypocalcemia.

Comment.—The diagnosis of hypocalcemia may be obscure unless the patient has tetany. When symptomatic hypocalcemia is discovered, follow-up studies should be obtained to document the response to calcium replacement therapy and to assess the serum magnesium concentration.

The total serum calcium is composed of the albumin-bound fraction and the free ionized fraction.[10] It is the latter that has physiologic significance, but it cannot be measured directly. Abnormally low serum albumin levels depress the total serum calcium content, but the ionized fraction remains normal. Thus in order to meaningfully interpret the total serum calcium, the serum albumin level should also be measured. For each gram of albumin below the normal range, the serum calcium level would be expected to be 0.8 mg/dL lower to maintain a normal free ionized calcium concentration. Additionally, in situations of low serum calcium content, symptoms and signs of "effective hypocalcemia" should be sought (e.g., Chvostek's sign, Trousseau's sign, prolongation of the QT interval) as a guide to the need for parenteral calcium therapy.

ABG analysis should also be obtained since alkalemia will lower the ionized calcium fraction by promoting calcium deposition into bone in exchange for hydrogen ion. Hyperventilation, by inducing a respiratory alkalosis (i.e., alkalemia), can also lower the ionized fraction and result in typical signs and symptoms of hypocalcemia.

The serum magnesium level should always be obtained in patients with hypocalcemia, especially in alcoholic patients because they are particularly prone to hypomagnesemia. Hypomagnesemia impairs the secretion of parathyroid hormone (PTH) in the face of hypocalcemia, as well as the action of PTH on bone.[11] Calcium replacement alone is insufficient treatment for hypomagnesemic, hypocalcemic patients because renal conservation of infused calcium is impaired in the absence of PTH.

Routine measurement of serum calcium levels has led to the increasingly frequent recognition of mild, asymptomatic hypercalcemia. Furthermore, patients who come to an ED with alterations of their mental status are occasionally noted to be hypercalcemic. Indeed, hypercalcemia should be suspected in every patient in a lethargic or comatose state, particularly those with a history of malignancy. Thyroid function should be evaluated in patients with an elevated calcium level because thyrotoxicosis may rarely cause hypercalcemia. Elevated PTH levels are useful in diagnosing hyperparathyroidism, but even in the presence of elevated PTH levels the possibility of other syndromes that cause hypercalcemia should be considered, especially malignancy.

In summary, patients with hypocalcemia should also have a determination of the serum magnesium concentration made. PTH levels are of limited usefulness in the differential diagnosis of hypocalcemia, but they may be of some use in hypercalcemic patients.

REFERENCES

1. American Diabetes Association: Bedside blood glucose monitoring in hospitals. Position statement—American Diabetes Association, *Diabetes* 16(suppl 2):38, 1993.
2. Stephens JM, Sulway MJ, Watkins PJ: Relationship of blood acetoacetate and 3-hydroxybutyrate in diabetes, *Diabetes* 20:485–489, 1971.
3. Hoekstra JBL, Van Rijin HJM, Erkelens DW, et al: C-peptide, *Diabetes Care* 5:438–446, 1987.
4. Kaplan MM, Utiger RD: Diagnosis of hyperthyroidism, *Clin Endocrinol Metab* 7:97–113, 1978.
5. Borst GC, Eil C, Burman KD: Euthyroid hyperthyroxinemia, *Ann Intern Med* 98:366–378, 1983.
6. Dorfman SG, Cooperman MT, Nelson RL et al: Painless thyroiditis and transient hyperthyroidism without goiter, *Ann Intern Med* 86:24–28, 1977.
7. Van Herle AJ, moderator: The thyroid nodule, *Ann Intern Med* 96:221–232, 1982.
8. Gwinup G, Johnson B: Clinical testing of the hypothalamic-pituitary-adrenocortical system in states of hypo- and hypercortisolism, *Metabolism* 24:777–791, 1975.

9. Carpenter P: Diagnostic evaluation of Cushing's syndrome, *Endocrinol Metab Clin North Am* 16:445–472, 1988.
10. Bringhurst FR: Calcium and phosphate distribution, turnover, and metabolic actions. In DeGroot LJ, editor: *Endocrinology,* vol 2, Philadelphia, 1989, WB Saunders, pp 805–843.
11. Rude RK, Oldham SB, Sharp CF et al: Parathyroid hormone secretion in magnesium deficiency, *J Clin Endocrinol Metab* 47:800, 1978.

Chapter 14

Gastrointestinal Testing

Sheldon Jacobson, M.D.

Patients who seek care in emergency departments (EDs) because of abdominal pain with or without nausea, vomiting, and diarrhea often have a condition that is difficult to diagnose efficiently. The difficulties in evaluating these patients stem in part from the large number of patients with similar symptoms who have relatively benign entities.[1] In several studies of ED patients seeking treatment for abdominal pain, approximately 40% do not have specific historical or physical findings or positive tests to justify a specific diagnosis. For the most part, these patients have benign conditions that usually resolve without a definitive diagnosis ever having been made. A small number of patients seeking treatment for acute abdominal pain, perhaps 10%, will have fairly obvious acute surgical conditions on initial evaluation. The remaining, 40% to 50% of patients will clearly appear ill, but will require laboratory testing and imaging studies to define the pathologic process.

For another group of patients who have jaundice and other signs and symptoms of hepatic dysfunction, the critical issue is to determine whether they have "medical" or "surgical" disease. Once this is resolved, further laboratory testing will help in the differential diagnosis of each type of jaundice. However, the specificity of the various liver function and viral serologic tests often is inadequate, and patients usually require an imaging procedure or liver biopsy before a definitive diagnosis can be established.

Before embarking on a course of diagnostic tests to sort out the various possibilities in the patient with abdominal pain, immediately life-threatening entities should be considered and excluded. These include cardiovascular emergencies such as myocardial infarction, ruptured aortic aneurysm, and aortic dissection and such obstetric or gynecologic crises as ruptured ectopic pregnancy and ovarian or tubal torsion. In a patient with chronic liver disease and sepsis, spontaneous bacterial peritonitis, hepatic encephalopathy, and gastrointestinal hemorrhage have to be considered.

Generally, there are six acute abdominal pain patterns:

1. The abrupt onset of localized abdominal pain associated with localized peritoneal signs (e.g., the patient with a ruptured viscus resulting from a perforated peptic ulcer, appendicitis, diverticular abscess, or ectopic pregnancy).
2. The abrupt onset of paroxysms of pain without localized abdominal findings (e.g., the patient with renal colic, small bowel obstruction, or biliary obstruction).
3. Vomiting with absent to minimal or moderate epigastric and left upper quadrant pain and tenderness (e.g., the patient with gastritis, gastric outlet obstruction, peptic ulcer disease, pancreatitis, biliary tract disease, or ischemic bowel syndrome).
4. The abrupt onset of nausea, vomiting, and diarrhea with a nonfocal abdominal examination (e.g., the patient with gastroenteritis or early appendicitis).

5. Epigastric and right upper quadrant pain and tenderness with or without vomiting (e.g., the patient with pancreatitis, biliary tract disease, or peptic ulcer disease.
6. Diffuse or localized lower abdominal pain of sudden onset in a woman during her reproductive years (e.g., the female patient with ectopic pregnancy, ruptured ovarian cyst, torsion of ovary/tube, pelvic infection, or mittelschmerz).

As a convenient way of categorizing and discussing gastrointestinal testing modalities, we consider separately the two groups of patients mentioned earlier, those who seek treatment for jaundice (with or without abdominal pain) and those who seek treatment for abdominal pain.

THE PATIENT APPEARING WITH JAUNDICE

CASE 14-1

A 46-year-old female was brought to the ED because of jaundice and the sudden onset of moderate epigastric, right upper quadrant, and periumbilical pain, which began the day before. The pain radiated around to the back and waxed and waned. Although the patient had similar pain intermittently for the previous 2 months, it was never as severe and the patient had never been evaluated by a physician for this problem. In addition to the pain, the patient also had moderate to severe pruritus without a rash for the past week. She denied fever and chills or nausea. Her last normal bowel movement was the morning of her ED visit. Past medical history was positive for cholecystectomy and type II diabetes mellitus. The patient had been taking alpha methyldopa for hypertension for the past year. She denied the use of alcohol, intravenous drugs, and risk factors for AIDS.

The physical exam revealed a stout, well developed woman in mild acute distress. She was afebrile with a pulse of 96/min, and a blood pressure of 160/100 mm Hg. The patient was moderately icteric. The cardiopulmonary examination was unremarkable. Her abdomen was scaphoid, soft with mild epigastric tenderness. There was no hepatomegaly.

The CBC revealed a Hct of 38%; a WBC of 11,800/mm^3 with 88% segs, 6% bands, and 4% eosinophils. Additional laboratory data revealed normal serum electrolytes and BUN with a glucose of 168 mg/dL. The total bilirubin was 16 mg/dL, and the direct bilirubin was 12 mg/dL. The delta bilirubin (see text) was 3.6 mg/dL, the ALT 68 IU/mL and the AST 48 IU/mL; alkaline phosphatase was 368 IU/mL, the protime was 14/12.6, the amylase was 180 IU/mL, and the lipase was 260 IU/mL.

CASE 14-2

A 46-year-old female alcoholic was brought to the ED because of jaundice, nausea, vomiting, chills and fever, and right upper quadrant pain for the past week.

The patient had been binge-drinking for 20 years and had 2 similar episodes of these symptoms in the past. The patient denied abuse of other drugs and denied taking prescription or nonprescription medications.

Physical examination revealed a chronically ill-appearing, jaundiced woman in moderate distress. She was febrile to 102° F and her respiratory rate was 22 breaths/min. Her pulse was 110/min and regular and her blood pressure was 98/60 mm Hg. There were telangiectasia and a few spider nevi on her face and upper chest. She had a liver span of 14 cm. The liver was smooth and tender. The spleen tip was palpable. The abdomen was protuberant and there was shifting dullness. Stool exam for occult blood was negative.

Laboratory testing revealed an Hct 30%; Hgb, 9.4 gm/dL; WBC, 3500/mm^3 with 88% polys and 5% bands; platelets 120,000 mm^3; BUN 4 mg/dL; and glucose 58 mg/dL. Electrolytes: Na 132 mEq/L; K 3.0 mEq/mL; and CO_2 28 mEq/mL. LFTs: total bilirubin 10.7 mg/dL; direct 8.4 mg/dL; ALT 320 IU/mL; AST 1020 IU/mL; AP 310 IU/mL; and amylase 180 IU/mL. Serum acetaminophen level was negative.

These cases are typical examples of patients seeking treatment for jaundice, upper abdominal pain, and fever, as well as other systemic signs and symptoms. As previously noted, the chief issue in the ED is to determine whether the jaundice is "medical" or "surgical," and diagnostic testing can be very helpful in resolving this issue. Imaging in these cases is also of major importance and is discussed in Chapter 20.

LIVER FUNCTION TESTS

The liver function tests (LFTs) usually available to the emergency physician include those for bilirubin, alkaline phosphatase, alanine aminotransferase (ALT, formerly known as SGOT) aspartate aminotransferase (AST, formerly known as SGPT), gamma glutamyl transpeptidase (GGT), and plasma ammonia levels. The prothrombin time and albumin concentration are also LFTs but are not discussed in this chapter (for a discussion of prothrombin time, see Chapter 12). The emergency physician should also be familiar with the serologic tests for viral hepatitis types A through E (see also Chapter 17), as well as the common hepatotoxins and the liver derangements they produce. The interpretation of these tests of liver function require a basic knowledge of liver physiology and pathophysiology, which are discussed only briefly in the text. More extensive discussions can be found in several recent reviews.[2, 3]

BILIRUBIN

Bilirubin[4] is an end-product of heme metabolism derived chiefly from the breakdown of aging red blood cells. Bilirubin is also produced from ineffective erythropoiesis in the bone marrow and from myoglobin and heme containing enzymes such as the catalase and P450 systems. In the liver, bilirubin is conjugated to monoglucuronides and diglucuronides via the glucuronyl transferase system, and the conjugated bilirubin is actively secreted into the bile. Conjugated bilirubin is also known as **direct-reacting bilirubin** because it reacts directly with the diazotization reagent in the absence of alcohol. Unconjugated bilirubin is known as **indirect-reacting bilirubin.** When serum levels of direct-reacting bilirubin are elevated above 1.6 mg/dL, bilirubin appears in the urine. In the presence of normal renal function, severe intrahepatic or extrahepatic obstruction to the normal excretion of conjugated bilirubin will result in the serum level peaking at 26 to 30 mg/dL. However, if renal insufficiency (or hemolysis) typically accompanies the obstruction, the level of bilirubin often greatly exceeds this range.[5] In contrast to the situation with elevated levels of conjugated bilirubin, even when serum levels of unconjugated bilirubin are markedly elevated, bilirubinuria is absent. In this condition, known as **acholuric jaundice**, the hyperbilirubinemia is usually caused by rapid red cell breakdown (hemolysis) or congenital or acquired defects in bilirubin transport into the hepatocyte or conjugation. Unconjugated bilirubin is lipid soluble and can pass through the blood-brain barrier. When unconjugated bilirubin levels are pathologically high in neonates, the neurologic condition known as *kernicterus* may result. Kernicterus was formerly a major cause of neonatal brain damage. In the full-term neonate, the exchange level (bilirubin level requiring exchange transfusion) is 20 mg/dL to 25 mg/dL,[6] and phototherapy should be started at the level of 15 mg/dL or greater.

Differential Diagnosis of Elevated Unconjugated Bilirubin

Gilbert's syndrome
Crigler-Najjar syndromes
Hemolytic anemia
Resolving hematomas
Transfusion of blood that is old and has a short survival time
Hemorrhagic pulmonary infarcts

Modified with permission from Wolf PL: Liver function. In Howanitz JH, Howanitz PJ, eds: Laboratory medicine test selection and interpretation, New York, 1991, Churchill Livingston.

Differential Diagnosis of Elevated Delta Bilirubin

Cholestasis, intrahepatic and extrahepatic
Neonates with physiologic jaundice
Gilbert's syndrome
Crigler-Najjar syndromes
Hemolytic anemia

Modified with permission from Wolf PL: Liver function. In Howanitz JH, Howanitz PJ, eds: Laboratory medicine test selection and interpretation, New York, 1991, Churchill Livingston.

Several congenital defects in bilirubin metabolism can cause hyperbilirubinemia:

Gilbert's syndrome, the most common congenital defect in bilirubin metabolism, is a mild defect in bilirubin uptake and conjugation without clinical significance. The defect in Gilbert's syndrome is aggravated by systemic illness and fasting.

The Crigler-Najjar syndromes, types I and II, are congenital defects associated with severe neonatal unconjugated hyperbilirubinemia.

The Dubin-Johnson and Roter syndromes are congenital defects in the secretion of conjugated bilirubin; here the defects *apparently* are in the active transport of conjugated bilirubin at the cannalicular pole of the hepatocyte. The alkaline phosphatase and other LFTs are usually normal in all of these conditions.

Delta bilirubin[4] is a compound formed when conjugated bilirubin binds covalently to albumin. It is determined as part of the total bilirubin level before fractionation. Delta bilirubin (see first box) is seen predominantly with prolonged intrahepatic and extrahepatic cholestasis and has a half-life in plasma similar to that of albumin and much longer than that of nonbound bilirubin.

Serum levels of conjugated bilirubin may be spuriously increased by the presence in the serum of the following drugs: PAS, levodopa, methyldopa, nitrofurantoin, and propranolol, which interfere with the chemical determination.[7]

Testing the urine for the presence of bilirubin may be useful as a quick method of determining whether a jaundiced patient has acholuric jaundice. The spot urine test by Miles laboratories (icto test) and the dipstick tests (Bililabstix, Multistix, Chemstrips) use diazotization methods. *False-positive urine tests for bilirubin are seen when rifampin, large amounts of phenothiazines, or phenazopyridines (Pyridium) are present. False-negative tests are seen when large amounts of ascorbic acid or salicylates are present in the urine together with bilirubin.*

Isolated high-serum levels of indirect-reacting bilirubin represent either hemolysis or a metabolic defect causing the deficient uptake or conjugation or bilirubin (see second box).

High levels of direct-reacting bilirubin (see box at right) signify either a failure of bilirubin secretion at the level of the hepatocyte, or cholestasis (medical jaundice), or obstruction of the biliary tree (surgical jaundice).

Differential Diagnosis of Elevated Conjugated Bilirubin

Cholestasis, intrahepatic and extrahepatic
Postoperative intrahepatic and extrahepatic cholestasis
Recurrent intrahepatic cholestasis during pregnancy
Dubin-Johnson syndromes

With permission from Wolf PL: Liver function. In Howanitz JH, Howanitz PJ, eds: *Laboratory medicine test selection and interpretation,* New York, 1991, Churchill Livingston.

Normal Ranges for Total Serum Bilirubin

Neonate, full-term cord blood	1.4 to 8.7 mg/dL
Neonate, days 1 to 5	1.5 to 12.0 mg/dL
Adults	0.2 to 1.2 mg/dL
NOTE: Adult conjugated bilirubin	<0.2 mg/dL

AMINO TRANSFERASES (TRANSAMINASES)

Alanine amino transferase (ALT)[7] previously termed serum glutamate-pyruvate transaminase (SGPT), is part of an enzyme system found in the microsomal fraction of the hepatocyte, in contrast to aspartate amino transferase (AST, formerly SGOT) which is found in both the cytosol and the mitochondria of hepatocytes. The greatest concentration of ALT is in the liver, with lesser amounts of ALT also found in the kidneys and the heart. The normal range of values is partly dependent on various analytic methods and approximates 10 to 40 IU/ml serum.

AST[7] is present in large concentrations in several tissues, including the liver, the heart, and skeletal muscle. Thus elevations of AST are less specific for liver disease than are elevations of ALT, and AST determinations offer little additional useful information except in two situations: (1) the reversal of the normal ALT/AST ratio in patients with alcoholic liver disease and, perhaps, (2) the continuous release of large amounts of mitochondrial AST in patients with massive hepatic necrosis. The adult reference range for AST is 10 to 40 IU/mL and varies with assay methodology. ALT elevations are typically seen only with hepatocellular diseases and injury.[1] In most cases of liver disease, AST will be elevated as well as ALT, but the ratio of ALT:AST will be >1. In contrast, in alcoholic hepatitis and massive hepatic necrosis, ALT:AST will be <1, apparently because of the greater release of hepatocyte mitochondrial AST.[1] By international agreement, enzyme activity is expressed as international units—IU/mL. One IU equals that amount of enzyme necessary for one micromole of substrate to be produced or consumed per minute.

ALKALINE PHOSPHATASE

Alkaline phosphatase (AP) is a monophosphatase that is concentrated on both the sinusoidal and canalicular borders of the hepatocyte. It is also found in portal and central vein endothelial cells within the hepatic lobule. Other sources of AP include bone (the osteoblast), gut, placenta, and lung. The structure of the enzyme differs according to the organ of origin, and these alkaline phosphatase isoenzymes can be separated by electrophoresis or by chemical means. Fractionation is seldom useful clinically in the ED. When the source of an elevated AP does have to be determined, the important differentiation is typically bone AP versus liver AP, and this differentiation can be easily accomplished by determining the **five prime nucleotidase test** (5′N) level or the **gamma glutamyl transpeptidase** (GTT) level. When the source of an elevated AP is the liver, 5′N and GGT will also be elevated. Conversely, when the source of an elevated AP is bone, 5′N and GTT will be normal.

Serum levels of AP are determined by a number of assays, and the normal reference range may vary in normal individuals because of age, gender, and pregnancy:

Normal Ranges for Serum Alkaline Phosphatase

Infants and children (1 to 12 years)	25 to 350 IU/mL
Adult men	25 to 100 IU/mL
Adult women	25 to 90 IU/mL
Adult women >70 years of age	29 to 120 IU/mL
Pregnant women	2 to 3 times normal at or near term, and can remain elevated for a month postpartum

NOTE: Normal adult range for 5′N is 2 to 17 IU/mL.

Clinical Significance of an Elevated Alkaline Phosphatase

Elevated levels of hepatic AP are found whenever there is obstruction anywhere in the biliary excretory system from the canaliculus to the ampulla of Vater. The elevation results from both regurgitation of AP into the blood and from increased synthesis of new AP, stimulated in some manner by the obstructing process. Intrahepatic infiltrative diseases that distort the lobule can increase the serum AP as a result of local canalicular obstruction (see accompanying box).

Bone AP is increased in any situation characterized by increased osteoblastic activity. Pulmonary, renal, and splenic infarction or inflammation may cause elevations in their respective AP isoenzymes. Carcinoma raises AP by three mechanisms: (1) production of ectopic AP, (2) invasion of liver and biliary tree, and (3) spread to bone with stimulation of osteoblastic repair.

Types of Hepatic Disease Associated with Elevated Serum Alkaline Phosphatase Level

Twofold increase
- Acute viral hepatitis
- Acute toxic hepatitis
- Acute alcoholic hepatitis
- Cirrhosis
- Acute fatty liver

Fivefold increase
- Infectious mononucleosis
- Postnecrotic cirrhosis

Tenfold increase
- Drug-induced cholestatic hepatitis
- Carcinoma of the head of the pancreas
- Choledocholithiasis

Fifteenfold to twentyfold increase
- Primary biliary cirrhosis
- Metastatic or primary carcinoma

Modified with permission from Wolf PL: Liver function. In Howanitz JH, Howanitz PJ, eds: *Laboratory medicine test selection and interpretation,* New York, 1991, Churchill Livingston.

The elderly, especially women, may occasionally have isolated elevations of AP that do not represent occult metastatic disease or chronic liver disease, and (usually) are of no clinical significance.

SERUM GAMMA GLUTAMYL TRANSPEPTIDASE

GGT[8] is an enzyme produced by the hepatocyte and is elevated in almost all types of hepatic and biliary tract disease. It's rise generally parallels and often precedes the rise of serum AP. However, this test is particularly sensitive in detecting early alcoholism, with or without obvious clinical liver disease. GGT is an inducible enzyme with a half-life of 26 days, and GGT levels are increased in patients taking phenytoin, phenobarbital, and several other commonly used medications (Table 14-1).

Normal Range of Gamma Glutamyl Transpeptidase

Male	9 to 50 IU/mL
Female	8 to 40 IU/mL

Table 14–1. Nonhepatobiliary Causes of Increased Serum Gamma-Glutamyl Transferase

Parameter	Magnitude of Increase*
Drugs	
Anticoagulants (e.g., coumarin)	Slight
Antihyperlipidemics (clofibrate)	Slight
Oral contraceptives (estrogens)	Slight
Analgesics (e.g., acetaminophen)	Moderate
Anticonvulsants (e.g., phenytoin)	Moderate
Antidepressants (e.g., cyclics)	Moderate
Barbiturates	Moderate
Alcohol	Moderate to marked
Disorders	
Diabetes mellitus	Slight
Hyperthyroidism	Slight
Kidney diseases	Slight
Neurologic disorders	Slight
Obesity	Slight
Pulmonary diseases	Slight
Rheumatoid arthritis	Slight
Hyperlipidemia	Slight to moderate
Myocardial injury	Slight to moderate
Exocrine pancreatic diseases	Moderate to marked
Malignancy	Slight to marked

*Slight increase: serum GGT <2X upper reference limit (URL); moderate: >2X to <5X URL; marked: >5X URL.

Modified from Wolf PL: Liver function. In Howanitz JH, Howanitz PJ, eds: *Laboratory medicine test selection and interpretation*, New York, 1991, Churchill Livingston.

PLASMA AMMONIA LEVELS

Plasma ammonia (NH_3) levels may be useful in identifying a hepatic etiology of an altered mental status (hepatic encephalopathy). An elevated NH_3 is an indicator of severe hepatic parenchymal derangements. NH_3 levels are also elevated with Reye's syndrome and those inborn errors of metabolism involving the urea cycle and related enzyme systems. NH_3 serum levels are also useful for monitoring patients during hyperalimentation and for documenting portosystemic shunting. Whether ammonia itself is the toxic substance that alters and depresses CNS function or is just a marker for other toxins remains somewhat controversial. However, clinical conditions such as gastrointestinal bleeding that increase ammonia load also aggravate the encephalopathy, and clinical measures that lower the ammonia level usually improve the patient's CNS function.

To obtain an accurate NH_3 level, blood should be collected in a heparinized or EDTA anticoagulated tube, transported to the laboratory on ice and analyzed promptly, as NH_3 levels rise rapidly on standing.

Normal Ranges for Plasma Ammonia Levels

Newborn	50 to 90 μg N/dL
0 to 2 weeks	79 to 129 μg N/dL
>1 month	29 to 70 μg N/dL
Adult	15 to 45 μg N/dL

TESTS FOR VIRAL HEPATITIS

When initial laboratory testing reveals LFTs consistent with acute hepatocyte inflammation or injury, the differential diagnosis includes toxic hepatitis, an insult related to shock and/or hypoxia, or acute viral hepatitis (see Chapter 17).

Used alone, there is no particular pattern of LFTs that can separate these entities. The typical LFT pattern[9] with hepatitis is (1) an ALT elevation 5 to 30 times normal, (2) a total bilirubin elevation of 5 to 10 mg/dL (with most of the bilirubin elevation consisting of the direct-reacting fraction), and (3) an alkaline phosphatase that is modestly ele-

Table 14–2. Serology of Viral Hepatitis

Serologic Marker	Interpretation
Hepatitis A	
IgM anti-HAV	Acute hepatitis A
IgG anti-HAV	Remote infection with immunity to hepatitis A
Hepatitis B	
HB_sAg	Acute or chronic hepatitis B (including carrier state)
IgM anti-HB_c	
High titer	Acute hepatitis B
Low titer	Chronic hepatitis B
IgG anti-HB_c	
Positive HB_sAg	Chronic hepatitis B
Negative HB_sAg	Previous exposure to hepatitis B
Anti-HB_s	Immunity to hepatitis B
HB_eAG	Acute hepatitis B; infectious state
Anti-HB_e	Convalescence or ongoing infection
HBV DNA	Ongoing infectious state

Table 14–2. Serology of Viral Hepatitis—cont'd

Serologic Marker	Interpretation
Hepatitis C	
Anti-HCV (ELISA) (RIA-I) (ELISA-II) RIBA-II)	*Chronic* hepatitis C infection (false-negative and false-positive results exist, especially false-positive results for autoimmune chronic hepatitis with the ELISA assay; later-generation tests are more specific).
HCV RNA (PCR)	*Chronic* hepatitis C infection
Hepatitis D	
IgM anti-HDV	
High titer	Chronic delta infection
IgG anti-HDV	
Low titer, IgM-negative	Prior delta infection
Hepatitis E	
Anti-HEV (Fluorescent AB assay) (Western blot assay)	Recent or remote hepatitis E infection (research use)
CMV	
IgM anti-CMV	Highly suggestive of active CMV infection
IgG anti-CMV	Fourfold rise in titer highly suggestive of active CMV infection
EBV	
IgM anti-VCA (viral capsid antigen)	Primary infection
IgG anti-VCA	Fourfold rise in titer diagnostic in reactivation infections
IgG anti-EA (early antigen)	Primary infection
EBV DNA (PCR)	Active primary or reactivation infection (research use)
Herpes simplex virus types 1 and 2	*Serology not useful at present*

Modified with permission from Hauptman W et al: *Hosp Med* Jan 1993, pp. 83–106.[34]

Table 14–3. Typical Features of Hepatitides A, B, C, D, and E

	Hepatitis Type				
Feature	A	B	C	D	E
Type of virus	RNA	DNA	RNA	RNA	?RNA
Age at onset	Childhood	Any	Any	Any	Adulthood
Oral transmission	+	+/—	?—	?—	+
Percutaneous transmission	Rare	+	+	+	—
Sexual transmission	+	+	—	+	?
Perinatal transmission	—	+	+/−	—	?
Mean incubation (days)	30	50	50	?	40
Viremia	Transient	Prolonged	Prolonged	Prolonged	?Transient
Fecal excretion of virus	+	—	—	—	+
Jaundice	—*	+/—	—	+	+
Mortality	Low	Low	Low	High	Moderate
Chronic carrier	—	+	+	+	—
Chronic hepatitis	—	+	+	+	—
Risk factor for hepatocellular carcinoma	—	+	+	?—	—

Modified from Hauptman W et al: *Hosp Med* Jan 1993, pp. 83–106.[34]
*Except in adults.

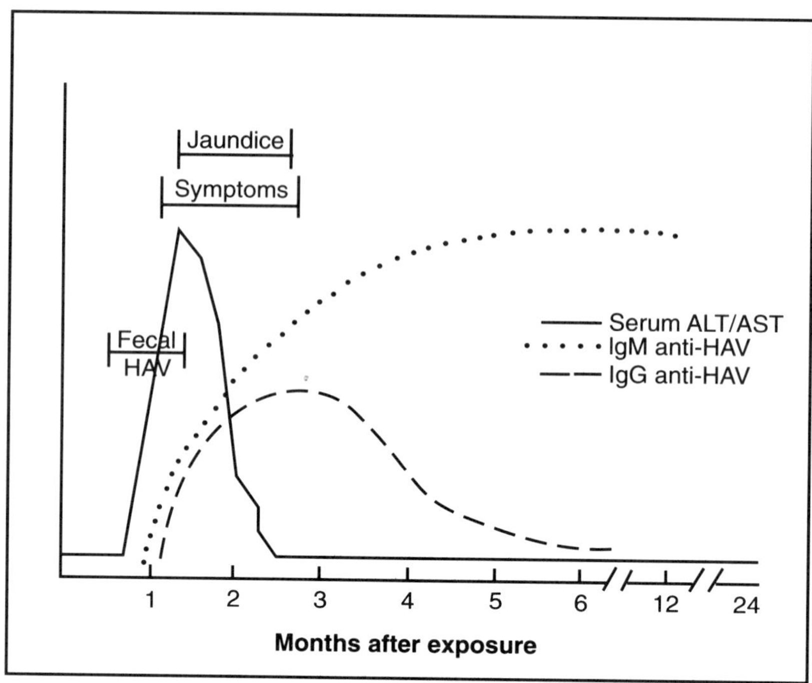

Fig. 14–1. Serologic course of hepatitis A virus infection. IgM anti-HAV appears in the blood during the acute infection and persists for several months after clinical onset. IgG anti-HAV is detectable concomitant with IgM anti-HAV and remains as a serologic marker of past HAV infection. (Adapted with permission from Hoofnagle JH: *Serologic diagnosis of acute and chronic hepatitis.* In Hepatology Update/Portal Hypertension: Viral hepatitis [postgraduate course of the American Association for the Study of Liver Disease], Slack, 1986, Thorofare, NJ. As it appears in Hauptman W et al: *Hosp Med* Jan 1993, pp. 83–106.[34])

vated to 2 to 3 times normal. However, a cholestatic picture with AP levels 5 to 10 times normal can also be seen with viral hepatitis, especially with hepatitis types A and E.

Serologic testing for hepatitis[10, 11, 12] is of secondary importance in the ED because there is usually a delay of a day or more before results are available and there are no immediate therapeutic advantages to the differentiation of the various viral hepatitides except for counseling and managing the patient's intimate contacts.[13] However, samples for serodiagnosis should be drawn in the ED to expedite the diagnostic process for later consideration (Table 14-2). Many of these patients will require written or telephone follow-up, and the case may need to be reported to the appropriate occupational health or public health authorities (see Chapter 22).

There are at least eight common hepatotropic viruses: hepatitis viruses A through E, herpes simplex virus (HSV), cytomegalovirus (CMV), and Epstein-Barr virus (EBV). Yellow fever virus is hepatotropic, but fortunately the disease is rare and limited to certain climates. Coxsackie viruses and adenoviruses can also be hepatotropic on occasion, but clinical liver disease is infrequent. The results of much research conducted in the past few decades has produced a broad, but often confusing, array of tests. Full serologic evaluation is available *clinically* for only hepatitis B. Partial serologic batteries are available for hepatitides A, C, and D. Serologic testing for hepatitis E virus has recently become available for clinical use. The typical serologic and clinical sequence of a hepatitis infection is for the viral antigen to appear first in the blood or secretions, followed by clinical symptoms, and, shortly thereafter, by jaundice. The serologic and clinical events for hepatitides A, B, C, and D are summarized in Figs. 14-1 to 14-5 and Tables 14-2 and 14-3. Knowledge of this sequence may allow the phy-

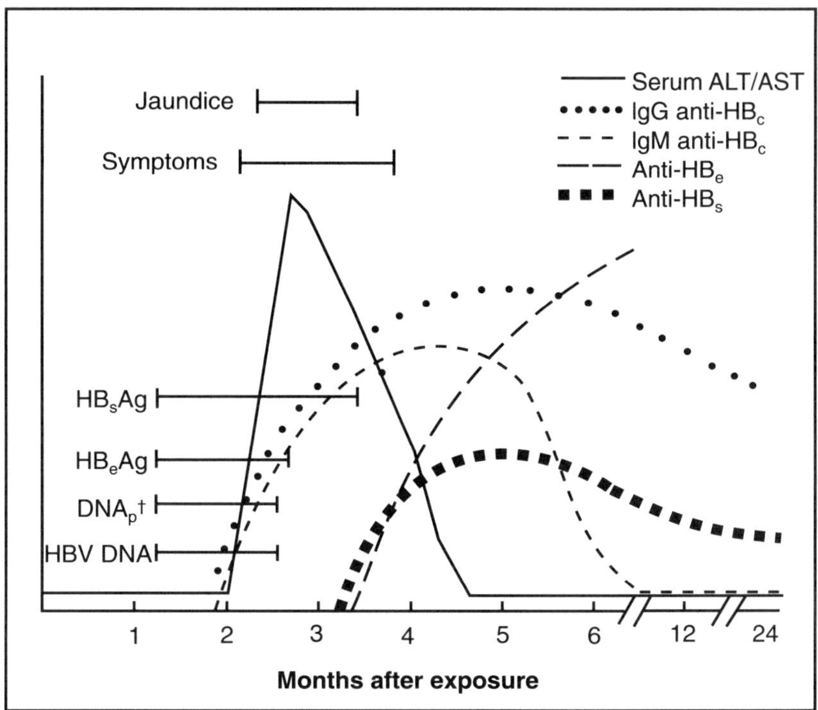

Fig. 14–2. Serologic course of acute hepatitis B virus infection. The diagnosis of type B hepatitis is usually made by finding HB_sAg in the serum. The presence of IgM antibody to hepatitis B core antigen (anti-HB_c), which appears approximately 8 weeks after infection, establishes the acuteness of HBV infection. HB_sAG appears in the blood about 6 weeks after infection and usually disappears by 3 months; persistence for more than 6 months implies chronicity. Anti-HB_s appears fairly late (some 3 months after infection) and persists; it accounts for recovery and immunity, although as many as one-third of HB_sAg carriers may at times have simultaneously detectable anti-HB_s. (Adapted with permission from Hoofnagle JH: *Serologic diagnosis of acute and chronic hepatitis.* In Hepatology Update/Portal Hypertension: Viral hepatitis [postgraduate course of the American Association for the Study of Liver Disease], Slack, 1986, Thorofare, NJ. As it appears in Hauptman W et al: *Hosp Med* Jan 1993, pp. 83–106.[34])

sician to diagnose not only the presence but also the stage of hepatitis, and possibly the exposure risk to others in close contact with the patient.

In viral hepatitis, the bilirubin typically peaks but does not plateau and the period during which infectious particles are found in the serum or other secretions typically lasts 1 to 3 months. When the bilirubin elevation plateaus and/or there is persistence of the infectious particles beyond 6 months, the patient is probably becoming a chronic viral carrier with a high risk of developing chronic active hepatitis. Of the various types of hepatitis, hepatitis C infection is most likely to result in a chronic carrier state and chronic active liver disease. Patients with chronic hepatitis B or C are also prone to develop cirrhosis and hepatoma. Chronic carriers of HBSag have a significant incidence of vasculitis as well.

In attempting to differentiate between an acute hepatitis B infection and a recrudescence of chronic hepatitis B, IgM anti-HBV testing is most useful; this test is positive early in the course of acute hepatitis B infection and usually becomes negative with chronic hepatitis B.

The current clinical test for hepatitis C is an anti-HCV assay. Development of anti-HCV is usually delayed by 5 to 20 weeks after the onset of clinical symptoms and LFT abnormalities. The new second-generation ELISA tests for HCAB are significantly more sensitive and specific and should make serologic diagnosis of hepatitis less problematic. In addition, HCAg can only be detected at present by the polymerase chain reac-

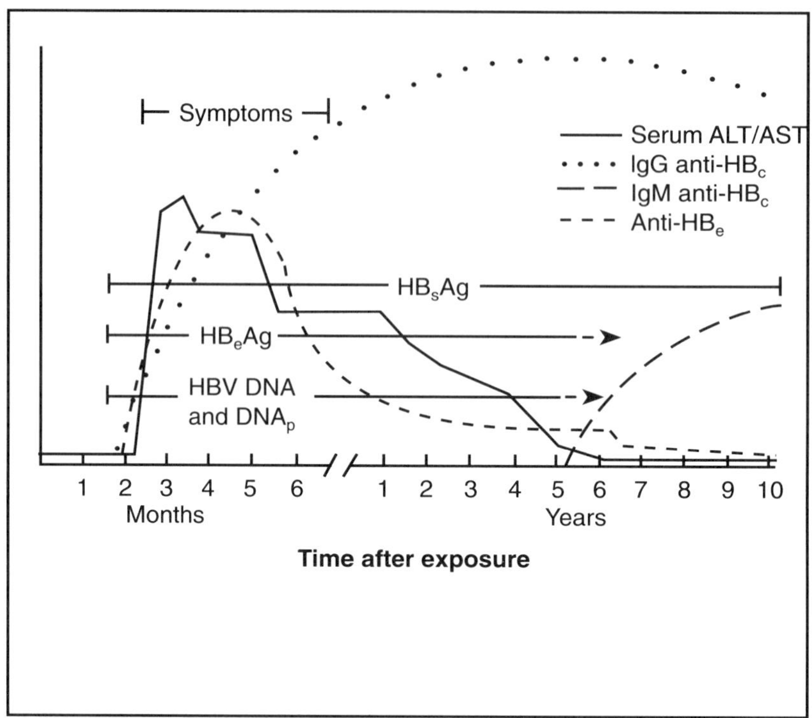

Fig. 14–3. Serologic course of chronic hepatitis B virus infection. The viral protein known as "e" antigen (HB$_e$Ag) correlates with ongoing viral synthesis and with infectivity. Persistence in the serum for more than 10 weeks strongly suggests development of chronic heptitis. Anti-HB$_e$ is generally a marker of relatively low infectivity. HB$_c$Ag cannot be detected in circulating blood, although anti-HB$_c$ can be detected. Persistence of IgM anti-HB$_c$ in the serum implies ongoing HBV-related disease, usually chronic active hepatitis. Low titers of IgG anti-HB$_c$ with positive anti-HB$_s$ mark hepatitis B infection in the remote past; higher titers of IgG anti-HB$_c$ without anti-HB$_s$ (and most often with HB$_s$Ag) indicate persistent viral infection. (Adapted with permission from Hoofnagle JH: *Serologic diagnosis of acute and chronic hepatitis.* In Hepatology Update/Portal Hypertension: Viral hepatitis [postgraduate course of the American Association for the Study of Liver Disease], Slack 1986, Thorofare, NJ. As it appears in Hauptman W et al: *Hosp Med* Jan 1993, pp. 83–106.[34]).

tion for hepatitis C viral RNA. This latter test is currently only available as a research tool.

Hepatitis E antigens and antibody tests are available in several research laboratories, and commercially available kits are under development. It is a fecal/orally spread disease found in the tropical regions of Asia and Africa and has also been reported in Mexico.

Hepatitis D is a superinfection that occurs in patients who are chronically HBag positive (chronic carriers or chronic active hepatitis patients). The delta hepatitis virus is an incomplete virus, requiring help from enzymes produced by the hepatitis B virus to become a complete infectious particle.

EBV hepatitis is seen with infectious mononucleosis and in immunosuppressed patients. In patients with acute EBV hepatitis, the presence of antibodies to EBV early antigen or IgM antibodies to EBV capsid antigen are helpful in confirming the diagnosis. The diagnosis of EBV hepatitis can be sustained in patients previously infected with EBV by the finding of a rising titer to EBV capsid antigen in patients who have had stable, positive titers previously.

CMV hepatitis can be community-acquired; however, most cases are seen in patients following multi-unit transfusions and is associated with immunosuppression. The diagnosis of CMV hepatitis can be made by liver biopsy and tissue culture. A rising titer of IGM antibodies to CMV by immunofluorescence may be useful in diagnos-

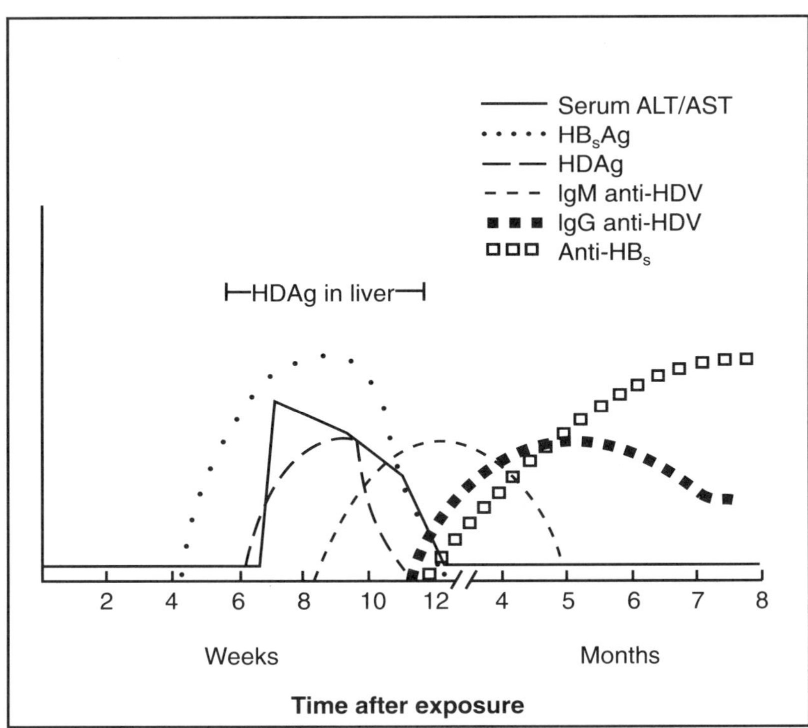

Fig. 14–4. Serologic course of hepatitis D virus infection simultaneous with acute hepatitis B. The diagnosis and monitoring of delta hepatitis hinges on detection of anti-HDV in the serum and serial titer measurements. HDAg may or may not be detected in serum. (Adapted with permission from Rizzetto M: The delta agent, *Hepatology* 3:733, 1983. As it appears in Hauptman W et al: *Hosp Med* Jan 1993, pp. 83–106.[34])

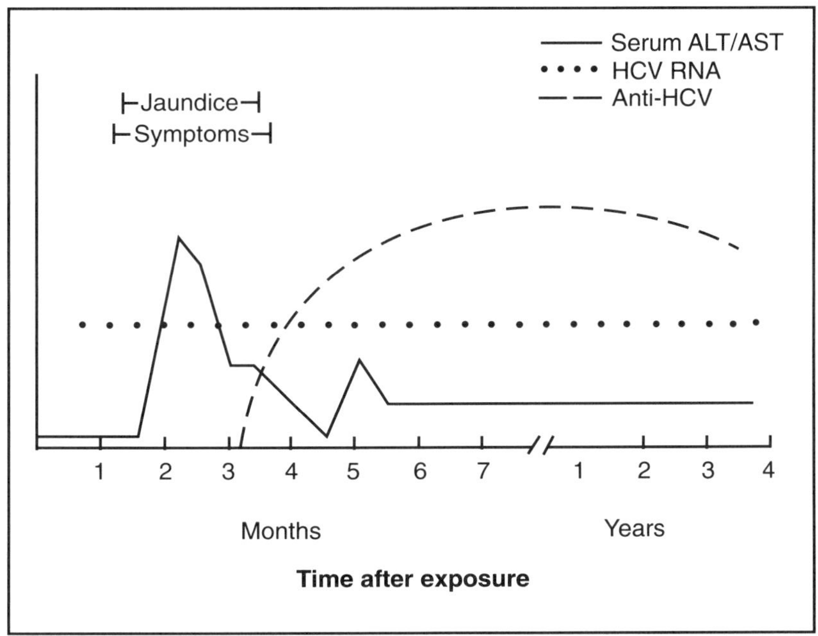

Fig. 14–5. Serologic course of acute hepatitis C virus infection progressing to chronic infection. Anti-HCV is detectable in more than three-quarters of posttransfusion hepatitis cases (acquired in the era before the availability of specific screening of donor blood and blood products). Because the antibody arises 3½ to 6 months after infection and 5 to 20 weeks after the onset of symptoms, presence of anti-HCV really serves to diagnose chronic rather than acute hepatitis C infection. In the near future, PCR may prove practical for detecting and quantitating HCV RNA in the serum. (Adapted with permission from *Seminars in Liver Disease* 11:78, Thieme Medical Publishers, 1991, New York. As it appears in Hauptman W et al: *Hosp Med* Jan 1993, pp. 83–106.[34])

ing primary infection, but the actual titer can remain elevated for prolonged periods following initial infection.

INTERPRETATION OF LIVER FUNCTION TEST PATTERNS

Interpretation of LFTs[14, 15] begins with classification of the patterns of tests into the following categories: (1) hepatocellular or hepatitic, (2) cholestatic, or (3) mixed pattern.

Hepatocellular or Hepatitic Pattern

Hepatocyte inflammation or necrosis results in an elevation of the ALT to levels 5 to 30 times normal while the bilirubin is elevated to 5 to 12 mg/dL. Almost all of the bilirubin elevation is direct reacting unless there is associated hemolysis; the delta bilirubin is low or absent from the serum. In massive hepatic necrosis, the rise in ALT can be even higher initially but will rapidly fall to low levels as the liver fails. There is a moderate (2 to 3 times normal) elevation of the AP. Possible causes of this pattern include acute viral and toxic hepatitis.[16] The causes of severe drug-related toxic hepatitis are listed in the accompanying box.

Common Drugs That Can Cause Hepatocellular Injury

Acetaminophen
Anesthetic agents
Isoniazid
Methyldopa
Nicotinic acid (niacin)
Penicillins
Phenytoin sodium
Procainamide HCl
Propylthiouracil
Quinidine
Valproic acid

Modified with permission from Herrera JL-:*Postgrad Med* 93(2), 1993.

Cholestatic Pattern

Failure or obstruction of bile secretion anywhere from the hepatocytes to the ampulla of Vater results in a cholestatic pattern consisting primarily of elevation of the conjugated bilirubin fraction and alkaline phosphatase.[17] The degree of bilirubin elevation depends on the length of time and degree of obstruction. In cases of sustained complete obstruction, the bilirubin will peak at a serum concentration of 20 to 26 mg/dL. The alkaline phosphatase is the most significant and characteristic abnormality in cholestasis, with levels up to 10 times normal when there is complete extrahepatic obstruction. The ALT is minimally elevated, and the delta bilirubin elevation is directly related to the completeness and duration of the obstruction.

Intrahepatic cholestasis can be caused by drug toxicity, hepatitis, alcoholic fatty liver, infiltrative diseases of the liver such as metastatic cancer and granulomatous dis-

Common Drugs That Can Cause Intrahepatic Cholestasis

Androgens
Chlorpromazine HCl
Clavulanic acid (Augmentin)
Diazepam
Erythromycin estolate
Estrogens
Haloperidol
Oral hypoglycemics
Penicillamine
Phenothiazines
Propoxyphene HCl

Modified with permission from Herrera JL: *Postgrad Med* 93(2), 1993.

eases, biliary cirrhosis, and cholestasis of pregnancy. Extrahepatic obstruction can be caused by tumor masses, biliary calculi or stricture,[18] biliary atresia, sclerosing cholangitis, and compression of the biliary tree by tumor in nodes of the porta hepatis. The drugs associated with a cholestatic pattern are listed in the accompanying box.

Mixed Pattern

The mixed pattern is unfortunately nondiagnostic and represents either a nonspecific liver insult caused by the indirect effects of severe systemic illness or intrinsic diseases of the liver and biliary tree. This pattern consists of mild-to-moderate (2-to-5 times normal) elevations of the bilirubin, AP and ALT. This pattern is most frequently seen in patients with acute and severe systemic disease such as sepsis and congestive heart failure, but the pattern is also consistent with chronic active liver diseases such as chronic active hepatitis and cirrhosis of various etiologies and stages.

Alcohol-related liver disease[19] can lead to a mixed pattern of LFT abnormalities, but the disproportionate elevation of the GTT and AST may be helpful. On occasion, the patient with a prolonged binge drinking habit can appear with a hepatitic pattern (alcoholic hepatitis) or a cholestatic pattern (alcoholic fatty liver syndrome). The imaging procedures and viral serodiagnoses will be negative, whereas the clinical response to abstinence and the results of a liver biopsy will be key to the definitive diagnosis.

CASE **14-1**-CONT'D

The initial laboratory tests were indicative of moderately severe cholestasis without significant hepatocellular damage (i.e., near normal transaminases). In addition, because *both* the amylase and the lipase levels were slightly elevated, attention was directed to a pancreatic lesion.

The provisional diagnosis in the ED was extrahepatic biliary obstruction, and the patient was admitted to the surgical service for further evaluation.

The differential diagnosis in this case was of intrahepatic versus extrahepatic cholestasis. The remarkable features of this patient's presentation included her epigastric pain and long duration of symptoms.

The patient had a subacute illness with an acute exacerbation. Although the complaint of acute pain might suggest a diagnosis of common duct stone, the history of similar milder episodes of pain over 2 months, the moderately deep jaundice, and the pruritus all point to a subacute or chronic picture. Carcinoma of the pancreas has become a common malignancy *and is said to occur more commonly in diabetics so this is still an important consideration. Toxic hepatitis is a significant complication of use of alpha methyldopa,* but the abdominal pain and the long duration of drug use makes this diagnosis less likely.

An abdominal CT and an ERCP were consistent with carcinoma of the head of the pancreas, which was confirmed at laparotomy.

CASE 14-2-CONT'D

Patient 2 was febrile and had a tender liver. She had a mixed clinical picture of active hepatic necrosis with an element of obstruction at presentation. The most serious acute prognostic entity to be ruled out is biliary obstruction associated with ascending cholangitis. Such patients rapidly succumb to gram-negative sepsis unless the obstruction is relieved.

Gallstones are said to occur more frequently in patients with chronic liver disease because of the lithogenic characteristics of their bile. Factors militating against biliary tract disease are the evidence of alcoholic liver disease and portal hypertension and the chronicity of the patient's presenting complaints. At this point, if the diagnosis still appears to be cholangitis, biliary imaging studies would be indicated, including cholescintigraphy and ultrasonography. Unfortunately, with this degree of liver dysfunction, cholescintigraphy may give false positive results, as the tagged anion may not be detected in the small bowel even with a patent common bile duct. Because it is a rather innocuous test, it was attempted in this patient, and a small amount of activity was seen in the small bowel. Ultrasound revealed normal common duct caliber and a normal gallbladder containing several large gallstones.

In this case antibiotic treatment was instituted and the patient was observed. The patient began to withdraw from alcohol on the day of admission and responded to intravenous lorazepam. Hepatitis serology tests were negative for acute viral hepatitis. The patient gradually improved, and liver biopsy performed on the tenth day of hospitalization revealed a complex picture of alcoholic hepatitis and fatty liver with centrilobular necrosis and Mallory's bodies.

THE PATIENT APPEARING WITH UPPER ABDOMINAL PAIN

Tests for Pancreatitis

The patient who comes to the ED with a chief complaint of upper abdominal pain is likely to have blood samples drawn early on for laboratory tests, and the serum amylase level is likely to be among the battery of tests requested to "rule in or rule out pancreatitis."[20, 21] The diagnosis of pancreatitis can be difficult to establish, and an elevated amylase level is often a helpful *final determinant* of the patient's diagnosis and management. Unfortunately, the serum amylase level is neither specific nor sensitive enough as a single test to establish or exclude a diagnosis of pancreatitis.

CASE 14-3

A 37-year-old male came to the ED because of epigastric pain of 2 days' duration. He had a long history of alcoholism; intravenous drug abuse; and recurrent admissions for abdominal pain, cutaneous abscesses, and minor and major trauma. Two years before he had undergone laparotomy and splenectomy following an abdominal knife wound, and HIV testing at that time was negative.

In the ED the patient was acutely ill, dehydrated, and retching intermittently. Temperature was 101° F rectally, respirations were 26/min, PR was 126, and BP was 90/60 mm Hg. The sclera were slightly icteric. The examination of the heart and lungs was unremarkable. The abdomen was distended, however, bowel sounds were present. There was diffuse abdominal tenderness most marked in the upper abdomen. A test for shifting dullness was positive. Laboratory data: Hct 42%; Hgb 13.3 gm/dL; WBC 14,500 mm^3 with a left shift; BUN 36 mg/dL; creatinine 1.6 mg/dL; Na 126 mEq/L; K 2.9 mEq/L; CO_2 17 mEq/L Cl 96 mEq/L; glucose 70 mg/dL; PO_4 2.0 mg/dL; Ca 7.6 mg/dL; albumin 2.6 gm/dL; total bilirubin 2.4 mg/dL; direct 2.0 mg/dL; ALT 128 IU/L; AST 125 IU/L; AP 352 IU/L; protime 14/12; amylase 1200 IU/L (lipase was not available). The chest film revealed cardiomegaly and a small left pleural effusion; a supine film of the abdomen revealed a ground glass appearance com-ascites. Several loops of air containing small bowel in the epigastric region were noted and said to be compatible with "sentinel loops."

The patient was admitted with a diagnosis of severe alcoholic pancreatitis. He was treated with nasogastric suction, analgesics, rehydration, and antibiotics. On the second day in the hospital the patient became hypoxic and developed a metabolic acidosis. Repeat films of his abdomen showed persistence of the sentinel loops. A chest radiograph was interpreted as compatible with ARDS. The ascites was sampled and the results were compatible with an exudate, but no organisms were seen on Gram stain.

AMYLASE AND MACROAMYLASE

The amylases are enzymes that can hydrolyze starch at the 1-4 positions; they are produced by several digestive organs and other tissues. The amylase molecule is a low molecular-weight protein of approximately 55,000 daltons, and it exists as two major isoenzymes along with several genetic variants that are relatively tissue specific. The serum level is maintained by a constant rate of production and renal clearance.[22] The kidney filters the molecule, but it is reabsorbed and degraded *in situ* within the nephron. Normally, very little active enzyme appears in the urine. This process, termed *nonexcretory clearance,* is also an important determinant of serum levels of other low molecular-weight proteins (e.g., insulin and lipase).

Although the highest concentration of amylase is in pancreatic tissue (amylase-P), large amounts are also found in the salivary glands (amylase-S). Several studies have demonstrated that in a significant proportion of alcoholic patients seeking treatment for abdominal pain and an elevated amylase level, it is the salivary amylase that is predominately elevated. The lungs and the liver have low concentrations of an amylase that has the same physical and chemical characteristics as salivary amylase. In the past, the fallopian tubes were said to be a source of elevated amylase in acute obstetric and gynecologic emergencies. However, in a recent study of such patients, no elevation was found.[22]

In acute and chronic pancreatitis, hyperamylasemia is caused by release of the enzyme into the circulation after absorption from sites in the pancreatic bed and peritoneum. The highest level of serum amylases are seen with pseudocyst formation and with pancreatic ascites (rupture of a pseudocyst).[23, 24] The clinical causes of pancreatitis are listed in the boxes on pages 260 and 261.

Several other conditions may be associated with hyperamylasemia, including diabetic ketoacidosis and malignancy. In these two situations, the hyperamylasemia is caused by amylase-S. Perforation, obstruction, or infarction of thc small bowel may permit leakage of intestinal pancreatic and salivary amylase through the damaged bowel wall, eventually gaining entrance to the circulation.

Hyperamylasemia is a frequent finding in renal insufficiency. It is presumably caused by the loss of the renal clearance mechanism. Conversely, pancreatitis is also a complication of uremia and can lead to renal failure, so that hyperamylasemia in a patient with uremia has to be considered in the context of the clinical situation. A small percentage of the normal population has hyperamylasemia without signs or symptoms of pancreatitis. This group has macroamylasemia. In macroamylasemia, the

Etiologies of Pancreatitis

I. Acute pancreatitis
- A. Biliary tract stones
- B. Tumor
  1. Pancreatic
  2. Ampullary
- C. Infection
  1. Mumps
  2. Coxsackie
  3. Mycoplasma
  4. Echovirus
  5. *Ascaris lumbricoides*
  6. *Clonorchis sinensis*
- D. Drugs
- E. Postoperative
  1. Common bile duct exploration
  2. Sphincteroplasty
  3. Distal gastrectomy
  4. Cardiopulmonary bypass
- F. Trauma
- G. Miscellaneous
  1. Postendoscopic retrograde cholangiopancreatography
  2. Metabolic
     - a. Hyperparathyroidism
     - b. Hyperlipidemia—types I, IV, V
     - c. Hypercalcemia
  3. Penetrating duodenal ulcer
  4. Connective tissue disorder
     - a. Systemic lupus erythematosus
     - b. Rheumatoid arthritis
     - c. Henoch-Schonlein purpura
     - d. Necrotizing angiitis
  5. Idiopathic
  6. Pancreas divisum
  7. Hereditary pancreatitis
  8. Scorpion bite
  9. Organ transplantation
     - a. Renal
     - b. Cardiac
  10. End-stage renal failure
  11. Outflow obstruction
     - a. Periampullary diverticulum
     - b. Duodenal Crohn's disease
     - c. Afferent loop syndrome

II. Chronic pancreatitis
- A. Ethanol abuse
- B. Malnutrition
- C. Obstruction
- D. Idiopathic

Modified from Steer ML: Acute pancreatitis. In Taylor MB, ed: *Gastrointestinal emergencies*, Williams & Wilkins, 1992, Baltimore.

Drugs Associated with Acute Pancreatitis

Definite	
Azathioprine	Sulfonamides
Thiazide diuretics	Tetracycline
Furosemide	Estrogens
Ethacrynic acid	Valproic acid
Probable	
Chlorthalidone	Methyl dopa
Procainamide	(Iatrogenic hypercalcemia)
Phenformin	L-Asparaginase
Equivocal	
Acetaminophen	Corticosteroids
Isoniazid	Propoxyphene
Rifampin	

From Steer ML: Acute pancreatitis. In Taylor MB, ed: *Gastrointestinal emergencies*, Williams & Wilkins, 1992, Baltimore.

amylase molecule is bound in a complex with immunoglobulin, and this significantly increases the molecular weight of the amylase moiety, decreasing its renal clearance and prolonging its half life. Macroamylasemia can be diagnosed directly by immunochemical means and indirectly by measuring the urinary amylase excretion, which is significantly reduced from the normal of 4 to 12 IU/hour to less than 4 IU/hour.

Several drugs can raise the serum amylase by a mechanism that has not been fully elucidated but is presumed to be chemically induced pancreatitis. These drugs include captopril, cimetidine, azathioprine, corticosteroids, estrogens, furosemide, oral contraceptives, sulfonamides, tetracycline, pentamidine, opioids, thiazides, and valproic acid.

A low serum amylase level occurs in the presence of pancreatic insufficiency and hepatic failure. Hyperlipemia with lactescent serum may interfere with some amylase assays, leading to falsely low values in cases of acute pancreatitis.

Normal Ranges of Serum Amylase

Newborn	5 to 65 IU/L
Adult	25 to 125 IU/L
Adult (>70 yrs age)	21 to 160 IU/L

The specificity and sensitivity of the amylase test for diagnosing pancreatitis[25, 26] has been difficult to establish because there is no "gold standard" test or imaging procedure that can be used for comparison. In several studies using clinical criteria and ultrasound, the sensitivity of the test is 70% to 80%, while the specificity is 65% to 75%. Thus the test is significantly better than chance alone in helping to make or exclude the diagnosis. However, the clinical assessment by an astute physician is still the most important factor in establishing the diagnosis of pancreatitis.

In an attempt to increase the specificity and sensitivity of laboratory testing for pancreatitis, two tests, the serum lipase and amylase isoenzyme determinations,[27, 28, 29] are used. These tests should help to define whether the hyperamylasemia is of pancreatic or salivary origin.

SERUM LIPASE

Lipase is a relatively small protein with a molecular weight of 48,000 daltons and is metabolized in a manner similar to amylase. Thus it is elevated in renal failure and can gain entrance to the blood stream in the compromised bowel via absorption across the peritoneum. It is present only in pancreatic tissue. Earlier assays for lipase activity lacked precision, and the test was virtually abandoned. However, the newer immunologic tests and the lipase fluorometric displacement assays have eliminated these problems.[30] In acute pancreatitis the sensitivity of lipase is approximately 80% to 90%, and the specificity is 90% to 100%. Recent studies using these tests have shown that the combined use of both amylase and lipase assays in the diagnosis of pancreatitis increases the specificity and sensitivity compared to either test used alone. The lipase assay is especially helpful in interpreting hyperamylasemia in alcoholic patients who have elevated salivary amylases and other possible causes for their abdominal complaints.

The amylase and lipase tests become positive within 24 hours of the onset of symptoms of pancreatitis with the lipase elevation, persisting several days longer than the hyperamylasemia. The levels of hyperamylasemia and hyperlipasemia are higher and persist longer with alcohol-related pancreatitis as compared with gallstone pancreatitis.

CASE 14–3—CONT'D

In addition to severe pancreatitis, the differential diagnosis in patient 3 should have included spontaneous peritonitis and other intraabdominal sepsis syndromes (including intraabdominal and pancreatic abscesses), ascending cholangitis, closed-loop intestinal obstruction, and perforation and penetration of a peptic ulcer.

The patient expired on the third day in the hospital and at postmortem examination was found to have a necrotic strangulated loop of proximal jejunum trapped by an adhesive band. The ascites was frankly purulent. There was a moderate degree of alcoholic cirrhosis, and changes of chronic pancreatitis were found.

This unfortunate patient with *chronic* pancreatitis entered with a picture entirely compatible with *acute* pancreatitis and, because of his presentation and the elevated amylase, other possible diagnoses were not considered further. In retrospect, the high amylase resulted from leakage of enzyme from the necrotic bowel.

On review of the patient's abdominal radiographs, the sentinel loops were fixed in position and were dilating progressively from day to day. Sentinel loops should not dilate progressively and should not remain fixed in one location.

When a patient deteriorates steadily, the diagnosis of pancreatitis should be confirmed surgically. Those patients who have a surgically correctable lesion can be diagnosed and treated, whereas those patients who have a hemorrhagic pancreatitis could benefit from drainage of the pancreatic bed or the occasional early pancreatic abscess.

Once a patient is labeled with a diagnosis by the emergency physician, it may not be reconsidered by the busy in-patient physicians until unusual and/or catastrophic events ensue. This "tyranny of labeling" can lead to the demise of the misdiagnosed patient. Thus the elevated amylase level was equated with the diagnosis of pancreatitis and further diagnostic workup ceased.

The use of predictive statistics are helpful in the clinical integration of a test result.[31, 32, 33] This interpretation of a result is greatly influenced by the pretest probability. Thus if the pretest probability of the patient having pancreatitis is high, and the test is positive, then the positive predictive value of an elevated amylase level is high. If the lipase is elevated as well, the positive predictive value of both tests used together is higher still. These high predictive values are not absolutely diagnostic, as they depend on the pretest probability, which is a clinically derived variable.

NOTE: I am grateful to Drs. Jerry Breslaw, Stanley Bauer, and Carl Teplitz for their critical reviews and suggestions for this chapter.

REFERENCES

1. Jacobson S: Evaluation of abdominal pain. In Harwood-Nuss A, Linden C, Steinbach G, Wolfson AB, eds: *The clinical practice of emergency medicine,* JB Lippincott, 1991, Philadelphia.
2. Middleton H, Cortess J: Normal liver function: a basis for understanding hepatic disease, *Arch Intern Med* 143:2291–2294, 1983.
3. Balistrari WF, Rej R: Liver function. In Burtis CA, Ashwood ER: *Teitiz textbook of clinical chemistry,* Philadelphia, 1994, W.B. Saunders.
4. Wolf PL: Liver function. In Howantiz JH, Howanitz PJ, eds: *Laboratory medicine test selection and interpretation,* Churchill Livingston, 1991, New York.
5. Fulop M, Katz S, Leurence C: Extreme hyperbilirubinemia, *Ann Intern Med* 122:254–258, 1971.
6. Rosenthal P, Sinatra F: Jaundice in infancy, *Pediatr Rev* 11:79–85, 1989.
7. Tiety NW: *Clinical guide to laboratory tests,* WB Saunders, 1990, Philadelphia.
8. Serum gamma glutamyl transpeptidase and chronic alcoholism: influence of alcohol ingestion and liver disease, *Digest Dis* 30(3):211–214. 1985.
9. Holt JT, Arvan DA: Acute viral hepatitis. In Griner PT, Panzer RJ, Greenland P, eds: *Clinical diagnosis and laboratory,* Yearbook, Chicago, 1986.
10. Kumar S, Pound DC: Serologic diagnosis of viral hepatitis, *Postgrad Med* 92(4):55–68, 1992.
11. Kumar S, Pound DC: Serologic diagnosis of hepatitis, *Postgrad Med* 92(4):59–62, 1992.
12. Hauptman W, Hitscherich R, Miskovitz P: Update and acute and chronic viral hepatitis, *Hosp Med,* pp. 3–106, Jan 1993.
13. Dindzans VJ: Viral hepatitis preexposure and postexposure proflylarsis, *Postgrad Med* 92(4):43–52, 1992.
14. Herrera JL: Abnormal liver enzyme levels. The spectrum of causes, *Postgrad Med* 93(2), 1993.
15. Herrera JL: Abnormal liver enzymes. Clinical evaluations in asymptomatic patients, *Postgrad Med* 93(2):119–130, 1993.
16. Done AK: The hepatotoxic presentation, *Emerg Med* pp 102–116, Nov 15, 1988.
17. Wilbur DC, Dean AA: Obstructive jaundice. In Griner PF, Panzer RJ, Greenlord P, eds: *Clinical diagnosis and the laboratory,* Yearbook, 1986, Chicago.
18. Kadakia SC: Biliary tract emergencies. Acute cholecystitis, acute cholangitis and acute pancreatitis, *Med Clin N Am* 77(5):1015–1036, 1993.
19. Magarian GJ, Lucas LM, Kumar KL: Clinical significance in alcoholic patients of commonly encountered laboratory test results, *West J Med* 156(3):287–294, 1992.
20. Steer ML: Acute pancreatitis. In Taylor MB, ed: *Gastrointestinal emergencies,* Williams & Wilkins, 1992, Baltimore.
21. Calleja GA, Bakin JS: Acute pancreatitis, *Med Clin N Am* 77(5):1037–1056, 1993.
22. Christensen H, Lansen MO, Schebye O: Serum amylase levels in gynecologic patients with acute abdominal pain, *Surg Gynecol Obstet* 175(4):355–356, 1992.
23. Winslet M, Hall C, London NJ, Neoptolemos JP: Relation of diagnostic serum amylase levels to aetiology and severity of acute pancreatitis, *Gut* 33(7):982–986, 1992.
24. Pieper-Bigelow C, Strocchi A, Levitt MD: Where does serum amylase come from and where does it go? *Gastroenterol Clin N Am* 19(4):793–810, 1990.
25. Hoffman JR, Jaber AJ, Schriger DL: Serum amylase determination in the emergency department evaluation of abdominal pain, *J Clin Gastroenterol* 13(4):401–406, 1991.
26. Stoler MA, Arvan DA: Acute pancreatitis. In Griner PF, Panzer RJ, Greenland P, eds: *Clinical diagnosis and the laboratory,* Yearbook, 1987, Chicago.
27. Pace BW, Bank S, Wise L, et al: Amylase isoenzymes in the acute abdomen: an adjunct in those patients with elevated total amylase, *Am J Gastroenterol* 80(11):898–901, 1985.

28. Lin XZ, Wang SS, Tsai YT, et al: Serum amylase, isoamylase, and lipase in the acute abdomen. Their diagnostic value for acute pancreatitis, *J Clin Gastroenterol* 11(1):47-52, 1989.
29. Leclerc P, Forest J: Variations in amylase isoenzymes and lipase during acute pancreatitis, *Clin Chem* 29:1020, 1983.
30. Gumaste DS: Serum lipase: a better test to diagnose acute alcoholic pancreatitis, *Am J Med* 92:239–242, 1992.
31. Mayewski RJ, Mushlin AI, Griner PL: Principles of test selection and use. In Griner PF, Panzer RJ, Greenland P, eds: *Clinical diagnosis and the laboratory,* Yearbook, 1987, Chicago.
32. Griner PF, Mayewski RJ: Principles of test interpretation. In Griner PF, Panzer RJ, Greenland P, eds: *Clinical diagnosis and the laboratory,* Yearbook, 1987, Chicago.
33. Suchman AL, Dolon JG: Adds and likelihood ratios. In Griner PF, Panzer RJ, Greenland P, eds: *Clinical diagnosis and the laboratory,* Yearbook, 1987, Chicago.
34. Hauptman W, Hitscherich R, Miskovitz P: Update on acute and chronic viral hepatitis, *Hosp Med* pp 83–106, 1993.
35. Ventrucci M: Update and laboratory diagnosis and prognosis of acute pancreatitis, *Digest Dis* 11(3):189–196, 1993.

Chapter 15

Dermatologic Testing and Skin Tests

Miguel R. Sanchez, M.D.

When evaluating a patient with a cutaneous disease of uncertain etiology, a physician must decide whether to treat for a presumed condition or to withhold therapy until the disease has been diagnosed by a dermatologist. In many cases, the diagnosis can be determined on the spot through simple tests. However, until expertise is developed, practitioners may lack confidence in their ability to perform these tests. With practice, competence can be acquired and results interpreted reliably.

PART I: DERMATOLOGIC TESTS

DIAGNOSTIC CLINICAL SIGNS

Diagnostic manipulations can improve diagnosis of certain skin diseases[1]:

- *Auspitz sign*—Discrete bleeding points appear when scales are scraped from a psoriatic lesion.
- *Nikolsky sign*—In patients with pemphigus or toxic epidermal necrolysis, firmly rubbing fingers through involved skin loosens the epidermis and results in superficial erosions.
- *Darier's sign*—Rubbing a lesion of urticaria pigmentosa (mastocytosis) produces a wheal.
- *Wart paring sign*—Paring down the hyperkeratotic surface with a rounded scalpel blade differentiates calluses from large warts since black or red points, which represent hemorrhages, are present only in warts.
- *Apple jelly sign*—Pressing a lesion of lupus vulgaris (cutaneous tuberculosis) with a microscopic glass slide changes its color to brown-yellow like apple jelly.
- *Vascular diascopy*—No blanching occurs if lesions of palpable purpura (vasculitis) or Kaposi's sarcoma are pressed with a microscopic glass slide.

MOLLUSCUM PREPARATION

Clinical differentiation of early lesions of molluscum contagiosum, comedonal acne, and flat warts can be difficult.

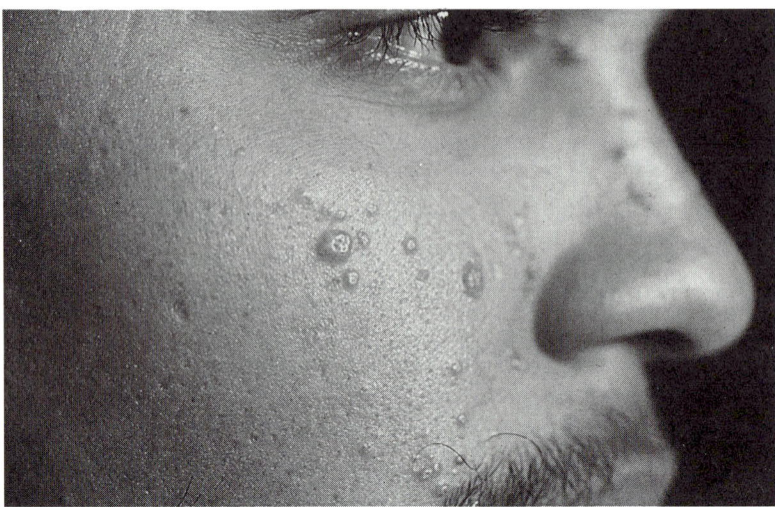

Fig. 15–1. Molluscum contagiosum.

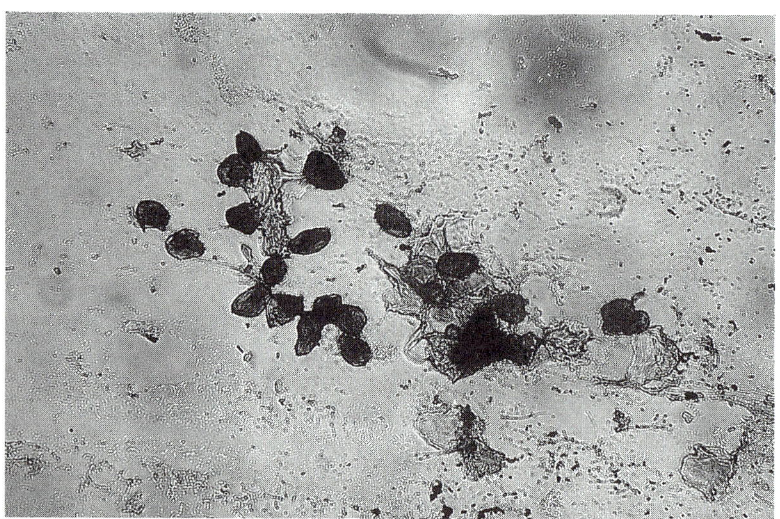

Fig. 15–2. Molluscum bodies.

CASE 15–1

A 34-year-old man infected with human immunodeficiency virus (HIV) has numerous small discrete, shiny, flesh-colored papules on his face and neck (Fig. 15–1). Despite treatment for acne, new lesions have erupted. What is your diagnosis?

Instructions

1. With a pointed (no. 11) scalpel blade puncture the lesion and loosen its contents. The inside of the lesion contains a small, firm, white "core" that resembles a small seed.
2. Extract the contents or "core" by pressing from the sides toward the center with the handle of the scalpel, by pressing down with a comedone extractor, or by curetting the entire lesion.

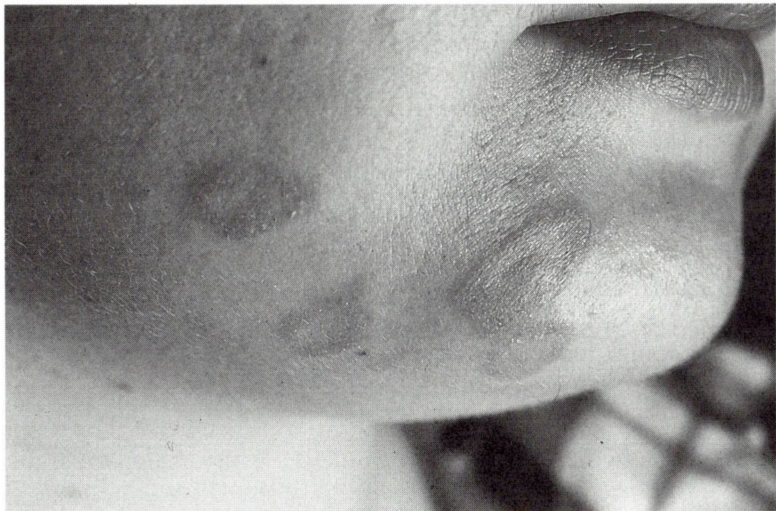

Fig. 15–3. Tinea faciei.

3. Crush the specimen between two glass microscope slides, allow to air-dry for 30 seconds, and colorize with Wright or Giemsa stain.

4. Examine under the microscope for molluscum (Patterson-Henderson) bodies, which are infected epidermal cells enlarged by abundant viral particles in the cytoplasm (Fig. 15–2).

Comments

Molluscum contagiosum is a cutaneous infection caused by a poxvirus. The lesions usually appear on the face, trunk, and extremities of otherwise healthy children or immunocompromised persons and on the genitals of sexually active adults. The round, well-demarcated dome-shaped papules may be flesh colored, white, or pink and have a characteristic dell or core. However, these umbilications are not always readily noted without a magnifying glass. The diagnosis of molluscum contagiosum can be immediately confirmed by microscopic examination of a smear prepared from the contents of the lesions.[2] Inside infected epidermal cells, the virus creates very large cytoplasmic inclusion bodies that can be demonstrated by examination with special stains. Widespread molluscum contagiosum is a sign of immunodeficiency, and patients with numerous lesions should be thoroughly evaluated.

POTASSIUM HYDROXIDE EXAMINATION

The diagnosis of dermatophyte infection can be readily established by mixing scales from a lesion with a solution of 10% potassium hydroxide (KOH), which dissolves keratin in the stratum corneum cells so that the microscopic detection of hyphae and spores is facilitated.[3]

CASE 15–2

Pruritic, well-circumscribed, erythematous, oval and round, annular plaques with fine scale at the periphery developed on the face of a 32-year-old female (Fig. 15–3). After application of a corticosteroid ointment, which was prescribed by her internist, the lesions have become larger and more numerous.

Instructions for Performing KOH Preparation

1. Remove creams or powders from the surface of the lesion with alcohol, and remove ointments with acetone.
2. Gently scrape the abnormal skin with a rounded-blade scalpel (no. 10 or 15), and collect the scales on a glass slide. The scaly border of the lesion is the best area to scrape. Organisms are more difficult to find in scrapings from inflamed skin and crusted surfaces.
   a. In bullous tinea, the roof of blisters should be cut with a scalpel or fine scissors and smeared on a glass slide.
   b. Nails should be clipped as far back as possible and the scale beneath the nail plate scraped off onto the slide with a scalpel blade or a chalazion curet. When subungual hyperkeratosis is not present, cut a piece of the abnormal nail with the scalpel blade into tiny fragments. In cases of paronychia, the inner edge of the nail fold is scraped.
   c. Scraping the surface of lesions of tinea capitis is not sufficient since the fungus can invade the hair exclusively. Hairs from affected areas must be plucked and examined.
3. Place two drops of a 10% KOH solution on the specimen and top with a plastic coverslip. The addition of dimethylsulfoxide (DMSO) or a dye such as chlorazol black to the KOH solution facilitates visualization of fungal structures but is not essential. If the specimen is too thick, let it stand for 15 minutes to allow the KOH to dissolve the scales and expose the hyphae.
   a. Nail particles are allowed to soak in KOH until the keratin is dissolved.
4. Heat the bottom of the slide with a match or cigarette lighter for 3 to 5 seconds but avoid boiling, which produces artifacts.
5. Examine the specimen under the 10× magnification objective, low-intensity light, and a low condenser. It is helpful to constantly adjust the fine focus knob in order to contrast the refractile hyphae against the background of cells (Fig. 15–4).
   a. When structures that resemble hyphae are visualized, confirmation with the 40× magnification objective is made. As the examiner becomes more experienced and confident, this step becomes unnecessary. Note that KOH is very damaging to the objective, so the lens must be cleaned after each use.

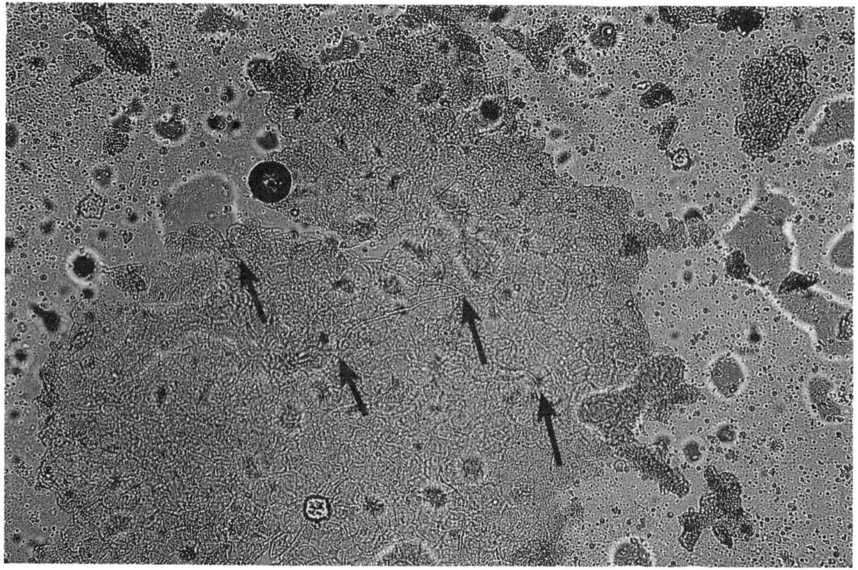

Fig. 15–4. Hyphae.

b. Hyphae are filaments that have uniform diameters, are usually straight although sometimes septate, often branch, and due to their length, extend across cells.
c. Trained examiners may be able to distinguish the pseudohyphae of *Candida*, which are long and uniform in diameter and have budding spores, from the hyphae of other dermatophytes, but a Gram stain better differentiates these organisms.
d. Inexperienced examiners are often confused by artifacts, especially lint and linear salt spicules caused by overheating. Salt spicules are crystalline, whereas lint is composed of large, linear structures with variable diameters and usually tapered or ragged ends (Fig. 15–5). Lipids around the periphery of cells create beaded lines that are commonly confused with hyphae and have been called "mosaic fungi"; however, these structures can be distinguished from hyphae because they do not cross cell walls (Fig. 15–6).
e. Chromomycosis can be diagnosed by removing the black dots, which represent

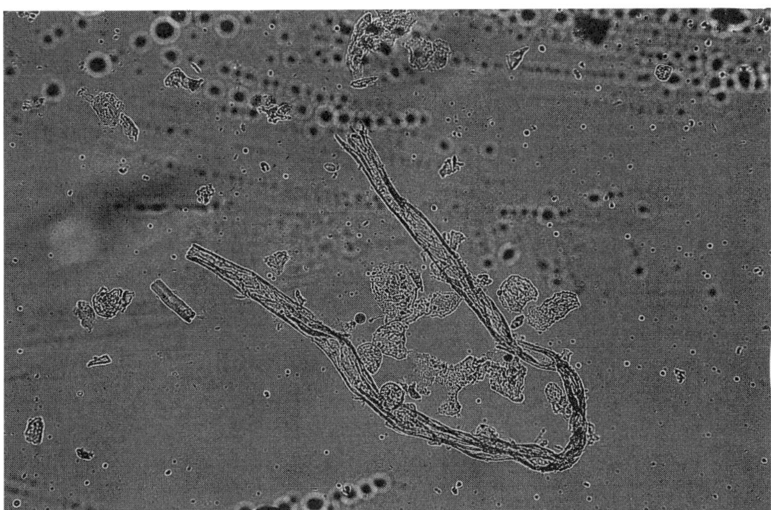

Fig. 15–5. Lint.

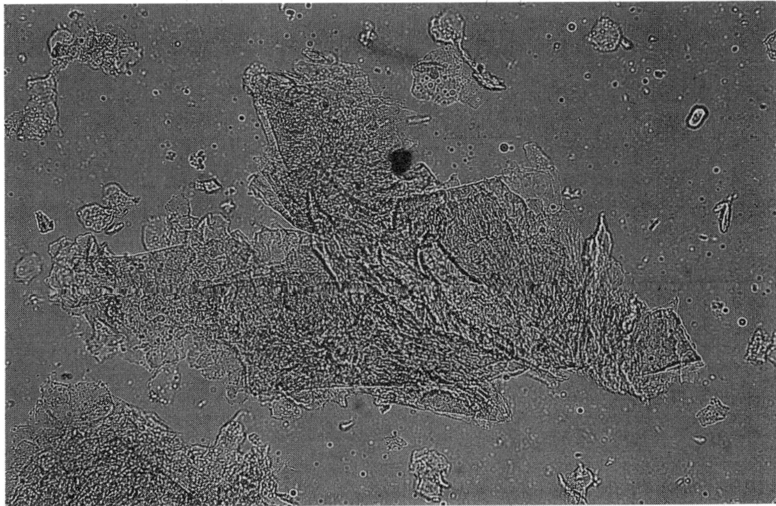

Fig. 15–6. Mosaic fungi.

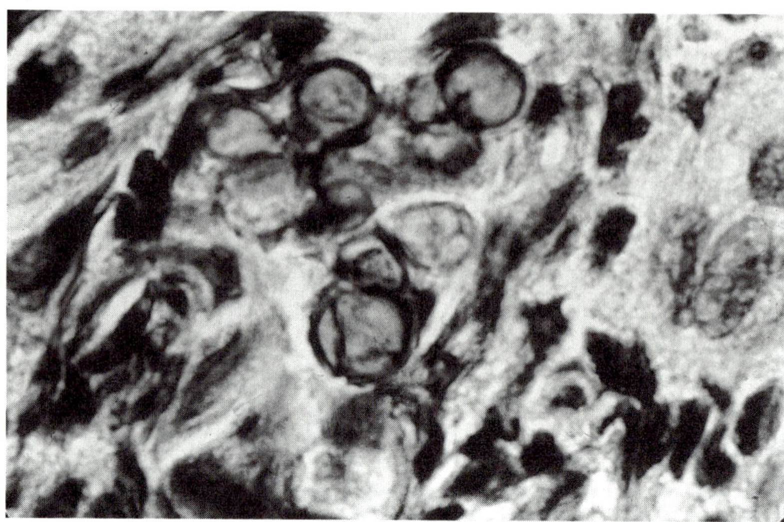

Fig. 15–7. Copper pennies.

old hemorrhagic microabscesses, from the lesion with a pointed (no. 11) scalpel blade. After the "black dot" dissolves with KOH, the spores, called *copper pennies* or *Medlar bodies* are readily visualized (Fig. 15–7).

f. The KOH preparation can also be used to diagnose fiberglass dermatitis in patients with intense itching. The skin is scraped and KOH examination reveals the straight, rigid-appearing spicules.

Special KOH Solutions

- Mix potassium hydroxide, 10 g, DMSO, 20 mL, and distilled water, 30 mL

or

- Dissolve 1 mg of chlorazol black E in 2 mL of DMSO and mix with 1 g of KOH in 20 mL of distilled water

or

- Purchase the commercially available preparation from Dermatologic Lab and Supply Co., Council Bluffs, Iowa.

Comments

Lesions caused by dermatophytic fungi can be pruritic or asymptomatic. The classic lesion is an erythematous plaque that over time expands at the periphery and clears in the center. As a result, the configuration resembles a large ring. The center of the lesion may become hyperpigmented or hypopigmented. The borders are slightly raised and sharply defined and may contain small papules, vesicles, or pustules. Topical corticosteroids initially improve the symptoms and appearance of tinea, but within days the lesions become more widespread and enlarge rapidly. Dermatophytes can be demonstrated by microscopic examination of scales dissolved in KOH. Annular lesions also occur in other cutaneous diseases such as granuloma annulare, sarcoid, urticaria, lupus erythematosus, Hansen's disease, and mycosis fungoides. Annular forms of eczema, lichen planus, erythema annulare centrifugum, pityriasis rosea, and secondary syphilis are often confused with tinea because the surfaces of the annular plaques are hyperkeratotic, although in contrast to dermatophytosis, scaling is not more pronounced at the periphery of the lesions in these diseases.

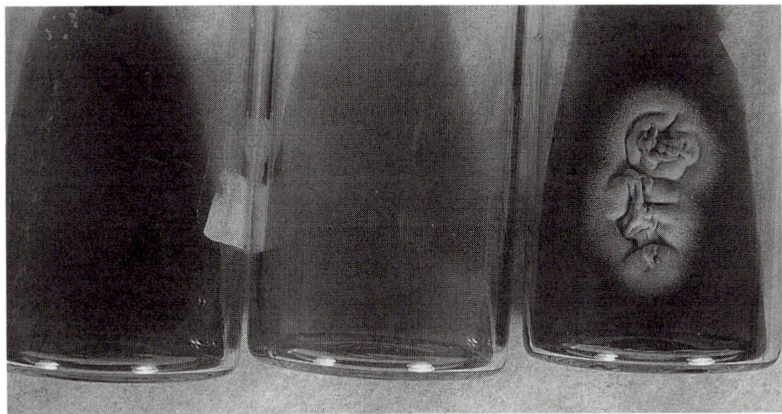

Fig. 15–8. Dermatophyte Test Media cultures.

The lesions of fungal infections may also be arcinate, vesicular, or pustular. Granulomatous, inflamed nodules, *Majocchi's granuloma,* may erupt on the legs of women who shave their hair. Because the fungus infects the deeper portions of the hair follicle, the diagnosis usually needs to be made by histopathologic examination of biopsied tissue.

FUNGAL CULTURES

Instructions

Wash the lesion only with water. Scales, blister roofs, nail debris, and hairs are collected as outlined for the KOH examination and directly deposited into a bottle containing fungal culture medium such as Sabouraud or preferably DTM (Dermatophyte Test Media).[4] The top of the bottle should be loosely screwed to allow the penetration of oxygen. The culture is incubated at room temperature. DTM contains chlortetracycline and gentamicin to prevent bacterial contamination, cycloheximide to inhibit the growth of molds, and phenol red, which turns the yellow media red within 14 days if the pH has been altered by a growing dermatophyte (Fig. 15–8).

Candida colonies grow within 1 week and have a characteristic tan or white, pasty appearance. In most cultures *Candida* is a contaminant and not the primary pathogen. Rarely, bacteria resistant to tetracycline and gentamicin turn the media red, so all positive cultures should then be sent to a mycology laboratory for identification of the organism.

Comments

Tinea of the scalp (capitis) occurs in children and immunocompromised adults. The lesions may be localized, scaly patches of alopecia with broken hair stubs, erythematous scaly papules and plaques, or kerions, which are boggy, tender, inflamed crusted plaques covered with follicular pustules and crust. The most common cause of "epidemic" tinea capitis is *Trichophyton tonsurans.* KOH examination demonstrates hyphae and spores around or within the infected hairs. Tinea barbae is characterized by papules and annular plaques or pustules and is usually caused by *T. mentagrophytes* or *T. verrucosum.*

The most common type of fungal infection is tinea pedis. In the intertriginous form, which is frequently caused by *T. mentagrophytes,* erythema, scaling, maceration, and fissuring develop between the toe webs. This fungus is usually cultured from the vesiculobullous form which first manifests as blisters on the soles, dorsa, and sides of the feet. In the papulosquamous or moccasin form, which is more often caused by *T. rubrum,* there is diffuse scaling throughout the soles and sides of feet. Identical vesicular and papulosquamous manifestations occur in tinea manuum. In young adults, the most common fungal infection is tinea cruris. Bilateral, macerated, erythematous, often pruritic plaques develop in the groin and extend toward the thigh. Initially, the entire surface of the plaque may be hyperkeratotic, but over time, scaling is only present along the advancing border. *Epidermophyton floccosum, T. rubrum* or *T. mentagrophytes* are frequently cultured.

In the nail fungal infection, *onychomycosis,* the nails are thickened and dystrophic with subungual keratotic debris, and white or yellow discolored nail plates. In HIV-infected patients, white onychomycosis, caused by *T. rubrum,* is often found. In contrast, in immunocompetent individuals white onychomycosis is caused by *T. mentagrophytes* and occasionally by *Candida albicans. T. rubrum* is more often cultured from hyperkeratotic onychomycosis. Chronic paronychia with erythema and inflammation around the nail folds is invariably caused by pathogenic *Candida* species. The lesion may become tender and purulent because of bacterial superinfection with *Staphylococcus aureus.*

SCABIES SCRAPING

Generalized pruritus is a common complaint that causes considerable distress to the patient. Evaluation of pruritus requires exclusion of skin diseases such as lichen planus, eczema, and drug eruptions. Patients with thyroid disease, biliary cholestasis, chronic renal failure, polycythemia vera, uncontrolled diabetes mellitus, drug hypersensitivity, reticuloendothelial malignancies, and HIV disease may have itching and excoriations, but no primary lesions.

CASE 15–3

Pruritic acuminate urticarial papules developed on the hands, interdigital webs, abdomen, penis, and axillae of a 30-year-old male (Fig. 15–9). Treatment with topical corticosteroids did not relieve the itching. How can you determine the cause of itching?

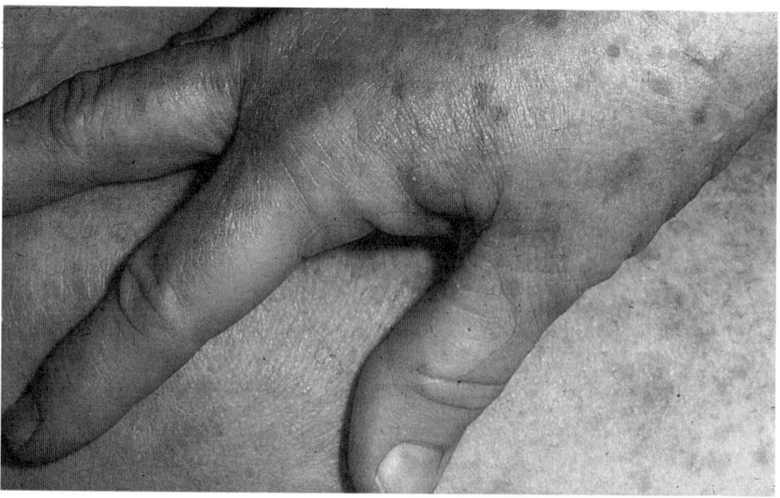

Fig. 15–9. Scabies.

Instructions

1. Look for burrows or vesicles. If none are found, select an unexcoriated, intact papule.
2. After a drop of immersion oil is applied onto the lesion, scrape the skin firmly with a rounded scalpel.
3. Place the specimen on a microscope slide and top with a coverslip.
4. Examine under low magnification for mites, the oval transparent eggs, and rectangular or irregularly shaped brown fecal material (Fig. 15–10).

Comments

Arthropod assault should be considered in all patients with intractable itching. Scabies is a common infestation caused by the mite *Sarcoptes scabiei,* which only infests humans.[5] This highly contagious infestation particularly afflicts homeless or institutionalized individuals and persons who share contaminated beds or clothing. The family members, sexual contacts, and health care providers of these patients can also become infested. The hyperkeratotic form on the hands and body folds, called Norwegian scabies, is caused by a rapid proliferation of mites in immunocompromised patients or the infirm elderly (Fig. 15–11).

The microscopic mite burrows into the skin of its host to feed and lay eggs. An intensely pruritic exanthem develops because of an allergic response to the mite and its waste products. Excoriated erythematous papules, patches, and plaques erupt anywhere in the body below the head, but particularly on the hands, genitals, axillae, and other body folds.[6] The face and scalp are often involved in infants but not in adults. Characteristically, burrows, which are long and narrow ridges with lengths between 0.5 and 1 cm, are present, especially on the hands.

EXAMINATION FOR LICE

Pediculosis pubis (pubic lice) is an infestation that is predominantly sexually transmitted. Pediculosis capitis (body lice) usually affects school-age children, the homeless, and institutionalized persons. Epidemics of scalp lice develop in schools and health care institutions.[7] Body lice predominantly infest undomiciled or schizophrenic individuals who, either for lack of access to baths or poor personal hygiene habits, infrequently shower and change their clothing. Lice infestation produces intractable pruritus over the involved areas. In pediculosis corporis the lice feed from the skin of body areas covered by clothing. Unlike scabies, in which burrows and a characteristic distribution of lesions are frequently seen, only excoriations are usually seen in pediculosis corporis.

Pediculosis capitis and pediculosis pubis can be diagnosed by examination for lice and eggs in scalp and pubic hair respectively. After parting the hair so that the underlying skin can be carefully visualized, the dark brown tiny ectoparasites are found stationary or crawling along the skin surface. A magnifying glass facilitates observation. The eggs (nits), which are white and oval, can be distinguished from lint or dandruff specks because they cannot be easily detached from the hair.

Instructions

The louse or a hair with the attached nit is plucked with fine forceps, placed on a microscopic slide, smeared with a drop of oil, topped with a coverslip, and examined under low (4 to 10×) magnification. The nits are dark, oval, smooth-walled, translu-

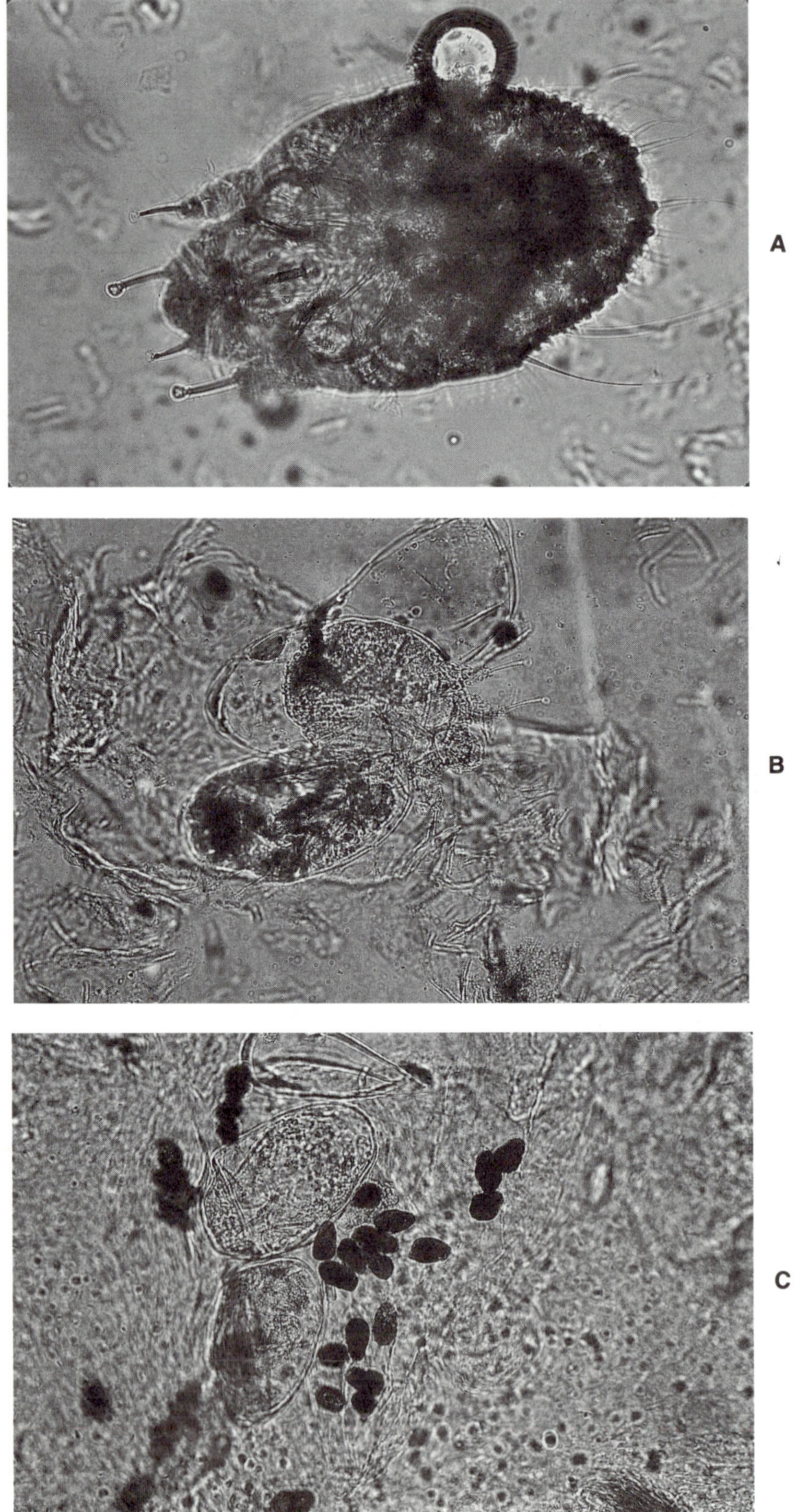

Fig. 15–10. A, Scabies preparation. **B,** Scabies emerging from egg. **C,** Scabies eggs and fecal material.

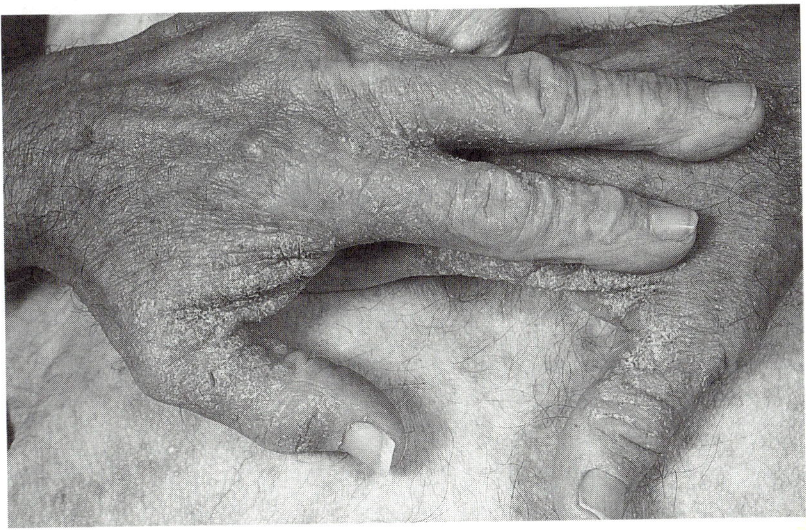

Fig. 15–11. Hyperkeratotic scabies.

cent bodies stuck to the hair (Fig. 15–12). *Phthirus pubis,* the pubic louse, is dark, broad like a crab, and only about 2 to 3 mm in size, whereas *Pediculus corporis,* the body and head louse, is lighter in color, thinner, and longer, measuring 3 to 4 mm (Fig. 15–13). Unlike other lice, the body louse is not usually found on the skin since it returns to the patient's garment as soon as it has fed. Therefore, patients with suspected pediculosis corporis should be instructed to remove their undergarments and clothing and to place them inside out on an examining table. The lice are found along the seams. The insect's three pairs of legs and blood meal through the peristaltic bowel are easily visualized under low power microscopy.

SLIT SMEAR FOR *MYCOBACTERIUM LEPRAE*

This test is done to rapidly diagnose borderline or lepromatous leprosy and to evaluate the response to treatment.[8] The test is usually performed on the earlobes or on lesional skin.

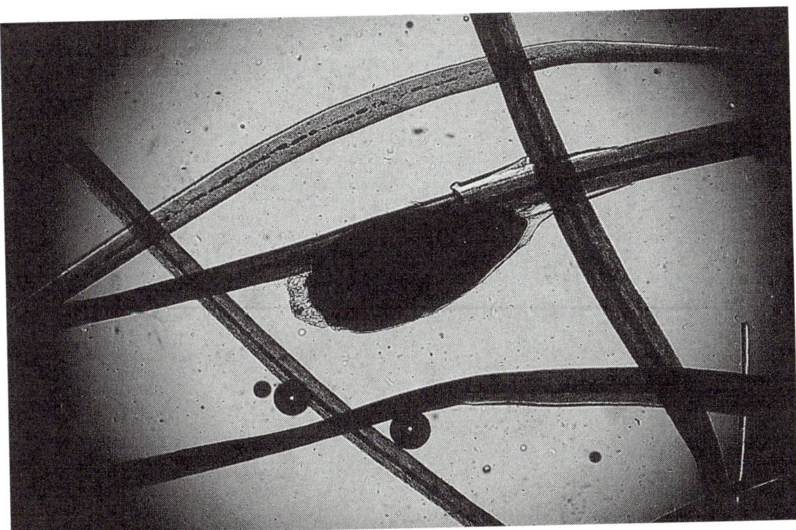

Fig. 15–12. Nits.

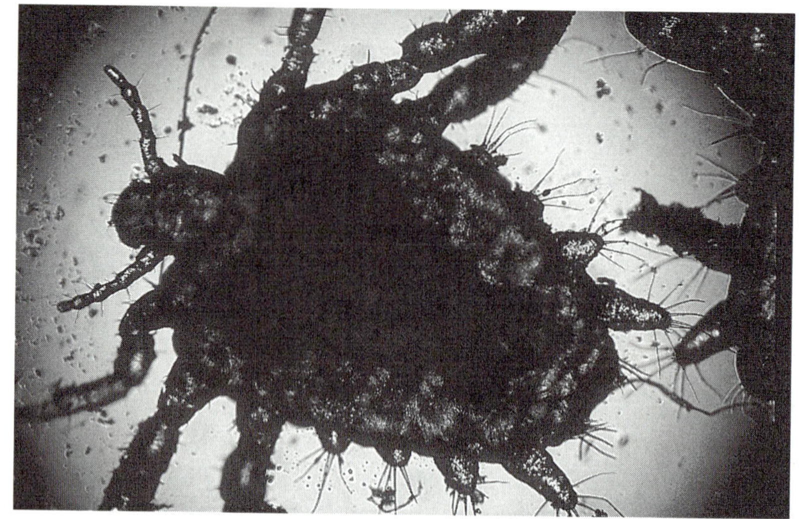

Fig. 15–13. *Phthirus pubis.*

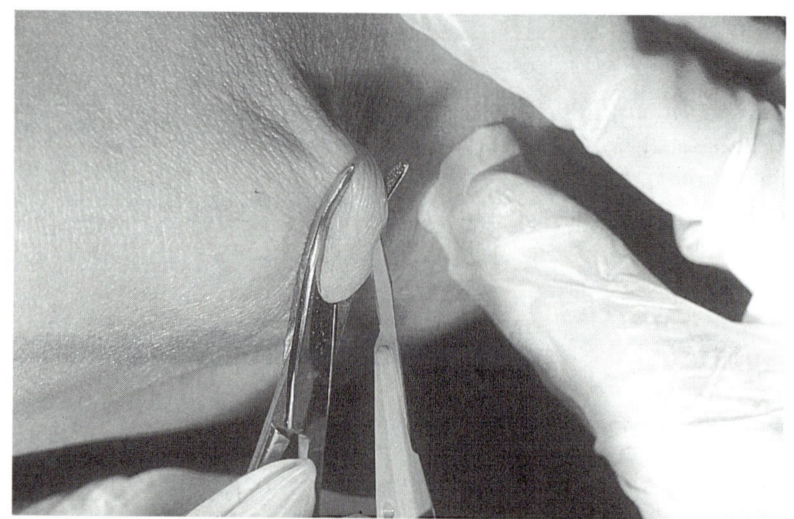

Fig. 15–14. Slit smear for leprosy.

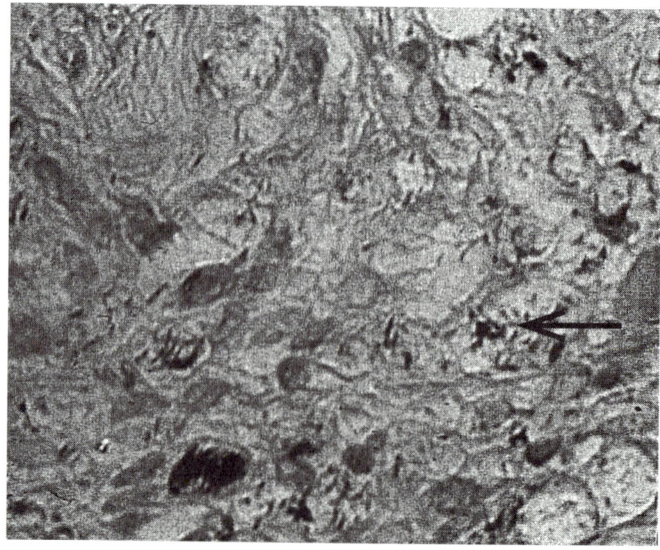

Fig. 15–15. *Mycobacterium leprae.*

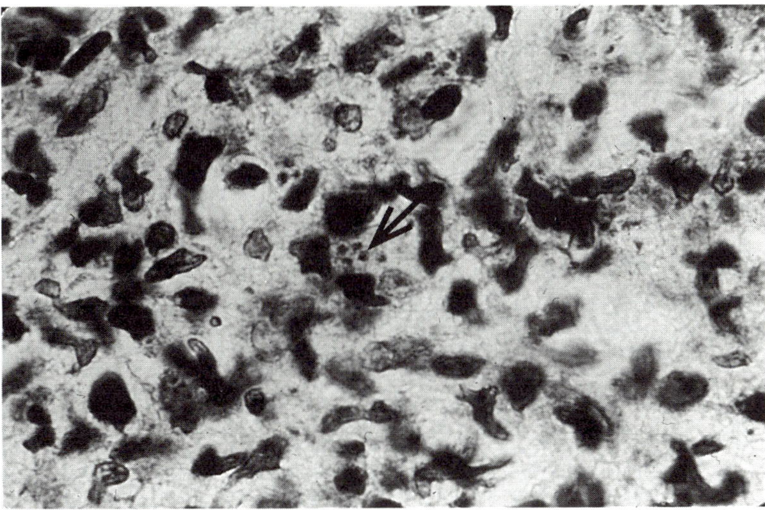

Fig. 15–16. Leishmaniasis.

Instructions

1. Pinch the skin very tightly between two fingers or with a clamp and make a superficial slit about 5 mm long and 3 mm deep with a rounded scalpel blade (Fig. 15–14).
2. Gently scrape the base and sides of the incision with the belly of the blade.
3. Smear the tissue pulp on a glass microscope slide.
4. Heat-fix and stain the tissue with Ziehl-Nielsen acid-fast stain.
5. Under oil immersion, examine for acid-fast bacilli, which appear as pink rods that are often clumped (Fig. 15–15).

TISSUE CRUSH FOR LEISHMANIASIS

Instructions

1. Take a punch biopsy of the lesion and cut a small piece longitudinally.
2. Send the larger skin piece for histopathologic examination. The crush preparation enables immediate diagnosis, but interpretation requires practice and experience and should be confirmed histopathologically.
3. Cut the epidermis from the smaller piece and then dissect away a portion of tissue about 1 mm^3 in size from the part of the dermis closest to the discarded epidermis. If a skin ulcer is present, tease out a piece of skin from the granulation tissue near the ulcer border instead.
4. Crush the tissue between two glass slides. Both slides will be smeared with the specimen.
5. Stain with Wright's stain and examine under the oil immersion objective of a microscope for large macrophages that contain organisms (Fig. 15–16).

In leishmaniasis the oval organisms have a dark nucleus and cytoplasmic vacuoles with dark-staining chromatin masses.[9]

TZANCK SMEAR

Herpes simplex or varicella-zoster virus infections are readily confirmed with this cytologic smear.[10]

CASE 15–4

A painful perianal ulcer developed in a 31-year-old man infected with HIV and has been enlarging for the last 4 weeks (Fig. 15–17). How can you establish the diagnosis?

Instructions

1. Scrape the sides of the ulcer. When blisters are present, one or more vesicles should be cleaned with alcohol and unroofed with a rounded scalpel blade or iris scissors. Scrape the inner portion of the blister roof and the blister base. Scraping is easier if the blister remains attached to the skin at a single point and is flipped over so that its inner portion faces up.
2. Smear the specimen on a microscope glass slide. If the inner surface is too difficult to scrape, gently smear the entire blister roof on the slide.
3. After air-drying, colorize the specimen with Wright, Giemsa, or Paragon multiple stains.
4. Examine under low-power magnification for multinucleated giant cells, which are huge cells that contain two or more large, hyperchromatic nuclei (Fig. 15–18). The presence of these cells establishes the diagnosis of herpetic infection. Multinucleated giant cells are more easily identified under the 40× magnification. Observation of acantholytic cells in a Tzanck smear from lesions of pemphigus vulgaris and mast cells in bullous mastocytosis may enable rapid diagnosis of these diseases. However, considerable experience is required and bullous skin diseases are better diagnosed by skin biopsy.

Comments

Although the diagnosis could have been eventually established with a skin biopsy or viral culture, only a Tzanck smear would have determined on the spot that the ulcer was caused by herpes infection.[11] The Tzanck smear is especially valuable in cases of suspected disseminated herpes simplex infection or varicella. However, the test cannot determine whether infection was caused by the herpes simplex or varicella-zoster virus. The presence of distinct crops of pruritic lesions at all stages of development and a lack of history of previous chicken pox would favor primary varicella, especially if the typical dermatomal distribution of herpes zoster or the characteristic appearance of grouped vesicles seen with herpes simplex is absent. Even when classic lesions are present, the diagnosis should be confirmed histologically with a Tzanck smear. Mucous membrane lesions, especially inside the mouth, are more common in varicella but may occur in any disseminated herpetic infection.

In immunocompromised patients with chicken pox, the blisters can be larger and hemorrhagic. Pneumonia, neurologic diseases, and gastrointestinal bleeding occur with greater frequency. Untreated, the mortality rate is as high as 71%.

Herpes Simplex and Varicella-Zoster Virus Cultures

Clean the surface of the vesicles with an antiseptic and rinse well with water. Cut and scrape the inner portion of the blister roof, or, if intact blisters are not present, scrape a nonimpetiginized erosion with a rounded scalpel blade and insert the spec-

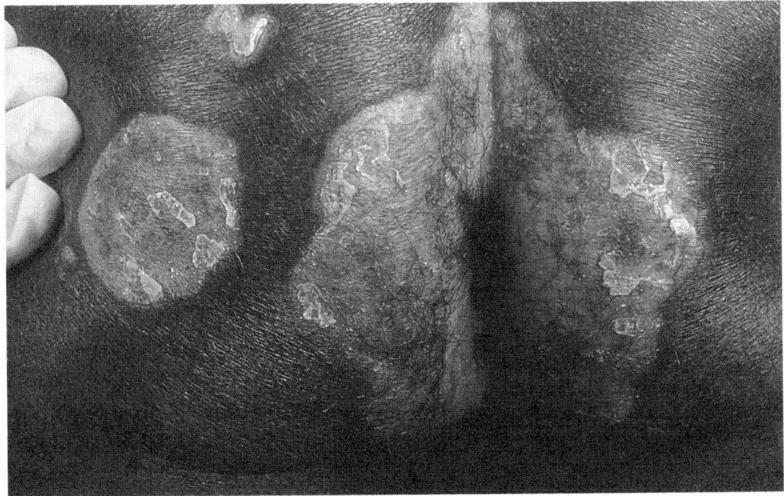

Fig. 15–17. Ulcerative perianal herpes.

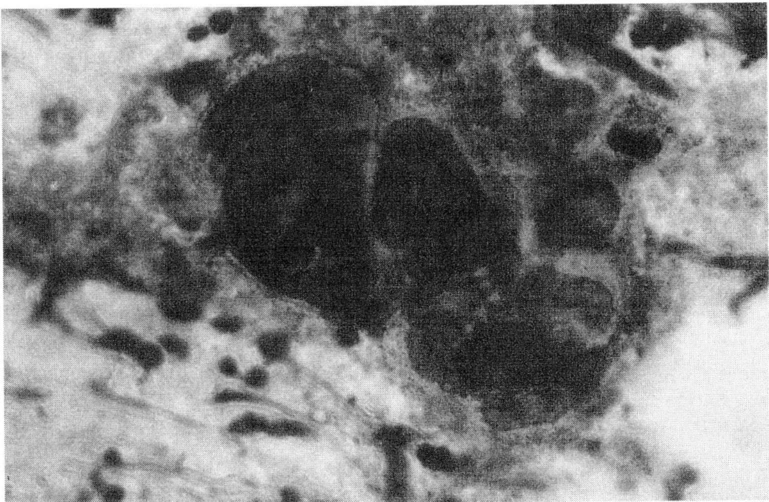

Fig. 15–18. Multinucleated giant cells.

imen into the liquid culture medium. The culture should be frozen if it cannot be rapidly transported to a laboratory.

WOOD'S LAMP EXAMINATION

Ultraviolet light with a wavelength of 365 nm emitted by a Wood's lamp facilitates the diagnosis of tinea, erythrasma, pigmentary disorders, and porphyria.[12]

CASE 15–5

Vesicles and erosions that healed with atrophic scars developed on the dorsa of the fingers, hands, face, and neck of a 31-year-old alcoholic man appearing older than his age. The skin of the hands is thickened, and hyperpigmented/hypopigmented patches and milia are noted on the involved areas of skin. The patient is otherwise in good health. How can the diagnosis be immediately confirmed?

Instructions

1. Collect a specimen of urine (about 5 mL) in a test tube.
2. Turn on the Wood's lamp and turn off the room light. The room should be completely dark, with doors, window shades, and curtains closed.
3. Hold the lamp 4 to 6 inches away from the urine sample, and note coral red fluorescence.

Comments

The patient has porphyria cutanea tarda (PCT). Although the clinical findings described are classic, more frequently patients have only some of these signs. The distribution of lesions on sun-exposed areas is characteristic. The diagnosis can be confirmed if Wood's light causes the urine to fluoresce red. The red fluorescence is due to the abnormal excretion of uroporphyrins. Normal urine fluoresces green. By acidifying the urine with hydrochloric acid or adding talc powder to the urine the sensitivity of this test is increased. In a random sample the test may be negative if the concentration of porphyrins in the urine is low, but most patients with active disease have total porphyrin urinary levels of 2 to 20 mg daily.

The test will also be positive in variegate porphyria. In PCT there is a hepatic deficiency of uroporphyrin decarboxylase, which in a 24-hour urine collection results in a uroporphyrin-to-coproporphyrin ratio of greater than 3. In variegate porphyria this ratio is less than 1.

Biopsy of a vesicle in PCT will show a subepidermal blister with irregular extensions of the dermal papillae into the blister cavity (festooning) and also characteristic pale, homogeneous, eosinophilic, periodic acid–Schiff (PAS)-positive, diastase-resistant material around the walls of superficial dermal vessels. Direct immunofluorescence can demonstrate IgG and sometimes IgM and complement within and around these vessels. Eruptions indistinguishable from PCT have been reported in patients receiving hemodialysis for renal failure; during ingestion of drugs, especially nalidixic acid, tetracycline, naproxen, and furosemide; and after exposure to chlorinated hydrocarbons such as hexachlorobenzene and dioxins.

Wood's light examination of skin and hair can be helpful in confirming the diagnosis of the following diseases.

Tinea Capitis

When invading scalp hairs, *Microsporum audouinii, M. canis, M. distortum,* and *M. ferrugineum* produce pigment that fluoresces bright yellow-green.[13] Hairs infected with *Trichophyton schoenleinii* fluoresce dull blue-white. Fluorescent lint is occasionally mistaken for fluorescent hairs but the lint can be shaken off. Fungi that cause "black dot" tinea capitis or that only invade the inner part of the hair follicle do not produce fluorescence. Fluorescence of hair is attributed to tryptophan metabolites.

Erythrasma

The scaly, erythematous, or pigmented patches and plaques of erythrasma are usually present on the groin, perianal area, toe webs, umbilicus, or axilla and are often confused with the lesions of fungal infection.[14] However, the disease is caused by the bacterium *Corynebacterium minutissimum,* which produces a porphyrin that fluoresces coral-red (Fig. 15–19). Since the substance is water soluble, the patient should not wash before the examination.

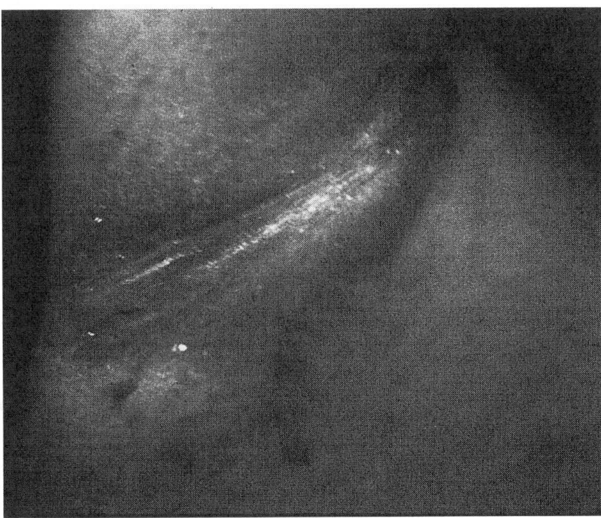

Fig. 15–19. Wood's lamp.

Pigmentary Disorders

Since melanin absorbs ultraviolet light, lesions with increased amounts of melanin in the upper layer of the skin, the epidermis, will become darker when irradiated with a Wood's lamp. However, since ultraviolet light does not penetrate deeply, the color of dermal hypermelanosis will not change perceptibly. This property helps to differentiate epidermal pigmentation, which responds to topical bleaching agents such as hydroquinone, from dermal pigmentation, which does not and requires laser treatment.

Areas with decreased melanin stand out against normal skin under Wood's light. This facilitates evaluation of the extent of vitiligo and the diagnosis of postinflammatory hypopigmentation, ash-leaf macules of tuberous sclerosis, indeterminate or tuberculoid Hansen's disease, albinism, and other diseases with hypopigmentation.

Pseudomonas aeruginosa Infection

This bacterium produces two pigments. Pyocyanin, a visible blue-green pigment, is quite noticeable in nail infections caused by this organism. Pyoverdin, which fluoresces bright aqua or yellow-green under Wood's light, facilitates the diagnosis of *Pseudomonas*-infected ulcers, erosions, and burns.

Tinea Versicolor

This dermatophytosis produces pink, tan, or hypopigmented patches with fine scales usually on the back and chest (Fig. 15–20). The diagnosis can be confirmed when the lesions fluoresce a golden-yellow color. However, this test should not substitute for microscopic potassium hydroxide examination; lesions in this disease are so loaded with the hyphae and spores of *Malassezia furfur* that the term "spaghetti and meatballs" is widely used to describe these structures under the microscope (Fig. 15–21).

Scabies

The diagnosis of scabies can be facilitated by painting the skin with a solution of fluorescein dye in glycerin and alcohol and then washing it off with water. This commercially available preparation penetrates the burrows, which under examination with Wood's light fluoresce a gray-white color, thereby increasing the chances of finding lesions with mites.

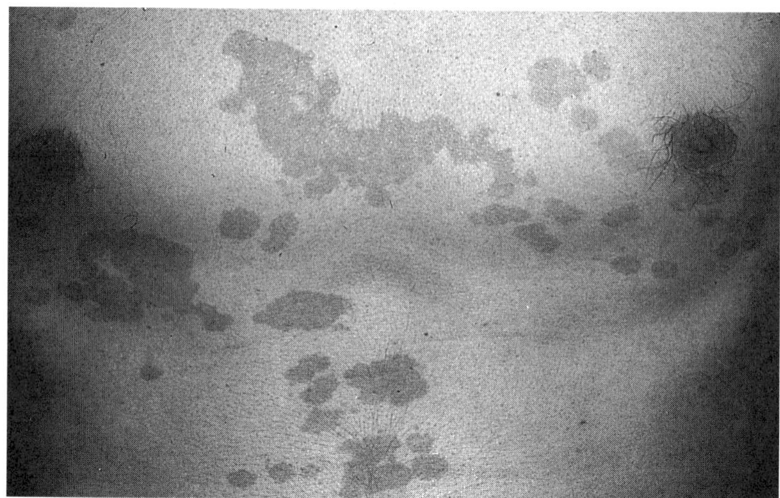

Fig. 15–20. Tinea versicolor: fine scales on chest.

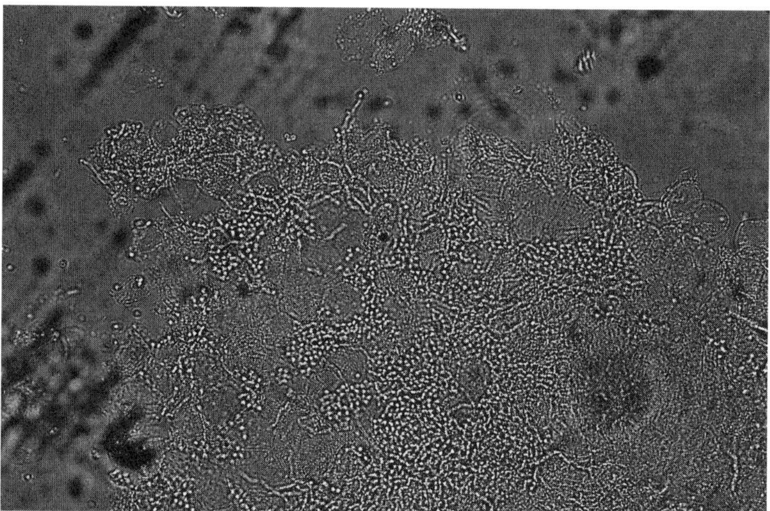

Fig. 15–21. Tinea versicolor: hyphae and spores.

Tetracycline Fluorescent Reaction

A patient treated with tetracycline derivatives for inflammatory acne may note yellow fluorescence of the lesions and nails while in an establishment with ultraviolet lighting such as a dancing club. Examination of the patient with a Wood's lamp confirms the finding, which can frighten the patient but only requires reassurance (Table 15–1).

PART II: SKIN TESTS

THE TUBERCULIN INTRADERMAL (MANTOUX) TEST

The tuberculin skin test involves a delayed hypersensitivity reaction that characteristically develops within 48 to 72 hours of injection of tuberculin protein in patients previously infected with *Mycobacterium tuberculosis*. Sensitivity to the test develops 2 to 10 weeks after the initial infection. Although false negative reactions have

Table 15–1. Fluorescent Reactions

Pathologic Process	Fluorescence
Infectious	
Erythrasma	Coral red
Tinea capitis	Yellow to pale green
Tinea versicolor	Golden yellow
Pseudomonas aeruginosa	Aqua, pale green
Noninfectious	
Hyperpigmentation	Dark brown
Hypopigmentation	Light tan or white
Depigmentation	White
Porphyria cutanea tarda	Pink to red (urine)

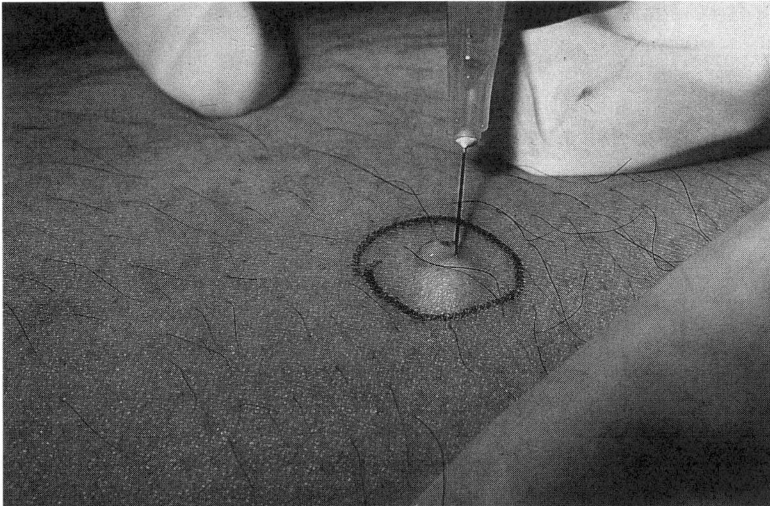

Fig. 15–22. Mantoux test for purified protein derivative.

been reported in up to 20% of patients with active tuberculosis, the tuberculin test remains the best diagnostic method for demonstrating infection with *M. tuberculosis.*[15] In order to obtain clinically reliable information, the test must be carefully administered and correctly interpreted. Multiple-puncture (tine) tests are still sometimes used for large-group screening, but positive results need to be confirmed with a Mantoux test (Fig. 15–22).

Instructions

1. Choose an area of normal skin on the volar surface of the forearm away from veins or cutaneous lesions.
2. Clean the skin with an alcohol wipe and allow a few seconds for the alcohol to evaporate.
3. Stretch down the skin to be injected with the thumb of the free hand.
4. Use a tuberculin syringe with a ¼- to ½-in, 27-gauge needle.
5. With the needle bevel directed upward, insert the tip of the needle just beneath the surface of the skin and inject 0.10 mL (5 tuberculin units [TU]) of purified protein derivative (PPD). Care must be taken to insert the needle superficially so that a 6- to 10-mm, discrete, pale elevation is produced.
6. Reexamine and palpate the area between 48 and 72 hours after placing the PPD

to determine induration. It is helpful to delineate the borders of the indurated area with ink (ball point pen).

7. Measure the area of induration transversely to the long axis of the forearm.

Interpretation of the Mantoux Test with 5-TU Tuberculin (PPD)

1. A reaction 15 mm or larger is classified as positive in
   a. Persons older than 35 years of age
   b. Persons previously vaccinated with bacille Calmette-Guérin (BCG) extract. The mean reaction of the Mantoux test is often less than 10 mm and wanes with time after BCG inoculation, so large skin reactions are considered indicative of infection with *M. tuberculosis.*
2. Reaction 10 mm or larger is considered to be positive in
   a. Intravenous drug users
   b. Residents of institutions (nursing homes, chronic care hospitals, prisons)
   c. Patients with diseases or conditions that increase the risk of developing tuberculosis, such as diabetes mellitus, immunosuppressive or corticosteroids therapy, hematologic and other malignancies, chronic renal failure, gastrectomy, jejunoileal bypass, and excessive weight loss
   d. All persons younger than 35 years of age with previously negative reactions
3. Reaction 5 mm or larger is considered to be positive in
   a. HIV-infected persons
   b. Persons at risk for HIV infection but unknown HIV serology
   c. Recent contact with infectious tuberculosis
   d. Persons with old healed tuberculosis in chest radiographs

ANERGY TESTING

Intradermal injection of a panel of standardized concentrations of antigens to which humans are often exposed evaluates a person's ability to mount an intact delayed hypersensitivity response. This is therefore a test of cell-mediated immunity.[16]

Table 15–2. Antigen Reactions

Antigen (Concentration)	Reaction Rate in Nonhospitalized Adults (%)
Candida (1:100 to 1:1000 wt/vol)	90
Tetanus (1:5 to 1:10 Lf/mL)	50-100
Mumps (standardized to 40 colony-forming units/mL)	65
Trichophyton (1:100 to 1:1000 wt/vol)	40
PPD* (5 to 250 tuberculin units)	30

**PPD,* purified protein derivative.

Instructions

1. With the technique previously explained for the placement of a PPD test, inject 0.10 mL each of *Candida,* tetanus, mumps, *Trichophyton,* and PPD antigens (Table 15–2) into a separate area of skin in the volar surface of the forearm.

2. A positive test response is classified as a 5- to 10-mm area of induration present 48 to 72 hours after injection of the antigen. Over 90% of patients should react to one or more antigens (see Table 15–2).

Reactivity is fairly consistent until 60 years of age, but then decreases appreciably to all antigens except PPD. In the absence of malnutrition, immunosuppressive therapy, advanced age, or obvious symptoms of a particular disease, lack of reactivity to an anergy panel should prompt evaluation for HIV infection, lymphoproliferative disorders, sarcoid and other granulomatous diseases, occult mycobacterial infection, lymphopenic states, and autoimmune diseases.

PATCH TEST

Patch testing is used to determine the cause of allergic contact dermatitis. Although the test is fairly simple to perform, experience in interpretation of the reactions is required. The allergen must be standardized as to concentration and vehicle in order to increase the number of positive allergy test reactions but reduce the frequency of irritant reactions due to inappropriately high concentrations.[17]

A tray with the 20 more commonly implicated antigens is available from Hermal Pharmaceutical Laboratories, Inc., in Delmar, New York (1-800-Hermal-1). More specialized trays (antimicrobials/preservatives, dental medicaments, organic dyes, perfumes, plastics, rubber, chemicals, photoallergens, pesticides, sunscreens, and plants) can be purchased from Ommiderm, Inc., Montreal, Canada (514-340-1114).

Do not test when there is active acute or severe contact dermatitis because the eruption can worsen or the other patches tested can become positive and lead to diffuse redness throughout the entire body area tested (angry back syndrome). Avoid testing patients for at least 1 week after discontinuation of systemic and topical corticosteroids to the body area on which the patches are applied.

Instructions

1. The area selected should be free of lesions. Hairs, if present, should be clipped. The back is the preferred location for patch testing.
2. Place the strip of Finn chambers on a table and apply about 0.5 mm of petrolatum-based allergen from a syringe into each chamber. For antigens in solution, place a filter paper disk in the chamber and apply one drop of solution on top.
3. Apply the Finn chamber strip to the upper part of the back or another body area and secure with Scanpor tape. If this equipment is not available, an amount of antigen to cover 1.0 cm^2 of skin surface is placed on a plastic adhesive strip, which is then applied to the skin and secured with occlusive tape.
4. With a marking pen write the number corresponding to each allergen on the skin next to the test area so that after the patches are removed, the site of each allergen is identified.
5. Instruct the patient not to shower or perform any exercise or work that will wet and loosen the patches.
6. Remove the patches in 48 hours.
7. Examine the skin after waiting 30 minutes in order to avoid pressure artifacts (Fig. 15–23).
8. Interpret according to the appearance of the patch (Table 15–3).
9. Evaluate the patient again 48 hours later since some allergens such as neomycin and organic dyes may not produce a reaction for 3 to 4 days after the patches are applied.

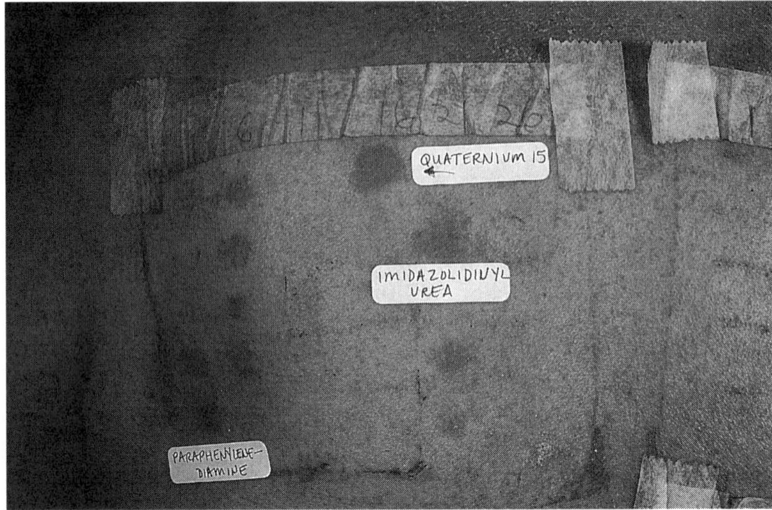

Fig. 15–23. Patch test.

Table 15–3. Patch Test Reactions

Reaction	Clinical Appearance	Allergy
Weak	Shiny, wet erythema, infiltration	+
Strong	Erythema with edema or vesicles	++
Extreme	Erythema spreads beyond the patch, bullae, erosions	+++
Indeterminate	Macular erythema	±
Irritant	Glazed or burned appearance, pustules, purpura, ulcer	−
Negative	Normal skin	−

False-negative responses are produced by low concentrations of the antigen, improper testing technique, early evaluation of the patches, low degree of sensitivity in the patient, a refractory allergic phase, or recent corticosteroid therapy. False-positive responses are due to prolonged patch testing, high concentration of the antigen, contamination of the allergen, use of an irritant substance to clean the location before the patch is applied, or testing on irritated skin.

Never test an unknown chemical. The substance could be extremely toxic to the skin. Cosmetic and personal care products can be applied to the skin directly. Soap and shampoos need to be dissolved 1:10 to 1:100 in water. Reference works such as Marks's *Contact and Occupational Dermatology* or Fisher's *Contact Dermatitis* should be consulted to determine appropriate concentrations of other substances.

Taping a piece of latex glove directly to the skin is not a specific test for latex hypersensitivity and can be dangerous in patients with latex contact urticaria. Patients suspected of being allergic to latex products should be patch-tested with the rubber chemicals included in the tray of common allergens.

SUMMARY

Patients with skin disease often seek treatment in emergency departments. When the cause of a skin disease is not obvious from visual inspection alone, a simple test can establish the diagnosis so that immediate and appropriate treatment can be initiated. Expertise in execution of the tests described in this chapter is essential for the emergency physician who evaluates and treats cutaneous disease. Similarly, familiarity with the techniques, capabilities, and limitations of skin testing will be of enormous benefit to the emergency physician in *initiating* a diagnostic evaluation. The resurgence of tuberculosis, particularly in immunocompromised patients, makes it extremely important for all emergency physicians to be knowledgeable in the proper techniques of performing a PPD test as well as the new guidelines for interpreting the results.

REFERENCES

1. Goldstein BG, Goldstein AO: *Practical dermatology*, St Louis, Mosby, 1992.
2. Epstein WL: Molluscum contagiosum, *Semin Dermatol* 11:184–189, 1992.
3. Brodell RT, Helms SE, Snelson ME: Office dermatologic testing: the KOH preparation, *Am Fam Physician* 43:2061–2065, 1991.
4. Rockoff AS: Fungus cultures in a pediatric outpatient clinic, *Pediatrics* 63:276–278, 1979.
5. Palicka P, Malis L, Samsinak K, et al: Laboratory diagnosis of scabies, *J Hyg Epidermiol Microbiol Immunol* 24:63–70, 1980.
6. Buntin DM, Roser T, Lesher JL, et al: Sexually transmitted diseases: viruses and ectoparasites, *J Am Acad Dermatol* 25:275–534, 1991.
7. Billstein S: Diagnosis and treatment of lice, J Sch Health 1977; 47:356–357.
8. Odinsen O, Nilson T, Humber DP: Viability of *Mycobacterium leprae:* a comparison of morphological index and fluorescent staining techniques in slit-skin smears and *M. leprae* suspensions, *Int J Lepr Other Mycobact Dis* 54:403–408, 1986.
9. Mengistu G, Akuffo H, Fehniger TE, et al: Comparison of parasitological and immunological methods in the diagnosis of leishmaniasis in Ethiopia, *Trans R Soc Trop Med Hyg* 86:154–157, 1992.
10. Oranje AP, Folkers E: The Tzanck smear: old, but still of inestimable value, *Pediatr Dermatol* 5:127–129, 1988.
11. Nahass GT, Goldstein BA, Zhu WY et al: Comparison of Tzanck smear, viral culture, and DNA diagnostic methods in detection of herpes simplex and varicella-zoster infection, *JAMA* 268:2541–2544, 1992.
12. Pariser DM, Caserio RJ, Eaglstein WH, editors: *Techniques for diagnosis skin and hair disease*, ed 2, New York, 1986, Thieme.
13. Prevost E: The rise and fall of fluorescent tinea capitis, *Pediatr Dermatol* 1:127–133, 1983.
14. Schlappner OL, Rosenblum GA, Rowden G, Phillips TM: Concomitant erythrasma and dermatophytosis of the groin, *Br J Dermatol* 100:147–151, 1979.
15. Neill MA, Mates S: Screening for tuberculosis: everything you already knew, probably forgot and meant to look up. *R I Med* 75:453–456, 1992.
16. Centers for Disease Control: Purified protein derivatives (PPD)—tuberculin anergy and HIV infection: guidelines for anergy testing and management of anergic persons at risk of tuberculosis, *MMWR* 40:27–32, 1991.
17. Marks JG, DeLeo VA, editors: *Contact and occupational dermatology*, St Louis, 1992, Mosby.

PART IV

Special Situations

Chapter 16

Evaluating Body Fluids

Theodore I. Benzer, M.D.
Katherine Leonard, M.D.
Frank Raymond, M.D.

The sampling and analysis of various body fluids is central to the evaluation of many patients in the emergency department (ED). Especially when infection is suspected, it is essential to obtain appropriate fluid samples to establish the correct diagnosis or identify a particular organism. Frequently, treatment can be instituted only after the diagnosis has been made by appropriate fluid analysis. This chapter reviews the tests that may be performed on fluid samples from the spinal canal, the pleural space, the peritoneal space, the vaginal cul-de-sac, and the joint space. The tests that can be obtained and/or performed by the physician in the ED are described in detail. Indications, contraindications, and complications associated with the procedures required to obtain the samples are reviewed; and the specificity, sensitivity, and diagnostic accuracy of the subsequent tests are discussed.

CEREBROSPINAL FLUID (LUMBAR PUNCTURE)

CASE 16–1

After attending a New Year's Eve party, a 14-year-old male came to the ED because he felt "disoriented." The triage nurse noted that the patient had alcohol on his breath. The patient was awake but stated that he felt "weak." Initial vital signs were as follows: systolic blood pressure by palpation, 70 mm Hg; pulse, 120/min; respirations, 40/min; temperature, 101.9°F. The patient was given high-concentration oxygen, IV access was obtained, and cardiac monitoring was initiated. Physical examination revealed a scant, generalized petechial rash with discrete areas of purpura. Neither nuchal rigidity nor focal neurologic deficits were present.

CASE 16–2

A two-week-old male infant was brought to the ED because of poor feeding and irritability. Past medical history was significant for a prenatal diagnosis of hydronephrosis and ureteropelvic junction (UPJ) obstruction. The patient had been taking amoxicillin until 2 days prior to the ED visit. Vital signs were as follows: temperature, 98.8°F; blood pressure, 78/50 mm Hg; pulse, 140 beats/min; respirations, 36/min. The patient appeared clinically well to the examiner, with no apparent abnormalities on physical exam.

A technique originating over 100 years ago, lumbar puncture (LP) is the procedure used by physicians to diagnose suspected bacterial or viral meningitis. It may also establish the diagnosis of subarachnoid hemorrhage. Although with increased availability the use of computed tomography (CT) and magnetic resonance imaging (MRI) has replaced LP as the initial diagnostic procedure in some clinical situations, LP remains an important diagnostic tool for a number of other neurologic entities including Guillain-Barré syndrome (GBS), multiple sclerosis, and other demyelination syndromes. This chapter examines the indications and contraindications for LP and, most importantly, the interpretation of the results of cerebrospinal fluid (CSF) testing.

Technique for Performing LP

Informed consent from the patient or guardian prior to performing LP is always desirable. However, most indications for LP constitute medical emergencies, and under these circumstances LP may be performed without formal consent if necessary. Alternatively, if an LP is not permitted, the patient may be treated empirically with antibiotics for suspected bacterial meningitis. In either case, the nature of the emergency situation as well as the need for immediate intervention should be meticulously documented in the patient's chart.

The technique for performing LP is well described in Roberts and Hedges.[1] However, two issues should be examined: First, the use of local anesthetic. Infiltration of the skin and subcutaneous tissue at the puncture site with lidocaine 0.5 to 1.0% (without epinephrine) has been the standard local anesthetic used in all age groups *except neonates.* However, Pinheiro et al.[2] have recently suggested that administering local anesthetic to neonates decreases their movement, which may be helpful in performing an LP. Although use of an emulsion of lidocaine and prilocaine, that is, a eutectic mixture of local anesthetics (EMLA), has been shown to be efficacious in children,[3] its delayed onset of action (>45 minutes) may limit its use in emergency situations. The second issue is position. Although placing the patient in the lateral recumbent position is standard practice and is the only reliable position for obtaining an opening CSF pressure reading, the *sitting* position or modified lateral decubitus position, with neck extended, may be preferable in neonates and young infants in an attempt to avoid airway obstruction and subsequent hypoxia.[4,5]

Infants and Children

LP is indicated for a child who has seizures and fever when the possibility of intracranial infection exits. The incidence of meningitis in children presenting with fever and seizures ranges from 1 to 5%.[6–8] Clinical findings consistent with meningitis may be subtle in children less than 18 months of age. LP is almost always indicated in patients with fever accompanied by seizures that are not easily classified as simple febrile seizures. Simple febrile seizures occur in the 6-month to 6-year age group and are characteristically nonfocal, self-limited, less than 15 minutes' duration, and accompanied by fever.

The diagnostic value of routine LP in children with orbital and periorbital cellulitis has recently been reviewed.[9] The study demonstrated that routine use of LP in these patients does not result in a higher incidence of diagnosing otherwise unsuspected meningitis. Thus, the need for the procedure in this setting should be individualized. Children with orbital and periorbital cellulitis due to *Hemophilus influenzae* type B appear to be at the highest risk for meningitis.

Bacteremia documented by positive blood cultures obtained during a recent ED visit warrants patient recall for LP unless the bacteremia is due to *Streptococcus pneumoniae* and the child is afebrile and well at the time of recall.

Fever and petechiae may indicate meningococcemia or other serious bacterial diseases *(H. influenza)*. Severity of disease from meningococcal infection ranges from bacteremia to sepsis with or without meningitis. LP results may provide prognostic as well as diagnostic information in meningococcemia; that is, meningococcemia in the absence of CSF pleocytosis (among other factors[10]) has been associated with poor outcome. Patients with significant thrombocytopenia (<50,000/mm^3) or a bleeding diathesis should be treated adequately for these problems and, if necessary, started on antibiotics empirically, before LP.

CASE 16–1 CONTINUED

Intravenous ceftriaxone was immediately initiated for the 14-year-old from the party. CBC revealed a platelet count of 52,000/mm^3; prothrombin time, 16.4/12.1 sec (control); partial thromboplastin time, 34.9/25.8 sec (control). Fresh frozen plasma (FFP) and a platelet transfusion were initiated. LP was performed only after correction of the thrombocytopenia and bleeding diathesis.

LP revealed the following: protein, 24 mg/dL, glucose, 74 mg/dL; simutaneously obtained serum glucose: 222 mg/dL. The CSF was opalescent and microscopic exam revealed: 27 WBCs; 50% polymorphonuclear (PMN) leukocytes. No organisms were noted on Gram stain, but *Neisseria meningitidis* was recovered from blood cultures on the following hospital day. The patient was treated with parenteral antibiotics and recovered uneventfully.

Comment.—Fortunately, this patient was managed appropriately and efficiently. Failure to examine the skin carefully, or attributing this patient's altered sensorium to alcohol use, could have delayed prompt diagnosis and treatment, possibly with catastrophic consequences.

Indications for Lumbar Puncture

Indications for LP depend on the patient's age, state of immunity, and overall clinical picture, although in all age groups, the most common indication is suspected meningitis.

A febrile pediatric patient of any age who appears toxic warrants an LP as part of a sepsis evaluation. The correct approach for infants who present with serious bacterial infections but with either no fever or with hypothermia may be problematic.

In neonates, LP is indicated as part of the evaluation for suspected sepsis. Despite the low risk of bacterial meningitis in well-appearing infants in this age group, most sources concur that all febrile (rectal temperature >100.5 F) infants less than 28 days of age warrant a complete sepsis evaluation, including LP, regardless of clinical and laboratory findings.[11]

CASE 16–2 CONTINUED

While awaiting disposition, this infant had a brief apneic episode. After the infant's breathing stabilized, a full sepsis evaluation was performed. LP revealed the following: purulent CSF; glucose, 10 mg/dL; protein, 250 mg/dL. Microscopic examination revealed 270 WBCs with 90% PMNs; numerous gram-negative rods were evident on Gram stain. CBC revealed a WBC of 12,700/mm^3 and a serum glucose of 60 mg/dL.

Antibiotics appropriate for suspected neonatal sepsis were initiated. Later *Escherichia coli* was recovered from initial cultures of the blood, CSF, and urine of this patient.

Comment.—This somewhat atypical case illustrates the subtle presentation of inadequately treated meningitis in a neonate. Neither fever nor the classic signs of meningitis were present on physical exam. The history of urinary tract abnormalities and prior antibiotic use coupled with a complaint of poor feeding and irritability warranted the sepsis evaluation even in the absence of fever.

A commonly encountered problem in pediatric patients is significant fever, >39°C, with no obvious source on physical examination. Patients are usually classified as "low risk" or "high risk" for bacterial sepsis based on WBC count (less than or greater than 15,000); urinalysis (positive or negative); character of stool (WBCs, blood, or mucus); and most important, the overall clinical picture.[11]

For young infants (30 to 90 days of age) with high fever and no obvious source on physical examination and who are judged to be at low risk for bacterial sepsis, LP should be performed prior to discharging the patient from the ED on outpatient antibiotic therapy. An LP in this situation helps preclude the possibility of inadequately treating meningitis.

For older infants and children (3 months to 36 months of age) with high fever and no obvious source, the decision to perform an LP should be based on the risk to the individual patient, taking into account the WBC count and clinical picture.

Adolescents and Adults

As in the pediatric patient, the most common indication for LP in adult and adolescent patients is suspected meningitis. LP is also helpful in establishing the diagnosis of demyelination syndromes such as multiple sclerosis (MS). A diagnosis of subarachnoid hemorrhage may be established by LP when CT scan is negative, equivocal, or unobtainable in a patient with a history and physical examination consistent with subarachnoid hemorrhage. A febrile adult patient with altered mentation and/or seizures may warrant LP following stabilization (including antibiotics) and CT scanning. *Therapeutic* indications for LP include treatment of pseudotumor cerebri and administration of intrathecal antibiotics and chemotherapy.

Risks, Complications, and Contraindications

A properly performed LP is considered a relatively safe procedure, with a serious complication rate that is probably less than 2%.[12]

Headache is the most common complication in adults and may occur in up to 25% of patients. Headache is rarely reported in children, although it may occur in this patient population as well. Post-LP headache is believed to be due to meningeal traction caused by decreased CSF volume.

Theoretically, patients with bacteremia or sepsis have an increased risk of developing meningitis as a *consequence* of lumbar puncture. However, no significant support for this possibility has been established.[13, 14] Other reported complications of LP include: backache, spinal epidural and subdural hemorrhages, intervertebral disc injury, vertebral body injury, radicular symptoms, and paresis. A late complication of LP is an epidermoid tumor, believed to result from an epidermal plug introduced into the subdural space as the result of using a nonstyletted needle.

Significant respiratory compromise can occur during LP particularly in acutely or chronically ill infants, as a result of airway compromise and other factors (see previous section). Hypoxemia during LP has been demonstrated in infants breathing room air compared to infants pretreated with oxygen.[15]

The most serious complication of LP is central or tonsillar herniation accompanied by neurologic deterioration. The actual incidence is probably less than 1%, but with a *reported* range of up to 12%.[12] Increased intracranial pressure may occur as a result of a space-occupying lesion as well as from acute bacterial meningitis. Children with acute bacterial meningitis may have significant elevations in CSF opening pressure.[16] Alternative diagnostic studies performed prior to LP do not always prevent this complication. In some instances, herniation following LP has occurred after a CT scan was obtained and interpreted as normal.[17] Both impending central and tonsillar herniation may cause neck rigidity that is clinically indistinguishable from the neck rigidity interpreted as a sign of meningitis.

A CT scan should be obtained (and if appropriate, antibiotics started prior to both CT and LP) in all patients who have significant changes in mental status, focal neurologic deficits, papilledema, head trauma, and in whom a space-occupying or other intracranial lesion is suspected. Papilledema may take 12 to 24 hours to evolve in the patient with an acute increase in intracranial pressure, and thus its absence does not imply lack of risk. If an LP *must* be performed even though intracranial hypertension is suspected, the incidence of complications may be avoided or diminished by using a small-gauge needle (no. 22) and withdrawing the smallest volume of fluid (1 mL) necessary. Half of a 1 mL specimen can be used for culture and the other half for an estimated cell count, followed by a Gram stain. This technique however, cannot be safely relied upon and other alternatives to LP should be carefully considered.

Other relative contraindications to LP include: platelet counts less than 50,000/mm^3, and abnormal coagulation profiles secondary to anticoagulation therapy or disseminated intravascular coagulation. These patients are at increased risk for spinal epidural hematoma, and LP should be deferred until bleeding diathesis is corrected. As mentioned, the patient should be treated empirically with antibiotics if necessary, while a correctable bleeding problem is treated. In stroke patients who require anticoagulation, the start of such therapy should be deferred 4 to 6 hours if possible after LP to prevent localized bleeding.

Skin infection overlying the site is an *absolute* contraindication to LP since organisms may be introduced by the spinal needle into the subarachnoid space. A lateral cervical or cisternal puncture utilizing fluoroscopic technique may be performed by appropriately trained personnel as a safe alternative to LP.

As previously stated, opening CSF pressure is reliably obtained only when the patient is in the lateral recumbent position. Normal initial pressures in infants, children, and adults range from 50 to 195 mmH_2O. In neonates, the range is from 80 to 110 mmH_2O. For pediatric patients, there is a method for estimating CSF opening pressure based on needle size, patient temperature, and the number of drops of CSF per second.[18]

Collection of Fluid

Three one-mL tubes of CSF should be collected for culture, chemistries, and cell count, respectively. A fourth tube may be useful for additional studies, such as viral studies and countercurrent immunoelectrophoresis (CIE) as dictated by clinical circumstances. CIE and latex particle agglutination can rapidly detect bacterial antigens in CSF and other body fluids, including antigens from those bacteria most commonly responsible for bacterial meningitis, such as *E. coli, H. influenza* type B, *S. pneumoniae,* group B streptococci, and *N. meningitidis.*

Cerebrospinal Fluid Analysis and Interpretation

Color

Normal CSF is colorless. A cloudy appearance, or turbidity, may signify the presence in the CSF of leukocytes (WBCs) ($>200/mm^3$), red blood cells (RBCs), ($>400/mm^3$), or significant concentrations of microorganisms.

A yellowish discoloration of the supernatant of a centrifuged CSF sample is referred to as *xanthochromia* and is most easily appreciated by holding the sample against a white background. True xanthochromia results from products of hemoglobin degradation, and occurs when erythrocytes have been present in the subarachnoid space for a minimum of 4 hours. Xanthochromia is most commonly seen in patients with subarachnoid hemorrhage, but may also occur in patients who have had previous "traumatic spinal taps." A yellowish discoloration of CSF (not xanthochromia) may also be seen in jaundiced patients, including neonates and premature infants; in patients who have systemic carotenemia; and in patients taking rifampin.

Cell Count and Differential

Normal CSF cell count is less than 5 WBCs/mm^3, of which 0% should be PMN leukocytes. Slightly higher absolute counts and a variation in the differential count may be seen in premature and term infants (mean 8 to 9 WBCs) and infants less than 1 month of age (up to 7 WBCs). Elevated CSF leukocyte counts are seen in all types of meningitis, as well as meningoencephalitis, neurosyphilis, meningeal carcinomatosis, brain abscess, and in some patients with seizures and fever but no other evidence of an intracranial infection.

Total (CSF) WBC count, and Differential

The differential white blood cell count may be helpful in distinguishing between bacterial and viral meningitis, a commonly encountered clinical dilemma. CSF leukocytosis in bacterial meningitis generally exceeds that seen in viral and other types of meningitis. Also, in bacterial meningitis, a predominance of PMN leukocytes prevails. Typical WBC counts in acute bacterial meningitis may exceed 1,000 WBCs/mm^3. In viral meningitis, CSF WBC counts are typically lower (hundreds/mm^3), and predominantly lymphocytic, although PMN leukocytes may predominate in early viral meningitis. Because of the significant overlap in total number and types of WBCs, it may be impossible to differentiate viral from bacterial meningitis based on cell count and differential alone. CSF glucose serum ratios and Gram staining used concomitantly may be helpful. When properly performed on a centrifuged specimen of CSF, Gram staining demonstrates a causative organism in 60 to 90% of patients with bacterial meningitis. False positive Gram stains may result from bacterial contamination of Gram stain reagents.

CSF Protein

Normal CSF protein concentrations obtained from LP range from 15 to 40 mg/dL. Normal neonates may have CSF protein elevations to 150 mg/dL, and infants less than 6 months of age may have CSF proteins as high as 60 mg/dL.

True elevations of CSF protein occur with all types of meningitis, neurosyphilis, late polyneuritis, intracranial or intraspinal bleeding, and demyelination syndromes; CSF protein elevation is thus a nonspecific finding. After a "traumatic LP," a 1 mg/dL elevation of protein per 700 RBCs may be seen.

CSF Glucose

Hypoglycorrhachia exists when the CSF glucose value is less than 60% of the simultaneously obtained serum value in euglycemic patients, and less than 40% of serum glucose in hyperglycemic patients. Abnormally low CSF glucose may result from altered glucose transport mechanisms in bacterial, fungal, and tuberculous meningitis.

India Ink Staining

India ink staining of CSF detects less than 30% of cases of cryptococcal meningitis on initial LP. Latex agglutination techniques for identification of cryptococcal antigen has a sensitivity up to 90%; serum cryptococcal antigen is helpful in suspected cases.

CSF Lactate Levels

The role of CSF lactate measurement in the diagnosis and management of meningitis had first been investigated over a decade ago.[19, 20] Increases in CSF lactate tend to parallel increases in CSF granulocyte counts. However, differentiating various types of meningitis by this means has not yet proven clinically useful. CSF lactate may be increased (>3 mmol/L) in tuberculous, bacterial, and partially treated bacterial meningitis.[21,22]

Other Tests

Myelin basic protein in CSF may be elevated during active periods of MS. CSF electrophoresis may demonstrate oligoclonal banding in up to 80% of patients suspected of having MS.

Low *CSF chloride* concentrations may support the diagnosis of tuberculous meningitis, if other clinical and laboratory data are consistent with this diagnosis. Acid-fast staining requires relatively large amounts of CSF (centrifuged to form a pellet, if possible) and may not reveal mycobacterial organisms in any case.

Methods for detecting bacterial antigens in CSF, such as CIE, *latex agglutination, and enzyme-linked immunosorbent assays (ELISA)*, are highly specific and useful in cases of inadequately treated meningitis where CSF cultures may be negative.

A positive *CSF VDRL*, when used in conjunction with the clinical presentation and serum treponemal testing, supports a diagnosis of neurosyphilis. Cytologic examination of CSF may be indicated for suspected central nervous system malignancy, although imaging techniques have replaced this procedure in most cases.

Common Difficulties in CSF Interpretation

Most difficulties in interpreting CSF results are related to traumatic LP, pretreatment with antibiotics, and (in children) fever and seizures.

Up to 20% of LPs are classified as traumatic. Traumatic LP precludes an accurate cell count necessary to diagnose meningitis and intracranial or spinal hemorrhage. Methods used to help differentiate traumatic from nontraumatic taps include the following:

1. Clinical observations during the procedure: CSF from traumatic LPs often clears visibly between the first and last tubes; cell counts should be performed on each tube. A failure to clear, is an inconclusive finding and cannot be used to exclude traumatic LP. A thin streak of blood may be observed flowing from the hub of the stylet in traumatic punctures and should be noted. The "ring sign" (peripheral concentric clearing of a drop of bloody fluid on a white sterile drape) suggests CSF admixed with blood from a traumatic tap.[23] Xanthochromia denotes bleeding into the CSF that has occurred from 4 hours to 10 days before the procedure. In contrast, when bloody CSF from a traumatic LP is centrifuged, the supernatant should be clear. Also, clotting of blood may be noted in traumatic LPs.

2. When the peripheral leukocyte and erythrocyte counts are normal, the ratio of RBCS to WBCs in traumatic LP is 700:1. The classic equation to correct for the presence of leukocytes introduced by trauma (true CSF WBC count = observed CSF WBC count − expected CSF WBC count due to trauma) has been shown to be of only limited value, especially in children with bacterial meningitis.

Partially Treated Meningitis

A significant number of patients receive antibiotics before the diagnosis of meningitis (see Case 16–2). Although Gram stain and culture may become negative, most cases of inadequately treated meningitis show no change in CSF cell count, glucose or protein, compared to untreated cases. Identification of the causative organism in these cases may be facilitated by testing for bacterial antigens using CIE, latex agglutination, or ELISA (see earlier section).

Febrile Seizures

CSF pleocytosis may result from febrile seizures in children without necessarily indicating the presence of intracranial infection.[24] Pediatric patients who warrant LP on clinical grounds with subsequent findings of CSF pleocytosis should be treated until all cultures are determined to be negative.

PLEURAL FLUID (THORACENTESIS)

CASE 16–3

A 65-year-old female came to the ED with dyspnea on exertion, bipedal edema, dry cough, and orthopnea. She denied chest pain, fever, chills, sputum production, drug or alcohol use. She admitted to cigarette smoking, but stated that she quit 10 years before. Her blood pressure was 100/60 mm Hg, pulse was 130/min and irregular, respirations were 32/min, and temperature was 36.1° C (97° F). Breath sounds were equal bilaterally but decreased at the bases, and fine rales were heard throughout. Jugular venous distension was noted and a summation gallop was heard. A posteroanterior (PA) chest radiograph revealed an enlarged heart and bilateral pleural effusions, with no evidence of focal infiltrates.

CASE 16–4

A 53-year-old male came to the ED because of progressive dyspnea, cough, and blood-streaked sputum. He had a 10-year history of sarcoid lung disease, for which he took prednisone. He denied fever, and stated that his purified protein derivative (PPD) test had been negative 1 year ago. When asked about weight loss or night-sweats, he stated that he had been gaining weight, and that he "sweats all the time." He denied smoking and illicit drug use, but admitted to drinking "socially." As part of his evaluation, a chest radiograph was obtained, which revealed bilateral hilar enlargement, a distinct right-sided pleural effusion, and left-sided blunting of the costophrenic angle.

Normally, the pleural space is only a potential one, in which a thin layer of fluid is physiologically present between the visceral and parietal pleura. When there is disruption of the normal forces which maintain this potential space, as in trauma, infection, inflammation, or neoplasm, pleural fluid can accumulate and may cause symptoms, especially if the collection is rapid and voluminous. Approximately one million patients develop pleural effusion in the United States every year.[25]

The practice of removing abnormal collections of fluid which have effused into the pleural space, a procedure known as thoracentesis, was first described in the medical literature by Hippocrates. In current practice, thoracentesis refers to the temporary placement of a needle or catheter in the pleural space for the diagnostic or therapeutic removal of fluid or air. Analyzing and interpreting pleural fluid in a logical, efficient and rapid, yet thorough manner enables the emergency physician to quickly arrive at the correct diagnosis (Fig. 16-1, pp. 304-305).

Evaluation of a Pleural Effusion

The first step in evaluating a pleural effusion is to obtain a history and perform a physical examination, with careful attention to the pulmonary and cardiovascular systems. If the clinical evaluation clearly indicates that the patient is in congestive heart failure (CHF) and the effusion is not large, no attempt at obtaining pleural fluid for analysis is necessary at this time; instead therapy directed at relieving the volume overload is indicated first. If the presentation is *atypical* (i.e., if there is a unilateral, unequal, or massive effusion; if the patient is experiencing pleuritic chest pain or fever; or if the effusion or symptoms persist despite appropriate therapy) a thoracentesis for direct fluid analysis is indicated. If the patient is already on a diuretic, however, one must remember that the effusion present in CHF, although typically a transudate, may be transformed into an exudate by diuretic therapy.[26]

Except when CHF is diagnosed clinically as described above, thoracentesis should be performed, when technically possible, on all newly identified effusions. Blunting of the costophrenic angles on a PA chest radiograph correlates with the presence of approximately 300 mL of fluid; blunting on lateral films can be seen when about 150 mL of fluid is present. A layering out of at least 10 mm of fluid must be visualized on lateral decubitus chest radiographs for the procedure to be performed safely at the bedside; less than this degree of layering indicates an amount of fluid that is technically difficult to tap, and either observation of the patient or ultrasound guidance for the tap is warranted, depending on the circumstances. A properly exposed decubitus radiograph can detect as little as 5 mL of pleural fluid.[27] Failure of an effusion to layer out suggests loculation, and in such a case it may be prudent to next obtain CT of the chest and/or perform the thoracentesis guided by ultrasound.

Appearance

The gross appearance of the pleural fluid may be clear, turbid, bloody, or chylous. Any specimen which appears bloody, should be centrifuged to determine its hematocrit. A hematocrit of less than 1% is not considered to be a significant finding, and may be due to the trauma of the thoracentesis. If the hematocrit is greater than 1%, malignancy, pulmonary embolism, or traumatic pleural effusion should be suspected. A concurrent peripheral blood hematocrit should be obtained; a pleural effusion hematocrit that is greater than 50% of the peripheral hematocrit is considered a hemothorax, and chest-tube drainage should be performed if the collection of fluid is large. In the absence of external trauma, aortic dissection should be suspected when the pleural effusion hematocrit approaches the value of the circulating hematocrit.

The supernatant of the pleural fluid should be inspected for cloudiness. If the fluid was originally turbid, but clears with centrifugation, one may proceed to chemical analysis of the specimen, because the cloudiness was undoubtedly due to cellular or particulate material. However, if the turbidity persists, the patient probably has chylothorax or pseudochylothorax. The two entities may be differentiated based upon history and examination of the sediment. Chylothoraces tend to be acute or traumatic. Pseudochylothoraces are usually related to the chronicity of the effusion. The presence of cholesterol crystals in the sediment, or a pleural fluid triglyceride level of less than 50 mg/dL also indicates a pseudochylothorax. A pleural fluid triglyceride level of greater than 110 mg/dL suggests a chylothorax.[25] For a triglyceride level between 50 and 110 mg/dL, a lipoprotein analysis of the fluid revealing chylomicrons helps establish the fluid as a chylothorax.

The odor of the fluid should be noted; a putrid odor suggests an infectious process, probably anaerobic, whereas an odor of ammonia or urine indicates urinothorax.

Transudate vs. Exudate—Chemical Analysis (see box)

The initial laboratory testing of the fluid should be aimed at differentiating a *transudate* from an *exudate.* Whereas a transudative effusion is simply an ultrafiltrate of the plasma due to hydrostatic forces, an exudative effusion signifies true pleural disease due to an inflammatory, infectious, or neoplastic processes.

Traditionally, there have been three absolute criteria for distinguishing a transudate from an exudate, as described by Light.[28] A fluid is an exudate if it is characterized by any or all of the following:

1. The pleural fluid protein divided by the serum protein is greater than 0.5.
2. The pleural fluid lactic acid dehydrogenase (LDH) divided by the serum LDH is greater than 0.6.

Differential Diagnosis of Pleural Fluid

Transudates

Acute atelectasis
Cirrhosis
Congestive heart failure (CHF)
Fontan procedure (procedure used to bypass a hypoplastic right ventricle in children)
Glomerulonephritis
Hypoproteinemia
Myxedema
Nephrotic syndrome
Peritoneal dialysis
Pulmonary embolism
Sarcoidosis (usually an exudate)
Superior vena caval obstruction
Urinothorax

Exudates

Amyloidosis
Asbestosis
Chronic atelectasis
Chylothorax
Collagen vascular diseases/drug-induced lupus
Dressler's syndrome (postcardiac injury syndrome)
Drug-induced pleural diseases (not of the drug-induced lupus type)
  Nitrofurantoin, Dantrolene, Methylsergide, Bromocriptine, Procarbazine, Amiodarone
Electrical burns
Endoscopic variceal sclerotherapy
Furosemide therapy
Gastrointestinal diseases
  Pancreatitis, hepatic abscess, splenic abscess
Hemothorax
Infectious diseases
  Lung abscess, bacterial pneumonia, tuberculosis, fungal infection, viral illness, *Rickettsiae* (Q fever), parasitic diseases
Lymphatic disease
Meigs' syndrome (benign ovarian tumor, ascites, and pleural effusion)
Neoplastic diseases
Pulmonary embolism
Pulmonary infarction
Radiation therapy
Sarcoidosis
Uremia

3. The pleural fluid LDH is greater than two thirds the normal upper limit of the serum LDH.

Valdes et al recently demonstrated in a series of 253 patients that cholesterol may be used as a reliable criteria for distinguishing a transudate from an exudate.[29] The patients' effusions were first classified as transudates, neoplastic exudates, tuberculous exudates, and miscellaneous exudates, using previously established criteria (i.e.,

LDH, protein, pleural biopsy, culture, and angiography). These patients were then reevaluated using various thresholds for cholesterol. The authors found that a pleural fluid cholesterol (PCHOL) of 55 mg/dL or less indicated a transudate with 91% sensitivity and 100% specificity. A ratio of pleural to serum cholesterol (PCHOL/SCHOL) of 0.3 or less likewise signified a transudate, with 92.5% sensitivity and 87.6% specificity. Using Light's three criteria (LDH ratios and protein ratio) collectively, achieved a 94.6% sensitivity and 78.4% specificity in this study. The use of cholesterol levels may augment or eventually supplant the traditional parameters of LDH and protein. However, until there is more experience with the use of pleural fluid cholesterol levels for differentiating exudates from transudates, it should not routinely be used as the sole criteria for making this distinction.

Physicians should avoid using a "shotgun" approach to ordering laboratory tests on pleural fluid: When a transudate is strongly suspected, 1 or 2 mL should be sent for LDH and protein (and perhaps cholesterol), and the remainder of the fluid held, pending the results. Studies suggest that once a transudate is identified by the above criteria, it is neither diagnostically helpful nor cost effective to submit the fluid for further analysis.[28,29] Almost all transudative pleural effusions are caused by either CHF or cirrhosis.

Pleural fluid protein and LDH are related to the degree of pleural membrane inflammation. In fact, LDH levels may be used to track the progression or regression of disease in the pleural space.[25, 28]

Other chemical criteria and cell counts are much less reliable in distinguishing between a transudate and an exudate, but may be helpful in separating and identifying specific *causes* of exudative effusions.

CASE 16–3 CONTINUED

Because of the large size of the effusion, thoracentesis was performed, and 300 mL of clear fluid was recovered. Some of the fluid was sent for protein and LDH measurements and both were less than one fourth of respective concurrent serum values. No further tests were performed on the pleural fluid. The patient was treated with intravenous furosemide, and soon began to diurese large volumes of urine, with partial improvement of her respiratory distress. Several days later, she felt much better, and the effusions were largely resolved.

Chemical Analysis

Amylase.—Levels greater than the upper normal limit for serum are significant, and may represent an esophageal tear, pancreatitis, pancreatic pseudocyst, or malignant pleural effusion.[30] A pleural fluid amylase level is important in identifying esophageal rupture; the presence of an acutely formed pleural effusion with a high level of the salivary isoenzyme of amylase is virtually diagnostic of esophageal rupture. Malignant effusions may also contain elevated salivary isoenzyme amylase levels,[31] but the clinical course is typically more indolent; in equivocal cases, the fluid pH helps to separate these two entities (see paragraph on pH that follows). Amylase isoenzymes are also useful for distinguishing effusions due to esophageal rupture and malignant effusions from the high amylase effusion that occurs with pancreatic disease. Serum isoenzyme levels should be measured as well.

Glucose.—Levels less than 60 mg/dL may be seen in tuberculous or parapneumonic effusions, rheumatoid effusion, malignant effusion, hemothorax, paragonimiasis, or Churg-Strauss syndrome. Glucose levels, however, are nonspecific, and higher values do not always exclude these diseases. Again, serum glucose levels should be measured concurrently, since abnormal serum glucose levels may affect pleural glucose values, and a very low or high pleural value may be the result of hypo- or hyperglycemia. Pleural glucose levels of less than 30 mg/dL help to distinguish rheumatoid pleuritis from lupus pleuritis: lupus effusions usually contain normal glucose levels. When a parapneumonic effusion has a glucose level of less than 40 mg/dL, chest-tube drainage should be performed.[30]

pH.—To obtain an accurate value, the pleural fluid specimen should be collected anaerobically in a heparinized syringe and transported on ice. A very acidic pleural fluid (i.e., pH < 6.0) strongly suggests gastric secretions in the pleural space, probably resulting from esophageal rupture or perforation. Surgical consultation and possibly intervention are required. Pleural fluid pH is also a useful parameter for determining if a chest tube should be inserted in a parapneumonic effusion: a pH value of less than 7.0 suggests an empyema or complicated parapneumonic effusion requiring drainage, whereas values above 7.20 may not need to be drained.[25] A pH less than 7.20 is also characteristic of systemic acidosis, tuberculous pleuritis, malignant pleural effusion, hemothorax, or paragonimiasis.[25] In rheumatoid pleuritis, the pH is usually less than 7.20 in contrast to lupus pleuritis, where the pH is usually above this level.[32] An alkaline pleural effusion may occur with *Proteus mirabilis* empyema and occasionally with CHF after diuretic therapy.

Adenosine Deaminase (ADA).—ADA has recently been shown to be a useful marker for diagnosing a tuberculous pleural effusion quickly and inexpensively. It may prove to be of value as a single test for use in remote regions which have a high prevalence of tuberculosis, and where other tests are not feasible because of their expense or lack of availability.[33] Levels of ADA greater than 70 U/L are indicative of tuberculous pleuritis, whereas levels of less than 40 U/L effectively rule out this diagnosis. At times, a patient with nontuberculous pleuritis will have elevated ADA levels (especially in lymphoma and empyema). However, large and small isoenzymes of ADA may be determined to distinguish tuberculous effusions from others: a tuberculous pleural effusion contains mostly the large isoenzyme, whereas effusions of other etiologies contain a predominance of the small isoenzyme.[34]

Gamma Interferon.—The presence of elevated levels has been shown to be unique to tuberculous effusions.[35, 36]

Tuberculostearic Acid (TBSA).—Detection of TBSA in CSF, sputum, and bronchial washings has been used successfully to establish the diagnosis of tuberculous meningitis and pulmonary tuberculosis. The use of TBSA for the diagnosis of tuberculous pleural effusion has been suggested. However, studies have shown it to be an unreliable parameter in *pleural fluid,* with both unacceptably high false-positive and false-negative results.[37]

Cell Counts

RBC Counts

See earlier on page 299.

WBC Counts and Differentials

A WBC count greater than 10,000 cells/mm^3 in a pleural effusion usually suggests an empyema or parapneumonic effusion.[28, 38, 39] An empyema is a primary infection of the pleural space, whereas a parapneumonic effusion is the result of inflammation of the pleura caused by an adjacent pneumonia. As with standard peripheral blood counts, specimens should immediately be transferred to a tube containing an anticoagulant, to prevent clotting or clumping of cells.

A predominance of PMN or neutrophil cells indicates acute pleural disease. An infiltrate and purulent sputum accompanying a neutrophilic effusion indicates a parapneumonic effusion; a neutrophilic effusion accompanied by an infiltrate, but without purulent sputum production, suggests pulmonary infarction.[40] Early tuberculous infection can cause a neutrophilic predominance in an associated effusion. When a neutrophilic effusion is present without an infiltrate or purulent sputum, one must suspect pulmonary embolism or digestive system and related causes (pancreatitis; subphrenic, pancreatic, splenic, or hepatic abscesses; endoscopic variceal sclerotherapy; esophageal perforation; recent abdominal surgery). Depending upon the clinical circumstances, a ventilation-perfusion scan and/or abdominal CT or sonogram should be performed.

A lymphocytic exudate is classically attributed to tuberculous effusions.[28, 38] However, lymphocytosis of the pleural fluid is not a constant finding in patients with tuberculous effusions. In one series, only 62% of patients had greater than 50% lymphocytes on initial examination of the pleural fluid, and 15% had greater than 90% PMN cells.[41] Nevertheless, the diagnosis of tuberculosis must be considered when a PPD-positive patient has an unexplained lymphocytic exudative effusion and such a patient should generally be treated with antituberculous medications even in the absence of direct identification of acid-fast bacilli (AFB).[42]

The most common cause of pleural fluid eosinophilia is the presence of blood or air in the pleural space. Other less frequent causes include benign asbestos effusion, drug reactions, paragonimiasis, and other parasitic diseases.[25, 38]

A predominance of *mononuclear cells* indicates chronic pleural disease such as malignancy and tuberculosis[38] and a pleural biopsy for culture and cytology is indicated.

If the above diseases have been excluded as the cause of a pleural fluid leukocytosis, consider fungal infection, collagen vascular diseases, and Dressler's (postcardiac injury) syndrome.

Bacteriology

Common organisms causing pleural effusions are the respiratory pathogens, which include *Streptococcus pneumoniae, Staphylococcus aureus*, the anaerobes, and *Mycobacterium tuberculosis*.[39, 40, 43] Aerobic and anaerobic cultures should be sent; Gram and acid-fast stains must be performed immediately, especially in the febrile or septic patient (see Chapter 6). When there is production of sputum, specimens should, of course, always be stained directly, as well as cultured. Tuberculous effusions are thought to result from a delayed hypersensitivity response to mycobacterial antigens in the pleural space, which probably enter through small subpleural foci of infection that rupture into the pleural space.[44, 45] This would account for the very low recovery of AFB from pleural fluid. Since pleural fluid staining and culture are usually not positive for AFB, pleural biopsy and culture are often required to confirm the diagnosis.[46] Tuberculous effusion is often present in the absence of other radiologic findings of active disease.[38]

A Gram-stained specimen and cultures should be obtained in all cases of rheumatoid pleuritis, since patients with rheumatoid pleuritis also have a high incidence of infected parapneumonic effusions.[25]

CIE is useful for identifying bacterial antigens in children with parapneumonic effusions. It is less helpful in adults, since in this population infections are often due to anaerobic organisms, which cannot be routinely identified with CIE.[25]

Cytology

The most common type of pleural malignancy is metastatic disease (predominantly from the colon and breast) followed by primary lung cancer. Primary pleural tumors are rare, the most common being malignant mesothelioma.[25] After all other tests have been performed or requested, the remaining fluid should be fixed in 50%

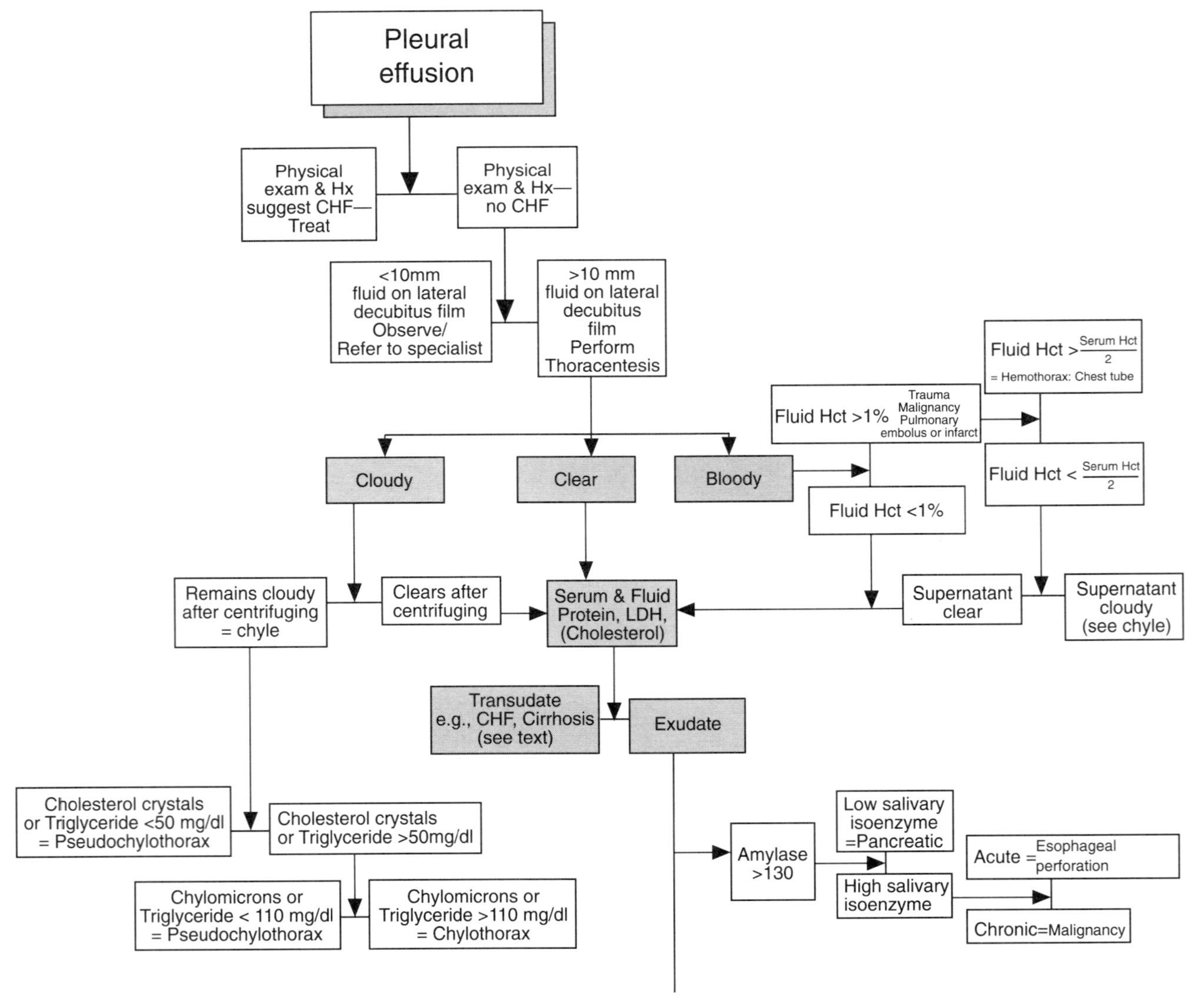

Pleural effusion
Physical exam & Hx suggest CHF—Treat
Physical exam & Hx—no CHF
<10mm fluid on lateral decubitus film Observe/ Refer to specialist
>10 mm fluid on lateral decubitus film Perform Thoracentesis
Cloudy
Clear
Bloody
Fluid Hct >1% Trauma Malignancy Pulmonary embolus or infarct
Fluid Hct > Serum Hct / 2 = Hemothorax: Chest tube
Fluid Hct < Serum Hct / 2
Fluid Hct <1%
Remains cloudy after centrifuging = chyle
Clears after centrifuging
Serum & Fluid Protein, LDH, (Cholesterol)
Supernatant clear
Supernatant cloudy (see chyle)
Transudate e.g., CHF, Cirrhosis (see text)
Exudate
Cholesterol crystals or Triglyceride <50 mg/dl = Pseudochylothorax
Cholesterol crystals or Triglyceride >50mg/dl
Chylomicrons or Triglyceride < 110 mg/dl = Pseudochylothorax
Chylomicrons or Triglyceride >110 mg/dl = Chylothorax
Amylase >130
Low salivary isoenzyme =Pancreatic
High salivary isoenzyme
Acute = Esophageal perforation
Chronic=Malignancy

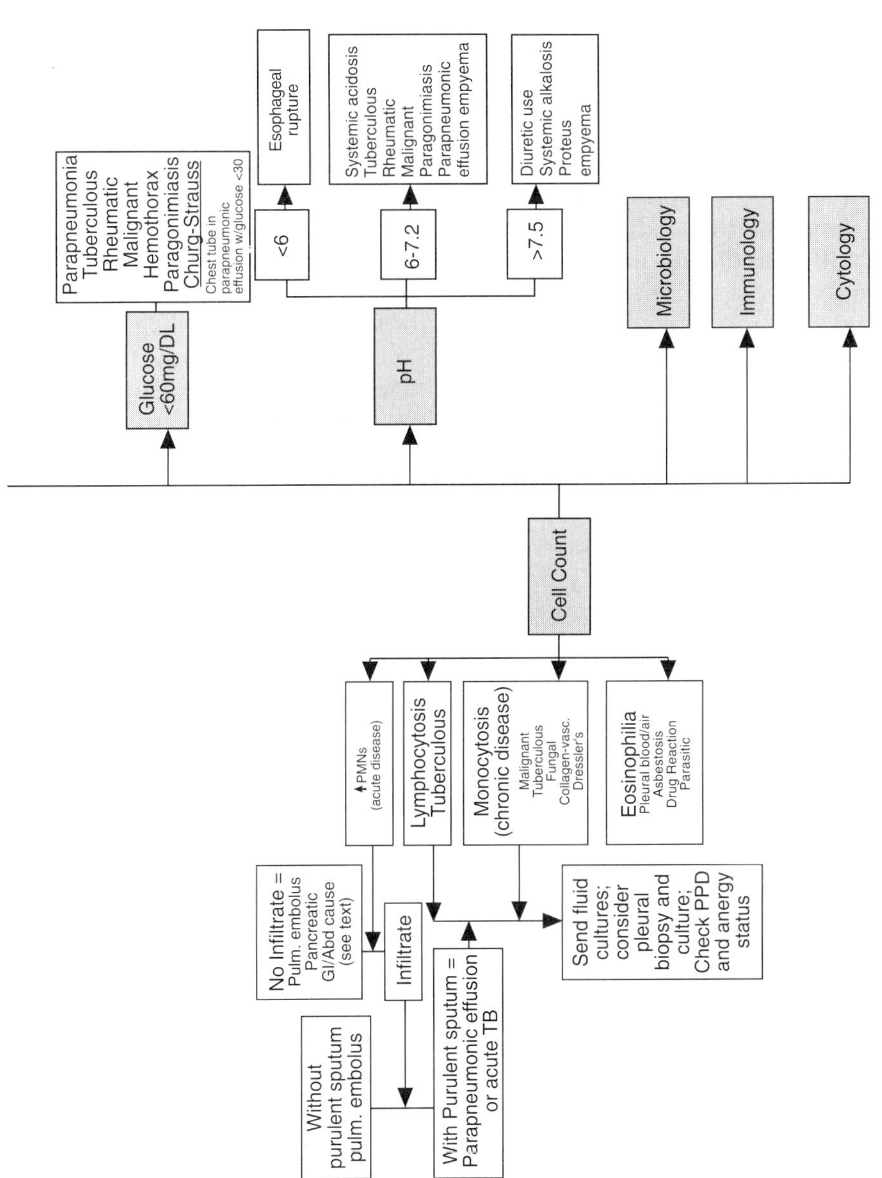

Fig. 16–1. Algorithm for pleural fluid analysis.

ethyl alcohol and sent to the pathology laboratory for cytospin/cell block. The greater the amount of pleural fluid that is sent for cytologic studies, the more likely that malignant cells will be detected.

Pleural fluid cytology is positive in 40% to 90% of patients with malignant processes involving the pleural space.[25] Unfixed specimens, or those standing for long periods before analysis, may yield false-negative results since cell architecture may be destroyed by autolysis. Effusions due to malignant processes that do not cause direct seeding of the pleura often yield negative cytology; such may be the case in tumor related lymphatic obstruction, postobstructive pneumonia, and atelectasis. Pleural biopsy may be necessary to establish a diagnosis when there is a suspicion of malignancy.[47]

Immunology

At some point during the course of the disease, rheumatoid pleuritis occurs in approximately 5% of patients with rheumatoid arthritis. The pleuritis usually occurs in the absence of rheumatoid lung disease. Rheumatoid factor is usually present in titers above 1:320, and the effusion may persist for weeks after the successful treatment of the disease.[32]

Pleural effusion occurs in about 40% of systemic and drug-induced lupus erythematosus.[25] Pleuritic chest pain is a consistent finding, and fever is common. In systemic lupus erythematosus, extrapulmonary manifestations can usually be identified before pleural involvement occurs. In drug-induced lupus pleuritis, a review of the patient's medications will reveal offending agents, such as isoniazid, hydralazine, phenytoin, procainamide, and chlorpromazine. Antinuclear antibodies (ANA) in the pleural fluid will confirm the diagnosis, when seen in titers of above 1:160, or a pleural fluid to serum ANA ratio greater than or equal to 1.[48] Certain drugs may cause an exudative pleural effusion, often via poorly understood mechanisms, which are distinct from the mechanism producing drug-induced lupus type (Fig. 16–1).

CASE 16–4 CONTINUED

The patient consented to thoracentesis, and 200 mL of slightly turbid, straw-colored fluid was removed. Both the fluid LDH and protein were found to be elevated beyond serum levels. Pleural fluid glucose was 75 mg/dL but concurrent serum levels were 210 mg/dL; pleural and serum amylase values were within normal limits. Pleural WBC count was 12,000/mm^3 with 75% mononuclear cells, and pH was 7.27. Pleural-fluid Gram and acid-fast stains showed no organisms; and cultures for aerobes, anaerobes, and tuberculosis were sent. Sputum Gram and acid-fast stains were performed, and (surprisingly) AFB were identified. The patient was then admitted to the hospital and started on appropriate antituberculosis medication.

PERITONEAL FLUID (DIAGNOSTIC PERITONEAL LAVAGE AND PARACENTESIS)

CASE 16–5

A 23-year-old female presented to the ED with severe abdominal pain after falling off a bicycle and striking a fence with her midabdomen. Her blood pressure was 90/60 mm Hg, pulse was 130/min, respirations were 24/min, and temperature was 98.8° F. The patient stated she was not pregnant, but urine testing yielded a positive result. Pelvic exam revealed the cervical os to be closed and there was slight cervical motion tenderness, but no blood was noted. Rectal exam was nontender, but revealed external hemorrhoids and heme-positive brown stools. Linear, patterned abrasions and ecchymosis were noted on abdominal examination, and there was diffuse tenderness and guarding, without rigidity or obvious peritoneal signs.

A pelvic sonogram was performed, and a single intrauterine pregnancy of approximately 6.5 weeks gestation was noted, with positive fetal heart movement and no intrauterine bleeding. A small collection of fluid was noted in the cul-de-sac. A nasogastric tube was inserted and clear, bile-stained fluid was recovered; urinary bladder catheterization yielded clear-yellow urine, negative for heme. Aside from a hematocrit of 30% and a hemoglobin of 9.5 mg/dL, blood tests were normal. The patient complained that her pain was getting worse.

Traumatic Peritoneal Fluid–Diagnostic Peritoneal Lavage

Blunt abdominal trauma can result in accumulations of blood or fluid in the peritoneal cavity. Because even small amounts are significant but not easy to aspirate, sterile solutions of Ringer's lactate or normal saline can be added and after mixing with the peritoneal fluid, subsequently removed for analysis. This technique, known as diagnostic peritoneal lavage (DPL), was introduced into routine clinical usage by Root et al in 1965.[49] Root's original technique of inserting a catheter percutaneously into the peritoneal cavity has since been refined, and today DPL is generally performed as an open procedure. When properly done, DPL is a safe and sensitive test for the diagnosis and management of abdominal trauma.

In the ED, DPL is performed most frequently to help diagnose intraabdominal injury resulting from blunt, or occasionally, penetrating trauma. However, DPL may also be useful or essential in diagnosing primary peritonitis (see p. 312) and, in settings other than the ED, various infectious, inflammatory, and surgical diseases affecting the contents of the peritoneal cavity. Culdocentesis is another route to obtaining peritoneal fluid, but because its use is directed at diagnosing a ruptured ectopic pregnancy, it is dealt with in a separate section of this chapter.

This section discusses the guidelines for the selection of patients in whom DPL is appropriate, the types of tests that may be obtained on the fluid, and the significance of the subsequent laboratory results.

Specificity and Sensitivity

Most recent studies report a 96% to 98% sensitivity and a 92% to 99% specificity for DPL.[50–52] Modified criteria for evaluating penetrating vs. blunt trauma further assist in the diagnostic value and accuracy of this test. Proper patient selection is the key to obtaining meaningful and useful results; the clinician should be aware of those clinical situations for which DPL is not the procedure of choice, along with the alternative studies available to quickly and accurately evaluate intraabdominal injury.

Indications

The chief value of DPL in abdominal trauma is to reduce the delay in detecting significant intraabdominal injury requiring surgery or, conversely, to obviate the necessity of performing a laparotomy with its attendant morbidity. Many sources report that in an awake and alert patient, abdominal examination alone can be 98% accurate in detecting the presence of an intraabdominal injury;[53] in other studies, the physical exam was far less reliable.[54] In any case, however, a physical exam is not a reliable indication of intraabdominal pathology in a multiply injured patient with an altered sensorium.

DPL is an operative procedure and will alter the subsequent examination of the patient. It should therefore be performed only if a positive test will be accepted as evidence that the patient requires celiotomy.

The mechanism of injury history and focused physical examination should quickly identify those patients for whom DPL would only delay required operative intervention and therefore should not be performed. A gunshot wound which penetrates the abdomen, for example, is considered to be an indication for immediate surgical exploration. Free air on an abdominal radiograph after blunt trauma also mandates laparotomy, although in the absence of other findings free air after penetrating (stab) injuries in the *anterior* abdomen does not necessarily require immediate exploration.[55] Progressive abdominal distention following trauma and gross blood in the gastrointestinal tract, as evidenced by hematemesis or hematachezia, are *contraindications* to DPL since operative celiotomy is mandatory and should not be delayed. Patients with multiple penetrating abdominal injuries and those who have obvious peritoneal signs related to trauma will also require immediate laparotomy.

In children with blunt abdominal trauma, CT is favored over DPL.[56] Any child to be evaluated by CT for blunt abdominal trauma should be stabilized, if necessary, with intravenous fluids and packed RBCs before the study. The inability to hemodynamically stabilize patients who do not have an identifiable source of blood loss is an indication for immediate surgical intervention. In children, the combination of hemodynamic instability (low trauma score, hypotension, hematocrit <30%) and a moderate to large, or expanding peritoneal fluid collection seen on CT, correlates well with the need for operative management.[57]

In those remaining patients whose history or examination after apparent or suspected abdominal trauma is unreliable, equivocal, or impractical to obtain the following criteria suggest the need for DPL[58]:

- Loss of consciousness
- Intoxication
- Unexplained hypovolemic shock that cannot be corrected with fluid resuscitation
- Head injuries accompanied by hypovolemic shock (head injuries alone are an unlikely cause of hypovolemia)
- Blunt abdominal trauma suggesting severe injury
- Blunt abdominal trauma with patterned ecchymoses/abrasions (e.g., from seatbelts)[59]
- Abdominal signs or symptoms of hypovolemia in a patient who jumped or fell from a significant height
- Flank wounds below the costal margin which penetrate the fascia on wound exploration
- Abdominal wounds penetrating the fascia on wound exploration
- Penetrating wounds to the chest below the fourth intercostal space. This type of wound should not routinely be explored in the ED since a pneumothorax may ensue. Routine laparotomy is sometimes recommended for detection of occult diaphragmatic laceration or hernias in these injuries.[60, 61]
- Fracture at or below the fourth rib accompanied by abdominal signs or hypovolemia
- Abdominal trauma for which laparotomy might otherwise be indicated in patients at high risk for general anesthesia because of serious concomitant medical problems

CT Versus DPL

With the increasing availability of CT, the possibility of obtaining the required information from a noninvasive procedure is very tempting. For this reason CT has supplanted DPL in many centers. CT should not, however, replace DPL when it is unlikely to provide the required information quickly enough. Many retrospective studies suggested that CT is both sensitive and specific, but no convincing *prospective* studies have been conducted to date.[62–67] The high sensitivity and specificity (both approaching 98%) of DPL on the other hand, has been well documented in prospective series.[68]

The minimum volume of blood in the peritoneal cavity required for detection by CT is about 100 to 200 mL, according to most sources,[69] DPL can identify as little as 50mL.[49]

CT studies of the abdomen require the use of oral and intravenous contrast material, which pose a risk for aspiration, allergic reaction, and renal compromise (especially in a hypoperfused kidney). In addition, a reliable study often requires a two- to three-hour waiting period to allow for intestinal transit of the oral contrast material. This time period may be further prolonged by conditions which delay gastric emptying (e.g., opiate use) or cause intestinal hypomotility (e.g., ileus).

An intoxicated or combative patient may be unable to remain motionless for the period required to perform the scan. At times, neuromuscular blockade to paralyze the patient, accompanied by intubation and pulmonary ventilation may be necessary to perform the study.

However, there are situations for which CT is either a helpful adjunct to or superior to DPL, such as in the evaluation of retroperitoneal and diaphragmatic injuries. CT can accurately demonstrate the anatomy of a lesion, localize collections of fluid, and possibly identify areas of hypoperfusion.[69–73] Contrast-enhanced computed tomography enema (CECTE) should be employed to evaluate the retroperitoneal colon in penetrating injuries, although its role in blunt trauma is not yet clear.[74]

With the growing availability of CT scanners located in close proximity to the ED, the "golden hour of resuscitation" need no longer be spent in a distant radiology suite. Furthermore, new spiral scanners dramatically reduce imaging time. The multitrauma patient often requires CT of the head and/or chest in addition to the abdomen; sometimes the whole body scan provides the most effective use of time and resources.

Contraindications

The only absolute contraindication to DPL is the presence of an existing indication for celiotomy.[58]

The main relative contraindication to DPL is a history or physical evidence of prior abdominal surgery (especially multiple surgeries) or adhesions. In these cases, sequestration of fluid in the abdominal cavity[50, 75] by loculations may result in a false-negative DPL.

Morbid obesity can make performing peritoneal lavage technically difficult, although the alternative study, abdominal CT, may not be an option for these patients, since many CT scanners are not made to withstand weights greater than 300 lbs.

Coagulopathies and anticoagulation treatment may result in extrinsic blood in the peritoneal cavity, even if not hemodynamically significant. Caput medusae seen in cirrhosis can extend across preferred incision sites.

Pregnancy, once considered a relative contraindication has been shown to present little danger when DPL is performed at the proper site.[76, 77] Conversely, radiologic studies are potentially harmful to the fetus and should therefore be avoided.

Risks and Complications

Properly preparing the patient by inserting a urinary catheter and nasogastric tube (unless contraindicated) minimizes risk, and is required for the proper interpretation of the lavage fluid. However, extreme care must be given not to "routinely" insert these tubes in the multiply traumatized patient. If maxillary trauma exists, a gastric tube should be inserted orally, not nasally, to avoid entering the cranium through a fractured cribriform plate. Likewise, disruption of the urethra should preclude the insertion of a Foley catheter. Blood at the urethral meatus, a high-riding prostate, or scrotal hematoma may indicate such an injury, and in this setting a suprapubic catheter should be inserted instead.[58]

Potential complications of DPL include:

- Urinary bladder laceration
- Small bowel laceration
- Wound dehiscence
- Wound infection
- Omental vessel laceration
- Evisceration of bowel
- No fluid return
- Fluid in chest

Interpretation of Findings (see box)

Specific criteria have been developed that define a positive DPL, which in turn indicate the need for surgical exploration of the abdomen. These criteria, based on the results of careful statistical analysis of clinical and experimental data,[49, 58, 73, 78–80] are:

- Aspiration of >5 mL of blood from the catheter
- Grossly bloody lavage fluid (cannot read newsprint through lavage tubing)
- RBCs >100,000/mm^3 in blunt trauma
- RBCs >50,000/mm^3 in penetrating trauma to the anterior abdomen[81–83]

A threshold value of 100,000 RBC/mm^3, was originally considered an indication of significant injury after blunt abdominal trauma. This value was then used for penetrating trauma as well, but more recent studies indicate that 50,000 RBC/mm^3 should be used as the criteria for surgical exploration after penetrating wounds of the anterior abdomen.

Retroperitoneal hematomas may be missed if the peritoneum remains intact,[58, 84] although, with time, RBCs may be detected in the lavage fluid because of diapedesis through the peritoneal membrane.[55, 58, 85] A negative lavage does not exclude damage to the aorta, vena cava, pancreas, kidneys and ureters, and portions of the duodenum and colon, all of which are in the retroperitoneum. Similarly, damage to the pelvic organs, which include the bladder, rectum, iliac vessels, and the female internal genitalia, may be missed.[75] To aid in the diagnosis of injuries to these organs and structures, a careful physical exam and wound exploration, with adjunctive tests such as

Positive DPL Findings[49, 58, 73, 78–83]

Aspiration of >5 mL of blood from the catheter
Grossly bloody lavage fluid (cannot read newsprint though lavage tubing)
RBC >100,000/mm^3 in blunt trauma, >50,000/mm^3 in penetrating trauma to anterior abdomen
WBC >500/mm^3
Recovery of lavage fluid through Foley catheter, nasogastric tube, or chest tube
Bile staining of lavage fluid
Contamination of lavage fluid with gastric or intestinal contents
Bacteria or vegetable fibers seen on Gram stain of lavage fluid
Amylase >175 Somogyi units/dL*

*Criterion varies from source to source–test now considered to be of questionable value.

CT, intravenous pyelogram, or retrograde cystogram, coupled with a high degree of clinical suspicion, will lead to the correct diagnosis. The mechanism of injury should suggest possible patterns of trauma: rapid deceleration and blunt trauma, such as in seatbelt injuries, can tear or devascularize portions of organs fixed behind the peritoneum. Penetrating wounds to the flank and back should be explored for their trajectory; those tracking anteriorly cause a greater degree of retroperitoneal organ involvement. Posterior fracture of a rib may lead to an injury sequestered in the retroperitoneum. Sequestration of a perforated or bleeding viscus in the chest through a diaphragmatic hernia may be missed on DPL; these injuries most commonly occur on the left side.[86–88] Chest radiography, along with auscultation and percussion findings help to detect this type of injury.

Pelvic fractures without other significant injury may produce a false-positive DPL due to diapedesis of RBCs into the peritoneal cavity.[55, 84]

Bleeding from the DPL incision site may contaminate the peritoneal cavity and lead to a false-positive result. Meticulous hemostatic technique should be observed; lidocaine with epinephrine should be used to help control bleeding. A detailed patient history (if possible) and a PT, PTT, and platelet count should be obtained.

- WBCs >500/mm^3

  To meaningfully interpret the WBC criteria, one must remember that 2 to 3 hours may be required for demargination and release of cells into the lavage fluid.[25] Patients whose cell-mediated immunity is defective (e.g., as a result of drug use, human immunodeficiency virus [HIV], chemotherapy, age) theoretically may not be able to mount an elevated WBC response characteristic of a positive DPL. Conversely, conclusions about the presence of WBCs in an otherwise benign lavage fluid should be made cautiously, since such an occurrence may be associated with false negatives.[89]

- Recovery of lavage fluid through a Foley catheter, nasogastric tube, or chest tube.[58]

  Aspiration of blood or lavage fluid from a Foley catheter may signify laceration or contusion in the urinary tract. Current investigations studying lavage fluid creatinine and urea to detect disruption of the urinary tract may ultimately result in helpful guidelines.[90] Blood or lavage fluid recovered from a nasogastric tube signifies gastrointestinal tract injury.

- Bile staining of lavage fluid[58]

  This finding indicates laceration of the liver or disruption of the hepatobiliary structures.

- Contamination of lavage fluid with gastric or intestinal contents

  This finding clearly indicates intestinal rupture or laceration.[58]

- Bacteria or vegetable fibers seen on Gram stain of lavage fluid

  Although signifying intraabdominal injury, the presence of this finding alone rarely justifies performing a laparotomy.[58]

- Pleural fluid amylase >175 Somogyi units/dL

An elevated pleural-fluid amylase alone does not constitute a positive lavage. The value of amylase levels as a criteria for a positive DPL is currently being questioned.[58] Serum amylase, on the other hand, as well as sequential peripheral hematocrit determinations should always be performed in the evaluation of abdominal trauma.

- Late complications of trauma missed by DPL include intestinal stricture formation resulting from devascularization or contusion of the bowel, and intestinal obstruction caused by hematoma formation in the bowel wall with occlusion of the lumen. Delayed intestinal rupture may occur in devitalized or ischemic tissue. A laceration of the small bowel may cause little or no recognizable bleeding and is a common cause of false-negative results. Any patient with an injury serious enough to require DPL should be admitted to the surgical service and observed for at least 24 hours, regardless of the results.

Discussion

Management of abdominal trauma is one of the most challenging diagnostic dilemmas that the emergency physician must face. Although CT is rapidly gaining popularity in many centers, DPL remains a proven standard, and often is still the preferred diagnostic test in evaluating abdominal trauma.

CASE 16–5 CONTINUED

Because of a high suspicion of intraabdominal injury, open DPL was performed. Lavage fluid was clear and contained 4,000 RBCs/mm^3 and 60 WBCs/mm^3, with an amylase of 12 U/dL. The patient was admitted to the surgical service for 24-hour observation, and discharged the following day with improvement of her symptoms.

Nontraumatic Peritoneal Fluid–Bacterial Peritonitis

The emergency physician is frequently required to evaluate the nontraumatic accumulation of peritoneal fluid, otherwise known as ascites. The most common causes of ascites include hepatic cirrhosis and malignancy. Additionally, patients requiring continuous ambulatory peritoneal dialysis (CAPD) have fluid iatrogenically placed in the peritoneal cavity, which at times must be analyzed. By far the most important disease process involving peritoneal fluid that must be diagnosed rapidly is bacterial peritonitis (BP), which can be further subclassified as spontaneous bacterial peritonitis (SBP) and secondary bacterial peritonitis.

SBP can be defined as infected ascitic fluid of cirrhotic patients, with no demonstrable primary source of infection. Although positive cultures are necessary to prove the diagnosis, it is rarely prudent to await their results before initiating appropriate antibiotic treatment.

When ascitic fluid becomes infected by contiguous spread from a primary source, or from a perforated viscus, this is considered a secondary form of bacterial peritonitis. Bacterial peritonitis resulting from contiguous spread that is not due to a perforated viscus is indistinguishable from SBP by ascitic fluid analysis, at least initially. However, correct diagnosis and specific treatment largely depend on identifying the primary source.

Gastrointestinal tract perforation into ascitic fluid with resultant peritonitis is *clinically* indistinguishable from SBP and secondary bacterial peritonitis by contiguous spread. In the case of perforation however, the ascitic fluid characteristics are distinct from these entities.

Although all of the aforementioned conditions that affect ascitic fluid are covered in this section, SBP is emphasized since prompt recognition and treatment in the ED may prevent death: often SBP is not clinically apparent, and the prognosis is extremely poor when SBP is untreated.

Prevalence and Prognosis

In the early 1970s, Conn and Fessel estimated the prevalence of SBP in cirrhotics with ascites to be 8%. In 1975, at the same institution, Correia and Conn[91] reported the prevalence to be 18%. Two prospective studies show an even higher prevalence, approaching 25%.[92, 93] The higher percentage in the later studies may be partially due to the increased clinical awareness and recognition of SBP and its various presentations.

Because of a 50% to 90% mortality,[92, 94, 95] the early recognition of SBP is extremely important, so that treatment can be initiated without delay. Appropriate and timely treatment does significantly increase survival.[94] According to Cummings, Hoefs, and Runyon[95] patients with a serum bilirubin >8 mg/dL and/or a serum creatine >2.1 mg/dL have the poorest prognosis and Attali et al[96] reported that a low pH (<7.15) of the ascitic fluid is a poor prognostic sign.

Clinical Diagnosis

Several large studies have shown that patients with SBP most commonly present with a temperature of 37.7° C (100° F) or above (67%), and abdominal pain (60%).[91, 92, 94, 97–99] Confusion or encephalopathy is seen in 57%. Abdominal tenderness and rebound are found in 50% and 42%, respectively. Diarrhea, hypotension, or hypothermia are found less frequently. However, symptoms may be minimal or absent in as many as one third of patients.[91, 92]

Appearance

The appearance of the ascitic fluid may be clear, cloudy, or bloody and is relatively unimportant in establishing the etiology of BP.

Cell Count

The main criteria for making the presumptive diagnosis of SBP or contiguous-spread BP in patients with chronic liver disease or cirrhosis is the PMN cell count: When the PMN cell count is >250 cells/mm^3, SBP should be the presumptive diagnosis and antibiotic treatment begun. Using this value has a sensitivity of 81% and specificity of 95%.[96, 100–103] Some authors use a PMN count of greater than 500 cells/mm^3 as the cutoff point, because it is about as sensitive and slightly more specific (97%)[96, 100–103] than a value of 250 cells/mm^3. The same studies that demonstrate the optimal PMN cutoff show that the total ascites-white cell count is not important; diagnosis and treatment is based solely upon the absolute ascites-PMN count. However, it should be noted, that Attali et al.[96] report that an elevated PMN is not diagnostic of bacterial peritonitis when ascites is due to carcinomatosis, tuberculosis, or pancreatic disease instead of cirrhosis.

The PMN threshold for treatment is the same for secondary BP due to contiguous spread as it is for SBP, although in this instance the obvious presence of a primary source of infection warrants specific treatment regardless of the fluid analysis. However, in many cases, it is impossible to differentiate between the two at the time of presentation. In a small retrospective study, Runyon and Hoefs[104] demonstrated that the two entities could be distinguished by the response of the PMN cell count to treatment. In SBP there was a rapid, exponential decline in the PMN cell count after appropriate antibiotic treatment was initiated; whereas in secondary BP due to contiguous spread, there was an actual rise in PMN count despite treatment.

Bacteriology

A definitive diagnosis of SBP is based on positive ascitic fluid cultures. In the larger series, organisms could be demonstrated in only one third of ascites specimens when Gram stain was performed on the fluid.[91, 92, 94, 97–99] About half of the concurrent blood cultures were positive, and in nearly all of them the same organism was cultured from the blood as from the ascitic fluid.

Microorganisms found in the gastrointestinal tract are the bacteria predominantly responsible for SBP, and infection is usually caused by a single organism (90%).[91, 94] Gram-negative bacilli are responsible for 70% of cases of SBP, with *E. coli* being the most common in this group (45%) followed by *Klebsiella pneumoniae* (10%). Gram-positive cocci account for approximately 20% of all cases of SBP, with *Streptococcus pneumoniae* being the most common (8%). Finally, anaerobes are found in 5% to 10% of infections, and are frequently encountered in polymicrobial infections.[91, 92, 94, 97–99]

There is an identifiable subpopulation of patients with chronic liver disease and ascites who present with a PMN count that is consistent with SBP, yet who are culture negative.[105] However the PMN count decreases after antibiotic treatment for SBP, suggesting that these patients indeed have infected ascites, and if left untreated may have developed culture-positive SBP. This phenomenon may result from suboptimal culture techniques and for that reason, inoculation of culture media at the bedside has been advocated as a way of increasing the diagnostic sensitivity of ascites cultures. Another possible explanation may be a low bacterial count in the ascitic fluid as suggested by the low yield of direct Gram staining in identifying organisms. Direct inoculation of blood culture bottles with at least 5 mL of fluid decreased the rate of culture-negative peritonitis in 1 study from 22% to 4%.[106]

In contrast to the monomicrobial infection usually seen in SBP and secondary BP that is caused by contiguous spread, the fluid obtained from patients with ascites who develop peritonitis from a perforated viscus demonstrates a polymicrobial flora on Gram stain and culture.[107] The criteria for diagnosing gut perforation into ascitic fluid is, however, based primarily upon chemical and radiologic data, as discussed below.

Chemical Analysis

Unlike fluids in other body compartments, the chemical composition of ascitic fluid in the peritoneal cavity does not change markedly as a result of infection.[94, 99] With the exception of BP caused by gut perforation, glucose, protein, and lactic acid dehydrogenase do not consistently change with the occurrence of BP and hence are not reliable predictors.

Ascitic pH, arterial to ascitic pH gradient, and ascitic lactate levels have all been studied as possible determinants of SBP.[96, 100–103] An ascitic pH of <7.35 has a sensitivity of 60% and a specificity of 96%; an arterial to ascitic pH gradient of >0.10 carries a sensitivity of 68% and a specificity of 98%. Ascites lactate level of >25 mg/dL is 81% sensitive and 93% specific. On the basis of these results, it is evident that these chemical criteria cannot supplant the PMN count as the standard for diagnosing SBP.[108]

In the presence of an elevated ascitic PMN count, antibiotic treatment clearly should not be withheld on the basis of normal ascitic pH and lactate criteria, because of their relatively low *sensitivity*. On the other hand, because of the high *specificity* of ascitic pH and lactate criteria, one might correctly diagnose and treat SBP early if these levels are abnormal, even if the ascitic PMN count is normal.

In contrast to other causes of BP, reliable chemical criteria have been established for identifying infection caused by gastrointestinal tract perforation into ascitic fluid.[107] At least two of the following three criteria must be satisfied: total protein concentration of over 1g/dL, LDH concentration of over 225 IU/L (or greater than the upper normal limit for serum), or a glucose concentration less than 50 mg/dL. When these criteria are met in a patient with ascites who is suspected of having a ruptured viscus, supine and upright radiographs of the abdomen should be obtained to identify free air under the diaphragm, and water-soluble contrast studies of the gastrointestinal tract should be performed.

Summary

Reynolds aptly stated that ascitic fluid is readily obtainable for analysis and SBP represents one of the few treatable aspects of advanced liver disease.[108] In the large prospective study of Pinzello et al.,[92] routine paracentesis of all patients with cirrhosis and ascites led to the identification and treatment of many patients with SBP who may otherwise have been missed. Conditions such as hepatic encephalopathy or gastrointestinal bleeding may in fact have been precipitated by sepsis due to SBP, which may be overlooked without ascitic fluid analysis.

Possible studies that can be done on ascites fluid and their positive values are:

- Culture and Sensitivity (C & S) (aerobic and anaerobic blood culture bottles injected with at least 5 mL fluid, done at bedside)
- PMN count >250 cells/mm^3
- Lactate >25 mg/dL
- pH <7.35
- arterial pH: ascitic pH >0.10
- Protein* >1 g/dL
- LDH* >225 IU/L (or > normal serum value)
- Glucose* <50 mg/dL

PERITONEAL FLUID FROM THE VAGINAL CUL-DE-SAC (CULDOCENTESIS)

CASE 16–7

At midnight, a 23-year-old female patient presented with nausea, vomiting, and pelvic cramps. Her initial blood pressure was 80 mm Hg by palpation but rose to 120 mm Hg systolic after 200 mL of normal saline was administered intravenously. On physical examination there was no vaginal bleeding, her uterus was normal sized and there were no masses palpable, but she had some left adnexal tenderness. Her initial hematocrit was 30% and a urinary pregnancy test was positive, but less than 50 units. The consulting gynecologist was 30 minutes from the hospital.

Culdocentesis is the procedure used to sample the fluid in the vaginal cul-de-sac. A needle is introduced through the posterior vaginal wall into the rectouterine pouch (the pouch of Douglas) and any fluid present is aspirated. In the past this technique was the standard approach to the diagnosis of ectopic pregnancy. Although mildly or moderately painful for the patient, the technique is simple and can be performed with a minimum of equipment and time. Romeo et al.[109] found that a positive culdocentesis combined with a positive pregnancy test, correlated with an ectopic pregnancy in 99.2% of cases. Even unruptured ectopic pregnancies frequently are associated with positive culdocentesis, and accounted for up to 60% of cases in the Romeo et al. study.[109] Sensitive measurements of urinary human chorionic gonadotropin (hCG)

*Request when gastrointestinal tract perforation is suspected (see previous section on bacterial peritonitis).

which can detect levels less than 50 IU, and new ultrasound techniques using transvaginal probes which can detect intrauterine pregnancies and adnexal abnormalities very early in pregnancy, have decreased the need for culdocentesis. An ectopic pregnancy can be virtually excluded by finding only an intrauterine gestational sac on ultrasound.* Alternatively, the finding of an adnexal mass combined with free fluid in the pelvis and a positive pregnancy test is highly indicative of a ruptured ectopic pregnancy. Vermesh et al.[110] have suggested that culdocentesis now has only a limited role in the evaluation of a possible ectopic pregnancy. They recommend instead using a combination of serum beta hCG testing and ultrasound (specifically transvaginal ultrasound). Laparoscopy is recommended in those patients who are symptomatic (i.e., who have abdominal pain and/or bleeding) with a positive pregnancy test and no definitive diagnosis on ultrasound.

Several other articles have addressed the use of culdocentesis in the evaluation of ectopic pregnancy.[111, 112] Krol and Abbott[111] recommend culdocentesis for those patients with a positive pregnancy test who are clinically stable with an indeterminate transvaginal ultrasound and those patients with a positive pregnancy test who have peritoneal signs but can be stabilized in the ED. Sauer and Rodi,[112] reporting on a large inner-city facility, are more liberal in their recommendations for culdocentesis. Citing the difficulty in obtaining ultrasound exams and problems with patient follow-up, they recommend culdocentesis for any patient with a positive pregnancy test and a high risk of ectopic pregnancy.

An excellent description of the technique of performing culdocentesis is provided in Roberts and Hedges.[113] Before performing the culdocentesis it is important to assemble all of the appropriate collecting tubes and media so that it is possible to gain the maximum amount of information from any fluid obtained, and the procedure, with its morbidity and risks, does not have to be repeated. These materials include:

1. Transport medium for culture and sensitivity of the fluid
2. An empty collection tube to observe (the specimen) for clotting of blood
3. A collection tube with anticoagulant to obtain hematocrit, Gram stain, and WBC determination of the fluid if needed.

Interpretation of Results

On gross observation, the results of a culdocentesis can be divided into five categories:

1. Nonclotting blood
2. Clotting blood
3. Serous fluid
4. Purulent fluid
5. No fluid or a dry tap

The most common reason to perform a culdocentesis is to determine if a patient has a hemoperitoneum from a leaking or ruptured ectopic pregnancy or a hemorrhagic ovarian cyst. Nonclotting blood obtained on aspiration is interpreted as a positive culdocentesis. There is some disagreement as to what constitutes a positive tap. Cartwright et al.[114] considered a positive tap to be more than 0.3 cc of nonclotting fluid with a hematocrit greater than 3%. More recently Vermesh et al.[110] used a hematocrit of 15% to indicate hemoperitoneum. Obtaining serous fluid is considered a negative tap. Large amounts of serous or serosanguinous fluid can indicate a ruptured ovarian cyst or inadvertent puncture of an intact cyst.[111] Purulent fluid is indicative of infection of which pelvic inflammatory disease, tubo-ovarian abscess, appen-

* See page 116.

dicitis, or ruptured diverticulitis are all possibilities to consider. When no fluid or clotting blood is obtained, the procedure is considered *nondiagnostic—not* not negative—and the physician should not let the results influence the decision making process. A recent study by Abbott et al[115] evaluated 65 patients with ectopic pregnancy, 43 of whom had culdocentesis performed on initial evaluation. The culdocentesis was negative (serous fluid) in 3 (7.0%) and indeterminate in 7 (16.3%). In other words, 23.3% of patients with an ectopic pregnancy initially had a negative or indeterminate culdocentesis. If the physician had been falsely reassured by a negative or indeterminate culdocentesis, these 10 patients would have had an increased risk of rupture. On the other hand, a positive culdocentesis combined with a positive pregnancy test is very strong evidence for an ectopic pregnancy. In the Romeo et al.[109] study of 133 patients with a positive pregnancy test and a positive culdocentesis, 132 (99.3%) had an ectopic pregnancy.

Contraindications and Complications

Culdocentesis should not be performed on patients who have had pelvic surgery in the past and may have adhesions and fixed pelvic organs. A mass in the cul-de-sac and a fixed, retroverted uterus are also contraindications to culdocentesis. A coagulopathy is considered a relative contraindication. Perforation of the uterus and the rectum occur with some frequency during the procedure but do not appear to cause serious morbidity.[111]

CASE 16–7 CONTINUED

Under the best of circumstances this patient would benefit from laparoscopy. The probability of ectopic pregnancy is high, and laparoscopy would enable the physician to diagnosis and possibly treat the problem. The emergency physician performed a culdocentesis on the patient, which yielded 5 mL of dark, nonclotting blood. The gynecologist then arrived and took the patient to the operating room for a laparotomy. The patient had a ruptured ectopic pregnancy.

SYNOVIAL (JOINT) FLUID (ARTHROCENTESIS)

CASE 16–8

A fifty-year-old male was brought to the ED by ambulance after falling in the street. The patient appeared unkempt and had the odor of alcohol on his breath. He stated that while walking, his right knee gave out and he fell to the ground. On physical exam the patient had a blood pressure of 130/85 mm Hg, a pulse of 110/min, respirations of 20/min, and a temperature of 38.4° C (101.3° F). The patient was coughing while being examined, and his respiratory exam revealed rales at the right base. His right knee was swollen and tender with a moderate effusion. There were scattered bruises on his lower extremities including the anterior right knee. A CBC, BUN, glucose and electrolytes, urinalysis, ECG, and radiographs of the chest and right knee were obtained. The WBC was 15,000/mm^3 with a left shift. The chest radiograph revealed a right lower lobe infiltrate, and the knee radiograph was reported as "negative for fractures."

The emergency physician must frequently evaluate a patient with a painful, swollen joint. Clinically distinguishing between the multiple disease processes that can lead to this condition is typically difficult or impossible. Frequently, however, a diseased joint has an increased amount of synovial fluid that can be easily withdrawn and analyzed. Such analysis may be invaluable in making a definitive diagnosis. Several of the most commonly affected joints (knee, wrist, and ankle) are amenable to arthrocentesis by the emergency physician. This section reviews the various tests that can be performed on the synovial fluid obtained.

Joint Fluid Aspiration Technique

The aspiration of fluid from a joint effusion can be performed in the ED by the emergency physician with a minimum of equipment and preparation. The approach to the most commonly affected joints can be learned with a little practice. Roberts and Hedges[116] present a clear, concise guide to the most commonly aspirated joints in the ED. Before performing the procedure, the emergency physician must insure that the following collecting tubes and culture media are available: red-topped (plain and sterile), lavender-topped (EDTA), and green-topped (sodium heparin) tubes for joint fluid samples and Thayer-Martin agar for gonococcal culture. This equipment must be available at the patient's bedside before beginning the procedure so that any fluid obtained can be fully analysed and the patient will not have to undergo a second aspiration procedure solely to obtain more fluid for a test that was neglected or forgotten the first time.

Arthrocentesis is usually a safe procedure, however several conditions can make the procedure hazardous.[116] The only absolute contraindication to arthrocentesis is infected, overlying skin and soft tissues. Performing arthrocentesis under these conditions risks transferring infection into the joint space. The presence of bacteremia is a relative contraindication, since a traumatic tap again risks introducing bacteria into the joint space. A coagulopathy is also considered a relative contraindication, but many clinicians therapeutically remove the blood from a tense, hemorrhagic effusion in a patient with hemophilia.

There are three broad categories for completely analyzing joint fluid: gross analysis, microscopic analysis, and chemical analysis.

Gross Analysis

The gross analysis of joint fluid includes the volume, color, clarity, and viscosity of the fluid and its ability to form a mucin clot.

The purpose of this gross analysis is to assign samples to one of five groups[117]: normal, noninflammatory, inflammatory, purulent, and hemorrhagic. This classification does not often lead to a specific diagnosis but does serve to limit the differential diagnosis and guide the further testing that will be done on the sample.

Volume

All joints contain some synovial fluid. Although it is impossible to withdraw normal synovial fluid from a small joint such as the great toe metatarsal-phalangeal joint, at least several drops of fluid may be obtained from a normal knee joint (the largest joint in the body). A large effusion may contain more than 100 mL of fluid.[118]

Color

Normal synovial fluid is colorless. An inflammatory fluid is xanthochromic from the breakdown of small amounts of heme pigment, whereas the presence of large numbers of leukocytes makes the fluid white. Bacterial infections also may impart characteristic colors to the fluid: *S. aureus* can impart a golden color, *Pseudomonas* a greenish tinge, and *Serratia* a reddish hue. A hemorrhagic effusion is red, but may appear to be bloodier than it actually is, unless a hematocrit is measured to establish the amount of blood in each sample. A very small amount of blood introduced by a traumatic tap also makes the joint fluid appear to be grossly bloody.

Clarity

Normal joint fluid is perfectly clear. The presence of cells in the fluid causes an inflammatory fluid to be translucent and a purulent or hemorrhagic fluid to be opaque.

Viscosity

Synovial fluid lubricates the joint during motion. The fluid contains hyaluronic acid, a glycosaminoglycan polymer which makes the fluid highly viscous. The viscosity of a sample can be estimated by measuring the distance that the fluid strings out before forming a drop when the fluid is transferred from one container to another. A highly viscous synovial fluid sample (similar to thick motor oil) can string out to 10 cm before forming a droplet. Normal and noninflammatory fluids have high viscosity. In contrast, the hyaluronic acid is degraded in inflammatory and purulent fluid and the viscosity is significantly decreased, causing the sample to form droplets like water.

Mucin Clot

The mucin clot is formed when the synovial fluid is mixed with several drops of glacial acetic acid. Intact hyaluronate forms a thick, white precipitate that holds together when shaken. Inflammatory and purulent fluids form a poor mucin clot which breaks into small particles when shaken.

Microscopic Analysis

Cells

Synovial fluid should always be submitted for cell count and differential WBC determination. Even if only a small sample of fluid is available, a single drop can be examined by wet prep for an estimate of WBCs and RBCs and this same slide can then be examined under polarized light for crystals (see below). The RBC count or hematocrit of the sample is a useful test to distinguish between pure blood and blood mixed with synovial fluid. The absolute WBC count, the percentage of PMN leukocytes, and the gross analysis of the fluid help further classify the sample into one of the major diagnostic groups (Table 16–1).

Shmerling et al.[119] determined the WBC count and differential on 100 synovial fluid samples obtained from patients who had the definitive diagnosis determined independently of the fluid results. The authors found that WBC counts greater than 2000/mm^3 effectively distinguished an inflammatory from a noninflammatory fluid (sensitivity, 0.84; specificity 0.84). The percentage of neutrophils greater than 75% also separated inflammatory from noninflammatory fluid (sensitivity, 0.75; specificity, 0.92).

Distinguishing septic from other inflammatory fluids, however, is more problematic using the WBC count and differential. Traditionally, a level of 50,000 cells/mm^3 has been used as a cut off for presumed septic arthritis[117] and studies have supported this view. Krey and Bailen[120] found that 70% of their patients with septic arthritis had a synovial fluid WBC greater than 50,000/mm^3. Similarly, Shmerling et al.[119] reported a median WBC of 60,500/mm^3 in their patients with septic arthritis; however, only 60% had counts above 50,000. More recently McCutchan and Fisher[121] reported that 68% of their patients with septic arthritis had WBCs below 50,000 cells/mm^3 and the median count was only 28,000 cells/mm.^{3} These findings suggest that even fluid that would be classified as "mildly inflammatory" by the above criteria should be evaluated for infection with glucose determinations, Gram stain, and culture, especially if infection is suspected clinically (such as in a patient with fever, elevated peripheral white blood count, immunocompromise, etc.).

Several factors may contribute to a relatively low synovial fluid WBC in septic arthritis, including underlying malignancy, steroid use, or an immunocompromised

Table 16–1. Analysis of Synovial Fluid

		Noninflammatory		Inflammatory			
Test Criteria	Normal	Degenerative Joint Disease	Traumatic Arthritis	Acute Gout	Acute Pseudogout	Rheumatoid/ Seronegative Arthritis	Purulent
Color	Colorless	Colorless	Xanthochromic/ bloody	Xanthochromic to white	Xanthochromic to white	Xanthochromic to white	White to cream colored
Clarity	Clear	Clear	Clear to opaque	Translucent to opaque	Translucent to opaque	Translucent to opaque	Opaque
Viscosity	High	High		Low	Low	Low	Very low
Mucin clot	Good	Fair/Good	Fair/Good	Fair/Poor	Fair/Poor	Fair/Poor	Poor
Leukocytes/mm^3	<200	<4,000	<4,000	2,000–50,000	2,000–50,000	2,000–50,000	5,000–50,000
% PMN's	<25%	<25%	<25%	>75%	>75%	50%–75%	>75%
Synovial glucose as % of serum glucose	95%–100%	95%–100%	95%–100%	80%–100%	80%–100%	~ 75%	<50%–100%
Crystals	None	None	(May contain fat droplets)	Needle shaped; negatively birefringent crystals	Rhomboid shaped; positively birefringent crystals	None	None

Data from Roberts JR, Hedges JR: Clinical procedures in emergency medicine, ed 2, Philadelphia, 1991, WB Saunders; and McCarty DJ: Arthritis and allied conditions, ed 12, Philadelphia, 1993, Lea and Febiger.

state.[121] Krey and Bailen[120] found large increases in synovial fluid WBC counts when the joints were retapped after a period of time, suggesting that early in the course of septic arthritis, WBC counts may be misleadingly low or that the immobility of a painful joint may allow the white cells to sediment in the joint and not be aspirated. The authors recommend that an attempt be made to mix the joint fluid within the joint before aspiration.[120]

Examination for Crystals

All inflammatory and purulent fluids should be examined for the presence of crystals. The finding of monosodium urate crystals (MSU) or calcium pyrophosphate dihydrate (CPPD) crystals virtually establishes the clinical diagnosis of acute gouty arthritis or pseudogout respectively, allowing the patient to be started on specific therapy and possibly avoiding an admission to the hospital for clinically suspected septic arthritis. Other crystalline or birefringent material besides MSU and CPPD can be found on examination. This material is either artifactual or contains crystals that only rarely cause symptoms of acute arthritis and is discussed only briefly.

The emergency physician can evaluate synovial fluid samples for the presence of crystals with the use of a polarizing microscope. Ideally, a well-equipped ED lab should have a polarizing microscope to enable the emergency physician to evaluate synovial fluid samples for crystals 24 hours a day. The number of crystals that can be identified in a sample declines with time.[122]

Crystalline material, especially MSU, can be seen with a regular-light microscope but definite identification is much easier with the use of a polarizing microscope. The polarizing microscope uses two polarizing filters and a red compensator filter. The lower polarizing filter is situated below the condenser and allows light to pass through only in parallel planes. The upper filter, called the analyzing filter is located above the objective lens and is rotated 90° with respect to the lower filter. When these filters are in place, no light can pass through the microscope and the field appears black. A sample containing birefringent crystals placed on the microscope stage is able to change the direction of the plane of polarized light passing through the polarizing filter and thereby allow some light to pass through the analyzing filter. Thus, the birefringent crystals appear white on a black background.

Additional information about the sample crystals can be obtained by using a first-order red compensator between the polarizing and the analyzing filter. This filter is marked with a line indicating the direction of the slow vibration. This line is marked with a "Z" or the Greek letter γ (gamma). With this filter in place, the field appears rose colored and birefringent crystals appear yellow or blue depending on their orientation to the z axis and whether they are positively or negatively birefringent. MSU is negatively birefringent. This means that when the long axis of the crystal is oriented parallel to the z axis of the red compensator, the crystal appears yellow in color. MSU crystals appear blue when oriented perpendicular to the z axis of the red compensator. In contrast, CPPD crystals are positively birefringent: They appear blue when viewed with their long axis parallel to the z axis of the red compensator and yellow when viewed perpendicular to the z axis.

To examine a sample of synovial fluid for birefringent crystals, the following technique should be used: Place a drop of synovial fluid on a clean microscope slide, place a coverslip on the sample and, if possible, seal the edges with clear nail polish to prevent drying of the sample and creation of crystalline artifacts; do not seal the slide if the same drop is needed for Gram stain (see next paragraph). The slide should first be scanned under low power (10×) with regular light to identify any obvious areas of interest containing WBCs or obvious crystals. These areas should be examined under high dry power (40×) using the polarizing and analyzing filters in place to identify any birefringent crystals which appear white on a black background. MSU crystals are needle like and can vary in size from barely detectable to 40 microns.[123] CPPD crystals can be needle like or rhomboidal and sometimes only weakly birefringent. Any crystals should be carefully examined with the red compensator in place and rotated to view them both parallel and perpendicular to the z axis of the filter. As noted, MSU crystals appear yellow when parallel and blue when perpendicular to the z axis, whereas CPPD crystals are blue when parallel to the z axis and yellow when perpendicular to the axis.

Gram Stain and Culture

Gram stain is one of the most important and specific tests that can be performed on synovial fluid. As noted above, even if only a small sample is obtained, one drop of fluid can be examined as a wet prep for crystals and this same drop can then be dried and fixed on the slide for Gram stain. Another drop can be sent for culture. If care is taken to avoid artifact (dirty microscope slide, contaminated staining reagents), the finding of bacteria on Gram stain is diagnostic of infection. Gram stain and culture should always be obtained on joint fluid even if another etiology is found for an inflammatory synovial fluid. Gardner and Weisman[124] reported 13 cases of pyarthrosis in patients with preexisting rheumatoid arthritis. Simultaneous gout and septic arthritis has also been reported.[125]

The most common bacterial cause of septic arthritis is *Neisseria gonorrhoeae* followed by *S. aureus.* Therefore, care should be taken to obtain cultures using Thayer-Martin culture media for *N. gonorrhoeae.* Gram-negative organisms can be found in the joint fluid of elderly patients, diabetics, and patients who use intravenous drugs. Unusual organisms, fungi, and mycobacteria are found more frequently now with the increase incidence of acquired immune deficiency syndrome (AIDS) and other immunocompromised states. The sensitivity of synovial fluid culture is low, however, and a negative result does not exclude infection.

Chemical Analysis

Glucose

A glucose determination simultaneously obtained on both the synovial sample and serum has long been advocated to help diagnose septic arthritis. Very low synovial glucose levels (50% of simultaneously obtained serum levels) have been found in patients with bacterial and tubercular arthritis. Rheumatoid arthritis may result in moderately reduced glucose levels. Shmerling, et al.[119] reported however, that when the synovial glucose level in 100 samples was analyzed, its sensitivity for distinguishing an inflammatory fluid was only 20% when a ratio of 0.75:1.00 of synovial fluid glucose to serum glucose level was used. Moreover, in their patients with septic arthritis, the serum glucose was normal in 50% of the cases. Because of these findings, the authors recommend that it is not necessary to obtain a synovial fluid glucose on routine samples.[119] If infection is considered, a synovial fluid glucose level should be sent. The diagnosis of septic arthritis should be seriously considered in cases where the synovial fluid leucocyte count is only moderately elevated, but the synovial fluid glucose is very low.

Protein

Although protein levels might be expected to be increased in inflammatory synovial fluid samples, Shmerling et al.[119] found in their study that the protein levels were constant among the various disease entities, including both inflammatory and noninflammatory joints. Therefore, like glucose levels, protein levels are not necessary or helpful in identifying the etiology.

LDH

In contrast to the recently available information downplaying the role of glucose and protein, LDH levels appear to be extremely useful in identifying an inflammatory fluid sample.[119] Using a value of >250 U/L Shmerling et al. found an 83% sensitivity and a 71% specificity for diagnosing an inflammatory arthropathy. An LDH level can be requested on a synovial fluid sample as it is routinely requested on serum, and the determination made by the regular chemistry lab of the hospital.

Other Chemical Tests

Many other chemical tests can be performed, including complement levels and various serologies, but none are used routinely on synovial fluid.

CASE 16–8 CONTINUED

The emergency physician drew blood cultures and then performed an arthrocentesis on the knee. Purulent fluid with a WBC count of 90,000/mm^3 and 90% PMN leukocytes was obtained. A Gram stain of the synovial fluid demonstrated rare gram-positive diplococci, identical in appearance to those seen on Gram stain of the patient's sputum. An orthopedic consultation was obtained in the ED and the patient was taken to the operating room for open drainage of the knee. The patient was subsequently treated in the hospital for pneumococcal pneumonia and septic arthritis with recovery of full right knee function.

Comment.— It is interesting to speculate what could have happened to this patient had the emergency physician focused his or her attention on the pneumonia and ignored or missed the knee problem. Perhaps the following scenerio might have ensued: the patient is admitted to the hospital with pneumonia. A sputum sample is obtained that shows many gram-positive diplococci. Blood cultures are obtained, the patient is placed on IV penicillin G, an ace bandage is placed on the knee. Over the next 3 days the patient continues to be febrile to 39.4° C (103° F). Initial blood cultures and sputum cultures are positive for *S. pneumoniae,* and subsequent blood cultures 3 days later are still positive for *S. pneumoniae.* When the right knee is reexamined on the fourth day, it is still swollen, warm, and quite tender and now has a tense effusion. The orthopedic surgeon who is consulted aspirates the knee joint and obtains purulent fluid. Gram stain of the joint fluid is positive for gram-positive diplococci. The patient is taken to the operating room for surgical drainage of the septic knee. The patient recovers slowly and is discharged with a painful knee that has limited function.

REFERENCES

1. Kooiker JC: Spinal puncture and cerebrospinal fluid examination. In Roberts JR, Hedges JR: *Clinical procedures in emergency medicine,* ed 2, Philadelphia 1991 WB Saunders.
2. Pinheiro JMB, Furdon S, Ochoa LF: Role of local anesthesia during lumbar puncture in neonates, *Pediatr* 91:379–382, 1993.
3. Halperin DL, Gideon K, Attias D, et al: Topical anesthesia for venous subcutaneous drug reservoir and lumbar puncture in children, *Pediatr* 84:281–284, 1989.
4. Gleason CA, Martin RJ, Anderson JV et al: Optimal position for a spinal tap in preterm infants, *Pediatr* 71:31–35, 1983.
5. Weisman LE, Merenstein GB, Steenbarger MC: The effect of lumbar puncture position in sick neonates, *Am J Dis Child* 137:1077–1079, 1983.
6. Joffe A, McCormick M, DeAngelis C: Which children with febrile seizures nedd lumbar puncture? *AJDC* 137:1153–1156, 1983.

7. Chessare JB, Berwick DM: Variations in clinical practice in the management of febrile seizures *Pediatr Emerg Care* 1:19–21, 1985.
8. Lorber J, Sunderland R: Lumbar puncture in children with convulsions associated with fever, *Lancet* 1:785–786, 1980.
9. Ciarallo LR, Rowe PC: Lumbar puncture in children with periorbital and orbital cellulitis, *J Pediatr* 122:355–359, 1993.
10. Emparanza JI, Aldamiz-Echevarria L, Perez-Yarza EG et al: Prognostic score in acute meningococcemia, *Crit Care Med* 16:168–169, 1988.
11. Baraff LJ, Bass JW, Fleischer GR et al: Practice guidelines for the management of infants and children 0 to 36 months of age with fever without source, *Pediatr* 92:1–12, 1993.
12. Marton KI, and Gean AD: The spinal tap: a new look at an old test, *Ann Intern Med* 104:840–848, 1986.
13. Shapiro ED, Nelson AH, Wald ER et al: Risk factors for development of bacterial meningitis among children with occult bacteremia, J Pediatr 109:15–19, 1986.
14. Krishna V, Liu V, Singleton AF: Should lumbar puncture be routinely performed in patients with suspected bacteremia? *J Natl Med Assoc* 75:1153–1157, 1983.
15. Fiser DH, Gober GA, Smith CE et al: Prevention of hypoxemia during lumbar puncture in infancy with preoxygenation, *Pediatr Emerg Care* 9:81–83, 1993.
16. Minns RA, Engleman HM, Stirling H: Cerebrospinal fluid pressure in pyogenic meningitis, *Arch Dis Child* 64:814–820, 1989.
17. Rennick G, Shann F, deCampo J: Cerebral herniation during bacterial meningitis in children, *Br Med J* 306:953–955, 1993.
18. Ellis RW, Strauss LC, Wiley JM et al: A simple method of estimating cerebrospinal fluid pressure during lumbar puncture, *Pediatr* 89:895–897, 1992.
19. Bailey EM, Domenico P, Burke CA: Bacterial or viral meningitis? Measuring lactate in CSF can help you know quickly, *Postgrad Med* 88:217–223, 1990.
20. Rutledge J, Benjamin D, Hood L et al: Is the CSF lactate measurement useful in the management of children with suspected bacterial meningitis? *J Pediatr* 98:20–24, 1981.
21. Conly JM, Ronald AR: Cerebrospinal fluid as a diagnostic body fluid, *Am J Med* 75:102, 1983.
22. Eross J, Silink M, Dorman D: Cerebrospinal fluid lactic acidosis in bacterial meningitis, *Arch Dis Child* 56:692–698, 1982.
23. Dula DJ, Fales W: The 'ring sign:' is it a reliable indicator for cerebrospinal fluid? *Ann Emerg Med* 222:718–720, 1993.
24. Portnoy JM, Olsen LC: Normal cerebrospinal fluid values in children: another look, *Pediatr* 75:484–487, 1985.
25. Light RW: Pleural Diseases, *Dis Mon* 38:261–331, 1992.
26. Chakko SC, Caldwell SH, Sforza PP: Treatment of congestive heart failure: its effect on pleural fluid chemistry, *Chest* 95:978–982, 1989.
27. Moskowitz H, Platt RT, Schachar R, et al: Roentgen visualization of minute pleural effusion, *Radiology* 109:33–35, 1973.
28. Light RW, MacGregor MI, Luchsinger PC, Ball WC: Pleural effusions: the diagnostic separation of transudates and exudates, *Ann Intern Med* 77:507–513, 1972.
29. Valdes I, Pose A, Suarez J, et al: Cholesterol: a useful parameter for distinguishing between pleural exudates and transudates, *Chest* 99:1097–1102, 1991.
30. Light RW, Ball WC: Glucose and amylase in pleural effusions, *JAMA*, 225:257–260, 1973.
31. Kramer MR, Cepero RJ, Pitchenik AE: High amylase in neoplasm-related pleural effusion, *Ann Intern Med* 110:567–569, 1989.
32. Halla JT, Schrohenloher RE, Volanakis JE: Immune complexes and other laboratory features of pleural effusions, *Ann Intern Med* 92:748–752, 1980.
33. Banales JL, Pineda PR, Fitzgerald JM, et al: Adenosine deaminase in the diagnosis of tuberculous pleural effusion: a report of 218 patients and review of the literature, *Chest* 99:355–357, 1991.
34. Ungerer JP, Grobler SM: Molecular forms of adenosine deaminase in pleural effusions, *Enzyme* 40:7–13, 1988.
35. Ribera E, Ocana I, et al: High levels of interferon gamma in tuberculous pleural effusions, *Chest* 93:308–311, 1988.

36. Barnes PF, Mistry SD, et al: Compartmentalization of CD4+ lymphocyte subpopulation in tuberculous pleuritis, J Immunol 142:1114–1149, 1989.
37. Tew WW, Chan CY, Kwan SY, Cheung SW, French GL: Diagnosis of tuberculous pleural effusion by the detection of tuberculostearic acid in pleural aspirates, *Chest* 100:1261–1263, 1991.
38. Light RW, Erozan YS, Ball WC: Cells in pleural fluid: their value in differential diagnosis, *Arch Intern Med* 132:854–860, 1973.
39. Bartlett JG, Gorbach SL, Thadepalli H, et al: Bacteriology of empyema, *Lancet* 1:338–340, 1974.
40. Light RW, Girard WM, Jenkinson SG, et al: Parapneumonic effusions, *Am J Med* 69:507–511, 1980.
41. Epstein DM, Kline LR, Albelda SM, Miller WT: Tuberculous pleural effusions, *Chest* 91:106–109, 1987.
42. Roper WH, Waring JJ: Primary serofibrinous pleural effusion in military personnel, *Am Rev Tuberc* 71:507–513, 1955.
43. Cowen ME, Johnston MR: Thoracic empyema: causes, diagnosis, and treatment, *Compr Ther* 16:40–45, 1990.
44. Leibowitz S, Kennedy L, Lessof MH: The tuberculin reaction in the pleural cavity and its suppression by antilymphocyte serum, *Br J Exp Pathol* 54:152–162, 1973.
45. Seibert AF, Haynes J, Middleton R, Bass JB: Tuberculous pleural effusion: twenty-year experience, *Chest* 99:883–886, 1991.
46. Bueno CE, Clemente MG, Castro BC, et al: Cytologic and bacteriologic analysis of fluid and pleural biopsy specimens with Cope's needle, *Arch Intern Med* 150:1190–1194, 1990.
47. Prakash URS, Reiman HM: Comparison of needle biopsy with cytologic analysis for the evaluation of pleural effusion: analysis of 414 cases, *Mayo Clin Proc* 60:158–164, 1985.
48. Good JT Jr, King TE, Antony VB, et al: Lupus pleuritis: clinical features and pleural fluid characteristics with special reference to pleural fluid antinuclear antibodies, *Chest* 84:714–718, 1983.
49. Root HD, Hauser CW, McKinley CR, et al: Diagnostic peritoneal lavage, *Surgery* 57:633–637, 1965.
50. Thal E, Shires G: Peritoneal lavage in blunt abdominal trauma, *Am J Surg* 125:64–70, 1973.
51. Fischer RP, Beverlin BC, Engrav LH, et al: Diagnostic peritoneal lavage. Fourteen years and 2586 patients later, *Am J Surg* 136:701, 1978.
52. Pachter HL, Hofstetter SR: Open and percutaneous paracentesis and lavage for abdominal trauma: a randomized and prospective study, *Arch Surg* 116:318, 1981.
53. Wisner DH, Chun Y, Blaisdell FW: Blunt intestinal injury—Keys to diagnosis and management, *Arch Surg* 125:1319–1323, 1990.
54. Burney RE, Mueller GL, Coon WW, Thomas EJ, Mackenzie JR: Diagnosis of isolated small bowel injury following blunt abdominal trauma, *Ann Emerg Med* 12:71–74, 1983.
55. Smedira N, Schecter WP: Blunt abdominal trauma, Emerg Med Clin North Am 7(3) Aug 1989.
56. Haftel AJ, Lev R, Mahour GH, et al: Abdominal CT scanning in pediatric blunt trauma, *Ann Emerg Med* 17:684, 1988.
57. Bowman LM, Bulas DE, et al. Blunt trauma in children: significance of peritoneal fluid, *Radiology* 178:185–188, 1991.
58. Ali J, Aprahamian C, Brown R, et al: Advanced trauma life support course: instructor manual, American College of Surgeons 111–125, 1989.
59. Appleby JP, Nagy AG: Abdominal injuries associated with the use of seatbelts, *Am J Surg* 157:457–458, 1989.
60. McCarthy MC, Gregory AL, Canal DF, Broadie TA: Prediction of injury caused by penetrating wounds to the abdomen, flank and back, *Arch Surg* 126:962–966, 1991.
61. Madden MR, Paull DE, Finkelstein JL, et al: Occult diaphragmatic injury from stab wounds to the lower chest and abdomen, *J Trauma* 29:292–298, 1989.
62. Marx JA, Moore EE, Jorden R, Eule J: Limitations of computerized tomography in the evaluation of acute abdominal trauma: a prospective comparison with diagnostic peritoneal lavage, *J Trauma* 25:933–937, 1985.

63. Davis RA, Shayne JP, Max MH, Woolfit RA, Schwab W: The use of computerized axial tomography versus peritoneal lavage in blunt abdominal trauma: a prospective study, *Surgery* 98:845–849, 1985.
64. Meyer DM, Thal ER, Weigelt JA, Redman HC: Evaluation of computerized tomography and peritoneal lavage in blunt abdominal trauma, *J Trauma* 29:1168–1172, 1989.
65. Frame SB, Browder IW, Lang EK, McSwain NE: Computed tomography versus diagnostic peritoneal lavage: usefulness in immediate diagnosis of blunt abdominal trauma, *Ann Emerg Med* 18:513–516, 1989.
66. Fabian TC, Mangiante EC, White TJ et al: A prospective study of 91 patients undergoing both computerized tomography and peritoneal lavage following blunt abdominal trauma, *J Trauma* 26:602–608, 1986.
67. Pagliarello G, Hanna SS, Gregory WD, et al: Abdominopelvic computerized tomography and open peritoneal lavage in patients with blunt abdominal trauma: a prospective study, *Can J Surg* 30:10–13, 1987.
68. Gomez GA, Alvarez R, Plasencia G, et al: Diagnostic peritoneal lavage in the management of blunt abdominal trauma: a reassessment, *J Trauma* 27:1–5, 1987.
69. Federle MP, Jeffrey RB: Hemoperitoneum studied by computed tomography.
70. Goldstein AS, Sclafani SJ, Kupferstein NH, et al: The diagnostic superiority of computerized tomography, *J Trauma* 25:938–945, 1985.
71. Federle MP: Computed tomography of blunt abdominal trauma, *Radiol Clin North Am* 21:461–475, 1983.
72. Federle MP, Goldberg HI, et al: Evaluation of abdominal trauma by computed tomography, *Radiology* 138:637–644, 1981.
73. Wing VW, Federle MP, et al: The clinical impact of CT for blunt abdominal trauma, *Am J Roentgenol* 145:1191–1194, 1985.
74. Phillips T, Sclafani SJ, Goldstein A, et al: Use of contrast-enhanced CT enema in the management of penetrating trauma to the flank and back, *J Trauma* 26:593, 1986.
75. Soderstrom C, Dupriest R: Pitfalls of peritoneal lavage in blunt abdominal trauma, *Surg Gynecol Obstet* 151:513–518, 1980.
76. Esposito TJ, Gens DR, Smith LG, Scorpio R, Buchman T: Trauma during pregnancy, *Arch Surg* 126:1073–1078, 1991.
77. Rothenberger DA, Quattlebaum FW, Zabel J, Fischer RP: Diagnostic peritoneal lavage for blunt trauma in pregnant women, *Am J Obstet Gynecol* 129:479–481, 1977.
78. Olsen WR, Redman HC, et al: Quantitative peritoneal lavage in blunt abdominal trauma, *Arch Surg* 104:536–543, 1972.
79. Engrav LH, Benjamin CI, et al: Diagnostic peritoneal lavage in blunt abdominal trauma, *J Trauma* 15:854–859, 1975.
80. Root H, Keizer P, Perry J: The clinical and experimental aspects of peritoneal responce to injury, *Arch Surg* 95:531, 1967.
81. Zappa MJ, Harwood-Nuss AL, Wears RL, Fallon WF: Objective determination of the optimal RBC count in DPL done for abdominal stab wounds, *J Emerg Med* 10:553–558, 1992.
82. Thal ER: Peritoneal lavage: reliability of RBC count in patients with stab wounds to the chest, *Arch Surg* 119:579–584, 1984.
83. Galbraith TA, Oreskovich MR, Heimbach DM, et al: The role of peritoneal lavage in the management of stab wounds to the abdomen, *Am J Surg* 140:4–6, 1980.
84. Hubbard SG, Bivans BA, Sachatello CR et al: Diagnostic errors with peritoneal lavage in patients with pelvic fractures, *Arch Surg* 114:844–847, 1979.
85. Smego DR, Richardson JD, Flint LM: Determinants of outcome in pancreatic trauma, *J Trauma* 25:771, 1985.
86. Probert WR Havard C: Traumatic diaphragmatic hernia, *Thorax* 16:99, 1961.
87. Morgan AS, Flanebaum L, Esposito T, et al: Blunt injury to the diaphragm: an analysis of 44 patients, *J Trauma* 26:565, 1986.
88. Freeman T, Fischer RP: The inadequacy of peritoneal lavage in diagnosing acute diaphragmatic injuries, *J Trauma* 16:538, 1976.
89. Parvin S, Smith DE, et al: Effectiveness of peritoneal lavage in blunt abdominal trauma, *Ann Surg* 181:255–261, 1975.
90. Rubin M, Blahd W, Stanisic TH, Meislin HW: Diagnosis of intraperitoneal extravasation of urine by peritoneal lavage, *Ann Emerg Med* 14:433–437, 1985.

91. Correia JP, Conn HO: Spontaneous bacterial peritonitis in cirrhosis: endemic or epidemic? *Med Clin North Am* 59:963–981, 1975.
92. Pinzello G, Simonetti RG, et al: Spontaneous bacterial peritonitis. A prospective investigation in predominantly nonalcoholic cirrhotic patients, *Hepatology* 3:545–549, 1983.
93. Kline MM, McCallum RW, Guth PH: The clinical value of ascitic fluid culture and leukocyte count studies in alcoholic cirrhosis, *Gastroenterology* 70:408–412, 1976.
94. Hoefs JC, Cannwati HN, et al: Spontaneous bacterial peritonitis, *Hepatology* 2:399–407, 1982.
95. Cummings D, Hoefs JC, Runyon BA: Determinants of hospital survival in patients with spontaneous bacterial peritonitis: multivariate discriminant analysis of prognostic factors, *Hepatology* 4(abstr):1071, 1984.
96. Attali P, Turner K, et al: pH of ascitic fluid: diagnostic and prognostic value in cirrhotic and noncirrhotic patients, *Gastroenterology* 90:1255–1260, 1986.
97. Conn HO, Fessel JM: Spontaneous bacterial peritonitis in cirrhosis: variations on a theme, *Medicine (Baltimore)* 50:161–197, 1971.
98. Weinstein MP, lannini PB, Stratton CW, et al: Spontaneous bacterial peritonitis, A review of 28 cases with emphasis on improved survival and factors influencing prognosis, *Am J Med* 64:592–598, 1978.
99. Runyon BA, Hoefs JC: Ascitic fluid analysis in the differentiation of spontaneous bacterial peritonitis from gastrointestinal perforation into ascitic fluid, *Hepatology* 4:447–450, 1984.
100. Stassen WN, McCullough AJ, Bacon BR, et al: Immediate diagnostic criteria for bacterial infection of ascitic fluid, *Gastroenterology* 90:1247–1254, 1986.
101. Yang CY, Liaw YF, Chu CM, Sheen IS: White count, pH and lactate in ascites in the diagnosis of spontaneous bacterial peritonitis, *Hepatology* 5:85–90, 1985.
102. Garcia-Tsao G, Conn HO, Lerner E: The diagnosis of bacterial peritonitis: comparison of pH, lactate concentration and leukocyte count, *Hepatology* 5:91–96, 1985.
103. Scemama-Clergue J, Doutrellot-Philippon C, et al: Ascitic fluid pH in alcoholic cirrhosis: a reevaluation of its use in the diagnosis of spontaneous bacterial peritonitis, *Gut* 26:332–335, 1985.
104. Runyon BA Hoefs JC: Spontaneous vs secondary bacterial peritonitis: differentiation by response of ascitic fluid neutrophil count to antimicrobial therapy, *Arch Intern Med* 146:1563–1565, 1986.
105. Runyon BA, Hoefs JC: Culture-negative neutrocytic ascites: a variant of spontaneous bacterial peritonitis, *Hepatology* 4:1209–1211, 1984.
106. Luce E. Nakagawa D, Lovell J, et al: Improvement in the bacteriologic diagnosis of peritonitis with the use of blood culture media, *Trans Am Soc Artif Intern Organs* 28:259–261, 1982.
107. Runyon BA, Hoefs JC: Ascitic fluid analysis in the differentiation of spontaneous bacterial peritonitis from gastrointestinal tract perforation into ascitic fluid, Hepatology 4:447–50, 1984.
108. Reynolds TB: Rapid presumptive diagnosis of spontaneous bacterial peritonitis (editorial), *Gastroenterology* 90:1294–1297, 1986.
109. Romeo T, Kadar N, et al: Value of culdocentesis in the diagnosis of ectopic pregnancy, *Obstet Gyecol* (4):519–522, 1985.
110. Vermesh M, Cracyzkowski JW, Sauer MV: Reevaluation of the role of culdocentesis in the management of ectopic pregnancy, *Am J Obstet Gynecol* 162(2):411–413, 1990.
111. Krol LV, Abbott JT: The current role of culdocentesis, *Am J Emerg Med* 10(4):354–357, 1992.
112. Sauer MV, Rodi IA: Utility of an algorithm to diagnose ectopic pregnancy, *Int J Gynecol Obstet* 31:29–34, 1990.
113. Braen GR: Culdocentesis. In Roberts JR, Hedges JR: *Clinical procedures in emergency medicine,* ed 2, pp. 936–941 Philadelphia, 1991, WB Saunders.
114. Cartwright PS, Vaughn P, Tuttle D: Culdocentesis and ectopic pregnancy, *J Reprod Med* 29:88, 1984.
115. Abbott J, Emmans LS, Lowenstein SR: Ectopic pregnancy: ten common pitfalls in diagnosis, *Am J Emerg Med* 8(6), 515–522, 1990.
116. Ezell SL, Kobernick ME, Benjamin GC: Arthrocentesis. In Roberts JR, Hedges JR: *Clinical procedures in emergency medicine,* ed 2, pp. 847–859 Philadelphia, 1991, WB Saunders.

117. McCarty DJ: *Arthritis and Allied Conditions,* ed 12, Philadelphia, 1993, Lea and Febiger.
118. Resnick D, Niwayama G: *Diagnosis of Bone and Joint Disorders,* ed 2, Philadelphia, 1988, WB Saunders.
119. Shmerling, et al: Synovial fluid tests; what should be ordered, *JAMA* 264(8):1009–1014, 1990.
120. Krey PR, Bailen DA: Synovial fluid leukocytosis: a study of extremes, *Am J Med* 67:436–442, 1979.
121. McCutchan HJ, Fisher RC: Synovial leukocytosis is infectious arthritis, *Clin Orthrop* 257:226–230, 1990.
122. Kerolous G, et al: Is it mandatory to examine synovial fluids promptly after arthrocentesis? *Arthritis Rheum* 32:271, 1989.
123. Gatter RA, Schumacher HR: *A practical handbook of joint fluid analysis,* ed 2, Philadelphia, 1991, Lea and Febiger.
124. Gardner GC, Weisman MH: Pyarthrosis in patients with rheumatoid arthritis, *Am J Med* 88:503–511, 1990.
125. Hamilton ME, et al: Simultaneous gout and pyarthrosis, *Arch Int Med* 140:917, 1980.

Chapter 17

Evaluating the Random Needlestick—AIDS and Hepatitis

Karen N. Hansen, M.D.

Gabor D. Kelen, M.D.

CASE 17–1

During a busy evening shift in an inner-city emergency department (ED), a female nursing assistant sustained a needlestick injury while attempting to recap a bloody needle. The source of the exposure was a cachectic-appearing white male who had apparent needle tracks from intravenous drug use. The incident occurred during attempted resuscitation of this patient, who sustained a cardiopulmonary arrest and died. The exposed nursing assistant was anxious but rational. The wound was a small puncture to her left index finger that bled slightly. Her most recent tetanus vaccination had been 3 years before. She had been given the last of her full three doses of recombinant hepatitis B vaccine a year ago but had never had her antibody status checked. She thought that she might be pregnant and was wondering whether she needed to start zidovudine (AZT, azidothymidine) therapy.

MANAGEMENT OF CASE

Following a percutaneous exposure, routine wound care and tetanus prophylaxis should be addressed. This exposed health care worker (HCW) had adequate tetanus immunity by history. Her wound should be well irrigated with water or saline.

The source should be tested for HIV if possible. In this case the source has died. Specific laws regarding consent for diagnostic serologic testing, especially for human immunodeficiency virus (HIV) vary by region. Even in the case of a deceased patient, the law may still require written consent from the next of kin in order to obtain an HIV test. If an autopsy is to be performed, additional information concerning exposure risks to the HCW may be available through direct communication with the medical examiner (see Chapter 23).

If it is not possible to test the source, management of the exposed HCW should proceed as though this high-risk source were known to be HIV positive. The exposed HCW should be tested for HIV soon after the exposure and then 6 weeks, 12 weeks, 6 months, and (if desired) 1 year later. She should be counseled to follow Public Health Service (PHS) guidelines to prevent HIV transmission in the unlikely event that she should seroconvert. She should be reassured that her risk for contracting HIV infection is low, but she needs to understand that it is not zero.

A pregnancy test should be done. If negative, possible use of prophylactic zidovudine should be discussed with the exposed HCW, and she should be informed about its potential risks and benefits. If the HCW is pregnant, zidovudine is not recommended.

The source should be tested for hepatitis B surface antigen (HBsAg) if possible. If this is not possible, this particular patient can be assumed to have been at high risk for infection. The exposed HCW should have her anti-HBsAg titer checked. If it is inadequate and the source tests positive for HBsAg (or his status cannot be determined), the exposed HCW should receive hepatitis B immune globulin (HBIG) and one hepatitis B vaccine booster dose.

Immune globulin (IG) administration for hepatitis C virus (HCV) prophylaxis is currently recommended if a source is known to have HCV or chronic non-A, non-B hepatitis. In this case, the source would have been at high risk for harboring HCV, and administration of IG may be of benefit. The source should be tested for HCV if possible because knowledge of a positive test will alert the HCW to the increased possibility for transmission. Treatment with IG need not depend on the results of this test, however, because a negative test for HCV does not rule out the presence of infection.

Follow-up in 48 to 72 hours should be arranged with the hospital's occupational health or employee health service. At this time, HIV, hepatitis B virus (HBV), and possibly HCV serologies can be checked, the HCW will receive appropriate HBV prophylaxis as warranted, and the need to continue zidovudine therapy, if initiated, can be discussed. In addition, psychological support and follow-up counseling should be available to the HCW as needed.

HISTORICAL BACKGROUND

Throughout the history of medicine, HCWs have been at risk for acquiring the infectious diseases of the patients whom they treat. However, by the second half of this century many previously common transmissible diseases had been in such decline that members of the health care community developed a sense of personal invulnerability to the diseases they were treating. This sense of security has eroded considerably since the first reports of occupationally acquired HIV.

Increasing attention is now being given to HCW risk for occupationally acquired infectious disease. HIV and hepatitis B and C viruses remain the primary concern, although a number of other infectious agents, including herpes simplex, varicella zoster, Epstein-Barr virus, cytomegalovirus, rubella, *Mycobacterium tuberculosis* (TB), *Neisseria meningitidis,* and *Salmonella,* may also be occupationally acquired. Of concern is the recent increase in TB infection, including multidrug-resistant strains, among HIV-infected patients and other groups.[1] However, TB is not known to be transmitted by needlestick. This chapter will specifically address HIV and hepatitis B and C risk to the HCW with a known or suspected needlestick exposure.

HUMAN IMMUNODEFICIENCY VIRUS

Epidemiology

Over 230,000 U.S. cases of acquired immunodeficiency syndrome (AIDS) have been reported to the Centers for Disease Control (CDC) since the disease was recognized, although most estimates now place the total number of HIV-infected persons (including those in whom an AIDS-defining illness has not yet developed) as well over 1 million.[2] Although the originally described cases of AIDS occurred almost exclusively among males who were either homosexual or intravenous drug users living in New York or California, recent data show dissemination of the epidemic to virtually all sectors of the population and all areas of the country.[3] Rates of reported AIDS cases are now increasing most rapidly among groups not previously felt to be at high risk: women and individuals whose only risk is possible heterosexual contact.[3]

In EDs, HIV serostatus cannot be reliably predicted on the basis of characteristics of age, race, sex, or clinical symptoms.[4] Although rates of HIV infection among ED patients may be higher in certain groups (e.g., young black males and those with identified risk), rates are significant across all demographic sectors, including those without risk factors.[4] Background rates of HIV among ED patient populations vary considerably. Inner-city EDs, specifically those on the East or West Coast, may see HIV seropositivity rates of 5% to 9% or greater.[5, 6] Rates in rural and suburban areas appear to be lower, possibly between 0.4% and 7%, but are likely increasing.[6, 7] All ED HCWs should assume that some of the patients they treat are HIV-positive, regardless of the site of practice or general patient demographics.

Questioning patients about their HIV status or risk factors has limited value when attempting to assess the potential risk to HCWs. In a series of serosurveys conducted in our inner-city ED, a large proportion of patients testing positive for HIV were themselves unaware of the infection.[4] Although most cases of HIV infection occur among patients with identified risk factors, a lack of risk factors for HIV does not rule out the possibility of infection. This was shown by one study in which rigorous risk factor assessment failed to identify 27% of those with unrecognized infection.[4] Even among patients who state that they have previously tested HIV negative, rates may be surprisingly high.[4]

Health Care Worker Risk

Because the proportion of AIDS patients who are HCWs (5.4%) is similar to that of the general population (5.7%),[8] it has been concluded that occupational transmission of HIV is not a major mode of spread into the health care community. However, HCWs with AIDS are more likely than other AIDS patients to lack identifiable risk factors for the disease (5.3% vs. 2.8%),[8] which leads to speculation that at least some of these individuals may have occupationally acquired infections.

The magnitude of the risk for occupational acquisition of HIV following an exposure to infected blood or body fluids and the factors contributing to this risk can be ascertained from documented case reports and surveillance studies. As of September 1993, the CDC[9] has reported only 39 documented cases of seroconversion among U.S. HCWs following occupational exposure to HIV-infected blood, bloody fluid, or concentrated virus. There are an additional 81 HIV-infected HCWs without other risk factors who have reported occupational exposures to blood or body fluids for whom seroconversion could not be documented. [9] Nearly all cases of documented seroconversion in exposed HCWs have occurred following percutaneous, mucous membrane, or nonintact skin exposure.[9, 10] Most (35/39, 90%) resulted from percutaneous injuries, primarily needlesticks.[9, 10]

There are numerous ongoing prospective surveillance studies of HCWs who have had percutaneous, mucous membrane, or cutaneous exposures to HIV-infected blood or bloody body fluids.[11, 12] Metaanalysis of these studies indicates the risk of HIV transmission following a single contaminated needlestick injury to be approximately 0.3% (6 of 1948 HCWs with 2042 total exposures).[11] No case of seroconversion has occurred among 668 HCWs who have been followed *prospectively* after sustaining a total of 1051 mucous membrane exposures or among 559 HCWs followed after a total of 2712 cutaneous exposures.[11]

Although the estimated rate of seroconversion following exposure may seem comfortingly low, there are reasons to believe that it may not accurately reflect the true risk. Follow-up for some patients reported in the surveillance studies may have been incomplete. Also, studies have documented that a significant number of HCWs, particularly physicians, fail to report their exposures[13, 14] and would therefore be missed in reporting surveillance data. Finally, individual events do not reflect a cumulative career risk. Wears et al.[15] have estimated the cumulative risk for an emergency physician practicing in a high prevalence area for 30 years to be as high as 1.4%.

Type of Exposure

Although HIV has been cultured from a wide variety of body fluids, documented HCW seroconversion has thus far only occurred following exposure to blood, bloody pleural fluid, or concentrated virus.[9, 10, 16] Transmission of HIV in nonclinical settings has occurred following exposure to semen,[17] vaginal secretions,[18] and transplanted organs and tissues,[19] all of which may be potential sources in health care settings as well. Because the risk of HIV transmission following exposure to nonbloody pleural fluid, peritoneal fluid, pericardial fluid, cerebrospinal fluid (CSF), synovial fluid, or amniotic fluid has not yet been determined, these should also be considered potential sources of infection.[10] Body fluids believed *not* to pose a risk for HIV transmission to the HCW include saliva, sputum, urine, vomitus, and feces.[10] However, in the relatively uncontrolled ED setting, the unanticipated presence of blood in any of these fluids may still place the HCW at risk.[10]

It has been suggested that an exposure involving a deep needlestick or a significant volume of injected blood would be more likely to result in the transmission of HIV. Theoretically, transmission would be more likely to occur with a larger viral inoculum. A higher concentration of viral particles is likely to be present in blood from HIV-positive patients who are symptomatic, particularly if untreated, than in patients who are asymptomatic or treated with AZT.[20] The relative contributions of these factors have not been defined, but it is also clear that seroconversion has occasionally occurred following apparently superficial needlesticks and without obvious injection of blood.[10, 16, 21]

Testing

There are four principal methods of testing for the presence of HIV infection: detection of antibody to HIV, viral culture, polymerase chain reaction (PCR) amplification of viral DNA or RNA, and detection of HIV-specific antigens. Viral culture and PCR are both currently too labor-intensive for routine use but are useful research tools. In certain cases PCR has been found to be positive before antibody seroconversion[22] and may therefore play a future role in early detection. Detection of viral p24 antigen can be a helpful guide for clinicians directing therapy of HIV-positive patients.[23] Although p24 antigen has been detectable in sera from some patients with early acute HIV infections,[24, 25] it is undetectable in 70% to 80% of asymptomatic HIV-positive patients and is therefore unsuitable as a screening test.[23, 26] At present, testing for antibodies to HIV remains the standard.

Testing for HIV antibodies generally employs an initial screening test, the enzyme-linked immunosorbent assay (ELISA). If repeatedly positive this will be followed by a confirmatory test, the Western blot (WB), or less commonly, indirect immunofluorescence assay (IFA). Each of these tests can be done on serum taken from a plain "red-topped" or "clotted" tube.

The ELISA tests for HIV antibodies by incubating patient serum with HIV antigens that are attached to a solid phase such as a microtiter plate well. The well is then washed, but any HIV antibodies will remain bound to the plate. Next, enzymatically labeled antibodies specific for human IgG are added to the wells. These will bind to the patient's HIV antibodies if present. In the final step, a substrate capable of changing color in the presence of the bound enzyme is added to the well, and the amount of color change is recorded as an optical density value. If a given sample produces a color change greater than a predetermined "cutoff" value, it will be read as a positive sample. Currently licensed ELISA preparations have been shown to have a minimum sensitivity of 99.0% to 99.5%[23, 27] and a specificity of approximately 99.8% if each initially reactive ELISA is repeated.[27] Reasons for a false positive ELISA include cross-reactive antibodies, autoreactive antibodies, heat inactivation of sera, severe hepatic disease, passive IgG administration, and certain malignancies.[23] Reasons for a false negative ELISA include B-cell dysfunction, hypogammaglobulinemia, and testing an infected individual before seroconversion.[23]

WB confirmation is reserved for sera repeatedly positive by ELISA because it has been shown to have an unacceptably high rate of falsely "indeterminate" results if used alone as a screen.[27] The WB is performed by incubating patient serum with a membrane strip containing separated HIV proteins. After washing the membrane, enzyme-linked (or radiolabeled) antibodies specific for human IgG are added, which can then be detected by colorimetric assay (or autoradiography). The resulting banding pattern is used to determine which HIV antigens were bound by antibodies from patient serum. WB scoring can be somewhat subjective[28] and depends on the number and combination of bands present that correspond to known HIV antigens. A test may have a positive, negative, or indeterminate result. An indeterminate test should be repeated. Retesting after 3 to 6 months may be considered for patients who have confirmed indeterminate WB or negative WB or ELISA results following an initially positive ELISA.[23] Patients without risk factors who remain WB indeterminate over a period of time are unlikely to be infected with HIV.[29] It is estimated that the sensitivity of WB is 96% or greater,[30] the specificity is 99.4%,[27] and the positive predictive value of the ELISA with WB confirmation is over 99%.[31]

IFA is sometimes used as a confirmatory test because it is rapid and accurate and requires less technical skill than the WB to perform. In this procedure HIV-infected cells are fixed on a slide. Patient serum is incubated with the cells to allow any anti-HIV antibodies to bind. The slide is washed and then incubated with fluorescent antibodies specific for human IgG. The slide is then viewed under a microscope and scored against positive and negative controls for the presence of fluorescent cells.

Although the available serologic tests for HIV are generally reliable, patients who have recently contracted the virus will test negative before the development of detectable levels of antibody. Antibodies to HIV can usually be detected about 6 to 12 weeks following infection[12] but may take longer.[32] It has been estimated that 95% of individuals who seroconvert following an exposure will do so within 6 months.[33] Although PCR,[22] p24 antigen,[24, 25] or viral culture[24 25] might be positive for some patients during this "window" period, no routinely available test can detect this state.

Several recently developed methods of HIV antibody testing may prove clinically useful in the future. Rapid ELISA-based HIV screening tests have been developed that produce results in approximately 10 minutes and have been shown to be quite accurate.[34] The use of rapid testing in the ED setting could be helpful in certain circumstances but would require extensive pretest and posttest counseling, patient consent, and strict confidentiality. Results would also require traditional ELISA and WB confirmation. ELISA-based tests for HIV antibodies in urine and saliva are currently under investigation and are achieving increasing accuracy.[35, 36] Although such tests may prove most helpful for population seroprevalence monitoring, it is possible that they will also become useful as clinical screening tools. Urine or salivary HIV tests would require the same counseling, consent, confidentiality, and confirmation as HIV tests performed on serum.

Management of Exposures

When an HCW sustains an occupational exposure to potentially infectious fluid, the HIV status of the source and the exposed HCW should be determined (Fig. 17–1). All testing should be done with the individual's consent, with confidentiality assured, and with appropriate pretest and posttest counseling. Testing practices must conform to all applicable federal, state, and local laws. If the source refuses testing or is unidentified, management strategy should be guided by the likelihood that this individual might harbor HIV based on risk factor analysis and the local prevalence of HIV. If the source tests HIV negative but is known to be at high risk for infection, the possibility that this patient is infected but has not yet seroconverted should be considered. Any HCW sustaining a significant exposure from a source who is HIV positive or whose status is undetermined but considered to be at risk for HIV should be tested at the time of exposure and at intervals of 6 weeks, 12 weeks, 6 months,[10] and if desired, 1 year later.[37] The exposed individual should be counseled to follow the guidelines recommended by the PHS for prevention of transmission of HIV,[38] including the practice of "safe sex" and avoidance of blood, semen, or organ donation. Women should be counseled to discontinue breast-feeding and to delay pregnancy until shown to be HIV negative at 6 months' follow-up. To date, all HCWs who have seroconverted following a documented exposure have done so within 6 months of the incident.[39] HIV-exposed HCWs can be entered into an ongoing nationwide surveillance study by calling the CDC at (404) 639–1547.

Data regarding the efficacy of AZT for prophylaxis after occupational exposure to HIV are inadequate, although several cases of failure of AZT to prevent seroconversion in significantly exposed individuals have appeared in the literature.[40–42] Because seroconversion following occupational exposure is a relatively rare event, thousands of subjects would be required in each arm of a prospective trial in order to prove or disprove the efficacy of prophylactic AZT.[39] We may therefore never know whether it is truly helpful. The potential use of AZT should be discussed with HCWs sustaining significant exposures to blood or other potentially infectious fluid from sources who are known or suspected to be HIV positive. The exposed HCW should be allowed to make an informed decision after receiving counseling regarding the potential risks and benefits of AZT treatment, taking into account the type and magnitude of their exposure. Because the human teratogenicity of AZT is unknown,[43] its use in pregnancy is not recommended. Data from animal studies suggest that retrovirus prophylaxis is most effective if administered within hours of an exposure.[43] Therefore, if treatment is chosen, it should be started immediately. The recommended dose is 200 mg, five to six times a day for 4 to 6 weeks.[43, 44]

HEPATITIS B

Epidemiology

An estimated 1 million Americans are carriers of HBV, and approximately 300,000 people are newly infected with HBV each year.[45] The failure of HBV rates to decline rapidly following the introduction of an effective vaccine is due mainly to failure of vaccination programs targeted for individuals (particularly intravenous drug users) at risk.[46] A recent study of our inner-city ED patient population revealed more than 5% to be actively infected with HBV as indicated by the presence of HBsAg.[47]

HCW Risk

Hepatitis continues to be a significant risk for HCWs. Each year approximately 12,000 HCWs become infected with HBV, 700 to 1200 of whom become chronic carri-

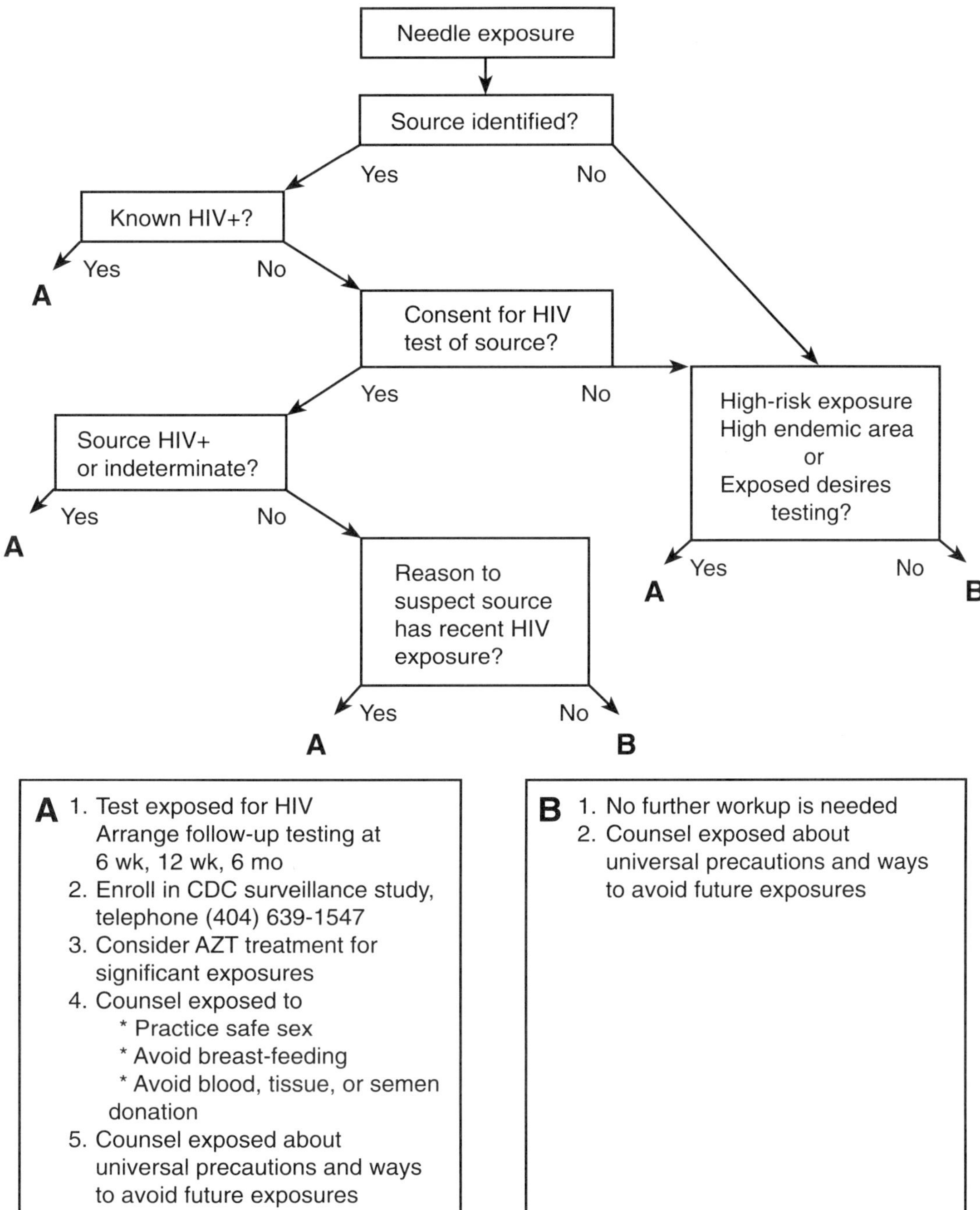

Fig. 17–1. Decision tree for needlestick exposure: human immunodeficiency virus *(HIV)* testing. *CDC,* Centers for Disease Control; *AZT,* zidovudine (azidothymidine).

ers and approximately 250 of whom die of complications of their disease.[10] At present, the threat of HBV to HCWs remains significantly greater than that of HIV since the number of HCWs who die each year of occupationally acquired HBV is many times greater than the number of HCWs known to acquire HIV. In contrast to HIV, the rate of transmission of HBV to a nonimmunized HCW following a percutaneous exposure may be as high as 30%[10] and apparently requires only minute quantities of blood or infectious fluid.[48] As with HIV, the body fluids felt to pose a risk for HBV transmission to HCWs are blood or any bloody fluid, semen, vaginal secretions, pleural fluid, peritoneal fluid, pericardial fluid, CSF, synovial fluid, and amniotic fluid.[10] In addition, HBV transmission has been documented following human bites, and animal research suggests that parenteral exposure to HBV-infected saliva may result in transmission.[10] Therefore, a bite or parenteral exposure to saliva from an HBV-infected person should also be treated as a potential exposure.

Testing

A number of reliable serologic tests have been developed to detect HBV infection and immunity status (Table 17–1 and 17–2). Each of these tests can be done on serum taken from a plain "red-topped" or "clotted" tube. The presence of HBsAg represents active infection, either acute or chronic, and thus indicates risk for an exposed HCW. HBsAg is detected by using either an ELISA similar to that used for HIV or a radioimmunoassay (RIA). Both tests are performed by using a solid phase with attached HBs antibodies to which a sample of patient serum is added. Any HBsAg present in the serum will be bound to the antibody complex. Enzyme-labeled (or radiolabeled) anti-HBs is then added to create an antibody-antigen-antibody "sandwich"

Table 17–1. Hepatitis B Virus Serologic Markers

Serologic Marker	Abbreviation	Significance/Comments
Hepatitis B surface antigen	HBsAg	Detected early in the course of HBV infection. Disappears with resolution of infection but remains detectable in patients with chronic infection. Presence of HBsAg in serum indicates presence of viral particles and therefore infectivity
Hepatitis B e antigen	HBeAg	Antigen closely associated with HBV nucleocapsid. A high serum titer of HBeAg correlates with HBV replication and infectivity
Hepatitis B core antigen	HBcAg	Commercial test not currently available
Antibody to HBsAg	Anti-HBs	Appears at resolution of HBV infection, after the disappearance of HBsAg. Indicates immunity to HBV either through prior resolved infection or vaccination
Antibody to HBeAg	Anti-HBe	Presence in the serum of an HBsAg-positive patient indicates a lower level of infectivity
Antibody to HBcAg	Anti-HBc	Indicates current or prior infection. Appearance of IgM anti-HBc occurs at the onset of clinical symptoms and correlates with the appearance of liver function abnormalities. Later IgM is replaced by IgG anti-HBc, which persists for life. Anti-HBc is detectable in the window period between the disappearance of HBsAg and the appearance of anti-HBs

Table 17–2. Test Comparison Chart

Test*	Sensitivity	Specificity	Complexity	Time	Cost
HIV: ELISA	++++ (99.0%–99.5%)	++++ (99.8%)	++	Days	$40-65
HIV: WB	+++ (96%)	++++ (99.4%)	++++	Days	$90–160
HBV: HBsAg (ELISA or RIA)	++++	++++	++	Days	$15–65
HBV: anti-HBs (ELISA or RIA)	++++	++++	++	Days	$15–65
HCV: anti-HCV	Unknown	Unknown	++	Days	$25-112

**HIV,* human immunodeficiency virus; *ELISA,* enzyme-linked immunosorbent assay; *WB,* Western blot; *HBV,* hepatitis B virus; *HBsAg,* hepatitis B surface antigen; *RIA,* radioimmunoassay, *HCV,* hepatitis C virus.

that is detectable by means of a measurable color change (or the presence of radioactivity). The number of such complexes can be quantified and correlates with the concentration of HbsAg in the serum.

The presence of HBs antibody indicates immunity to HBV, acquired either through prior resolved infection or immunization. Antibodies directed against hepatitis B core antigen (HBcAg) develop early in the course of HBV infection, generally persist for life, and indicate either current or prior infection. The presence of anti-HBc indicates natural exposure because immunization does not result in the development of anti-HBc. Anti-HBs and anti-HBc antibodies are detected by ELISA or RIA with the "sandwich" method similar to that described above.

Management of Exposures

The need for HBV prophylaxis following an exposure is based on knowledge of the immunity status of the exposed HCW and the infectivity of the source (Fig. 17–2). If the exposed HCW has been vaccinated and is known to have had an adequate anti-HBsAg titer within the past 2 years, no treatment is needed.[45] Likewise, if the source of the exposure tests negative for HBsAg, no further treatment is needed. If the exposed HCW has been fully or partially vaccinated and the antibody response is unknown or has not been tested within 2 years, a serum sample should be sent for anti-HBsAg titer. All HCWs exposed to an HBsAg-positive source and who have an inadequate antibody response or have never been vaccinated require the administration of HBIG and one dose of hepatitis B vaccine.[45] In all situations, HCWs who have not received or completed HBV vaccine should be encouraged to do so.

Hepatitis B Virus

All HCWs at risk for occupational exposure should receive hepatitis B vaccine. The currently licensed recombinant vaccine consists of HBsAg that has been produced in common baker's yeast; it therefore conveys no risk of HBV, HIV, or other infection[46] and is considered safe for use in pregnant women.[46] Following three doses of deltoid intramuscular vaccine, more than 90% of healthy adults mount an adequate antibody response[49] that imparts virtually complete protection against HBV infection.[49]

HEPATITIS C

Epidemiology and Risk

HCV is now recognized to be the major etiologic agent of non-A, non-B hepatitis.[50] It has recently been cloned,[51] and an assay for anti-HCV antibodies has been developed.[52] In a recent study in our inner-city ED, the rate of HCV infection among ED patients was found to be extraordinarily high. Anti-HCV antibodies were detected in 18% of all patients, 51% of all black males between 35 and 44 years of age, and 83% of all intravenous drug users.[47] The risk of occupational acquisition of HCV for HCWs is unknown, although cases of documented transmission have been reported.[53, 54]

Testing

Testing for antibodies to HCV employs the same immunologic techniques used for HIV and HBV. HCV antigens cloned in yeast are bound to a solid phase for use in an ELISA or similar test to detect anti-HCV antibodies.[52] Blood drawn for HCV testing should be sent in a "red-topped" or "clotted" tube.

The currently available HCV tests are imperfect because the development of anti-

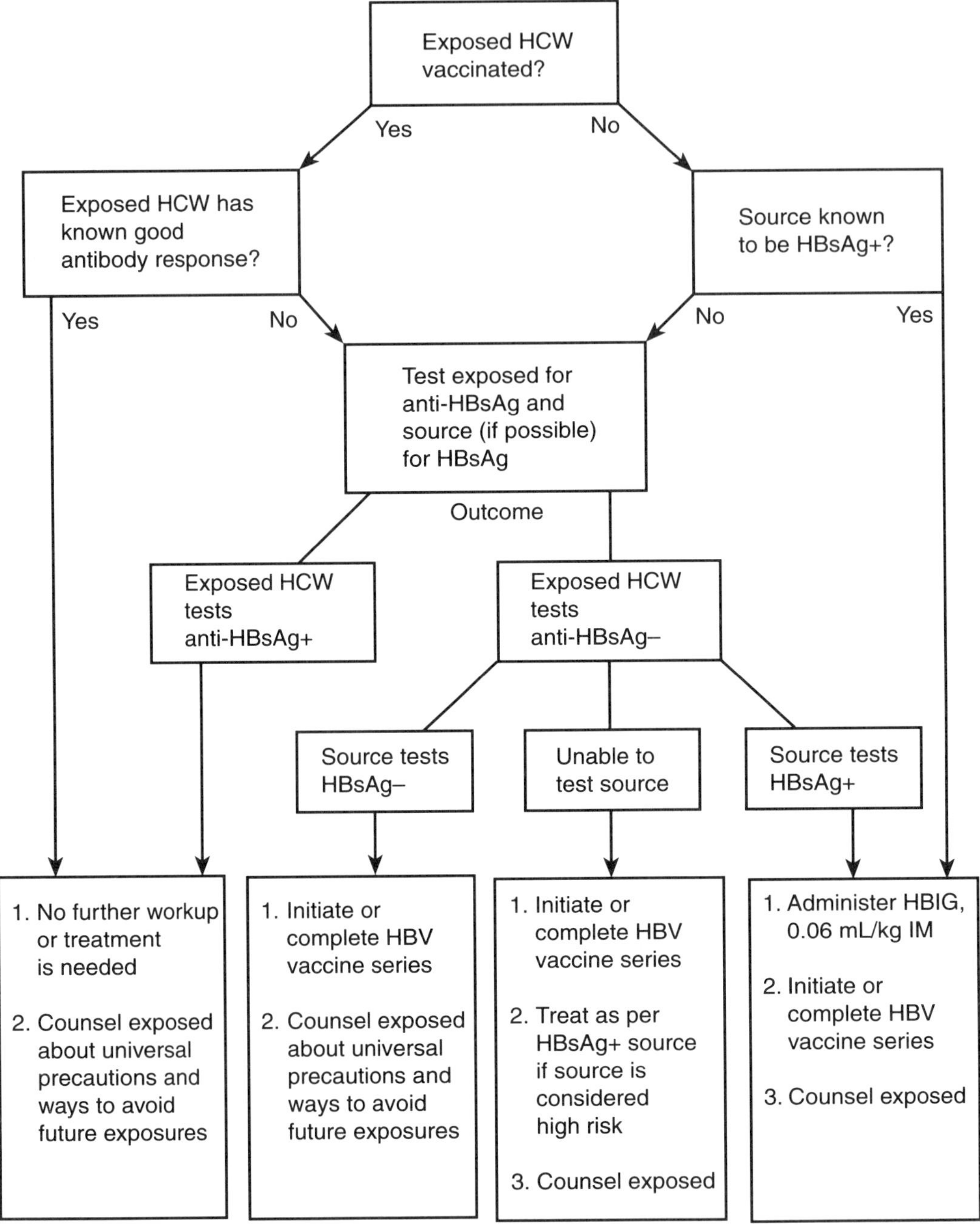

Fig. 17–2. Decision tree for needlestick exposure: hepatitis B virus *(HBV)* testing. *HCW,* health care worker; *HBsAg,* hepatitis B surface antigen; *IM,* intramuscularly.

bodies to HCV is delayed for an average of 22 weeks after exposure and 15 weeks after development of the initial symptoms.[50] Infectivity likely precedes seroconversion, as evidenced by documented transmission of HCV following the transfusion of blood initially screened as negative for anti-HCV antibodies.[50] Some patients remain seropositive for HCV, whereas others lose antibody to HCV after a period of time. Whether the presence or persistence of anti-HCV antibodies always indicates potential infectivity is unknown[50, 55, 56] and will require further investigation. Because of these limitations, it is not currently possible to determine the precise sensitivity or specificity of these assays.

Management of Exposures

Because it is possible that a source testing negative for HCV is nonetheless infectious, no specific recommendations currently exist regarding testing for HCV following an occupational exposure. However, it may be helpful to test the source for HCV when possible because knowledge of a positive test may alert the exposed HCW to the increased possibility of HCV transmission.

In situations where an exposure involves a source known to harbor HCV or is found to test positive for HCV, administration of IG, 0.06 mL/kg intramuscularly, may be of possible benefit.[45] It is also reasonable to administer IG to an exposed HCW if the source has identified risk factors for HCV. For an exposure involving an unknown source it may be reasonable to administer IG if it seems likely, based on what is known about local rates of HCV infection, that the HCW has been exposed.

PREVENTION

At present our best defense against occupationally acquired blood-borne infections lies in strict compliance with the principles of universal precautions as outlined by the CDC.[57] Under these guidelines, HCWs should consider all blood, CSF, and pleural, pericardial, peritoneal, amniotic, or synovial fluid to be potentially infectious regardless of the source. In the relatively uncontrolled ED setting, *all* body fluids should probably be considered potentially infectious because of the possibility of admixture with blood.[10] Barrier precautions are recommended for all situations when the possibility for contact with a potentially infectious fluid occurs.

Unfortunately, the greatest risk for nosocomial transmission of HIV or HBV stems from exposures due to needlesticks or other sharp implements, which are not generally prevented by the use of barrier precautions. It appears that many of these percutaneous injuries are preventable.[58, 59] Inexperienced HCWs, both physicians and ancillary staff, seem to be at particular risk for percutaneous exposure.[14, 59] Several studies have shown that one of the most common causes of needlestick injuries is attempted recapping of an uncovered needle.[14, 58, 59] Another large group of potentially preventable needlesticks occurs either during needle disposal or as a result of improper disposal.[58, 59] Improved design of the barrier devices and sharp implements used in the practice of medical care may eventually reduce the incidence of HCW exposures. Even when this is accomplished, however, all HCWs will need to exercise educated caution and follow existing recommendations in order to minimize personal risk.

REFERENCES

1. Centers for Disease Control: Nosocomial transmission of multi-drug resistant TB to health-care workers and HIV infected patients in an urban hospital—Florida, *MMWR* 39:718–722, 1990.
2. Centers for Disease Control: HIV prevalence estimates and AIDS case projections for the United States: report based on a workshop, *MMWR* 39:5, 1990.
3. Centers for Disease Control: The HIV/AIDS epidemic: the first 10 years, *MMWR* 40:358–360, 1991.
4. Kelen GD, DiGiovanna T, Bisson L et al: Human immunodeficiency virus infection in ED patients: epidemiology, clinical presentations, and risk to HCWs. The Johns Hopkins experience, *JAMA* 262:516–522, 1989.
5. Kelen GD, Johnson G, DiGiovanna T et al: Profile of patients with human immunodeficiency virus infection presenting to an inner-city emergency department, *Ann Emerg Med* 19:963–969, 1990.
6. Marcus R, Bell DM, Culver DH et al: Frequency of emergency care providers' contact with

blood of patients infected with human immunodeficiency virus, *Ann Emerg Med* 19:454, 1990 (abstract).

7. Baraff LJ, Talan DA, Torres M: Prevalence of HIV antibody in a noninnercity university hospital emergency department, *Ann Emerg Med* 20:782–786, 1991.
8. Centers for Disease Control: Update: acquired immunodeficiency syndrome and human immunodeficiency virus infection among health-care workers, *MMWR* 37:229–234, 1988.
9. Centers for Disease Control: Health care workers with documented and possible occupationally acquired AIDS/HIV infection, by occupation, reported through September 1993, United States, *HIV/AIDS Surveillance Report, Third Quarter Edition* 5:13, 1993.
10. Centers for Disease Control: Guidelines for prevention of transmission of human immunodeficiency virus and hepatitis B virus in health-care and public-safety workers, *MMWR* 38:6, 1989.
11. Henderson DK, Fahey, Willy M et al: Risk for occupational transmission of human immunodeficiency virus type 1 (HIV-1) associated with clinical exposures, *Ann Intern Med* 113:740–746, 1990.
12. Marcus R: The Cooperative Needlestick Surveillance Group: Surveillance of health care workers exposed to blood from patients infected with the human immunodeficiency virus, *N Engl J Med* 319:1118–1123, 1988.
13. Tandenberg D, Stewart KK, Doezema D: Under-reporting of contaminated needlestick injuries in emergency health care workers, *Ann Emerg Med* 20:66–70, 1991.
14. Mangione C, Gerberding JL, Cummings SR: Occupational exposure to HIV: frequency and rates of underreporting of percutaneous and mucocutaneous exposures by medical house-staff, *Am J Med* 90:85–90, 1991.
15. Wears RL, Vuckich DJ, Winton CN et al: An analysis of emergency physicians' cumulative career risk of HIV infection, *Ann Emerg Med* 20:749–753, 1991.
16. Oksenhendler E, Le Roux JM, Rabian C: HIV infection with seroconversion after a superficial needlestick injury to the finger, *New Engl J Med* 315:582, 1986 (letter).
17. Stewart GJ, Tyler JPP, Cunningham AL et al: Transmission of human T-cell lymphotrophic virus type III (HTLV-III) by artificial insemination by donor, *Lancet* 2:581, 1985.
18. Ziegler JB, Cooper, Johnson RD et al: Postnatal transmission of AIDS-associated retrovirus from mother to infant, *Lancet* 1:896, 1985.
19. Quarto M, Germinaro C, Fontana A et al: HIV transmission through kidney transplantation from a living related donor, *N Engl J Med* 320:1754, 1989.
20. Ho DD, Moudgil TM, Alam M: Quantitation of human immunodeficiency virus type 1 in the blood of infected persons, *N Engl J Med* 321:1621, 1989.
21. Centers for Disease Control: Apparent transmission of human T-lymphotrophic virus type III/lymphadenopathy-associated virus from a child to a mother providing health care, *MMWR* 35:75–79, 1986.
22. Loch M, Mach B: Identification of HIV-infected seronegative individuals by a direct diagnostic test based on hybridisation to amplified viral DNA, *Lancet* 2:418–421, 1988.
23. Davey RT, Vasudevachari MB, Lane HC: Serologic tests for human immunodeficiency virus infection. In DeVita VT, Hellman S, Rosenberg SA, editors: *AIDS: etiology, diagnosis, treatment, and prevention,* Philadelphia, 1992, JB Lippincott, pp 141–155.
24. Clark SJ, Saag MS, Decker WD et al: High titers of cytopathic virus in plasma of patients with symptomatic primary HIV-1 infection, *N Engl J Med* 324:954–960, 1991.
25. Stramer SL, Heller JS, Coombs RW et al: Markers of HIV infection prior to IgG antibody seropositivity, *JAMA* 262:64–69, 1989.
26. Alter HJ, Epstein JS, Swenwon SG et al: Prevalence of human immunodeficiency virus type 1 p24 antigen in U.S. blood donors—an assessment of the efficacy of testing in donor screening, *N Engl J Med* 323:1312–1317, 1990.
27. Centers for Disease Control: Update: serologic testing for antibody to human immunodeficiency virus, *MMWR* 36:833–840, 1988.
28. Consortium for Retrovirus Serology Standardization: Serological diagnosis of human immunodeficiency virus infection by Western blot testing, *JAMA* 260:674–679, 1988.
29. Jackson JB, MacDonald KL, Cadwell J et al: Absence of HIV infection in blood donors with indeterminate western blot tests for antibody to HIV-1, *N Engl J Med* 322:217–222, 1990.

30. Schwartz JS, Dans PE, Kinosian BP: Human immunodeficiency virus test: evaluation, performance and use, *JAMA* 259:2574–2579, 1988.
31. Centers for Disease Control: Recommendations for prevention of HIV transmission in health-care settings, *MMWR* 36:2–18, 1987.
32. Ranki A, Krohn M, Allain JP et al: Long latency period precedes overt seroconversion in sexually transmitted human-immunodeficiency-virus infection, *Lancet* 2:589–593, 1987.
33. Horsburgh CR, Jason J, Longini IM et al: Duration of human immunodeficiency virus infection before detection of antibody, *Lancet* 2:637–639, 1989.
34. Kelen GD, Bennecoff TA, Kline R et al: Evaluation of two rapid screening assays for detection of human immunodeficiency virus-1 infection in emergency department patients, *Am J Emerg Med* 9:416–420, 1991.
35. Connell JA, Parry JV, Mortimer PP et al: Preliminary report: accurate assays for anti-HIV in urine, *Lancet* 335:1366–1369, 1990.
36. Behets FM, Bazepeyo E, Quinn T et al: Detection of salivary HIV-1–specific IgG antibodies in high-risk populations in Zaire, *J Acquir Immune Defic Syndr* 4:183–187, 1991.
37. Baraff LJ, Schringer DL et al: Management guidelines for health care workers exposed to blood and body fluids, *Ann Emerg Med* 20:1341–1350, 1991.
38. Centers for Disease Control: Public Health Service guidelines for counseling and antibody testing to prevent HIV infection and AIDS, *MMWR* 36:509–515, 1987.
39. Gerberding J: Postexposure management of health care workers occupationally exposed to HIV. In DeVita VT, Hellman S, Rosenberg SA, editors: *AIDS: etiology, diagnosis, treatment, and Prevention,* Philadelphia, 1992, JB Lippincott, pp 550–555.
40. Lange JMA, Boucher CAB, Hollak CEM et al: Failure of zidovudine prophylaxis after accidental exposure to HIV, *N Engl J Med* 322:1375, 1990.
41. Looke DFM, Grove DI: Failed prophylactic zidovudine after needlestick injury, *Lancet* 336:1280, 1990 (letter).
42. Durand E, LeJeunne C, Hughes FC: Failure of prophylactic zidovudine after suicidal self-inoculation of HIV-infected blood, *N Engl J Med* 324:1062, 1991.
43. Centers for Disease Control: Public Health Service statement on management of occupational exposure to human immunodeficiency virus, including considerations regarding zidovudine postexposure use, *MMWR* 39:1–14, 1990.
44. Henderson DK, Gerberding JL: Prophylactic zidovudine after occupational exposure to the immunodeficiency virus: an interim analysis, *J Infect Dis* 160:321–327, 1989.
45. Centers for Disease Control: Protection against viral hepatitis: recommendations of the Immunization Practices Advisory Committee (ACIP). *MMWR* 39:2, 1990.
46. Centers for Disease Control: Update on hepatitis B prevention, *MMWR* 36:353–360, 1987.
47. Kelen GD, Green GB, Purcell RH et al: Hepatitis B and hepatitis C in emergency department patients, *N Engl J Med* 326:1399–1404, 1992.
48. Gerberding JL, Hopewell PC: Transmission of hepatitis B without transmission of AIDS by accidental needlestick, *N Engl J Med* 312:56, 1985 (letter).
49. Centers for Disease Control: Hepatitis B virus: a comprehensive strategy for eliminating transmission in the United States through universal childhood vaccination, *MMWR* 40:13, 1991.
50. Alter HJ, Purcell RH, Shih JW: Detection of antibody to hepatitis C virus in prospectively followed transfusion recipients with acute and chronic non-A, non-B hepatitis, *N Engl J Med* 321:1494–1500, 1989.
51. Choo Q-L, Kuo G, Weiner AJ et al: Isolation of a cDNA clone derived from a blood-borne non-A non-B viral hepatitis genome, *Science* 244:359–362, 1989.
52. Kuo G, Choo Q-L, Alter HJ et al: An assay for circulating antibodies to a major etiologic virus of human non-A, non-B hepatitis, *Science* 244:362–364, 1989.
53. Seef LB: Hepatitis C from a needlestick injury, *Ann Intern Med* 115:411, 1991 (letter).
54. Kiyosawa K, Sodeyama T, Tanaka E: Hepatitis C in hospital employees with needlestick injuries (brief report), *Ann Intern Med* 115:367–369, 1991.
55. Esteban JI, Gonzales A, Hernandez JM et al: Evaluation of antibodies to hepatitis C virus in a study of transfusion-associated hepatitis, *N Engl J Med* 323:1107–1112, 1990.
56. Farci P, Alter HJ, Wong D et al: A long-term study of hepatitis C virus replication in non-A, non-B hepatitis, *N Engl J Med* 325:98–104, 1991.

57. Centers for Disease Control: Update: universal precautions for prevention of transmission of human immunodeficiency virus, hepatitis B virus, and other bloodborne pathogens in health-care settings, *MMWR* 37:377–388, 1988.
58. Jagger J, Hunt EH, Brand-Elnaggar J et al: Rates of needle-stick injury caused by various devices in a university hospital, *N Engl J Med* 319:284–288, 1988.
59. Hochreiter MC, Barton LL: Epidemiology of needlestick injury in emergency medical service personnel, *J Emerg Med* 6:9–12, 1988.

Chapter 18

Basic Concepts for Using Radiologic Studies

Richard A. Rosen, M.D.
Leon J. Feldhamer, M.D.
Wayne J. Olan, M.D.
William A. Weiner, D.O.

Depending somewhat on the location (urban medical center, rural community hospital, etc.) and the time of day, the role of the emergency physician often must include the preliminary interpretation of appropriately obtained radiologic studies. Therefore it is essential that emergency physicians understand the basic concepts underlying the different types of radiologic studies available. It is also essential for the emergency physician to approach specific clinical problems logically, from a radiologic perspective regardless of where and when they present.

An additional problem affecting the radiologic evaluation of emergency patients is the redistribution of acute care patients resulting from hospital overcrowding. Emergency physicians now frequently evaluate and treat patients long after they would ideally have been transferred to an intensive care unit, coronary care unit, or operating room. Because of the development of an "ED ward," emergency physicians must evaluate disease processes which were previously addressed only on an inpatient service. The distinctions between emergency department radiology and acute care radiology are disappearing.

Because of the expanded use and increasing complexity of problems encountered in the ED, defining the types of examinations appropriate to this setting is essential. Clearly, not all patients who come to the ED have emergent problems, and the radiologic examination of patients who do not require an immediate study can delay the examination of others who do.

Conversely, there are patients who are *too sick* for radiologic studies. Such patients may be unable to tolerate the examination, especially studies such as computed tomography (CT) or magnetic resonance imaging (MRI), or they may require immediate treatment without delay for further evaluation. Clinical recognition of these patients is mandatory; they do not belong in a radiology suite.

This chapter presents the different types of radiologic examinations and their applications. Chapter 19 discusses recommended approaches to specific clinical problems.

SELECTING EXAMINATIONS

The decision of which radiologic study to obtain should be based on a series of specific questions. The first and most important question is the one to be answered by the study: the more precisely the question is framed, the better the chance that the right examination will be chosen to answer that question. For example, "abdominal pain," is not a question, nor is it adequate information for choosing the optimal imaging examination. With so many other more sophisticated modalities available, there are few logical indications for a plain film abdominal study. However, only meaningful clinical information can help the radiologist decide whether a particular patient would benefit from that examination; or if CT, ultrasonography, a radionuclide study, or angiography would be more helpful.

The problem becomes more complex when the patient's condition makes it difficult to narrow the clinical possibilities. This situation would apply to patients who are unable to give an adequate history or who are not responsive, as well as to patients whose problems are complicated by underlying disorders. The findings in critically ill elderly patients, for example, may be less striking than in younger adults. Persons with diabetes may have less pain or less of a temperature elevation than one would normally associate with a serious or catastrophic illness. Compromised patients may also be more prone to the complications of radiologic procedures, whether it be an increased susceptibility to serious adverse effects from an iodinated contrast medium, as is the case with persons with diabetes mellitus, or the possibility of aspiration, which is more likely to occur when oral contrast is administered to individuals with neurologic problems. It is extremely important, therefore, that in addition to the specific question, the radiologist receive information about complicating factors so that one of the least dangerous options can be chosen, even if the study ultimately performed is not the optimal diagnostic choice.

DESCRIBING THE PROBLEM

Although the specific clinical question is an important guide to the choice of radiologic examination, complete information about the situation may be necessary in choosing and interpreting the studies. For example, knowing the mechanism of an injury is usually as important as knowing that an injury has occurred. The kinds of soft tissue and bony injuries associated with inversion injuries of the ankle differ significantly from those that follow eversion; and the type and location of a traumatic aortic injury may depend on the direction from which the victim was struck. Commonly, multiple examinations are requested for trauma patients with no more history than, "Rule out fracture." The radiologic examinations performed under these circumstances may not answer the clinical questions. A properly performed study is designed to show a particular area, and if the technologist does not know which one is of greatest concern, that area may appear in the corner of a radiograph. The yield is much greater when the specific site of injury is indicated on the request form.

CHOOSING THE STUDY

The choice of an examination, then, depends on certain clinical considerations which allow the requesting physician to frame the specific question which the radiologic (or other) examination is supposed to answer. The examination chosen must certainly have the *potential* to answer that question, but that is not enough. The study must also have a reasonable *likelihood* of doing so. Gallstones are sufficiently calcified to be seen on plain abdominal radiographs only about 15% of the time. Consequently, an abdominal radiograph usually does not adequately answer the question of whether or not the patient has cholelithiasis. Ultrasonography, however, demonstrates over 95% of gallstones, and this examination is therefore a far better choice.

In choosing the proper investigation various considerations should be balanced. Can a particular examination answer a specific question? Is it *likely* to do so? Are there other studies which can supply the information? Which one is safest? Which one is least expensive? Which is available when needed? With which one does the hospital staff have the most experience? Will one of these studies interfere with another necessary test? (For example, a barium enema makes an angiographic procedure difficult or impossible to perform until the barium has been evacuated.) Weighing factors such as these insures that the choice of examination is the careful judgment it should be, not merely a mechanical one.

The consequences of a wrong choice should not be overlooked: in addition to delaying the performance of the correct examination for a particular patient, an unnecessary study of that patient may delay the performance of a necessary one for another patient. This is an especially severe problem when resources are limited. If there is only one technologist or one CT machine, only one study can be done at a time. Ideally, it will be a necessary one. Similarly, unnecessary risks or expenses may be eliminated by choosing a simpler way to solve a problem. Finally, the wrong study can create misleading information. For example, the fact that gallstones are not seen on a particular abdominal film does not exclude such a diagnosis since, as mentioned, the vast majority of gallstones cannot be seen on this type of examination.

RISKS OF RADIOLOGIC EXAMINATIONS

Although they do not occur commonly, some additional problems are associated with radiologic examinations, and the emergency physician should keep them in mind. One of the most significant problems is the potential for aggravating a patient's injury by improper immobilization during a study. Clearly manipulating the head or neck of an individual with a cervical spine injury can have catastrophic consequences. Such patients, as well as those who are medically unstable, should always be immobilized and accompanied to the radiology department by someone competent to supervise and care for them if a problem arises.

There is a small but finite risk from radiologic contrast media, especially to patients with diabetes mellitus, renal disease, cardiovascular disease, or allergies. Many patients experience some adverse effects from the contrast material which may include a feeling of warmth, a bad taste, and nausea. Common *allergic* manifestations include pruritus and hives. More severe allergic reactions include bronchospasm, vascular collapse, and cardiac arrest. Deaths occur in approximately one out of 25,000 to 100,000 examinations depending on patient selection and type of contrast medium used, but less severe problems are not infrequent. Two important nonallergic sequelae relate to increased cardiovascular load brought on by a very hypertonic material and toxic effects on the kidneys which are more severe in persons with diabetes mellitus, especially when they are dehydrated. On occasion, a dehydrated patient with multiple myeloma will also suffer renal damage secondary to protein precipitation in the kidneys following contrast administration. It is important to note that the introduction of nonionic contrast media to replace (in some or all cases) the ionic materials used heretofore, has significantly reduced the number of problems; however, reactions, even fatal ones, may still occur.

One other risk of a radiologic examination over which there is a great deal of anxiety is the very small potential for genetic damage from radiation exposure. However, when the radiologic examination is properly chosen and performed, the health risk to an individual is far less than the risk of not performing it. Of course, improperly chosen studies, no matter how low the risk, should not be done.

UNNECESSARY EXAMINATIONS

Many radiologic requests are for examinations which need not, and therefore should not, be done in the ED. Although many of these studies are of no direct risk to the patient, they delay the performance of definitive procedures and this places the patient at some risk. A typical example is the abdominal radiograph requested for a patient with acute appendicitis. Very often, a clinician comfortable with his or her clinical impression nevertheless hopes to see an appendicolith to clinch the diagnosis. Unfortunately, however, the likelihood of such a finding is less than 10%, and the absence of an appendiceal stone does not in any way mitigate the results of a properly performed history and physical examination. The time required to perform the examination and to interpret the radiograph only delays the patient's trip to the operating room. Similarly, since the presence or absence of abnormalities on a chest radiograph rarely proves the presence or absence of an aortic dissection or injury, spending time performing a study or arguing over the results of what is often an inconclusive supine chest radiograph only delays definitive studies such as CT or angiography and/or medical or surgical treatment.

Another type of unnecessary examination is the one requested to answer an unnecessary question. "Is there a rib fracture?" is a question best answered by obtaining rib radiographs. But for the patient with chest pain following trauma to the upper thorax, it is usually far more important to learn if there is a pneumo- or hemothorax, a pulmonary contusion, or an injury to the aorta. Just as chest radiographs are not satisfactory to evaluate ribs, rib studies do not ordinarily help answer questions about the lungs, pleura, or mediastinum. Treatment of rib fractures is usually symptomatic, whether the fractures are seen or not. More active intervention is required for a pneumothorax or torn aorta and the proper question therefore usually deals with these problems, not with rib fractures. Obtaining rib studies may also delay critical therapy. Of course trauma to the lower ribs requires a different analysis: an early indication of possible significant injury to the spleen or liver is fracture of several ribs in those areas. Once again, it is apparent that the best choice of a diagnostic (or therapeutic) study must be based on a thoughtful consideration of the goals of the examination.

"Routine" examinations should also be avoided. These include studies such as the preoperative chest radiograph, the routine admission chest radiograph, and the abdominal radiograph requested for any patient with any abdominal complaint. In the absence of a clinical history or findings of chest disease, the preoperative or admission radiographs provide very little information that alters patient management immediately, except perhaps in areas where tuberculosis is prevalent. The same is true of abdominal radiographs for which no specific question has been formulated. The logic of a "baseline film" is similarly questionable if no thought has been given to its ultimate use. Aside from the expense, performing unnecessary studies also delays the management both of the patients involved, as well as of others waiting for examination.

PORTABLE RADIOLOGIC STUDIES

Of particular importance in the choice of examinations is the proper use of nonstandard studies. One of the most common nonstandard studies requested is the bedside examination, usually a chest study, using portable radiologic equipment. Although such examinations may be crucial in the management of some critically ill patients who cannot be transported to the radiology department without significant risk, the radiographs obtained require more time to perform, are far more expensive, and are inferior in quality to those which can be obtained using fixed equipment and standard positioning. The portable chest radiograph is usually done in the anterior-posterior projection with a short tube-to-film distance, resulting in increased magnification and distortion. Portable machines usually require longer exposures to obtain equivalent density, and often patient motion compromises the examination. Moreover, because of the limitations imposed by positioning the patient in a *bed,* standardized views often cannot be obtained. These are only a few of the many difficulties caused by the use of this type of equipment, but they illustrate why radiologists prefer not to do portable studies unless they are absolutely necessary. Unfortunately, portable studies are often requested merely for staff convenience or to obtain faster service.

SPECIAL CONSIDERATIONS

Some specific considerations relate to particular patient groups such as pediatric patients. Because the younger patients are at risk for the potentially (but rarely) deleterious effects of radiation for more years than older patients, it is good practice to limit these examinations in children even further. In some clinical situations, this may mean that the problem should be managed without radiologic studies whenever possible, to limit the extent of any studies performed and/or to avoid follow-up examinations when not essential. Also, some standard examinations may require different techniques and views in children because of different age-dependent disease patterns, as well as the inability of the young patients to cooperate fully. Finally, because normal development governs the appearance of many structures, especially bones, it is often important to get radiographs of a clinically normal area to compare with the abnormal one. By studying both extremities when only one is injured, the stage of development of the epiphyses can be determined and the mistake of confusing a normal growth plate with a fracture can be avoided.

Similarly, when pregnant patients are examined, the risk to the fetus should also be considered. Generally speaking, the radiation risk of an appropriate radiologic study to mother or fetus is far less than the risk of the disease for which the study has been requested. Studies that do not require ionizing radiation, such as ultrasonography, are desirable whenever they can be used—especially for pregnant women with abdominal or pelvic disease.

WORKING IN YOUR HOSPITAL

Finally, emergency physicians must always base the choice of radiologic procedures on the policies, strengths, and weaknesses of their particular radiology departments. No two departments function in exactly the same manner. Many departments distribute a manual which describes the facilities and the hours that certain services are provided, as well as providing suggestions for the sequencing of examinations in various circumstances. In addition, individual staff members can advise the emergency physician on examination choices in particular clinical circumstances or for particular types of problems or areas of the body. The recommendations made in this chapter and the next are meant only as a general guideline, to be used especially at those times when a radiologist is not immediately available for consultation.

AVAILABLE IMAGING MODALITIES

Plain Film Radiographic Studies

Although the plain film radiographic study was once the only tool available for the evaluation of patients with emergent problems; in the last three decades it has been supplemented by a variety of imaging procedures using ionizing radiation as well as ultrasound and magnetic fields. Nonetheless, the plain film radiograph remains the "backbone" of patient evaluations, with the other modalities providing useful "appendages." Standard plain film radiographic studies are generally available at all times, wherever emergency medical treatment is given, whereas more specialized examinations may only be performed on a more limited basis. The plain film radiograph may be obtained either in the department or at the bedside—a distinct advantage over fixed equipment like CT, MRI, and much of the available ultrasonography and nuclear medicine machinery.

Plain film radiographic studies are usually the first, and often the only ones necessary for evaluating most emergency problems. While specific positioning considerations are beyond the scope of this chapter, a few basic points should be borne in mind. Most importantly, the chest examination, the study most frequently obtained, is properly performed with the patient standing. For a variety of reasons, recumbent studies of the chest are almost always technically inferior to erect studies and yield less information. Not every patient can cooperate fully, however, and supine chest radiographs are frequently necessary. Awareness of the limitations of recumbent radiographs, prevents unreasonable expectations.

Inability of the patient to cooperate affects the performance of other examinations as well. Motion can degrade the radiographic image to the point at which it is uninterpretable. Thus, it is futile to request studies on a patient who is flailing about or otherwise unable to remain still. Since most examinations are done, or can be done, with the patient supine, few are compromised by a patient's inability to stand or assume an uncomfortable position. With the use of cross-table, lateral, or other projections, most studies can be done with the patient lying down. But patient motion in this position too can destroy an otherwise satisfactory study.

Linear Tomography

Linear tomography is a technique that uses a tube and a film cassette which move in opposite directions to provide a single-plane view of an object rather than a full-thickness view. The plane that is in focus is the one at the level of the rotational axis of the tube and film, and the thickness of the "slice" is inversely related to the distance the tube and film move. If the tube and film do not move, the object's full thickness is seen. As the motion increases, the slice thickness diminishes.

As with plain film radiography, the utility of linear tomography has decreased significantly in recent years. CT has all but replaced linear tomographic studies, but useful information can still be obtained by this method in certain circumstances. In patients with fractures parallel to the plane of a CT slice, linear tomography may better demonstrate the extent of the fracture and the degree of fusion. Linear studies of the orbits and facial bones may provide a good deal of information in situations or at times when CT is not available. Renal outlines are often well seen with tomography, either with or without the introduction of intravenous contrast. Notwithstanding these specific instances, linear tomography does not have much utility in most emergent situations.

Contrast Procedures

Contrast procedures can demonstrate anatomic features (e.g., the patency and integrity of viscera and blood vessels) or physiologic function (e.g., the excretory ability of the urinary tract) not detectable on plain film radiographs and therefore provide a valuable supplement to initial examinations. These studies, which use radiopaque contrast materials, may be useful in evaluating acutely injured or ill patients, and can be performed in most radiology departments 24 hours a day. Contrast examinations rely on normal (or abnormal) physiology to transport the materials to specific locations thereby making visible those structures not ordinarily seen well enough for radiologic evaluation. The materials administered may be air, iodinated contrast media, and barium preparations.

Because some of the most devastating conditions with which patients present to the ED result from trauma, the most significant of contrast procedures performed there are usually vascular studies. These include central vascular studies, to determine the presence or absence of aortic of other major vessel injury, as well as peripheral and proximity studies. Interventional procedures may also be performed to stop hemorrhage (e.g., embolization of bleeding vessels), drain obstructed urinary and biliary systems, drain abscesses, detect pulmonary embolism, and guide the placement of vena caval filters to prevent repetition, detect aortic dissections, demonstrate the path of perforating injuries (intraperitoneal and otherwise), etc. By the time most of these procedures are underway, the patients have usually been admitted; however, the rapid decision to perform the appropriate procedure is often the responsibility of the emergency physician.

Another common use of iodinated contrast material is in the excretory urogram, also known as the intravenous urogram (IVU) or intravenous pyelogram (IVP). This examination can demonstrate the ability of the kidneys to concentrate and excrete contrast, as well as the anatomy of the urinary tract itself. In cases of abdominal trauma, when urinary tract injury is possible, urography may provide rapid anatomic information. In addition, before nonurinary tract emergency surgery, it may be necessary to demonstrate the function and anatomy of urinary structures. Obstruction, most often by an acute stone, is another frequent reason for an emergency urogram. Finally, many departments routinely obtain a single abdominal radiograph following angiography or a CT contrast study of an area other than the abdomen (see later section) to demonstrate the urinary tract. Such a radiograph provides additional information, which may be of some value immediately or in the future, without subjecting the patient to an additional exposure to contrast material. Moreover, if the patient has a reaction to the contrast material in the initial study, this bonus radiograph may turn out to be the only study of the urinary tract obtainable.

One additional procedure that employs iodinated contrast is myelography (with or without CT). The study may be required to elucidate the cause of acute cord compression. For other indications, myelography can usually be scheduled rather than performed as an emergency study.

Barium sulfate is a contrast medium which has a long history of safe use in evaluating the gastrointestinal (GI) tract. Although not usually appropriate for the evaluation of ED patients, the occasional cases for which it's use is reasonable include examinations for a foreign body in the esophagus (usually food), evidence of GI tract perforation due to trauma or from other causes, bowel obstruction, and identifying bowel when unusual gas patterns are encountered (e.g., hiatus hernia or gastric volvulus). A barium examination may be undertaken as a combined diagnostic and therapeutic procedure in babies with intussusception. Barium may also be given (in very dilute form) when it is necessary to fill the GI tract to differentiate the bowel from other structures on abdominal CT.

Barium is an extremely safe material, and its use is rarely a problem. However, there are occasions, especially in acutely ill patients, when iodinated materials should be used in examinations ordinarily requiring barium. The most common example is when bowel perforation, and/or subsequent bowel surgery, is a consideration. Because "spilled" barium will not be resorbed as will a water-soluble contrast medium, the barium may persist in the chest or abdomen indefinitely after it escapes the GI tract. Although persistent barium is generally benign, granuloma formation and fibrosis in response to its presence occasionally causes problems in the peritoneum or mediastinum.

Irrespective of the type of contrast material used, the barium enema examination itself poses some definite, if uncommon, risks. The most serious of these is perforation of the colon, which can happen with inflamed or obstructed bowel, or because of trauma from placement of the enema tube itself. Approximately one death in 50,000 barium enemas occurs secondary to this complication.

Angiography

Angiography, the study of the vascular system by the introduction of iodinated contrast material, is of great value in the examination of many of the most critical patients in the ED—those who have suffered major trauma. The direct visualization of the arteries and veins permits the diagnosis of vessel displacement (by hematomas), injury, and leakage. The information cannot be obtained without some risk however, since the possible adverse effects of contrast material, as well as the invasiveness of vascular catheterization, must be recognized. Although these complications are uncommon, vascular spasm, thrombosis, embolization, and damage can occur and increase morbidity. In addition, the studies may be lengthy and require the presence of physicians and technical staff not initially on premises.

Notwithstanding these cautions, angiography can provide lifesaving information in a number of circumstances such as vascular injury, blood loss, and aneurysms (including dissections). Studies of the pulmonary venous system are often obtained in patients with pulmonary embolism. However radionuclide lung scans are less invasive and less expensive and can often answer the question without the need for pulmonary angiography (see Chapter 19).

The individual who performs the angiographic procedure (i.e., the interventional radiologist) is often able to provide therapeutic as well as diagnostic services. Among the emergency procedures that may be indicated are the embolization of bleeding vessels, the placement of vena caval filters, the dilation of strictured vessels, and the drainage of abscesses and obstructed urinary and biliary systems.

Nuclear Medicine

Nuclear medicine examinations (radionuclide studies, isotope scans) provide an additional option in some acute situations. The preparations used are not toxic, as iodinated contrast media may be, nor are they associated with hypersensitivity reactions. Although some clinicians are concerned about radiation from the materials used, generally the patient receives no more radiation than from a comparable study using x-rays and frequently is exposed to less radiation.

Because these materials may be used by the body in physiologic processes, they can provide both anatomic and functional information. Nuclear medicine studies have a limited role in the ED, however, because most of the problems solved using radionuclides are not emergent, and because nuclear medicine testing is, in most institutions, only available during daytime hours. Nonetheless, in a few circumstances critical information may be provided by isotope scans which can directly affect acute care.

The most common acute situations for which a radionuclide study may be indicated are pulmonary embolism and acute cholecystitis. In the former situation pulmonary blood flow and the distribution of ventilated air can be followed and compared. The comparison of these two, the V/Q scan, allows determination of the likelihood of pulmonary embolism. The other common problem, acute cholecystitis, can be evaluated by the use of materials which are secreted by the liver into the biliary system. Hepatic imido diacetic acid (HIDA) scans (see Chapter 20) use this mechanism to determine whether there is obstruction of the cystic duct.

Two less common problems for which radionuclide investigation may be extremely helpful are testicular torsion and complications caused by Meckel's diverticulum. When the blood flow to the two testes is compared, torsion may be diagnosed if the blood flow to one has been decreased or eliminated. The frequent presence of ectopic gastric mucosa in a Meckel's diverticulum may be the essential clue to its presence in a patient with intestinal bleeding. Preparations of pertechnitate (a technetium-99m compound) are secreted by gastric cells and may be demonstrated on a scan (see Chapter 20).

Ultrasonography

Ultrasonography is one of the most rapidly proliferating imaging tools available in most hospitals. It is a highly desirable technique because it does not require the use of ionizing radiation, making it an ideal method for the investigation of pregnancy and its complications as well as for problems in infants and children. The ability of ultrasound to discriminate between different types of tissues, to identify fluid collections and their locations and interfaces between structures, and to demonstrate "stones," (whether calcified or not) give ultrasound wide applicability in acute situations. Unfortunately, however, these studies are frequently nondiagnostic. One technical consideration is the presence of gas or bone overlying structures of interest. The interface between soft tissue and gas or bone reflects sound waves. Patients with large amounts of gas in their intestines, resulting from the primary problem or secondary to air swallowing, may not be good candidates for this examination, since structures behind the gas (or behind bone) will be obscured. Large amounts of subcutaneous fat may also create a problem since the fat may conceal other structures. Lack of sufficient training in this modality may also lead to serious misdiagnosis.

In the hands of experienced sonographers, ED utilization of ultrasound is appropriate for a wide variety of situations, with ectopic pregnancy and other complications of pregnancy among the most important. In addition, ultrasound may be the first radiologic modality to choose for such abdominal conditions as masses and fluid collections, cholelithiasis, hematuria, and abdominal aneurysms. Because of the broad range of accessible anatomy and potential disease processes that can be diagnosed with this tool, some authors consider ultrasound the best technique with which to begin evaluating the ambiguous "acute abdomen," provided that the pattern of gas distribution is not in question. Pericardial effusion and other vascular problems are also amenable to ultrasound assessment.

Doppler (blood flow) studies may be useful in patients with presumed deep vein thrombosis, penetrating injuries, or testicular torsion as well as for the evaluation of blood flow in the neck and abdomen.

Computed Tomography

Computed tomography (CT, CAT SCAN) has become an essential tool for the proper evaluation of many acute clinical problems. CT has achieved importance because of its ability to "see" more than the human eye can appreciate, and to display what it sees in planes different from the ones demonstrated by plain film radiography. Although plain film examinations usually present a summation of information through the entire thickness of the patient, CT can isolate thin cross sections of the patient and identify structures at a particular level. The information thus obtained can be displayed as cross sections or "reconstructed" in coronal, sagittal, or oblique plains. Some units can even perform three-dimensional reconstructions of the information obtained by CT. Thus, CT demonstrates relationships of different structures *to each other* far better than plain film radiography can.

The information displayed on a CT scan is also more detailed than can be recognized on plain film radiographs. Ordinarily, four different kinds of radiodensities: air, fat, water and calcium (metal) densities can be identified on plain film radiographs. In CT, the electronic receptors (which "see" the transmitted x-ray photons) and the computer which evaluates the information received from them can not only differentiate these densities easily but can also discriminate much more subtle density differences and display them on the terminal or on film. Also unlike ultrasonography, CT is not adversely affected by bone, gas, and fat. Thus on CT, minor soft tissue differences never before visible can be appreciated, like those between grey and white matter in the brain. For those reasons CT has become the primary diagnostic modality in the evaluation of head injury and stroke, frequently obviating the need for dangerous and technically difficult vascular studies of the brain.

The same ability to discriminate among similar radiodensities makes CT an important modality for evaluation of other areas, especially the abdomen. The minor differences between such structures as the kidneys, liver, gallbladder, and pancreas are not detectable by ordinary radiography, but are obvious to the photoreceptors and the computer. With the addition of oral contrast material, the intestine becomes visible and intravenous contrast demonstrates the vascular system.

In the ED, CT is particularly valuable in evaluating certain kinds of trauma, especially in areas such as the spine and hip where demonstrating cross-sectional relationships may be critical in evaluating the primary problem and potential complications. CT also may be helpful in planning possibly complex surgery for the restoration of normal or functional anatomy. Certain vascular problems such as aneurysms and leaks may also be studied by CT. While arteriography is often required in these situations, CT is more often available in many centers and is less invasive. Other uses of CT in the ED include the evaluation of the abdomen for abscess collections and pancreatic disease. In regard to the injured patient, however, it must be emphasized that while many other radiologic studies can be performed with the patient remaining on the same stretcher that brings him to the radiology department, to do a CT scan, the patient must be moved onto the CT table. Therefore, the clinician must be convinced before moving the patient that if there is a possibility of a spinal injury the technique used for moving the patient will not exacerbate it. Finally, it must be emphasized that because CT is an expensive study it should not be viewed as a screening procedure, but should be used as part of a well-thought-out plan to obtain the information needed, and simpler and/or less expensive alternatives for obtaining this information should be considered.

Magnetic Resonance Imaging

MRI is the newest and most expensive of the major imaging modalities. It is therefore less likely to be available to the ED than are the other modalities thus far described. MRI works by entirely different means than other imaging tools, employing magnetic fields rather than ionizing radiation to provide information. By the use of both magnetic and radio-frequency fields, MRI can provide a "proton map" which, after computer processing, yields images similar in appearance to those of a CT examination. The information on MRI images however, is quite different. The protons detected by MRI are actually hydrogen nuclei, and the resulting images demonstrate the various tissues in a manner which reflects the amount of water (which contains most of the body's hydrogen) in them, as well as the local physicochemical environment. Different tissues have different characteristic patterns, both in their normal and abnormal states, and these differences are completely independent of "density" as reflected on radiographs.

Although the literature describing the capabilities and applications of MRI is increasing rapidly, the place of MRI in medical practice is already very significant. However, MRI is not yet commonly used in emergency situations. As was the case with CT, most of the early development has been in the area of intracranial pathology and spinal problems; orthopedic disease is another area frequently studied by this technique. Currently, the best use for MRI is in orthopedic studies of soft tissues, tendons, ligaments, muscle, and menisci; these problems rarely require examinations that cannot be scheduled. Some exceptions to this general rule involve the spinal cord when compression or other traumatic damage may justify an emergency examination. Similarly, vascular trauma may justify such studies since MRI has the ability to image the vascular system without the use of contrast media or the need for technical expertise to deliver it to specific sites. The frequency with which patients who require such urgent studies also require monitoring, life support, or are agitated, unstable, or otherwise incapable of tolerating such a lengthy study, however, mitigates against the use of this modality. The strength of the magnetic field around the unit could affect life support machinery.

Other Studies

Additional radiologic procedures are available, but most have little application to emergency situations. A single exception perhaps, is the occasional need for *sinography* or *fistulography* to determine the source of drainage of pus in a febrile patient or to follow a knife wound to determine its extent, but these problems can often be investigated by other modalities such as CT.

SUGGESTED READINGS

Harris HJ, Jr, Harris WH, Novelline RA: *The radiology of emergency medicine,* ed 3, Baltimore, 1993, Williams and Wilkins.

Keats TE: *Emergency radiology,* ed 2, Chicago, 1989, Year Book Medical Publishers.

Keats TE: Emergency department radiology, *Radiol Clin North Am* 30:2, 1992.

McCort JJ, Mindelzun RE: *Trauma radiology,* New York, 1990, Churchill Livingstone.

Mirvis SE, Young JWR, editors: *Imaging in trauma and critical care,* Baltimore, 1992, Williams and Wilkins.

Chapter 19

The Radiologic Evaluation

Richard A. Rosen, M.D.

Leon J. Feldhamer, M.D.

Wayne J. Olan, M.D.

William A. Weiner, D.O.

From a radiologic standpoint it makes sense to divide emergency department (ED) patients into two categories: those who have experienced trauma and those who have not. EDs are already frequently organized this way to staff and equip the department to deal with these problems appropriately.

Because the radiologic evaluation must be governed by the clinical problem, the differences between these two types of patients play an important part in the choice of particular radiologic studies. The organization of this chapter is therefore based on this division: trauma is considered first, starting with life-threatening situations, and is followed by less urgent trauma. Nontrauma emergencies are then reviewed. In both cases, clinical problems are organized by body region *or* organ system. For example, following blunt abdominal trauma, consideration must be given at times to various problems localized to one area. Conversely, in evaluating a positive stool guaiac, consideration must be given to diseases of the entire intestinal tract, from the nose and mouth to the anus, and including the head, neck, chest, and abdominal organs, but limited to consideration of the enteron and the structures which can bleed into it. Since this chapter contains three separate reviews of certain areas or organs, it may be necessary to read more than one section to obtain a complete evaluation of a single problem.

TRAUMA PATIENTS

Life-Threatening Situations

Patients with life-threatening trauma are difficult to manage because of the wide range of injuries that may be present and the speed needed to manage them. The initial evaluation, or "primary survey," is *clinical*; radiologic studies are initiated only during the "secondary survey" and typically include the protocol of standard radiographs obtained on all multiply injured individuals. Because some significant injuries may be overlooked even in the conscious patients, these radiologic studies should generally be performed on all such patients irrespective of clinical findings. Of course, in unstable patients the need for definitive treatment takes precedence over even the most basic radiologic studies. Radiographs of the cervical spine, chest, and abdomen/

pelvis are most likely to provide the greatest amount of significant information about emergent situations in the least amount of time. The abdominal radiograph should cover the abdomen down to the inferior margin of the symphysis pubis, including the acetabula and femoral heads. Additional views of the thoracic and lumbosacral spine should be considered as well, if there is any clinical suggestion of spinal injury.

On the basis of clinical and radiologic assessment, the patient may be classified by degree of stability and the likely location of the most significant injury. Further imaging decisions are made on the basis of this information.

Stability

The two most common causes for the rapid demise of a patient who presents to the ED after trauma are intracranial damage and massive blood loss. If blood loss does not result from a visible external wound or an obvious source such as an extremity that has enlarged visibly, it may be occurring in the chest or abdomen/pelvis. The initial protocol survey radiographs may provide a clue to that source. The chest radiograph may show a pleural fluid collection or a finding such as mediastinal widening or blurring of the aorta, which might suggest aortic damage. The abdomen/pelvis radiograph may demonstrate fractures that by their configuration, suggest a mechanism of injury and a possible location of the bleeding site, for example, pelvic or abdominal. The best method of evaluating possible intraabdominal bleeding may be difficult to determine. Although peritoneal lavage or taking the patient directly to the OR may be necessary for the unstable patient, CT, especially using the newer high-speed units, is also a relatively rapid, noninvasive method for evaluating possible intraabdominal bleeding.

Site of Injury

In addition to the level of stability, the primary and secondary surveys are likely to suggest the area(s) in which serious damage has occurred. The algorithms for evaluation generally depend on the designation of the most significant injuries. If they appear to be intracranial, further evaluation may have to await a neurosurgical procedure to manage the problem. As is noted later, however, certain steps can be taken while the patient is being prepared for surgery to speed the postoperative management of other injuries.

The Cervical Spine

Radiologic examination of the cervical spine should begin with a horizontal-beam (cross-table) lateral radiograph, which can be performed without touching the patient. This is very often the initial protocol radiograph of the secondary survey. The film should be examined carefully for evidence of prevertebral swelling, alignment of the vertebrae, the presence of a normal (0 to 3 mm) space between the anterior ring of C1 and the odontoid, disc space narrowing, and evidence of subluxation or rotation of vertebrae and fracture, whether of the body or posterior elements. A common problem encountered in this examination is failure to visualize the lower cervical spine and the cervicothoracic junction. Because of the frequency of significant fractures and subluxations in this region, the study cannot be considered complete until this area is seen and cleared. Gentle traction on the arms while the lateral radiograph is being performed often solves the problem; however it may be necessary to perform an overexposed lateral radiograph centered on C7 to visualize it. These radiographs may not be pleasing aesthetically, the upper spine appearing "burnt out," but if C7 and T1 can be evaluated, the study has accomplished its purpose. A careful search for evidence of both fractures and abnormalities of alignment must be made.

Anterior subluxation due to bilateral facet dislocation is an extremely serious injury with a high incidence of cord damage. The lateral view demonstrates anterolisthesis of 50% or more. In addition to frank subluxation, however, unilateral facet dislocation is an important, although somewhat less common flexion-rotation injury. C4-C6 are the most common areas affected. Radiologic examination shows an anterior subluxation that is always less than half the vertebral body width with the dislocated facet anteriorly positioned. On anteroposterior (AP) views, spinous process rotation to the side of dislocation can be seen. Careful evaluation of the soft tissues anterior to the spine is important since widening of these tissues, representing bleeding, may be the only clue to a serious injury.

Although the radiologic findings may be minimal, the teardrop fracture-dislocation is the most severe axial loading-flexion injury and is extremely unstable. Often only flexion of the cervical spine and a small triangular fragment of the anteroinferior margin of one of the cervical vertebrae are present. This injury is usually a lower cervical spine injury and often results either from diving into a shallow pool or from using the head as a battering ram—typically in football. Complete ligamentous disruption may accompany this finding leading to subluxation and cord compression. Because a history may not be available in these individuals, all unconscious near-drowning patients should be considered to have such a fracture and treated accordingly. A hyper-*extension* teardrop fracture may also occur with rupture of the anterior longitudinal ligament and a typical triangular bone fragment. This lesion, although not as immediately life threatening as the flexion variety, and usually having a completely different history, is nevertheless potentially unstable and should be immobilized before further evaluation.

Attention is often not focused on this area, but great care should be taken in the evaluation of C1, a common location for a burst or Jefferson fracture (see Fig. 19–1), which results from axial loading. Although these are unstable, neurologic symptoms are uncommon because the fragments are displaced away from the cord. At lower cervical levels, burst fractures are more likely to be symptomatic and to predispose to cord damage since posterior displaced fragments are likely to cause cord compression. They should, therefore, be viewed as life-threatening injuries with a significant risk of paraplegia.

Another of the cervical injuries that should be treated as unstable is the "hangman's" fracture (Fig. 19–2), which usually includes the pedicles and pars interarticularis of C2 with an associated traumatic spondylolisthesis. The fracture results from a combination of hyperextension and axial compression. In the past, this fracture was the cause of death by hanging. Currently, when seen in the ED as a result of automobile trauma, the injury may be less severe, possibly unaccompanied by neurological findings. It should, nonetheless, be considered unstable.

Approximately 80 to 90% of significant abnormalities can be identified on a technically satisfactory lateral view alone. Therefore after a review of this radiograph demonstrates no significant abnormality, cassettes may be carefully placed under the spine for the AP and odontoid (open-mouth) views to complete the study. The odontoid view is required in order to evaluate C1–3 in the frontal projection since the mandible and occiput are superimposed on the upper cervical spine on the standard AP view. Jefferson fractures may first be appreciated on this projection by the displacement of one or both lateral masses of C1 by more than 7 mm from the odontoid. Tomography, either linear or computed, should be performed when a question of injury remains following these views, when additional injuries are sought in addition to one(s) already identified, or when mapping of the location of multiple fragments is important as in a Jefferson fracture. Because of the horizontal orientation of the CT view, some transverse vertebral body fractures may not be recognized without sagittal (or three-dimensional) reconstruction, a procedure not often performed under emer-

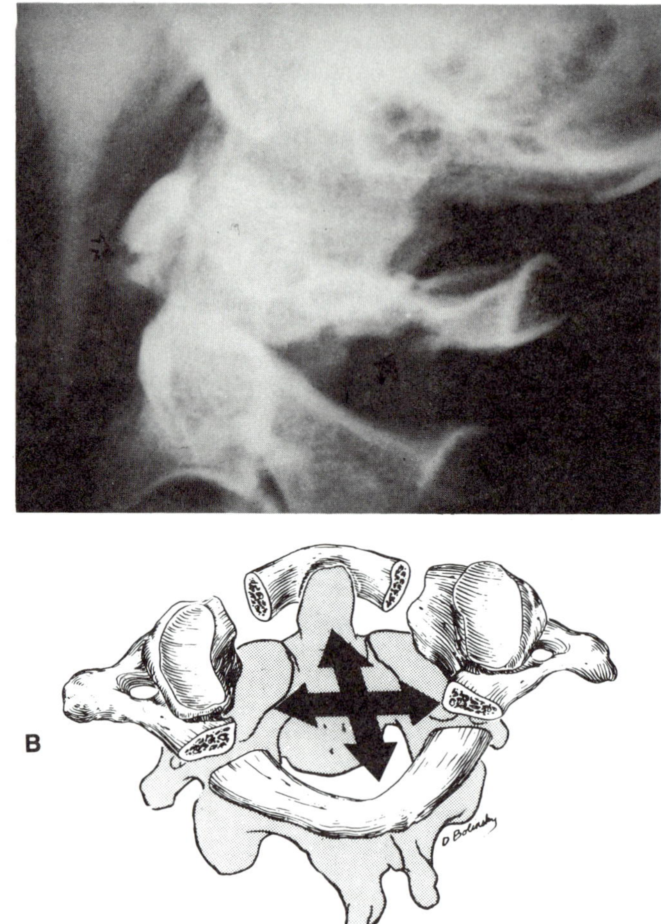

FIG. 19-1. Jefferson fracture. **A,** Lateral radiograph shows fractures of the anterior arch *(open arrow)* as well as the posterior arch *(solid arrow)*. **B,** Schematic drawing of Jefferson fracture. (From Rosen P, Doris P, Barkin R et al: *Diagnostic radiology in emergency medicine,* St Louis, 1992, Mosby, p 236.)

gency circumstances. Great care will be required when transferring the patient from the stretcher to the CT table.

After exclusion of a fracture or obvious subluxation by plain film radiography and CT, the suspicion of injury may still remain and warrant further evaluation. Soft tissue injuries such as damage to ligaments and tendons, will not be apparent on the studies already undertaken, but may contribute to instability of the cervical spine. Therefore, techniques that demonstrate such abnormalities should be considered at this time. Flexion and extension lateral views may be used to demonstrate excessive motion, which indicates injury of supporting soft tissues. However, it must be remembered that these views are performed to demonstrate *instability,* a situation that may lead to cord injury. Therefore, it is imperative, that only voluntary flexion and extension by the patient is allowed, not forced motion by a technologist or other staff member, and only in the presence of an individual who is qualified to supervise a patient with an unstable cervical spine.

When there is a possibility of injury within the neural canal (direct cord damage, bleeding, or disc herniation), a study of this region may be required. Magnetic Resonance Imaging (MRI) is highly sensitive and is being used increasingly to evaluate the cord and neural canal in such critical situations as cord transection or hemorrhage.

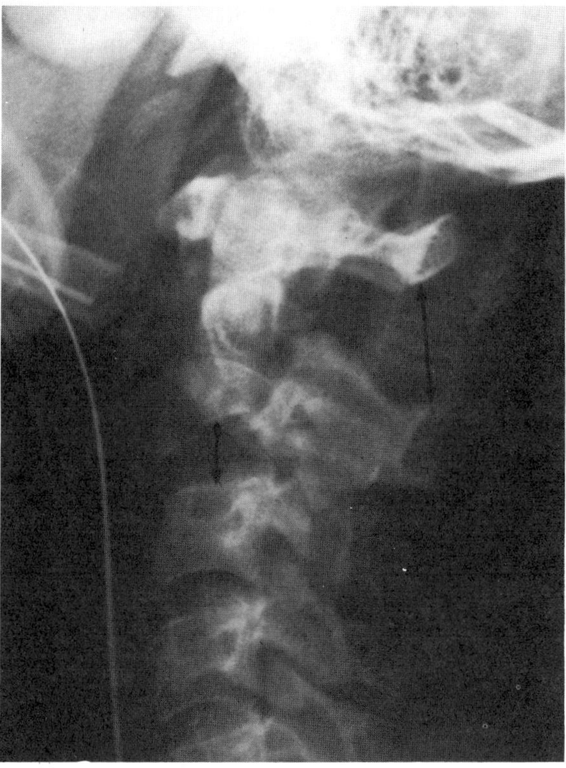

Fig. 19–2. Hangman-type fracture. Lateral radiograph shows disruption of the posterior arch of C2 extending into the body. There is widening of the disk space *(short double arrow)* and also widening of the interspinous space between the posterior arch of C1 and the spinous process of C2 *(long double arrow).* (From Rosen P, Doris P, Barkin R et al: *Diagnostic radiology in emergency medicine,* St. Louis, 1992, Mosby, p 237.)

Unfortunately, the constraints imposed by the limited availability of MRI, as well as the frequent presence of electronic and mechanical equipment attached to the patient currently restrict the use of MRI in an emergency. Nevertheless, because of the frequency and seriousness of associated ligamentous injuries associated with spine trauma, MRI should be obtained if at all possible. Myelography, though not as sensitive as MRI, is an acceptable substitute in many institutions and typically is performed as part of a CT study rather than using plain film radiography, since CT is more sensitive and requires less patient manipulation.

The Thoracic and Lumbosacral Spine

Although damage to the thoracolumbar spine and the cord and nerves it contains are less likely to be life threatening than damage to the cervical spine, the morbidity of such injuries warrants a similar degree of care in dealing with these patients. During an automobile crash the seat-belted patient may flex forward rapidly, causing vertebral compression. This occurs most commonly at or near the thoracolumbar junction in adults, and at T4, T5, and L2 in children. Superior endplate involvement is also common. Transverse vertebral flexion-distraction fractures ("Chance fractures") may also occur in this situation, as may a variety of flexion-rotation injuries including fractures, disc disruptions, and ligamentous disruptions with or without subluxations.

A variety of other mechanisms of injury must also be considered: "Jumpers" who land on their feet transmit a great deal of force to the spine, and vertebral fractures are common in this group. Fractures secondary to lateral bending, shearing or hyperextension as a result of a fall are subject to both bony and ligamentous injuries, with and without subluxations. In the presence of either clinical complaints or neurologic findings suggesting such a problem, or of an abnormality on either the chest or abdomen/pelvis radiographs, additional studies should be performed to clarify the situation, and the patient should be treated as if a fracture or subluxation is present until proved otherwise. CT, with or without intrathecal contrast, and MRI are indicated in this situation for reasons similar to those for the cervical spine.

The Neck

Penetrating injuries of the neck, usually caused by knives or bullets, are relatively common ED problems. The neck contains critical vascular structures as well as the airway and upper esophagus, all in close proximity to each other. As is the case with other critical injuries, the unstable patient belongs in the operating room (OR) not the radiology department. The stable patient, however, will require further studies before management decisions can be made. Clinical evaluation of the airway is part of the primary survey; but with penetrating injuries of the neck, even if the patient lacks symptoms, the neck vessels and esophagus should be evaluated. A four-vessel angiogram, including delayed radiographs for visualization of venous structures is currently the most reliable means for determining the integrity and patency of the vessels as well as for determining if there is any extrinsic mass (hematoma) displacing or compressing them.

Studies of the cervical esophagus are less reliable. Water-soluble contrast studies may demonstrate a leak. However, there is a high false-negative rate for this study as well as for endoscopy. The combination of the two is better than either alone, but if clinical suspicion remains even after the two negative studies, consideration should be given to repeating one or both after observing the patient for several hours. The water-soluble contrast media are very irritating and, if aspirated, may induce a chemical pneumonitis.

Fracture of the larynx should be diagnosed clinically and an airway established without awaiting any radiologic studies.

The Chest

Apart from an intracranial lesion, one of the most devastating problems which can be encountered in the multiple injured patient is massive hemorrhage. The vast majority of persons with rupture of the aorta or other major vessel do not survive long enough to reach the ED, but many of those who do will have a chance of surviving if they are rapidly diagnosed and treated. For this reason, the screening supine AP radiograph taken as part of the secondary survey may play a critical part in the management of these patients. If the patient is stable, the mediastinum is distinct and not widened, and there is no evidence of pleural fluid, the possibility of a ruptured aorta is remote. If, however, the examination is equivocal or positive, further evaluation should be undertaken, the extent and nature of which depends on the patient's clinical state.

The simplest additional view to obtain is the semi-erect or erect frontal radiograph. The ability to perform this study, however, may be limited by the possibility of spine injury or shock. If there are no clinical contraindications, the head of the bed or stretcher may be raised to approximate the position for an upright radiograph and the mediastinum can be reevaluated. While such projections are not the equivalent of a proper PA view, they do overcome some of the problems that characterize the supine view. If these views demonstrate the presence of mediastinal bleeding, and the patient is stable, aortography should be performed. In the presence of equivocal findings on the plain film radiographs, dynamic CT with contrast may be used to demonstrate aortic injury. Although dynamic CT is a very reliable study, a few reports of missed diagnoses have led some authors to obtain aortographic examination when there is a strong clinical suspicion of aortic rupture despite negative studies. Irrespective of other considerations, the unstable patient with a presumed aortic rupture should go straight to the operating room without any delays in the radiology department.

Other thoracic findings which may be appreciated on the posttrauma radiologic examination of the chest include pneumothorax, pulmonary contusion (hemorrhage), rib fractures, radio-opaque foreign bodies and, in the case of penetrating trauma, evidence of the bullet or knife track. In considering a possible pneumothorax, a lateral view or a decubitus view may be of value. Although either of these radiographs only rarely demonstrates pleural air which is not visible on the AP radiograph (or erect PA radiograph if this can be obtained), the lateral or decubitus radiographs may confirm a suspected diagnosis, clarify its extent, or demonstrate the concomitant presence of fluid.

Of all the possible findings noted above, the one that is probably least important is a rib fracture. Although the secondary effects of rib fractures (hemothorax, pneumothorax, etc.) are likely to be clinically important, the fractures themselves generally only require symptomatic therapy unless there is a flail chest, a finding which should be suspected clinically. If, however, it is important to document the condition of the ribs, a rib series consisting of AP and oblique views should be obtained. Since this examination is aimed at demonstrating bone rather than the lungs and vascular structures, the technique used is likely to be very different from that employed for soft tissues, even the AP radiograph; for this reason it is difficult to use the rib radiographs to evaluate the lungs and heart. Conversely, a report of "No rib fractures seen" on a chest radiograph is almost meaningless since a chest radiograph is not adequate to exclude a fracture.

The Abdomen

Blood loss into the abdomen presents a very different problem from blood loss into the chest. The supine abdomen/pelvis radiograph is often very helpful, especially with a lateral view to localize a bullet or other foreign body, but is nonspecific. Indeed, in some centers no protocol radiograph of the abdomen is taken. In the unstable patient, peritoneal lavage is often the most rapid means of making the diagnosis of intraperitoneal bleeding, and the finding generally warrants immediate surgery without further studies. Some surgeons even omit lavage and perform abdominal explorations in all patients with penetrating abdominal wounds. Localization radiographs for foreign bodies may be performed in the OR.

In order to determine the extent of patient injuries, the evaluation of blunt trauma in the stable patient should be undertaken with specific questions in mind. Is there any evidence of vascular injury, with or without free peritoneal fluid? Has there been damage to a parenchymal organ? Has there been a perforation of the bowel? The single examination best suited to answer all these questions is CT. Some preparation is required, however, in order to maximize the yield of the study. To differentiate unopacified bowel from fluid collections, it is important to give the patient contrast material orally or through a gastric tube early since it takes an hour or more to fill the small bowel. Contrast administered directly by rectum opacifies the colon. Intravenous contrast is important to visualize and evaluate the aorta and the other major vascular structures, and also to demonstrate the patency and function of the urinary tract. Free air, either intra- or retroperitoneal, is usually obvious on this study, even in relatively small amounts. Conversely, it may be impossible to appreciate free air on a standard supine abdominal radiograph. Such a finding, in the absence of penetrating trauma, indicates bowel rupture and the need for surgery. Likely sources of retroperitoneal air are the duodenum and colon. A careful evaluation for blood around the aorta as well as around parenchymal organs provides a quick answer to questions about the most serious traumatic lesions. Free intraperitoneal blood should be sought as well. Lower rib or transverse process fractures increase the likelihood of splenic or hepatic injury.

The status of the urinary tract is demonstrated by the completeness of the nephrogram (opacification of renal parenchyma) as well as evidence of excretion of contrast medium into the collecting systems, ureters, and bladder. Absence of nephrograms bilaterally may indicate systemic hypotension, while absence on one side is more suggestive of damage to the ipsilateral renal artery. Leakage of contrast (extravasation of urine) around the ureters is an extremely important, although sometimes subtle finding. Similarly the finding of contrast around the kidneys and bladder indicates a breach in one of these organs. Since the bladder may rupture intraperitoneally as well as extraperitoneally, contrast should be sought between or around some of the loops of bowel bordering on the bladder. However, because the intraperitoneal space is ordinarily free, the contrast may spread out rapidly or become diluted by peritoneal fluid, thus making its identification very difficult. The spine should be carefully evaluated, even in the absence of specific symptoms. A retrograde urethrogram should be performed before catheterization in all patients suspected of having lower urinary tract injury. Catheter insertion can exacerbate a urethral injury, making a partial tear complete, and introducing bacteria to the periurethral tissue. Injury to the posterior urethra most often occurs in adult males in a motor vehicle accident, with or without associated pubic fractures. Children may injure the anterior urethra in bicycle accidents.

After continuity of the urethra is established, retrograde cystography can be used to accurately diagnose bladder rupture. Findings of bladder rupture depend upon the location of the tear. Peritoneal tears cause extravasation into the peritoneal cavity, which causes contrast to outline the serosa of the bowel or the dependent portions of the peritoneal cavity. These collections of contrast have smooth margins of the structures they outline as opposed to the more irregular appearance of extraperitoneal contrast. These injuries may be much more obvious on a retrograde study than on CT.

Penetrating wounds of the abdomen may require a different approach. Peritoneal lavage is an excellent and quick test for intraperitoneal penetration in the case of an anterior stab wound. Another approach is the injection of water-soluble contrast into the wound site followed by a supine abdominal film to look for intraperitoneal spread of the material. If the wound is posterior, the use of lavage is less helpful since a negative study cannot be used to determine if there is retroperitoneal damage. Contrast enhanced CT should be performed in these patients.

The initial abdomen/pelvis radiograph may disclose bony injuries which require further investigation. Pelvic fractures may be associated with vascular injuries or rupture of the bladder or urethra. Pelvic CT should be considered for clarification of the nature of the fractures, especially those in the area of the acetabulum, although fracture repairs are usually less urgent than organ or vascular injury. Evidence of pelvic vascular injury, either on the CT examination or, in the unstable patient, based on the appearance of the pelvic fractures, should be followed by either angiography or immediate exploration. Transcatheter embolization of bleeding vessels may allow for the stabilization of the patient before surgery, or even obviate the need for surgery, and this technique should be used if indicated and if available.

The leading cause of fetal death in cases of maternal trauma is maternal hypotension, not fetal injury. For this reason, the unstable patient does not belong in the radiology department, because the delay in therapy caused by the exam can do the greatest harm. The second most frequent cause of fetal demise following injury is placental separation. Sonography, although imperfect, is the best modality for evaluating this problem. Liquid blood or an echogenic clot may be detected between the placenta and uterine wall. However, because the echogenic clot may have an echogenicity similar to the placenta, the abnormal thickness of the placenta may be the only diagnostic finding. If vaginal bleeding is present, all of the blood may escape, making it impossible to determine whether the placenta which is juxtaposed on the uterine wall is attached or not. In this case, monitoring of fetal heart rate is the most valuable index of fetal well-being and if fetal hypoxia cannot be corrected, only emergency cesarean section will preserve fetal viability. Other abnormalities such as fetal fractures, traumatic uterine perforation, or spontaneous perforation during pregnancy can also be diagnosed sonographically.

CT is the study of choice for evaluating suspected abdominal trauma in victims of child abuse. Intravenous contrast-enhanced CT scans using high volume bolus injection, allow accurate demonstration of solid organ rupture, intraperitoneal hemorrhage, retroperitoneal hemorrhage, or organ devascularization. Hematomas or gas in retroperitoneal locations are easily identified. Hematomas and organ lacerations appear as low-attenuation areas relative to the adjacent enhanced organ parenchyma. Bowel wall hematomas are also readily identified. An alternative method to evaluate possible duodenal hematoma, which may result from automobile trauma, is an upper gastrointestinal series.

Because many patients have damage to more than one organ or region, the radiologic approaches must be modified for the specific clinical situation. For example, when CT of both head and abdomen are required, the study of the head is generally performed first. If there is evidence of intracranial bleeding and the study of the abdomen is aborted so that the patient can be taken directly to the OR, it is still possible to perform peritoneal lavage and obtain a portable film urogram in the OR. If there is concern about a vascular injury, it is even possible to do a single film angiogram to assess major damage. On the other hand, however necessary these shortcuts may be in critical situations, they pose a risk for missed findings or errors. Shortcuts do not substitute for formal radiologic examinations and these should be done as soon as the patient can tolerate them.

The Diaphragm

Although laceration and rupture of the diaphragm are common, *direct* diagnosis is often extremely difficult. These injuries may be assumed with penetrating injuries of the chest below the level of T4; but with blunt injury, the guidelines are less clear. Lavage may introduce air into the peritoneum and cause a pneumothorax visible on a chest radiograph. Even if a radiologic study does not produce a positive finding of peritoneal injury, a negative study does not exclude a diagnosis of diaphragmatic damage. Poor delineation of the diaphragms (more often the left than the right) on the chest radiograph is a suggestive finding, and the presence of bowel in the chest is definitive. This more reliable finding can be seen on the left side on the plain film radiograph, but care should be taken not to confuse an elevated diaphragm with a bowel herniation. A contrast study may be necessary to differentiate between these possibilities. Since the colon may herniate without stomach involvement, the contrast should be followed through the bowel if gastric position does not confirm the diagnosis.

Injury of the right diaphragm, though fortunately a less serious problem, is much more difficult to diagnose because the liver prevents bowel from herniating into the chest. Haziness of the right diaphragm may suggest this occurrence. On occasion, a radionuclide scan of the liver will demonstrate an abnormality of the dome which suggests its herniation through a narrow opening.

The Extremities

Apart from vascular damage and blood loss, injuries of the extremities are not immediately life threatening. Fat embolization, which may occur at the time of trauma or some time thereafter, is unlikely to pose a problem for the patient in the first few days since the clinical syndrome results not from the actual embolization, but from the formation of free fatty acids after the marrow fat is metabolized by pulmonary lipase. The free fatty acids are toxic to alveolar membranes and result in a chemical pneumonitis.

Vascular injury is a more immediate problem, whether or not it is apparent. In the presence of a penetrating injury and clinical evidence of damage to a vessel, the surgeon will probably want to explore the limb promptly. Although an angiographic study may be desirable to facilitate the surgery, most surgeons will operate immediately without further studies. However, when clinical evidence is equivocal, angiographic findings concerning the presence and extent of damage can affect the decision to operate.

Evaluating the patient who has a blunt or penetrating injury in the "proximity" of a major vessel, but who has no clinical evidence of vascular damage is problematic and controversial. Although many surgeons favor vascular studies on all such patients, the yield is relatively low (10% to 15%) and there does not seem to be an increase in morbidity if there is a delay of up to 24 hours before the study is performed. This delay is important because it permits the evaluation of more serious problems first and because it allows the study to be done under controlled conditions rather than as an emergency study in the middle of the night. In the interim, some screening by conventional ultrasound and Doppler pressure and flow studies can be performed and in some instances obviate the need for angiography.

Non-Life-Threatening Injuries

When the patient's condition is stable, the evaluation and treatment may be undertaken for those injuries not previously sought or identified but considered of secondary importance. The following section discusses these injuries as isolated problems. However, combinations of injuries may alter the evaluation and treatment options. An erect Waters view of the sinuses, for example, cannot be obtained on a patient in a Stryker frame.

Facial Bones

The leading causes of facial bone fractures are assault and motor vehicle accidents. Most radiology facilities have a standard facial bone series usually including a Waters view (occipitomental), a Caldwell view (PA), and lateral views. As is the case elsewhere, however, the best examination is the one directed at the specific question to be answered. In the case of the facial bones, the examination is governed by the particular bone or structure that is suspect. In all instances the studies suggested presuppose prior clearance of the cervical spine since moving the patient will be necessary to obtain some of these views.

The Orbits

The walls and rims of the orbits are composed of components from multiple facial bones. The most common locations for orbital fractures are (1) the floor of the orbit which is formed from the roof of the facial bone, and (2) the medial wall or lamina papyracea, the thinnest wall of the orbit. Orbital fractures may be isolated or they may be components of more complex facial injuries. Initial examination should include a Waters view and oblique views of the orbit(s). Direct radiologic signs of orbital fracture consist of bone fragmentation, bony depression, and soft tissue prolapse through the orbital floor. Secondary signs include orbital emphysema (which indicates fracture into an air-containing sinus) and sinus opacification, especially evidence of free fluid on the erect Waters view. Soft tissue prolapse through the orbital floor (hematoma, orbital fat, or herniated muscle) can be confused with concurrent, but unrelated sinus disease on plain films. The threshold for performance of a CT examination should be extremely low since CT can help differentiate the prolapsed contents, especially when herniated muscle or muscle entrapment is suspected. It will also permit much more precise mapping of bone fragments, which makes surgical decisions considerably easier. Since CT has replaced linear tomography for evaluation of the orbit and other facial bones, linear tomography should only be performed if CT is unavailable.

The Zygomas

Trauma to the zygomatic bones can be isolated or associated with other facial injuries. Because the zygoma is part of a ring, fracture usually occurs in at least two places. This may involve the arch of the bone, or it may consist of a complete separation of the malar eminence at the zygomaticofrontal suture, the zygomaticotemporal suture, and the zygomaticomaxillary suture. This combination is commonly known as a tripod injury. Plain film studies best designed to visualize the zygoma are the Waters, Towne (frontooccipital) and base (submentovertex, tangential zygomatic arch, "jug-handle") views. Zygomatic injuries, and the extent of depression or displacement, are usually easily recognized on this series, although infrequently CT is required for the diagnosis. CT is also useful when an associated facial injury is suspected.

The Maxilla

Isolated maxillary fractures are uncommon, accounting for less than 5% of midface fractures. The maxillary bones provide bony support for the face, forming the lateral walls of the nasal cavity and the anterior hard palate as well as maxillary alveolus. They also form the orbital floor and medial portion of the infraorbital rim and thus are frequently involved in orbital as well as tripod fractures. Maxillary bones participate in the classic Le Fort fractures (Fig. 19–3), which are complex injuries involving not only the maxilla but the orbits, zygomatic arches, and pterygoid plates. These fractures are typically unstable and require careful evaluation for surgery. CT examination is needed to supplement the plain film study. Three-dimensional reconstruction from CT studies is useful in sorting out these complex injuries.

The Mandible

Mandibular fractures are common, typically resulting from a direct blow. The mandible is firmly attached to the skull bilaterally at the temporomandibular joint and behaves as a bony ring. Fifty percent of mandibular fractures are bilateral or are associated with temporomandibular joint dislocations. The majority of mandibular fractures occur in the body and angle; injuries to the symphysis and ramus occur less frequently. Plain film examination should include a PA view of the mandible, oblique views of the two sides, and a steep Towne view to demonstrate the ramus and the temporomandibular articulation. Some radiology departments can perform panoramic views which can be a great help in demonstrating the mandible free of other overlying structures. For this projection, as well as for occlusal views, it may be necessary to refer the patient for dental examination. Indeed, the relationship of mandibular fractures to the teeth should always be noted. Communication with a tooth root converts a mandibular fracture into an open injury.

The Nasal Bones

The nasal bones are the most frequently fractured portion of the facial skeleton. A transverse fracture isolated to the nasal tip is the most common type and is best eval-

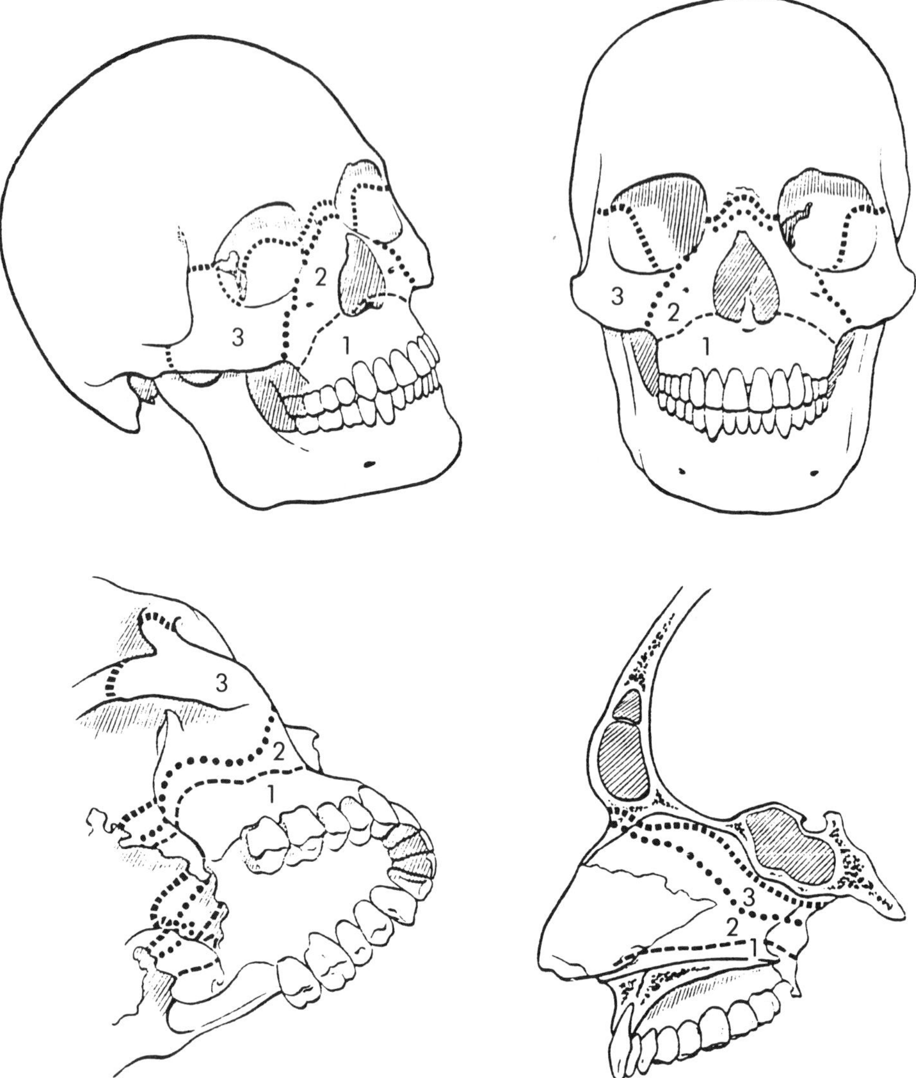

Fig. 19–3. Le Fort I fracture on the level of the nasal floor *(1)*; Le Fort II through the nasal bones, infraorbital rims, and maxilla *(2)*; and Le Fort III through the frontozygomatic suture, orbits, and the zygomatic arch *(3)*. (Used with permission from Dingman RO, Natvig P: *Surgery of facial fractures,* Philadelphia, 1964, WB Saunders.)

uated by an underpenetrated, coned-down lateral view. Less common, longitudinal nasal bone fractures occur and must be differentiated from normal grooves of the nasomaxillary suture and nasociliary nerve. These grooves are more irregular and less lucent than a fracture line. A Waters view may be helpful in visualizing a longitudinal fracture disrupting the nasal arch and any deviation of the bony nasal septum. It should be noted that studies of the nasal bones are of questionable value, since closed treatment usually suffices.

The Spine

The absence of an immediately identifiable life-threatening injury initially is no guarantee that a significant spinal injury does not exist. A more systematic review can be obtained in the radiology department once the patient is stabilized. As was the case during the survey of the mandible, plain film radiography is the starting point for the evaluation. If the earlier initial radiographs were technically adequate, only supplementary studies need be obtained at this point; but if less than ideal views were obtained, they should be repeated. Once again, CT and CT myelography as well as MRI should be considered. MRI permits noninvasive evaluation of the intervertebral disks, ligamentous injury, and relationships of vertebral fragments to the spinal cord. To assess anatomic stability, it is extremely important to evaluate the anterior and posterior longitudinal ligaments and annulus fibrosis in addition to more easily seen bony structures. Distinct patterns on MRI differentiate acute cord hemorrhage, spinal cord edema, and contusion. In addition, late complications such as syringomyelia are well evaluated by MRI. Indications for MRI include clinical evidence of spinal cord injury without osseous findings, a fracture-dislocation considered insufficient to cause the observed symptoms, and the clinical progression of symptoms that cannot be accounted for by simpler examinations. MRI cannot be used on patients who have cardiac pacemakers, cerebral aneurysm clips, or claustrophobia. Nonmagnetic support-system equipment now available allows MRI evaluation of many of these critical patients.

The Cervical Spine

Evaluation of the initial plain radiographs requires examination of alignment, bone integrity, joint spaces, and soft tissues. The lateral view is used to look for a smooth curve along the anterior margins of the vertebral bodies, the posterior margins, and the base of the spinous processes (spinolaminal line). Children in particular may present with a pseudosubluxation at C1–C2 and C2–C3. An intact spinolaminal line indicates the ligamentous laxity is physiologic.

Oblique views show the posterior elements of the vertebrae including the neural foramina. If the patient cannot be moved for standard oblique views, the technologist may be able to obtain studies by angling the tube and adjusting the position of the tube and film without moving the patient. The same is true if the remainder of the cervical spine exam is normal and the open-mouth view is inadequate. It may be helpful to perform angled or obliqued views of the area. This often permits adequate visualization of the odontoid.

Flexion and extension views of the cervical spine are reserved for patients with abnormal alignment. Abnormal alignment may be caused by positioning as well as by muscle spasm or instability. Since the first examination is likely to have been performed with the patient wearing a collar, or with the head supported by the stretcher, a true neutral lateral view will not have been obtained and straightening or flexion of the spine may be suggested on the radiographs. If the patient's condition permits an upright lateral radiograph with the collar removed, this view may demonstrate that alignment is normal.

Flexion Injury

While flexion injuries of the cervical spine are often extremely unstable, some compression fractures may not be associated with significant neurological problems. In addition, hyperflexion fracture of the spinous process, the "Clay Shoveler's" fracture (Fig. 19–4), is a stable injury without significant sequelae. This injury usually involves C6, C7, or T1. Nonbony injuries may also be present. Hyperflexion sprains present with focal symptoms. On radiological examination there may be focal kyphosis, mild anterolisthesis, and a widened posterior and narrowed anterior disk space. If the diagnosis of instability cannot be established, the best additional views *(when possible and under close supervision)* are upright-lateral and flexion and extension views. The diagnosis of "whiplash," a hyperextension-hyperflexion injury typically following an automobile accident, should only be made after more serious structural damage has been excluded.

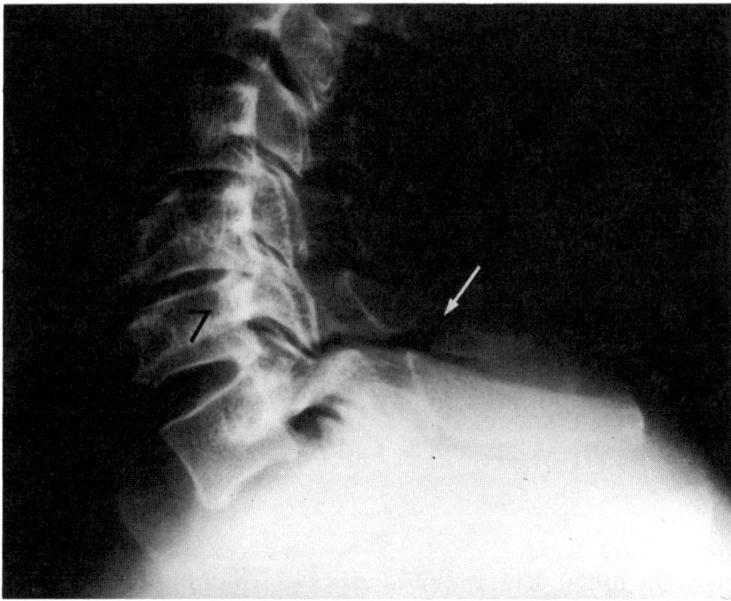

Fig. 19–4. Clay shoveler" fracture of the spinous process of C7 *(arrow).* (From Rosen P, Doris P, Barkin R et al: *Diagnostic radiology in emergency medicine,* St. Louis, 1992, Mosby, p 239.)

Hyperextension Injuries

Hyperextension of the cervical spine places major stress on the posterior elements leading to fractures of the posterior ring and spinous process. Because these are adjacent to the cord, all posterior fractures should be viewed as unstable. However, muscle sprains may be present without bony injury. Hyperextension injuries often occur with blows to the face and forehead and are usually accompanied by fractures of these areas.

Thoracolumbar Spine

In addition to the more serious thoracolumbar injuries, simple compression fractures, traumatic spondylolysis, disc herniations, and soft tissue injuries may occur. Oblique views, especially of the lumbosacral spine, may be useful, particularly to evaluate the pars interarticularis (for fracture) and the neural foramina. Flexion, extension, and lateral flexion radiographs may be used to determine range of motion and stability of the spine. The same cautions that pertain to the rest of the spine should be considered here, although the likelihood of serious damage is not nearly as great. MRI is an excellent modality for evaluation of the ligaments and muscles around the spine as well as the intervertebral discs. Although CT myelography may also be used for disc evaluation, MRI, if available, is preferred.

Sacrum and Coccyx

Even though fractures of the sacrum and coccyx may be associated with spinal or pelvic injuries, they are often overlooked. On plain film radiographs the presence of bowel and stool overlying these structures makes evaluation difficult. Lateral and angled views of the sacrum are sometimes useful but not definitive. Linear tomography in the lateral projection may offer some help as will CT, especially if multiplanar or three-dimensional reconstruction is available.

The Extremities

Much more common than spinal injuries are fractures and dislocations of the extremities. Typically, the radiologic evaluation of the extremities is straightforward, consisting of right-angle views, usually AP and lateral, of the affected areas. In some cases, different views such as internal and external rotation views of the shoulder or AP and oblique views of the ribs are indicated. In all cases, the radiographs obtained should be of adequate quality to evaluate the soft tissues as well as the bones, since the presence of joint effusion, swelling, soft tissue air, or foreign bodies provides valuable diagnostic information. Not all foreign bodies however, are visible by radiologic examination, and failure to identify such foreign bodies does not exclude their presence. This is especially true of wood, glass, plastic, and graphite.

A combination of frontal and lateral plain film views is a good way to begin a skeletal study but specific areas and specific diagnoses require unique examinations. In the case of a suspected fracture that cannot be visualized by plain film radiography, a radionuclide bone scan performed 1 or 2 days following the trauma may demonstrate the fracture. These studies are quite sensitive and are almost always positive within this period if there is a fracture. Conversely, a negative radionuclide scan 3 days after injury virtually excludes a fracture. Bone scanning is especially important in the evaluation of possible child abuse. A good screening procedure is to request a total body scan followed by plain film radiographs of suspicious areas.

Special consideration should be given to fractures in children for other reasons. Because the appearance of the bones differs greatly based on age and stage of development, as well as on a wide range of normal variants, it may be necessary to obtain comparison radiographs of the asymptomatic side to get a sense of what is normal for that particular child at that age. Even if the sides are not identical, the child's own anatomy and development will probably be the best control available. In addition, developing bones are subject to different kinds of injuries from those which are more mature. Open epiphyses are prone to fractures, and such fractures may have very serious implications if healing of such a fracture leads to premature epiphyseal closure. Children's bones are also more elastic than those of adults and therefore fractures have a different appearance. Fractures through children's bones are often incomplete, either without a distinct fracture line or with one that does not cross the bone. "Greenstick" and "torus" fractures are examples of this type of injury. Bowing of these elastic bones ("plastic deformity") may also occur and the bone may heal with the bowed shape causing functional problems.

Shoulder

Because obtaining internal and external rotation views may worsen the damage caused by trauma, an alternate approach is necessary. A lateral view of the shoulder (transthoracic lateral) is often difficult to evaluate because the target anatomy is obscured by the ribs, spine, and the other shoulder; therefore, an oblique view is preferable. A useful projection is the lateral scapular view ("Y view") which is taken in the axis of the body of the scapula. Consequently, the humeral head should be superimposed on the glenoid making the evaluation for dislocation simple. While an anterior dislocation of the humerus is easily recognized both clinically and on a standard radiograph, a posterior dislocation may be more subtle. The Y view gives direct information regarding this possibility.

If acromioclavicular separation is suspected, the examination should include both sides, since a comparison of the two may make diagnosis easier. AP radiographs both with and without 5 pound weights in each hand should accentuate any separation. The important finding is an increased distance between the acromion and clavicle superoinferiorly, not laterally. Although capsular and ligamentous injury may be suspected on plain film radiographs, they are best diagnosed by arthrography or by MRI.

Elbow

Internal and external rotation views may demonstrate a radial head fracture not seen on the standard series. If an elbow effusion is present, there is about a 50%

chance of a fracture, whether it is seen or not. In adults, the radial head is the usual site. The supracondylar area of the humerus is more commonly affected in children. If a fracture is suspected but not demonstrable on plain film radiography, it may be useful to treat the patient as if a fracture is present and obtain a radionuclide scan or repeat plain film examination in 7 to 10 days when bone resorption should make a fracture line more obvious.

Forearm

Isolated fractures of the radius and ulna are the norm. However, an association of a fracture of either of these bones with a second fracture or dislocation at the joint proximal or distal to the fracture is also common. For this reason it is important to see both the elbow and wrist when examining a forearm fracture. This will help in the diagnosis of a Monteggia fracture (ulnar fracture with a radial head dislocation [Fig. 19–5]) or a Galeazzi fracture (radial fracture with distal ulnar dislocation [Fig. 19–6]).

Wrist and Hand

A lateral view of the wrist is very helpful in evaluating the relationship of the carpus to the distal radius. Lateral views of the hand are typically less useful to accompany the frontal view because of the numerous overlying bones which may obscure any pathology. For this reason an oblique view of the hand with the fingers separated is preferable.

Injuries of the ligaments and cartilages of the wrist may be effectively visualized by MRI as is the case with these tissues elsewhere. Three-compartment arthrography, although more invasive than MRI, is more likely to demonstrate ligamentous disruption.

Pelvis

The pelvis is a ring structure and, like a doughnut, is rarely broken in only one place. If one fracture is found, a thorough search for another fracture, or a disruption of the symphysis pubis or of one of the sacroiliac joints is mandatory. Similarly, ischial fractures are rarely isolated. Finding a second ischial fracture, however, should be considered the same as finding one fracture of the entire pelvic ring, and a search for a second pelvic fracture should be undertaken.

Examination of the sacroiliac joints is usually unsatisfactory on the standard AP

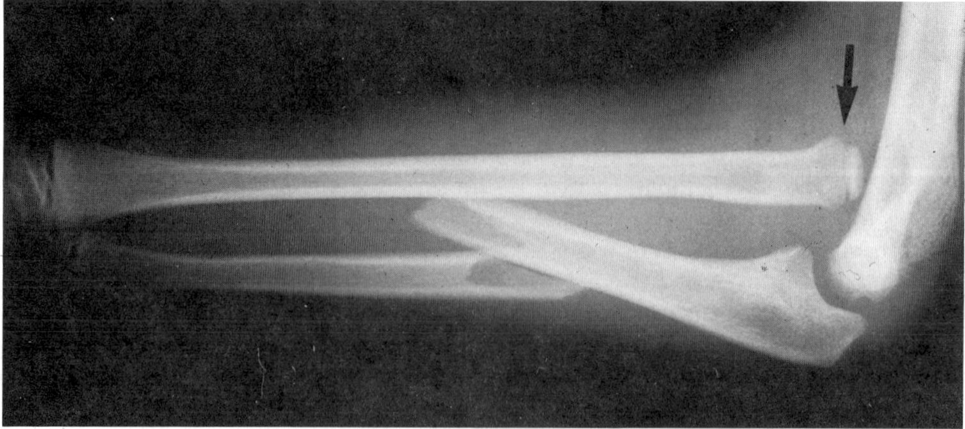

Fig. 19–5. Monteggia fracture, lateral view. A fracture of the proximal ulna is demonstrated along with anterior dislocation of the radial head *(arrow).* (From Rosen P, Doris P, Barkin R et al: *Diagnostic radiology in emergency medicine,* St. Louis, 1992, Mosby, p 170.)

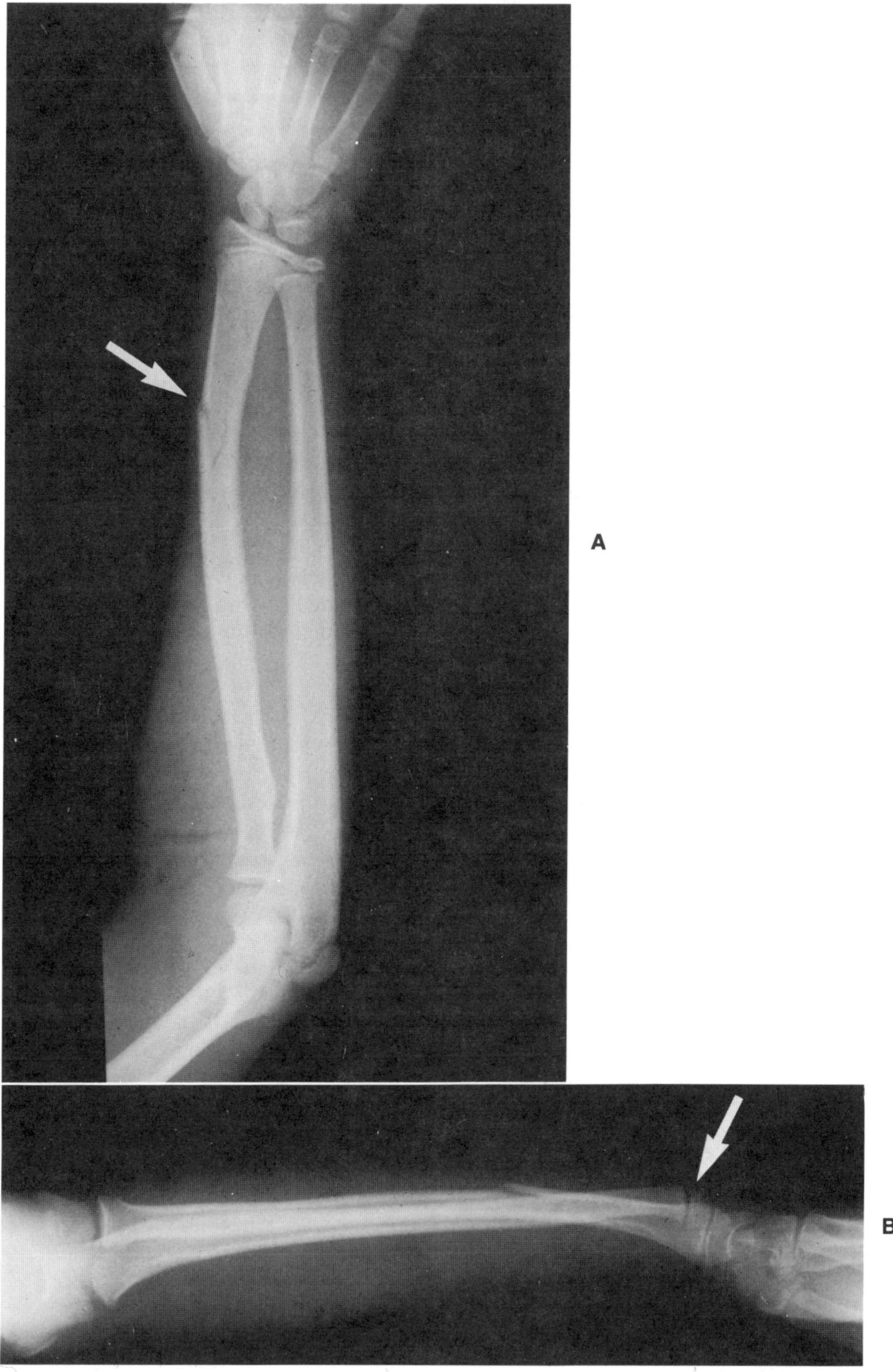

Fig. 19–6. Galeazzi fracture. **A,** AP view. This fracture involves a break at the junction of the middle and distal thirds of the radius *(arrow)* with disruption of the distal radioulnar ligaments. **B,** Lateral view. Note subluxation of distal radioulnar joint *(arrow).* (From Rosen P, Doris P, Barkin R et al: *Diagnostic radiology in emergency medicine,* St. Louis, 1992, Mosby, p 171.)

film of the pelvis. (A lateral view of the pelvis is rarely taken since it is ordinarily not revealing.) Because of the angle of the joints, the SI joints in a prone patient are oriented in the same direction as the diverging x-ray beam and they can be better seen on this projection. An alternative is to obtain oblique views of the joints with the patient supine.

Fractures of the acetabular area are extremely difficult to sort out on plain film radiographs because of the complex anatomy of the anterior and posterior pillars. CT examination permits the identification of the fracture fragments, including any which are intraarticular, and guide the orthopedic management.

Hip

A lateral view is extremely important in the evaluation of a fracture or dislocation, but it should be obtained without moving the patient so as not to increase the damage. It can be taken with the normal hip in flexion and raised above the tabletop while using a horizontal (cross-table) beam.

Knee

AP and lateral views are adequate in most situations; however the addition of tangential ("skyline" or "sunset") views helps in the evaluation of the patella. A tunnel view may help if an intraarticular bony fragment is sought. To best demonstrate the head of the fibula and the proximal tibiofibular joint, an oblique view with the lower leg internally rotated is helpful. Ligamentous and cartilaginous injuries are common but not visible on plain film radiography. MRI, which is extremely sensitive in these situations, has supplanted knee arthrography.

Ankle

Ankle injuries frequently result in multiple fractures or in a combination of bony and ligamentous injury. Moreover, the fibular fracture in an *eversion* injury may be several centimeters proximal to the ankle. Thus it is important to see the distal third of the fibula in patients with ankle injuries. Oblique views are useful for visualizing the ankle and the knee. Avulsion fractures of the base of the fifth metatarsal are associated with *inversion* ankle injuries. An oblique view of the foot demonstrates this to advantage.

Calcaneus

Calcaneal fractures often result from jumps or falls and should be suspected in such injuries along with spinal fractures. A tangential calcaneal view should be taken in addition to a lateral view.

NONTRAUMA PATIENTS

Although the radiologic evaluation of emergency patients who have not suffered trauma is in many ways similar to the evaluation of injured patients, additional studies are done for nontrauma patients, which are more specific for "medical" emergencies.

Facial Bones

Paranasal Sinuses

Because of the possible consequences of acute sinusitis, emergency evaluation is sometimes necessary, especially when sphenoid cells are involved. The minimum examination in this situation is an erect Waters view to demonstrate the maxillary antra and the frontal sinuses. If the study is done with the mouth open, the sphenoids may be seen. Otherwise an erect lateral view should be obtained as well. A Caldwell view will be necessary if visualization of the ethmoids is required. In the presence of clinical evidence of acute sinusitis, air-fluid levels, which indicate free fluid, are diagnostic. Free blood may have the same appearance and is an important finding in persons who have suffered trauma. Mucosal thickening or masses within the sinuses suggest chronic inflammation. A completely opacified sinus, especially a frontal cell, raises the possibility of a mucocele. Evidence of bony expansion around the lesion supports this diagnosis.

Mastoids

Since mastoiditis is not a radiologic diagnosis, there is no reason to request an examination of the mastoids in the ED.

Cervical Spine

Plain film radiography of the spine remains the first choice in the evaluation of neck pain or torticollis. Positioning of patients with nontraumatic neck pain is considerably easier than after trauma, and the entire examination may be performed immediately without review of the first radiograph. Because nerve root compression is a common cause of neck pain, especially pain radiating to the arms, oblique views should be obtained. To fully evaluate patients with rheumatoid arthritis, it is important to obtain an adequate study of the odontoid. Since such patients may have atlantoaxial involvement with instability, they should be examined with this possibility in mind. When a cervical disk herniation is a consideration, CT (myelography) or MRI may be used.

Osteomyelitis of the spine as well as other bones is becoming an increasingly common problem because of the prevalence of intravenous drug use and HIV infection. In these patients, its clinical and radiologic patterns are far more varied than in the past. Because of the morbidity associated with bone infection, rapid diagnosis and therapy are important. However, disease findings may not be seen on plain film radiographic films for at least 10 days to 2 weeks and even then the manifestations may be nonspecific, although significant damage has already occurred. Radionuclide bone scan is a rapid, relatively inexpensive study for the early diagnosis of osteomyelitis. Although bone-seeking radiologic agents simply identify areas of increased turnover, in the appropriate clinical setting they can assist in rapid diagnosis. If confirmation is needed, an additional study can be performed using gallium or indium-labeled white cells, since these agents localize at the site of infection. However, these studies take longer to perform and are more expensive than studies with technetium and should not be the first examinations performed in this situation.

Thoracolumbar Spine

Strains, sprains, and disk disease present the majority of problems in both the cervical and thoracolumbar spine. Degenerative disease is also extremely common in this area, but it is difficult to correlate this finding with specific symptoms. The most common reason given for a request for lumbosacral spine radiographs is "low back pain." Such pain may originate in the aorta, pancreas, urinary tract, and pelvic and abdominal organs, as well as in the spine, and routinely obtaining spinal radiographs in these patients is expensive and unproductive. Although difficult to define, specific justification for a radiologic examination in the ED might include neurologic findings, radiation of pain, and clinical findings suggesting either osteomyelitis or tumor of the spine.

The initial radiologic survey should include AP and lateral views of the symptomatic area, with a coned-down lateral view of the lumbosacral junction, if disease is suspected at this level. Although oblique views are useful in evaluating the lumbar spine for spondylolysis, this defect is not likely to occur in the thoracic spine, and oblique views are rarely useful in evaluating this portion of the spine. Because abnormalities of the sacroiliac (SI) joints may present as low back pain, SI joint views may be required. The indications for radionuclide scanning, CT, CT myelography, and MRI are the same as for the evaluation of the cervical spine.

Although extremely uncommon, cord or cauda equina compression can be catastrophic and requires urgent evaluation and decompression. Among the causes are acute disk herniation, tumor, and other sources of vertebral collapse, including trauma and infection. In the past, the "gold standard" examination in this situation was myelography, alone or as part of a CT study. MRI can demonstrate the location of the problem and the cause of the compression, as well as its effect on the cord and nerve roots. For these reasons, and because it is simpler and safer, MRI is now the examination of choice.

Neck

Soft tissue radiographs are essential to the management of airway compromise in the neck. These films evaluate epiglottitis effectively and noninvasively. A lateral neck radiograph shows the air column, the swollen epiglottis and aryepiglottic folds, and subglottic edema. The referring physician should always accompany the patient to Radiology in the event that an emergency intubation or cricothyrotomy is necessary.

Radiodense foreign bodies, such as chicken bones, may be detected on a lateral neck radiograph. Fish bones are usually radiolucent and not seen on the study. Complicating the situation further is the sensation of a "stuck" bone, resulting from its earlier passing.

Another radiolucent foreign body commonly encountered is food, especially meat, caught in the cervical airway obstructing air flow. If the foreign body reaches the cervical or thoracic esophagus, a contrast esophagram may be performed. Care should be taken not to induce aspiration of the contrast medium; the iodinated materials are extremely toxic to the lungs and barium is a safer material. Once the foreign body has been located and removed, it is worthwhile to consider repeating the esophagram to determine whether inflammation or tumor may have caused a preexisting narrowing of the esophagus, that prevented the food from passing.

Chest

Radiologic studies of the chest are more standardized than those of other regions and are well known to the clinician. The best examination for almost any chest complaint warranting a study consists of an erect PA and a left lateral radiograph (Fig. 19–7). Since the study is best performed while the patient is inspiring deeply, its usefulness will be limited by the patient's ability to do so. A technically satisfactory study provides excellent visibility of the heart and lungs with minimum magnification and distortion.

Unfortunately, not all patients can cooperate for this examination, and for very sick patients the best study obtainable may be a supine AP radiograph. On this view, the diaphragms tend to be higher, since gravity does not aid in lung expansion, and therefore lung visualization is often poor. The heart and mediastinal structures are magnified since the radiograph is taken at 40 to 48 inches instead of the standard 6 feet, and the pulmonary vessels appear engorged because of greater hydrostatic pressures compared to a patient who is upright. Nevertheless, a properly performed AP examination is usually satisfactory for the clinical management of the emergency patient.

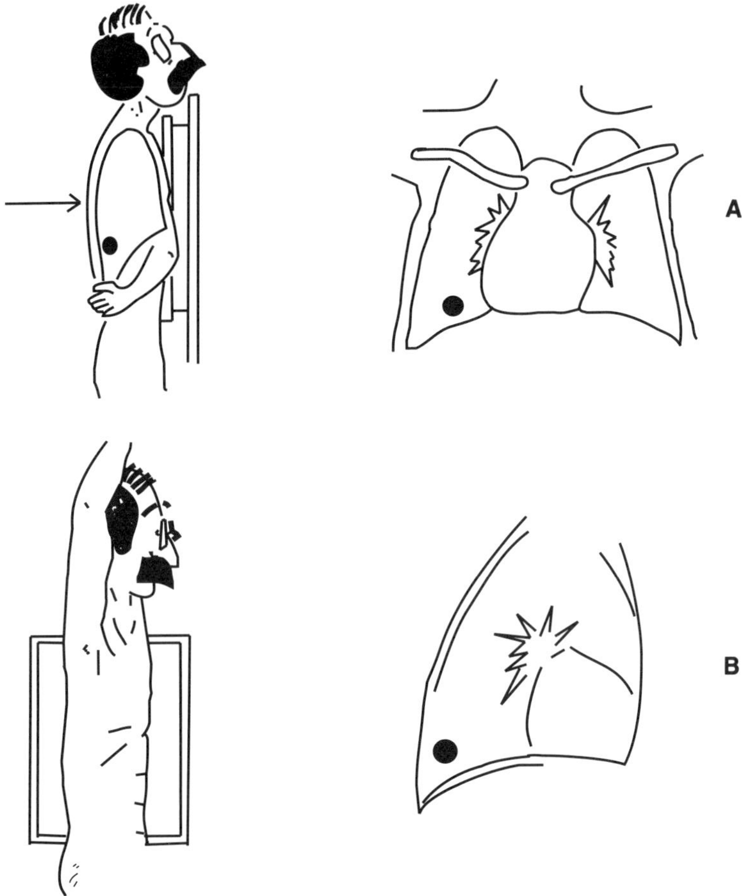

Fig. 19–7. Commonly used projections for chest radiography. **A,** Posteroanterior projection, **B,** lateral projection. Although a left lateral is routine and is illustrated here, a right lateral might be chosen on some occasions for evaluation of a right-sided abnormality. A right lower lobe mass is shown to demonstrate how a typical pulmonary density might appear on the different views.

Except for infants, the radiologic examination of the chest in pediatric patients is similar to the examination in adults, although many centers do not obtain lateral radiographs for this group because of the low yield. For infants, the study often consists only of a supine AP radiograph because other views may be difficult to obtain. A horizontal-beam ("cross-table") lateral view is often very helpful when looking for a pneumothorax in an infant.

Although the standard examination can answer almost all of the clinical questions raised during the emergency chest evaluation, additional views may be useful in particular situations. These situations are usually defined by the specific findings sought, rather than by a particular disease. The discussion that follows, therefore, focuses on the best methods for demonstrating these findings.

Pulmonary Densities

It is unusual for a significant pulmonary density, infiltrate, or mass to be present if there is no indication of it on the standard PA and lateral views. Therefore, it makes neither medical nor economic sense to order a "routine" apical lordotic view to screen for tuberculosis. Such a view, which allows visualization of the lung apices without overlying clavicles and upper ribs (Fig. 19–8), should be obtained only when there is

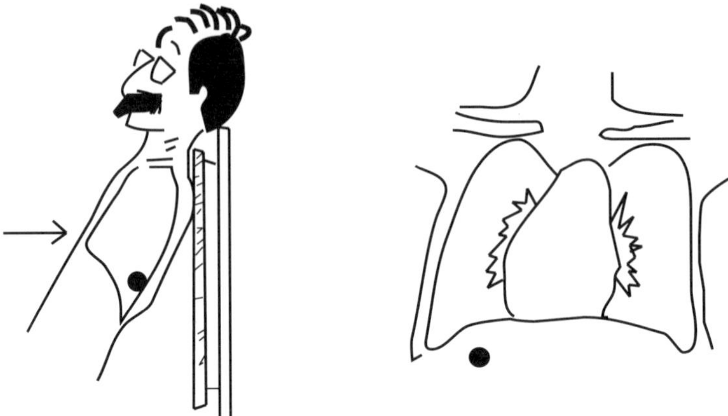

Fig. 19–8. Apical lordotic projection.

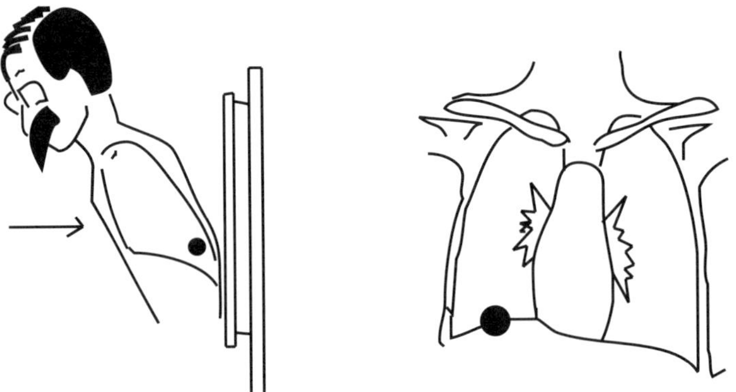

Fig. 19–9. Kyphotic projection—has its greatest application for posterior basal densities.

an ambiguous finding on the initial study (PA and lateral radiographs). The lordotic view is taken with the patient's thoracic spine hyperextended, whereas the kyphotic film is taken with the patient flexed forward. The kyphotic view (Fig. 19–9) shows the lung bases posteriorly, especially those areas that are ordinarily hidden by the diaphragmatic domes on the frontal view. The upper portion of the chest is somewhat distorted on this view. As is true of the lordotic view, the kyphotic radiograph should only be obtained to clarify findings already noted on another study.

Oblique views (Figs. 19–10, *A* and *B*) occasionally help localize a density seen in only one view, either the PA or the lateral. By noting the direction of movement of the density relative to structures whose location is known (e.g., the spine) the position of the density in question can be determined. Oblique views also provide additional perspective of an already identified mass.

The lateral decubitus view may be very helpful in demonstrating the pulmonary parenchyma when other methods are unsuccessful because of the patient's inability to expand the lungs fully. It is difficult to evaluate pulmonary processes on the side of the body on which the patient is lying, because the lung has a relatively small volume. The relative overexpansion of the raised lung, however, displays the pulmonary parenchyma quite well. The raised lung is also clearly seen because in this position much of the blood flow is shunted away from it. This shunting away of blood may determine the degree to which "vascular shadows" are responsible for a finding of a pulmonary density because the vessels will change in appearance while other densities will not.

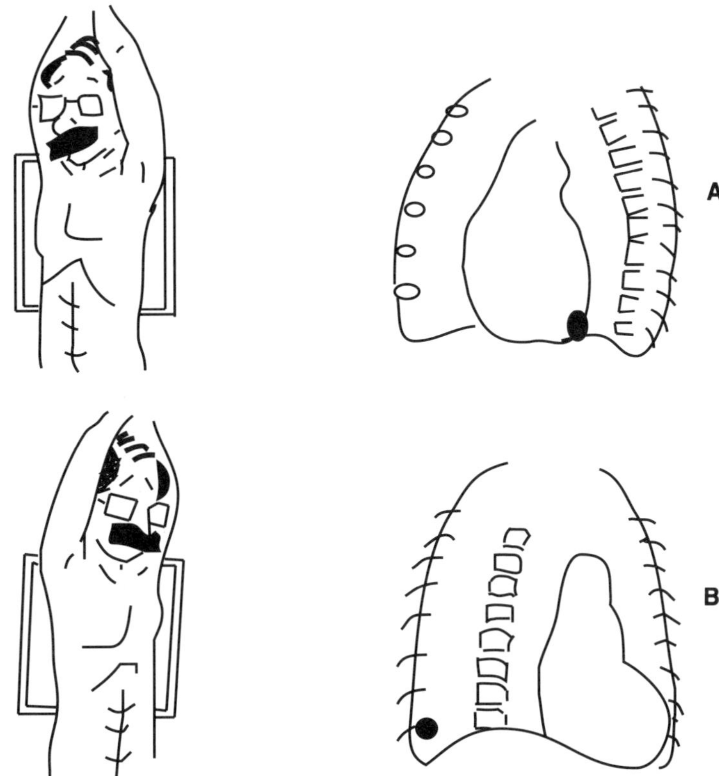

Fig. 19–10. A, Right posterior oblique. A similar appearance may be noted on a left anterior oblique position. **B,** Left posterior oblique, the equivalent of the right anterior oblique.

CT and MRI can provide additional information about the nature and number of pulmonary masses, as well as the character and possible cause of interstitial disease. However, they are rarely indicated in the ED.

Pleural Fluid

Apparent elevation of the diaphragm, especially when accompanied by a concave "meniscus" where the diaphragm meets the chest wall, suggests the possibility of pleural fluid. The decubitus views are the best choice for differentiating free fluid from fixed pleural fibrosis, loculations, or diaphragmatic elevation. In addition, the decubitus position may allow unseen fluid to "layer out" along the chest wall where it will be easily identified. Because of the way fluid may be distributed inferior to the lung on erect radiographs, several hundred milliliters of fluid may be present but not seen without additional radiographs. Properly positioned decubitus views may be used to demonstrate far smaller volumes—as little as a few milliliters under experimental conditions.

Although the viewer's attention is ordinarily attracted to the dependent side in the search for fluid, the raised side should be checked as well. The goal of decubitus views is to change the appearance of the costophrenic angle. It does not matter whether a clear angle becomes blunted and fluid layers out when the patient changes position or whether a blunted angle becomes clear. In both instances the change indicates movable fluid. Since the dependent side may be more difficult to evaluate because of interference from overlying sheets and the mattress, it may be helpful to look for clearing on the (raised) side with the blunted angle. Decubitus views are labeled by the side that is dependent. A right lateral decubitus radiograph is taken with the right side down. The request for a right-sided decubitus radiograph to evaluate a possible left-sided effusion may seem incorrect unless the purpose of the particular projections is understood.

CT is very sensitive to the presence of pleural fluid, and this finding may be noted on a CT examination obtained for another purpose. An attempt to diagnose or exclude pleural fluid, however, is not an adequate reason to perform a CT.

Pneumothorax

Horizontal-beam radiographs are the most sensitive for demonstrating pleural air, and the erect PA chest view is the best study to demonstrate pneumothorax (and for pneumoperitoneum since the air rises to the inferior margins of the diaphragm). Since small amounts of air paralleling the upper chest wall and apex may be difficult to see, obtaining an expiratory view may help. Decreased lung volume causes the extrapulmonary air to occupy a greater percentage of thoracic volumes and appear more obvious. Decubitus views may also help by shifting the air from the apex to the lower lateral chest wall. The nondependent side in these patients is the one of interest.

Tension pneumothorax, accompanied by compromise of functional pulmonary volume and compression of mediastinal vessels, is a life-threatening emergency. Radiologic examination will demonstrate complete absence of lung on the involved side and displacement of the mediastinum contralaterally. Because of the life-threatening nature of this problem, if the diagnosis is suspected clinically, a tube thoracostomy should be performed before obtaining any radiologic views.

Pulmonary Blood Flow

The recognition of pulmonary embolism is one of the most difficult clinical challenges a physician must face. Although history and laboratory findings may suggest the diagnosis, the findings vary widely. The standard chest radiograph may demonstrate hilar prominence, apparent discrepancies in pulmonary blood flow, diaphragmatic elevation, infiltrate (pulmonary infarction), or pleural fluid (pulmonary infarction), but more typically the radiograph will be normal or nondiagnostic. Both clinical and radiologic findings may overlap in cases of asthma and other types of obstructive pulmonary disease. The "gold standard" imaging examination for demonstrating blood flow is pulmonary angiography. However, radionuclide studies, especially the combination of vascular perfusion and ventilation (V/Q) scans, have become the standard screening procedure for most patients. Angiography, which is more invasive and time consuming, should be reserved for ambiguous situations following lung scanning and for those cases when immediate surgery is planned and the surgeon needs a "road map."

When the most likely source of a pulmonary embolus is venous thrombosis in the deep veins of the legs, compression ultrasonography and Doppler studies should be performed to verify this possibility. Radionuclide and contrast venography may also be considered for this purpose. However, all of these studies are best delayed until the emergency situation has been resolved.

Evidence of cardiac failure is provided by standard views of the chest, which can demonstrate pulmonary vascular engorgement, usually secondary to cardiac failure. Although the degree of cardiac failure may be quantified by the size of the hilar and peripheral vessels, the hilar vascular angle, and the distribution of vessels through the lungs, the *clinical* assessment of cardiac failure is the best guide for patient management.

Aortic Integrity

Aortic dissection, like aortic rupture, can result in rapid exsanguination and obstruction of arteries that branch from the aorta (e.g., the carotids and vertebrals), causing ischemia of the organs served by these vessels. The diagnosis of aortic dissection, once considered, must be evaluated expeditiously. The suggestion of mediastinal widening in a patient with chest or back pain may trigger concern about a dissection but is not a reliable finding, especially on recumbent radiographs.

Echocardiography may directly demonstrate a dissection at the aortic root, as well as aortic regurgitation or pericardial fluid, if these accompany the dissection. Contrast-enhanced CT, particularly with dynamic imaging, is an excellent method for demonstrating luminal narrowing by subintimal collections. Contrast may also be demonstrated on both sides of the flap. Note should be made of blood surrounding the aorta, which is a sign of rupture.

Aortography for dissection, like pulmonary angiography for pulmonary embolism, is the definitive examination if other studies are nondiagnostic or if precise information is necessary for surgery. However, since aortography is both hazardous and time consuming, patients with actual or possible dissections should be taken to the intensive care unit or operating room as soon as possible. When the dissection extends into the abdomen, evaluation by ultrasound may be useful; however, overlying gas-filled bowel, may interfere with this study.

Airway Compromise

Foreign bodies within the trachea or main bronchi, as well as strictures, masses, or extrinsic compression, may compromise air flow which in turn may be physiologically significant or may simply cause audible wheezing. High-kilovoltage (kv) chest radiographs may demonstrate deviation of the trachea but rarely resolve questions concerning specific tracheal lesions. Mediastinal CT is a very sensitive technique for evaluating the mediastinum, and both intratracheal and extratracheal lesions are well seen on this study. Multiplanar reconstruction to image the trachea along its axis will further delineate areas of narrowing. The CT studies should be done with intravenous contrast since a "mass" in the mediastinum may be a vascular structure.

Foreign bodies are usually suggested by the history and may be treated with bronchoscopy following plain film radiography. In children, the history may be less clear, and a foreign body should be suspected. A persistent infiltrate, an area of apparent emphysema, or a deviated mediastinum should also suggest the possibility of a foreign body. Inspiratory and expiratory radiographs, or chest fluoroscopy, may demonstrate differential aeration of the two lungs, that is, lobes or segments that do not expand and areas that, on expiration, do not empty. A ventilation lung scan may be used to demonstrate areas that are not being ventilated properly.

Mediastinal Widening

In addition to aortic dissection, causes of mediastinal widening include mass lesions of the mediastinum, which also may present acutely and be suspected from the initial chest radiographs. In particular, tumors compressing the superior vena cava may present acutely and require urgent therapy. As noted above, contrast-enhanced CT is a rapid and sensitive examination for evaluation of mediastinal masses.

Cardiomegaly

A basic component of the interpretation of the PA chest radiograph is determining cardiac size. Although this measurement is much more difficult to obtain when the examination is performed on a supine patient, a reasonable assessment can usually be made. However, the underlying cause of the enlargement is more difficult to determine. In addition to wall thickening and chamber dilation, the appearance of a large heart can be caused by pericardial effusion. Since acute effusion raises the possibility of tamponade, a rapid diagnosis is important. Echocardiography can differentiate between cardiac and pericardial causes rapidly and precisely. In addition, this modality characterizes valvular disease very well.

Abdomen

Generalized Abdominal Pain

In evaluating acute abdominal pain, the emergency physician is faced with a large and often confusing array of diagnostic procedures, each supplying different information. Often a good history, a physical examination, and routine laboratory tests can localize the source of the pain to a region or an organ system, or even a specific diagnosis (see Chapter 14). Unfortunately, when the history, physical, and laboratory tests are not diagnostic, radiologic examinations yield very little information. However, if a study is done, the initial views should be an upright PA chest radiograph and a supine abdominal radiograph (Fig. 19–11). If an erect chest radiograph cannot be obtained, a supine AP view is usually adequate. These studies can be done rapidly and they are readily available, inexpensive, and noninvasive.

Chest radiographs may demonstrate empyema, lower lobe pneumonia, or Boerhaave's syndrome, which occasionally simulates an intraabdominal process. An elevated hemidiaphragm or tiny lucencies overlying the dome of the diaphragm can suggest a subphrenic abscess. An upright chest radiograph is also the most sensitive view for demonstrating free intraperitoneal air, which is almost pathognomonic for intestinal perforation.

Except in cases of urinary tract stone or bowel dilatation secondary to intestinal obstruction or adynamic ileus, plain film abdominal radiographs are rarely of diagnostic value. The vast majority of abdominal problems may be associated with abnormalities visible on radiographs, but these problems present no specific or diagnostic findings that would indicate the use of plain film radiography rather than a more specific radiologic modality. Biliary calculi and appendicoliths may be seen in a small minority of cases; however, these diagnoses are better made by other means as noted in the next section.

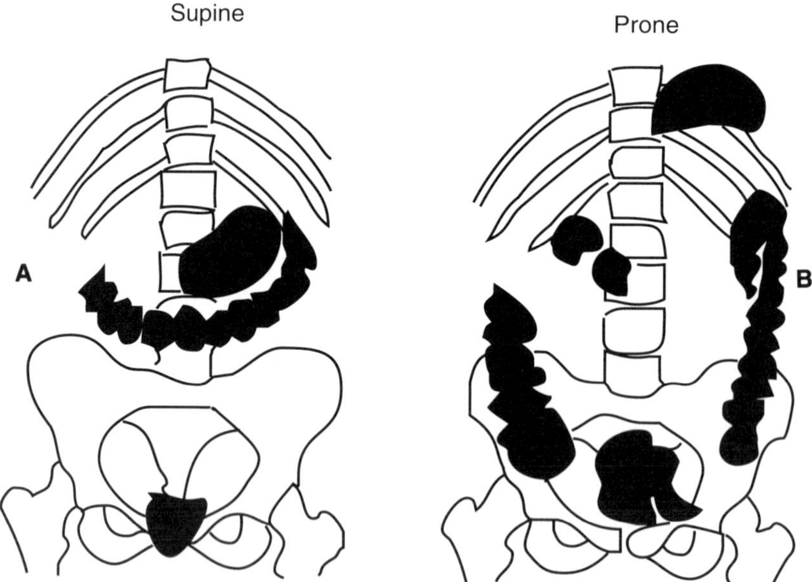

Fig. 19-11. Normal gas distribution on abdominal radiographs. **A,** Supine abdomen (AP projection). Gas is seen in the transverse portion of the stomach in the midline and to the left (body and antrum). Colon gas is primarily in the transverse colon, part of the sigmoid and rectum. **B,** Prone abdomen (PA projection). Distribution of gastric air is now more lateral and posterior in fundus and at pylorus. Gas is also seen in the duodenal bulb. The ascending colon is now gas-filled as is the midsigmoid.

Peritonitis

Since peritonitis can be diagnosed clinically with a high degree of confidence and since patients with peritonitis may require immediate surgery, the information gained by a radiologic investigation is usually not worth the treatment delay. Nevertheless, in some ambiguous situations a *limited* radiologic evaluation may be useful.

An upright chest radiograph is the most sensitive view for demonstrating free intraperitoneal air, which is almost pathognomonic for intestinal perforation. A supine AP chest radiograph may be useful in the overall evaluation of the patient but is very insensitive to intraabdominal air. For this reason, when an upright chest radiograph is not possible, a left-lateral decubitus view of the *abdomen* should be obtained, preferably after the patient has been lying on his left side for 10 to 15 minutes.

The supine abdominal radiograph, although frequently abnormal in patients with peritonitis, is rarely useful in management, since the findings are usually nonspecific. Although this view may confirm the presence of peritoneal fluid, adynamic ileus, or massive amounts of extraluminal gas (as noted earlier, the left-lateral decubitus is far more sensitive), these findings are usually suspected before the study is undertaken. Much less frequently, the radiograph may demonstrate an unsuspected foreign body, biliary calculi, an appendicolith, or air in the wall of the bowel or the portal venous system, indicating bowel infarction. The possibility of demonstrating such an unsuspected finding, however, is a weak justification for the study, and other modalities should be considered in the face of a diagnostic dilemma.

Intestinal Obstruction/Adynamic Ileus

Plain film abdominal radiography is the best initial study for evaluating the possibilities of intestinal obstruction or adynamic ileus. Analysis of intraluminal gas distribution and lumen size on plain films is an excellent method of diagnosing and roughly localizing intestinal obstruction. The hallmark of obstruction on plain radiographs is gas-filled, dilated bowel proximal to the point of obstruction, accompanied by gasless bowel distally. This appearance may take several hours to develop, and serial radiographs will be necessary to establish the diagnosis. Occasionally the bowel proximal to the obstruction will be filled with fluid, making the diagnosis on plain film radiographs difficult. Adynamic (paralytic) ileus is also characterized by air in the bowel. However, in contrast to intestinal obstruction, the anatomic localization is not related to any single point in the enteron behind which gas is caught and beyond which it is not found. Instead, the gas may be scattered in a nonanatomic pattern, or it may be localized to several loops of bowel in a specific region of the abdomen, reflecting irritation by an inflamed structure nearby. For example, inflammation of the body and tail of the pancreas may cause dilatation of the stomach, proximal jejunum and colon, whereas intervening small bowel may appear normal.

One frequently held misconception is that air-fluid levels indicate obstruction. On the contrary, they form any time air and fluid are present in the same viscus and are visible on horizontal beam radiographs. Although air-fluid levels may be seen in patients with bowel obstruction, they also occur in adynamic ileus. These levels may also be seen in the small bowel, which normally contains air and fluid, especially after the patient has swallowed a large amount of air while drinking carbonated beverages or eating food or as the result of pain, or apprehension, or even mouth-breathing secondary to nasal or respiratory problems.

Occasionally the plain film abdominal radiograph may also demonstrate the cause of the obstruction or ileus. Detection of air over the inguinal canal suggests an incarcerated hernia; a gas-filled loop in the typical "coffee bean" configuration indicates a close-loop obstruction such as a volvulus or internal hernia; the finding of biliary air and a right-lower-quadrant calcification indicates a gallstone ileus.

Intussusception is a possibility in an infant or young child with bloody diarrhea and crampy pain, in whom a right-sided abdominal mass may be palpable. Plain film radiographs may appear normal or may show a soft tissue mass in the right abdomen with a convex upper margin outlined by air. Because the clinical presentations and the plain film findings are often atypical, the possibility of intussusception should not be excluded without a definitive study. A barium enema can be both diagnostic and therapeutic if the examiner is able to nudge the intussuscepted bowel retrograde to its normal position.

Complete obstruction in a newborn raises the possibilities of bowel atresia, stenosis, or a meconium ileus. Within the first few months of life, additional causes of obstruction include hypertrophic pyloric stenosis, which can be demonstrated by ultrasonography, and Ladd's bands, which are associated with a malrotation of the bowel.

Adynamic ileus may be accompanied by an appendicolith, pancreatic calcifications, and a suggestion of a mass or gallstones in the usual location. Each of these accompanying findings suggests the respective organ as the source of the ileus.

Oral contrast administration may be needed to define the level of obstruction or the specific lesion. However, the use of oral barium is contraindicated in cases of what appears to be low, small bowel obstruction, until the possibility of a colonic lesion has been excluded. If the lesion is in the right colon, a situation that may simulate small bowel blockage, barium that enters the colon proximal to the obstruction will desiccate and become impacted above the lesion, complicating the obstruction. If plain film radiography demonstrates a low, small bowel obstruction, a study of the large bowel should be performed to exclude a right colon lesion before giving oral barium. If an oral barium study is done, suctioning as much intestinal gas and fluid as possible will result in the most rapid study and most accurate results.

Water-soluble contrast agents such as Gastrografin can be used to delineate obstruction at the level of the stomach or duodenum, but they are of no use in evaluating more distal small bowel obstruction because these agents mix with the large amounts of fluid either already in the bowel or drawn into the bowel by the agents themselves. By the time water-soluble contrast material reaches a lesion in the jejunum or ileum, it may be so diluted as to be useless diagnostically.

Contrast enemas, using either barium or a water-soluble agent, can define the level and nature of a colonic obstruction, as well as rule out a cause in the large bowel. The possibility of Ladd's bands associated with a mid-gut volvulus in an infant can often be verified by a colon study that demonstrates the malrotation found in these patients. As is true for orally administered contrast, barium is preferred unless there is a good reason not to use it. Fear that a compromised bowel may perforate, spilling barium (and feces) into the peritoneum with resulting granuloma formation or other complications, should mitigate against the performance of *any* study.

Intestinal Ischemia and Infarction

Intestinal ischemia often presents with vague symptoms and is a difficult diagnosis to establish. Whether arising from arterial or venous disease or resulting from slow flow, intestinal infarction can be catastrophic if not treated promptly. Unfortunately, radiologic findings by all imaging modalities are nonspecific. However, although neither is dependable alone, plain film radiography combined with CT can make this diagnosis, each having approximately a 35% sensitivity. Using both modalities together, about two thirds of cases can be diagnosed radiologically. Adynamic ileus is a frequent though nonspecific plain film finding associated with intestinal infarction. However if wall thickening develops, causing separation of the gas in adjacent loops, the diagnosis of ischemia should be suggested. Intramural hemorrhage causes a scalloping of the wall referred to as "thumbprinting," which is visible if there is air in the lumen. Serial radiographs may show one or more dilated loops whose configuration dose not change. Air in the bowel wall indicates that some necrosis has already occurred. If the diagnosis is evident on plain film radiographs, a CT scan is not necessary, thus saving valuable time. However, if the diagnosis is not established by plain film radiography, the same signs may be found on CT. Portal venous gas, for example, is better visualized on CT than by plain film radiography.

Findings on contrast examinations are similar to those on plain film radiography, except that the bowel lumen is outlined by positive contrast (barium) instead of negative contrast (gas). A barium enema is very sensitive in detecting colonic ischemia. Findings include spasm, wall thickening, and thickening of the folds, which can progress to create either a "picket fence" appearance or thumbprinting. If infarction is suspected, however, the additional information obtained from barium enema is not worth the risk of perforation and subsequent spilling of barium and feces into the peritoneal cavity.

Mesenteric angiography can demonstrate mesenteric arterial or venous obstruction, and in slow flow states may demonstrate vascular spasm. If the patient is not in shock or septic, pharmacologic agents can be instilled through an intravascular angiographic catheter in an attempt to reverse thrombosis or vasoconstriction before the bowel necroses.

Sonography is not generally helpful in diagnosing intestinal ischemia. Duplex Doppler sonography, although theoretically useful for diagnosing intestinal vascular disease has, in practice, proven to be disappointing. It is extremely time consuming, highly operator dependent, and even in the best of hands, often nondiagnostic.

Right Upper Quadrant Pain

The common complaint of right upper quadrant (RUQ) pain suggests a complex differential diagnosis (see Chapter 14). In addition to the possibility of acute cholecystitis which may necessitate immediate surgical intervention, right-sided pyelonephritis, pancreatitis, peptic ulcer disease, liver abscess, and inflammatory processes originating elsewhere in the abdomen or even the chest must be considered. RUQ pain is also a symptom of hepatitis; ascending cholangitis; and subphrenic, subhepatic, or intrahepatic abscess formation. Many of these entities, such as hepatitis, have no specific radiologic findings and in these cases, the diagnosis must be based on clinical and laboratory information.

The most frequent findings on chest and plain film abdominal radiographs have already been discussed. Additionally, the presence of air bubbles may signify an abscess, and air in the gallbladder lumen or wall may indicate an infection in that organ. If the greatest clinical concern is the possibility of acute cholecystitis, however, the plain films are unlikely to be useful and a radionuclide study should be obtained.

A dIsIDA scan uses intravenously administered technetium-99m (^{99m}Tc) labeled d-Isopropyl Imido Diacetic Acid (dIsIDA) with scanning of the RUQ at frequent intervals. These studies are generically known as "HIDA" scans since dIsIDA is one of the *H*epatic *I*mido *D*iacetic *A*cids. In the absence of biliary obstruction, the dIsIDA flows rapidly through the biliary tree and the common hepatic duct into the cystic duct, gallbladder, and common bile duct, eventually passing into the duodenum and the remainder of the bowel. In the presence of biliary obstruction, the dIsIDA diffuses throughout the biliary tree, moving distally to the level of blockage. Early in the study, the hepatic anatomy is well visualized and parenchymal lesions may be identified. Later imaging demonstrates the biliary tree and bowel. Absence of radionuclide in the bowel accompanied by activity in the biliary tree indicates common bile duct obstruction. If only a portion of the biliary tree is visualized, this may indicate obstruction at the junction of the visualized and nonvisualized portions. Although obstruction can be accurately diagnosed, the cause of obstruction is not revealed. Such obstruction is often the only radiologic sign of ascending cholangitis.

In the clinical setting being discussed, visualization of the entire biliary tree, without visualization of the gallbladder, within 2 hours of an injection, is diagnostic of acute cholecystitis with a positive predictive value of 95 to 99%. A frequent explanation for a false-negative study is a gallbladder which is overfilled with bile before the examination, leaving no room for the dIsIDA. This is most likely to occur when the patient has fasted for a prolonged period before the examination, and the error can be avoided by pretreating the patient with cholecystokinin (CCK). A negative study is equally accurate in ruling out acute cholecystitis. Occasionally, the filling of the gallbladder may be delayed, which is usually indicative of chronic cholecystitis.

Ultrasound provides primarily anatomic information about those structures not obscured by overlying bone or gas. Duplex Doppler and color Doppler sonography may provide physiological information as well. Certain crystalline structures such as stones, whether calcified or not, are highly reflective of sound waves, and ultrasound is an excellent means of demonstrating them. Plain film radiography demonstrates only those gallstones with enough calcium to stand out from surrounding structures. Such stones comprise about 15% of all gallstones. Even CT, which can detect slight calcification, is relatively insensitive here, demonstrating only about 75% of gallstones, whereas sonography demonstrates 98% of all stones. The few false-negative studies occur when patients are obese or gassy, or when there is a single stone impacted within the neck of the gallbladder or cystic duct.

Sonography of the RUQ can usually demonstrate the gallbladder, portions of the liver, right kidney, and the intrahepatic and extrahepatic biliary tree, as well as free or loculated fluid collections. Sonography may also demonstrate the pancreas if the patient does not have too much bowel gas. As noted, this study can accurately diagnose cholelithiasis. Occasionally, in acute cholecystitis, if the process is far enough advanced, sufficient edema in the gallbladder wall will be present to be detected sonographically. This "halo" sign is specific for acute cholecystitis. Air in the wall of the gallbladder, although diagnostic of acute cholecystitis, can be misinterpreted as loops of bowel obscuring the gallbladder. Other findings, which are less diagnostic, include a thickened wall, echogenic bile, or pericholecystic fluid. The "sonographic Murphy sign," pain on compression of the gallbladder during the study, is subjective and not always reliable. In most cases of early acute cholecystitis, sonography is nonspecific. Since gallstones are very common, their presence is frequently coincidental and this finding alone cannot be used to establish a definitive diagnosis.

A dIsIDA scan is more sensitive and more specific than sonography for diagnosing acute cholecystitis. Acute common bile duct obstruction is also more accurately diagnosed with a nuclear scan. However, the sonogram is indicated for patients who have significant elevation of bilirubin, whose nuclear scan results are equivocal or contrary to clinical impression, or when nuclear scans are unavailable.

CT provides an anatomic view of RUQ, information similar to that provided by sonography. Since the presence of the liver provides an acoustic window in the RUQ, the quality of sonograms in that area is uniformly high. For this reason and because sonography is more sensitive in demonstrating calculi, CT is rarely indicated in the evaluation of acute RUQ upper pain. If biliary obstruction is present, however, CT is more capable of demonstrating the cause of the obstruction since the dIsIDA study can only document the obstruction, not identify it, and the Ampulla of Vater is a structure only infrequently seen on sonography.

Acute Pancreatitis

Pancreatitis is principally a clinical diagnosis. Conventional radiography is notoriously inaccurate for diagnosing pancreatitis. Plain film radiographs may reveal a localized or generalized paralytic ileus. Although a mass may be demonstrated, no determination can be made from the plain film as to whether the mass is in fact a pseudocyst. Peritoneal or pleural fluid may also be detected by plain film radiography and help establish the diagnosis. If acute pancreatitis is superimposed on chronic pancreatitis, pancreatic calcifications may be demonstrated. However these calcifications may be an incidental finding when a patient seeks treatment for a different abdominal emergency, and the mere presence of such calcifications alone cannot be used to establish the diagnosis of *acute* pancreatitis.

Although sometimes helpful in confirming the clinical impression of pancreatitis, sonography of the pancreas is rarely indicated in the ED. A patients with acute pancreatitis usually has an adynamic ileus, which obscures the pancreas sonographically. Even if the pancreas could be visualized, the accuracy of sonography is limited, especially when acute pancreatitis is superimposed on chronic pancreatitis. In cases of suspected gallstone pancreatitis, however, sonography is the study of choice to determine if gallstones are present, and whether the common duct is dilated.

Later in the course of the disease, sonography is extremely helpful in diagnosing and following the development of pseudocysts, the major complication of pancreatitis. However, pseudocysts can become infected or erode into vessels, two major complications that are difficult to diagnose with sonography alone.

CT is more sensitive than sonography in diagnosing pancreatitis and associated retroperitoneal and mesenteric inflammatory changes. Although less readily available and more expensive than sonography, CT is more sensitive for demonstrating pseudocysts. Another serious complication of pancreatitis is a pancreatic abscess, which usually appears on CT as a peripancreatic fluid collection. This abscess is indistinguishable from an uncomplicated pseudocyst except in the unusual case in which gas is demonstrated within it. The complication of pancreatitis associated with the highest mortality is acute pancreatic infarction. This can be diagnosed accurately using dynamic, contrast-enhanced CT. The infarcted portion of the pancreas, will not be enhanced by contrast administration, indicating that it has been devascularized.

Peptic Ulcer

Most peptic ulcers can be detected using fiberoptic endoscopy, or contrast radiography with barium. Single-contrast barium studies are significantly less sensitive then endoscopy. However, *double-contrast* radiography is almost as sensitive as endoscopy in demonstrating ulcers and is faster, less expensive, and less hazardous to the patient. Nevertheless, radiographic studies should never be relied on to differentiate benign from malignant lesions.

Gastrointestinal Hemorrhage

Gastrointestinal hemorrhage can be catastrophic, and rapid therapy may be life saving. In order to institute the proper therapy, the cause and the location of the bleeding must be determined quickly. The major imaging tools useful in diagnosing the cause and location of gastrointestinal bleeding are radionuclide imaging, angiography, and endoscopy. Coagulopathies, which may cause gastrointestinal bleeding, should be investigated before the radiologic evaluation.

Radionuclide imaging is useful for detecting and localizing colonic bleeding, using ^{99m}Tc, pyrophosphate-tagged red cells or a ^{99m}Tc-labeled sulfur colloid scan. In an actively bleeding patient, radionuclide imaging can detect and localize active colonic bleeding of as little as 0.15 mL/min. This is ten times more sensitive than angiography and much less invasive. Imaging after injecting these agents will demonstrate the entire pool of circulating blood. Any blood containing radionuclide that is outside the vascular system will be detectable as a hot spot.

The major difference between sulfur colloid and tagged red cells is that sulfur colloid is removed from the blood rapidly by the liver, thereby reducing the background blood-pool radiation. This accentuates the signal from any blood in the bowel lumen. The disadvantage of sulfur colloid imaging is that the uptake of radionuclide in the liver may obscure bleeding in the hepatic flexure.

Although more invasive than radioisotope imaging and less sensitive for the demonstration of lower intestinal bleeding, angiography is indicated in cases of significant intestinal bleeding if the patient is hemodynamically stable. The major advantage of angiography is that it offers the best opportunity for treatment as well as diagnosis. Arterial feeders of a bleeding point can be embolized, and varices can be sclerosed with ethanol. Patients undergoing angiography must have normal coagulation profiles. A major disadvantage of angiography is that the patient must be bleeding at a rate of at least 1 to 2 mL/min (slightly less with digital subtraction techniques) for the bleeding to be detected. Also, angiography is relatively invasive. Nevertheless, angiography is a far less invasive therapy than surgical control of bleeding.

Barium studies and/or endoscopy are indicated when the bleeding has subsided, and in cases of minor bleeding, to demonstrate a lesion that could be a source of bleeding. Esophageal varices, peptic ulcers, and tumors are the most common upper intestinal sources of bleeding; whereas diverticula, angiodysplasia, and tumors predominate in the colon. After bleeding has stopped, it may be impossible to prove that a particular lesion was the actual cause. Barium studies are contraindicated in the presence of active heavy bleeding because the studies delay definitive diagnosis and therapy, and because the presence of blood can obscure the lesion. Moreover, the presence of barium may preclude successful angiography, isotope scanning, or endoscopy.

Extraintestinal sites of bleeding include the nasal and oral cavities, the pharynx, and the esophagus. Acute bleeding from the nose, mouth, and pharynx are easily recognized. However, evaluation of the esophagus may be difficult. Radionuclide imaging and angiography may demonstrate such sources of bleeding as varices or Mallory-Weiss esophageal lacerations. However, esophagoscopy is most likely to provide the specific diagnosis rapidly. Much less frequently, the source of bleeding may be from a biliary tract lesion or from perforation of the aorta into the duodenum, a complication of aortic grafting.

Bowel Perforation

Intestinal perforation may result from trauma, foreign body ingestion, peptic ulcer disease, obstruction or perforating tumor, abscess, recent surgery, radiation, or other iatrogenic causes. As in other situations, plain film radiography is indicated as the initial examination primarily because of its noninvasive nature, availability, and rapidity. Horizontal-beam radiographs are very sensitive in detecting free air which accompanies most gastric or colonic perforations. However, the diagnosis of small bowel perforation, which frequently does not result in the presence of free intraperitoneal air, often requires the use of oral contrast agents. Although water-soluble agents can be used to study the *proximal* small bowel, dilution of the contrast material by fluid in the lumen renders them less useful than barium suspensions for studying the mid and distal bowel.

Splenic Infarction

Splenic infarction may occur in the presence of a thromboembolic condition such as atrial fibrillation. Such patients often present with acute left-sided abdominal pain. During the first 24 hours after the infarction, no structural changes occur. Therefore, any imaging modality demonstrating only morphology, such as sonography, cannot be used to make this diagnosis. However, a ^{99m}Tc-labeled sulfur colloid scan of the liver and spleen will clearly demonstrate a defect in the splenic image corresponding to the avascular segment. Similar information could be obtained using dynamic contrast-enhanced CT. However, CT is more invasive, more expensive, and more prone to failure because of inadequate or improperly timed injection.

Intraabdominal Abscess

Plain film radiography is usually inadequate to diagnose intraabdominal abscess that may occur as a result of bowel perforation, extension of such inflammatory processes as diverticulitis or appendicitis, or after surgery or penetrating injury. Plain film radiographs may suggest the diagnosis by demonstrating a collection of bubbles in what appears to be an extraluminal location, but otherwise this examination is inadequate.

CT has had a great impact on the evaluation and management of intraabdominal abscesses, accurately detecting the presence of collections of pus in the abdomen and precisely characterizing their geometric relationships to surrounding structures. Because of its excellent contrast resolution, pus can be accurately differentiated from a solid mass or phlegmon. Intravenous contrast is not required to make this distinction. The degree of localization of the abscess and the number and nature of loculations can be shown. This information determines whether the abscess is amenable to percutaneous drainage under CT guidance. If so, the CT-guided drainage can be therapeutic, and aspiration and culture can be diagnostic. If percutaneous drainage is impossible, CT can be useful to direct surgical drainage.

Accurate CT of the abdomen requires adequate preparation. An abscess appears as a collection of fluid and possibly some gas. This is exactly the same as the appearance of a loop of bowel; in fact, most mistakes in CT diagnoses of abscesses result from confusion of abscess with bowel because of inadequate bowel opacification. It is therefore imperative that the patient be prepared before CT by flooding the gastrointestinal (GI) tract with oral contrast to differentiate bowel from extraluminal collections. Because of the high contrast resolution of CT itself, the contrast material, whether a water-soluble medium or barium, is very dilute and quite innocuous. Unfortunately it is often difficult for sick patients to tolerate the large volume required for optimal studies.

The accuracy of CT is decreased if the abscess communicates with the GI tract. CT is incapable of differentiating infected fluid from uninfected fluid, except in the rare cases when gas is present in the (infected) collection. For this reason, CT cannot differentiate pancreatic pseudocyst from abscess, and cannot be used to determine which of many fluid collections may be infected.

In the improperly prepared patient, ultrasonography (like CT) has limited value in evaluating intraperitoneal abscesses because the abscesses resemble loops of bowel. Unlike CT, however, there is no ultrasonographic GI contrast material to enhance the ability of sonography to distinguish abscesses from bowel. An additional problem in obtaining useful abdominal sonograms is that the visualization of intraperitoneal structures is often obscured by bowel gas or by gas in the abscess itself.

Radionuclide scanning with gallium-67 citrate is useful in the evaluation of many inflammatory and neoplastic conditions. Intravenously injected tracer doses of gallium are concentrated in the liver, colon, and in tumors or areas of acute inflammation. Scintiphotography 24 to 96 hours after its administration delineates areas of active inflammation or infection. This study is very useful in localizing the source of a septic process especially when no localizing signs are elicited clinically. Gallium scanning can be used in the initial stages of the diagnostic evaluation to direct the investigation to the proper area and imaging modality and to increase the sensitivity of other imaging modalities by focusing attention on the pathologic area. It can verify the findings from other radiologic studies by determining whether a collection of fluid is infected or not; when multiple fluid collections are demonstrated, the gallium scan can determine which is (are) infected. Gallium scanning has almost a 90% sensitivity in detecting localized abscesses and, like almost all scintigraphic scans, is an innnocuous procedure, with virtually no complications.

The usefulness of gallium scanning in the abdomen is limited by interference from bowel and liver excretion. Subtraction techniques using simultaneous imaging with ^{99m}Tc dIsIDA is helpful in reducing this interference. More often, however, it is necessary to wait a day or two following administration of the gallium to increase the ratio of specifically localized radionuclide to the background. For this reason, at the first indication that a particular patient may require gallium for the localization of an obscure infected site, the radionuclide should be given, rather than waiting to see if other modalities are successful. If the collection is localized before the time of the gallium scan, it can simply be omitted. Conversely, if other studies fail to resolve the problem, it will not be necessary to wait additional time before scanning the patient. Gallium scans are not as useful in patients who have recently undergone surgery, because the surgical site will demonstrate increased activity. Additionally, therapy with systemic antibiotics can cause false-negative scans.

Scanning with indium^{111}-labeled white blood cells is replacing gallium for evaluation of intraabdominal infections. Unlike gallium, indium is not excreted in the colon and therefore abscesses are not obscured or mimicked by colonic activity. However, indium scanning does share the other limitations of gallium.

Upper Urinary Tract Obstruction

Acute urinary tract obstruction is most often the result of renal stones and is one of the few acute abdominal problems for which the supine abdominal radiograph is an ideal first study. Since 80% to 85% of urinary calculi are radioopaque, plain film abdominal radiography, demonstrates the majority of stones. Radiographs taken to detect calculi should be performed using low energy technique (70 to 80 kVp) to maximize stone visibility. On occasion, sonography may be used as the initial study to demonstrate urinary tract calculi because it is the least invasive study capable of doing so. However, sonography is less sensitive than plain film radiography in detecting radioopaque stones. Stones in the collecting system that are too small to shadow will blend in with the surrounding echogenic renal sinus structures, and stones can be missed in the ureters when these are completely obscured by surrounding bony structures and bowel gas.

Upon diagnosing a stone, many urologists do not perform any more studies but instead treat the patient with fluids and analgesics in the expectation that the stone will pass. If further information is required, intravenous urography is performed to demonstrate radiolucent stones as well as other causes of obstruction *intrinsic* to the urinary tract, such as a stricture or a tumor. However, *extrinsic* causes of obstruction cannot be directly evaluated by the urogram.

Other studies may provide supplementary information. Ultrasonography is exceptionally sensitive for demonstrating the presence and amount of pyelocalyceal dilation. However, the amount of dilation does not always correlate with the degree of obstruction. In the absence of obstruction, dilation of the renal collecting system can result from infection, residual dilation from previous obstruction, or from acute diuresis. In addition, other conditions such as parapelvic cysts or papillary necrosis may mimic pyelocaliectasis sonographically. Therefore, although sonography is sensitive, its specificity is limited.

Since radionuclide scans are *functional* studies, they are more specific than sonography for demonstrating obstruction. Agents such as ^{99m}Tc-labeled diethylenetriamine-pentacetic acid (DTPA) that are excreted into the urine can be used for evaluation of obstruction and drainage as well as for the precise assessment of the excretory function of the kidneys, not only "globally" but in different areas of the parenchyma. These agents can be used to determine and follow the effects of an obstruction as well as its presence. The disadvantage of radionuclide imaging is its inability to demonstrate the cause.

Bladder Outlet Obstruction

Obstruction of the lower urinary tract in males is almost always a result of prostatic hypertrophy. This and other causes of outlet obstruction are accurately evaluated by sonography, which can display the size of the prostate and pre- and postvoid bladder volumes. Other abnormalities such as bladder wall tumors or bladder calculi can be accurately detected by sonography. No other imaging modality can evaluate these conditions as rapidly, safely, and accurately.

Urinary Tract Infection

Imaging procedures are not ordinarily required to diagnose urinary tract infections except to detect complicating lesions such as obstruction or abscess.

Sonography is a readily available, noninvasive, and accurate means of identifying these complications and can also be used to guide percutaneous drainage or nephrostomy if required. If sonography is unavailable, CT can also detect these problems and it too can be used to guide percutaneous drainage. CT with contrast is better than sonography for differentiating hydronephrosis from parapelvic cyst, However, CT is more invasive and expensive. Some abscesses are indistinguishable from cysts on CT. Although this problem happens less frequently with ultrasound, it can occur when the abscess arises from spread of infection to a preexisting cyst. In this case, radionuclide scanning using gallium-67- or In^{111}-tagged white cells will help differentiate noninfected cysts from infected ones.

Acute Appendicitis

Acute appendicitis is usually a clinical diagnosis and appropriate surgical therapy should not be delayed by radiologic studies. However, some cases present atypically and require radiologic investigation. Moreover, other illnesses that may mimic appendicitis, such as pelvic inflammatory disease or inflammatory bowel disease, may be diagnosed by imaging studies. If a radiologic study is undertaken, plain film radiography should be the initial examination because of its rapidity and safety. Occasionally in adults, and frequently in children, an appendicolith is present, which may help establish the diagnosis. Moreover, the presence of an appendicolith in the clinical setting of appendicitis is associated with a high incidence of perforation. Other indirect evidence of appendicitis includes a soft tissue mass, peritoneal fluid, abnormalities of the cecum, and, very rarely, free air.

Until recently, barium enema was the only useful adjunct to plain film radiography for the radiologic diagnosis of acute appendicitis. A barium enema may demonstrate inflammatory changes of the ascending colon or an indentation on the cecum caused by an inflammatory mass or abscess. However, these are relatively late findings. Barium enema is contraindicated if there is any evidence of perforation.

In advanced cases of appendicitis, CT is more sensitive than either plain film radiography or a barium enema in demonstrating an abscess or inflammatory mass. CT allows direct visualization of these processes while conventional radiography relies on indirect evidence of effects on surrounding structures. CT is valuable in accurately distinguishing an inflammatory mass from an abscess collection. If pus is detected, CT can be used to guide percutaneous drainage. In addition, early on, CT is capable of demonstrating the inflammatory changes in the surrounding fat that, although they will not establish a precise diagnosis, can help by identifying the location of the process. Although the accuracy of CT in diagnosing acute appendicitis in equivocal cases is very good, it is expensive, moderately invasive, and time consuming, and therefore should not be used routinely in the diagnosis of uncomplicated acute appendicitis.

Recently, sonography has been advocated for suspected appendicitis cases where physical exam and plain film radiography are equivocal. The technique involves compression of the iliac fossa with the ultrasound transducer to displace intervening bowel. This requires a high level of patient cooperation and examiner skill and may be quite painful. The study is one of the most operator-dependent of ultrasonographic procedures, with a success rate that varies greatly from one sonographer to another. Commonly, the appendix cannot be identified, resulting in a negative sonogram. Finding an edematous, incompressible appendix, an appendicolith, or, in more advanced cases, a periappendiceal abscess is considered to be a positive exam. When the sonogram is not useful in evaluating the appendix, it can be used to confirm or exclude the presence of other entities that can mimic appendicitis. This must be done with caution, however, since inflammatory fluid from acute appendicitis can spread to adjacent structures, imitating the appearance of an inflammatory process arising from that structure. For example, inflammation from appendicitis can spread to the pelvis creating a sonographic appearance identical to pelvic inflammatory disease.

Female Genital Tract

Ultrasonography is the mainstay in the radiologic diagnosis of female pelvic pathology. Because interposing bowel can be displaced from the pelvis by filling the urinary bladder, the pelvic structures can be uniformly demonstrated and evaluated sonographically. Unlike studies requiring ionizing radiation, sonography is readily available, accurate, and safe and therefore can be used without concern for a developing fetus. However, sonography does not obviate the need for clinical and laboratory evaluation.

Ectopic Pregnancy

Although an ectopic pregnancy can sometimes be directly visualized sonographically, many ectopics cannot be identified before they rupture. The most sensitive means of diagnosing an ectopic pregnancy involves the combined use of sonography and the quantitative measurement of the beta subunit of human chorionic gonadotrophin (β-hCG). A β-hCG level indicating pregnancy together with a sonogram showing no intrauterine pregnancy, suggests an ectopic pregnancy. Conversely, except for pregnant women using fertility drugs who may have multiple and heterotopic pregnancies, a sonogram demonstrating an intrauterine pregnancy virtually excludes an ectopic.

Transabdominal sonography is able to resolve an intrauterine gestational sac reliably 6 weeks after the last menstrual period (4 weeks after fertilization), when β-hCG levels are about 6500 mIU/mL (of the second international standard). Transvaginal sonography is reliable at 5 weeks, when β-hCG levels are around 600 mIU/mL. Before 5 weeks, the sac is microscopic and cannot be demonstrated sonographically. Consequently, sonography at this stage is incapable of differentiating ectopic from intrauterine pregnancy.

The combination of sonography and plain film radiography may locate a "missing" intrauterine device (IUD) string. Sonography readily demonstrates the presence of an IUD in the endometrial cavity. The IUD is strongly echogenic, and the configuration of the echoes is determined by the geometry of the IUD. The most commonly seen IUD today, the Lippe's loop, creates a characteristic dashed line of bright echoes in the midsagittal plane. Plain film radiographs can be used to demonstrate an IUD within the abdomen or pelvis. If no IUD can be seen on the plain abdominal film, then it must have fallen out. If the IUD is detected on the plain film abdominal radiograph, but is not in the endometrial cavity on sonography, then it must have perforated.

Other Gynecologic Problems

Sonography is often helpful in establishing the diagnosis of pelvic inflammatory disease (PID), demonstrating free peritoneal fluid and ovarian swelling in acute PID, and hydrosalpinx, and pelvic adhesions in patients with chronic inflammation. As noted previously, contiguous spread of inflammatory processes from adjacent organs, such as appendicitis or diverticulitis, can cause identical findings; and sonography alone cannot be relied on for a definitive diagnosis. The main use of sonography in these patients is to detect the presence of a complicating tuboovarian abscess and to evaluate the efficacy of the treatment by demonstrating adequate resolution.

The diagnosis of endometriosis is chiefly clinical, based on the cyclic nature of the pain. Sonographic findings are nonspecific, consisting of fluid, adhesions, and complex masses. Sonography is useful in assessing the extent of the disease and evaluating the success of therapy. Another cause of pelvic pain, for which sonography can be extremely helpful in the diagnosis, is an ovarian cyst. Although the presence of a cyst alone can cause pain, pain is more frequently caused by complications such as rupture, hemorrhage, or torsion. Sonography clearly demonstrates the presence of ovarian cysts. Hemorrhage can be spontaneous or secondary to torsion. In either case, sonography demonstrates echogenic material within the cyst, and rapid enlargement if a recent prior scan is available. A ruptured cyst can often be inferred from the presence of large amounts of free fluid, without other visible pathology.

Male Genitalia

The most common causes of acute scrotal pain and swelling are testicular torsion, inflammation, trauma, and tumor. Because acute torsion is an emergency requiring rapid diagnosis and intervention to preserve the viability of the testicle, the focus of the diagnostic evaluation of an acutely painful swollen testicle is to determine whether or not torsion is present.

Nuclear scintigraphic studies demonstrating blood flow to the testicle have been the mainstay in the diagnosis of torsion. Scintiphotography of the groin area during the initial arterial distribution, and later in the static phase after injection of a blood pool agent, accurately distinguishes torsion from other scrotal pathology. Nuclear scanning is rapid and relatively noninvasive (see Chapter 20).

Sonography with color flow and pulsed Doppler is also used to diagnose torsion. Ultrasonography with color flow Doppler is the definitive imaging technique for diagnosing torsion.

The Extremities

Apart from trauma and vascular emergencies there are relatively few emergencies involving the extremities. Standard views on plain film radiography can generally answer most questions.

As noted previously, osteomyelitis cannot be diagnosed early by plain film radiography. Bone scanning, especially if followed by a gallium or indium study, will allow an earlier diagnosis. MRI is also a useful though expensive tool. Bone scanning can also be used to differentiate soft tissue infection from osteomyelitis. A three-phase study permits the separate evaluation of soft tissues, blood pool, and the bone itself.

The diagnosis of arthritis is usually clinical, using laboratory methods as well. Although radiographs may be helpful in late stages, a specific clinical diagnosis can usually be made before specific bone changes can be seen.

Ultrasonography may be a useful tool in the investigation of some intraarticular processes, especially in the pediatric population. It can reliably identify effusions and synovitis, as well as unossified cartilage. This is extremely important in the evaluation of congenital hip dislocation. Cystic lesions such as a Baker's cyst are also well demonstrated using ultrasound.

Avascular necrosis of bone, especially Legg-Perthe's disease, may require more than plain film radiography for a definitive diagnosis. Theoretically, a radionuclide scan should demonstrate the devascularized area; however, that early finding may not be present when the patient is examined. MRI, should be considered for further evaluation, although not as an emergency procedure.

• • •

The imaging of patients in the ED may play a critical part in their successful management, especially if it can be accomplished rapidly and safely. The most important considerations in achieving this goal relate to patient selection and the careful definition of the specific questions which need to be answered. Understanding the capabilities and the limitations of these procedures contributes immeasurably to choosing appropriate studies.

SUGGESTED READINGS

Atlas SW: *Magnetic resonance imaging of the brain and spine,* New York, 1991, Raven press.

Dalinka MK, Orthopedics, *Radiol Clin North Am,* 28(2), 1990.

el Ferzi G, Ozuner G, Davidson PG et al: Barium enema in the diagnosis of acute appendicitis, *SGO* 171:40–42, 1990.

Enzmann DR, DeLaPaz R, Rubin JB: *Magnetic resonance of the spine,* St. Louis, Mosby, 1990.

Galli RW, Spaite DW, Simon RR: *Emergency orthopedics: The spine,* Norwalk, 1989, Appleton and Lange.

Gillies C: The x-ray diagnosis of fractures, *Clear Images,* Jan. 1990, pp. 25–34; April 1990, 44–49; Aug. 1990, pp. 45–50.

Harris JH, Jr, Edeikin-Monroe B: *The radiology of acute cervical spine trauna,* ed 2, Baltimore, 1993, Williams and Wilkins.

Harris HJ Jr, Harris WH, Novelline RA: *The radiology of emergency medicine,* ed 3, Baltimore, 1993, Williams and Wilkins.

Keats TE: *Emergency radiology,* ed 2, Chicago, 1989, Year Book Medical Publishers.

Keats TE, editor: Emergency department radiology, *Radiol Clin North Am* 30(2), 1992.

Kelly J, Raptopuolos V, Davidoff A et al: The value of non-contrast-enhanced CT in blunt abdominal trauma, *AJR* 152:41–48, 1989.

Lerner RM, Mevorach RA, Hulbert WC et al: Color doppler US in the evaluation of acute scrotal disease, *Radiology* 176:355–358, 1990.

McCort JJ, Mindelzun RE: *Trauma radiology,* New York, 1990, Churchill Livingstone.

Mettler FA, Guiberteau MJ: Tumor and inflammation imaging. In *Essentials of nuclear medicine imaging,* ed 3, WB Saunders, 1991, Philadelphia.

Mindelzun RE, McCort JJ: Acute abdomen. In *Alimentary tract radiology,* ed 4, Margulis AR, Burhenne HJ, editors: Mosby, 1989, St. Louis.

Mirvis SE, Young JWR, editors: *Imaging in trauma and critical care,* Baltimore, 1992, Williams and Wilkins.

Modic MT: Imaging of the spine, *Radiol Clin North Am,* 29(4), 1991.

Murphey MD, Batnitskym S, Bramble JM: Diagnostic imaging of spinal trauma, *Radiol Clin North Am,* 27:855–872, 1989.

Pathria MN, Petersilge CA: Spinal trauma, *Radiol Clin North Am,* 29:847–865, 1991

Sartoris DJ: Musculoskeletal trauma, *Radiol Clin North Am,* 27(5), 1989.

Schultz RC: *Facial injuries,* Chicago, Year Book Medical Publishers, 1988.

Smith R, Copely DJ, Bolen FH: ^{99m}Tc RBC scintigraphy: correlation of gastrointestinal bleeding radtes with scintigraphic findings, *AJR* 148:869–874, 1987.

Wing VW, Federle MP, Morris JA et al: The clinical impact of CT for blunt abdominal trauma, *AJR* 145:1191–1194, 1985.

Young JWR, Resnik CS: Fracture of the pelvis: current concepts of classification, *AJR* 155:1169–1175, 1990.

Chapter 20

Nuclear Medicine in the Emergency Department

Harold L. Mignott, M.D.

Nuclear medicine scanning can be a useful tool to help diagnose a number of acute disease processes frequently seen in the emergency department (ED) such as pulmonary embolism, cholecystitis, testicular torsion, and gastrointestinal bleeding.

The accuracy of these tests, however, in large part depends on whether they are used in the correct clinical context. This chapter will attempt to show the utility of nuclear scans for diagnosing each of the above disorders in the ED.

PULMONARY EMBOLISM

CASE 20–1

A 28-year-old female who had a spontaneous vaginal delivery 2 weeks before admission came to the ED with complaints of sudden onset of pleuritic chest pain associated with shortness of breath.

On examination, her blood pressure was 120/70 mm Hg; pulse, 100/min; respirations, 20/min and temperature 99° F. Her examination was otherwise unremarkable, including clear lungs and normal cardiac findings. Initial laboratory evaluation included an arterial blood gas (ABG) determination on room air; pH of 7.45; pCO_2, 35 mm Hg; pO_2 85 mm Hg; and HCO_3^-, 21. Chest radiographs showed no active disease.

Comment.—This patient's clinical presentation is highly suggestive of pulmonary embolism. Supporting data include the history of a recent delivery and the clinical findings of tachycardia and tachypnea. The relatively normal blood gas results do not rule out pulmonary embolism. (Nor does a low pO_2 establish the diagnosis.) Therefore additional information is required before the diagnosis of pulmonary embolism can be established or eliminated.

The "gold standard" of tests for pulmonary embolism is pulmonary angiography, but this is an invasive test that exposes the patient to the risk of bleeding, an allergic reaction to contrast media, and the possibility of acute renal failure, especially in older patients with diabetes mellitus and renal insufficiency. Therefore, a ventilation-perfusion (V/Q) scan would be requested first (Fig. 20–1). The V/Q scan is not a perfect test but, if used correctly, can be helpful in avoiding an invasive procedure.

The test is done in two parts. The perfusion scan is done via injection of radiolabeled albumin aggregates followed by lung imaging with a gamma camera. An abnor-

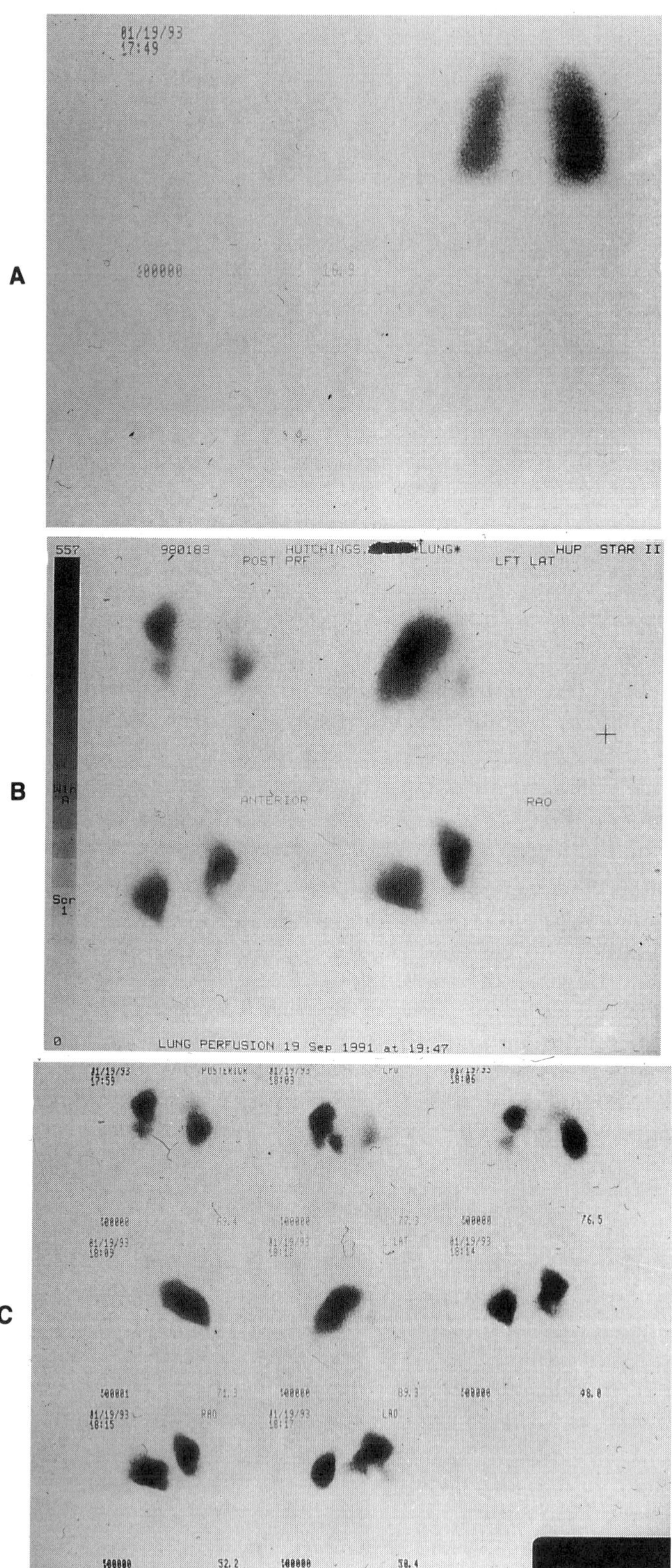

Fig. 20–1. High probability ventilation-perfusion scan in a postoperative patient. Note the multiple perfusion defects with a normal ventilation scan.

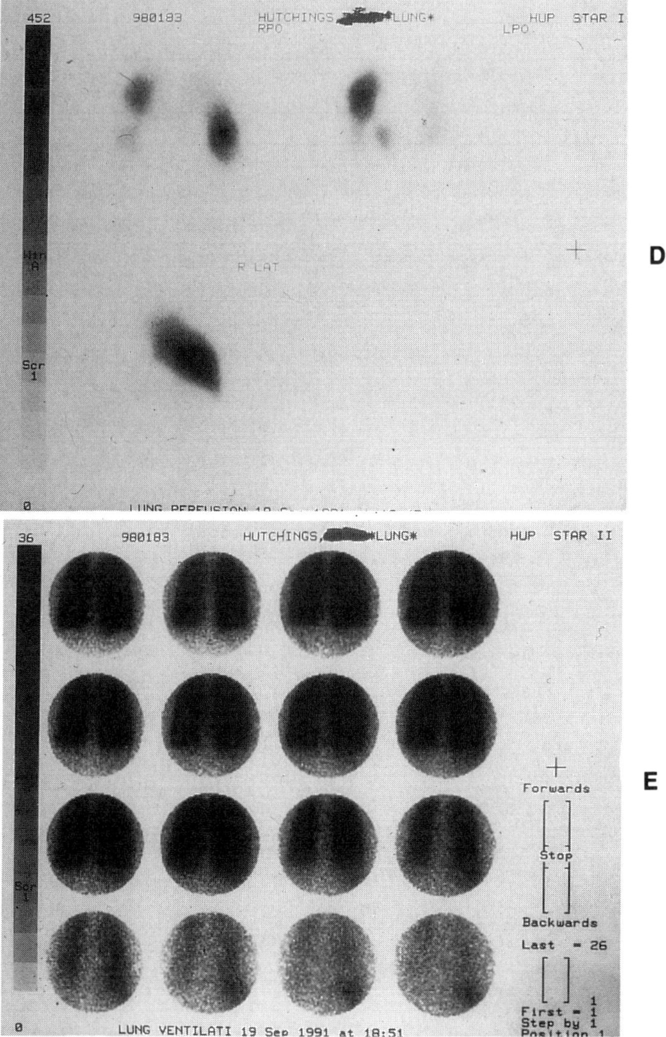

Fig. 20–1, cont'd. See opposite page for legend.

mal perfusion scan is classified by the presence or absence of defects and the number and size of any defects present.

The second portion of the test is the ventilation scan. The patient inhales radiolabeled inert gases, most commonly xenon-127. Images of the lungs are then obtained in the view that best corresponds to the perfusion defect.

The V/Q scan is then interpreted as "high probability," "intermediate probability (indeterminate)," "low probability," or normal. A *high-probability scan* is defined as two or more segmental perfusion defects without matching or corresponding ventilation defects or, alternatively, one large, segmental, isolated perfusion defect.

An *intermediate-probability scan* has segmental perfusion defects with matching ventilation defects or perfusion defects in an area that is abnormal on the chest x-ray film. A scan that cannot be clearly placed in the categories of high or low probability but is not normal is placed in the category of intermediate probability.

A *low-probability scan* is one with subsegmental perfusion defects or perfusion defects corresponding to an abnormality on chest x-ray.

A *normal scan* is a scan with no perfusion defects.

Table 20–1. Probability of Pulmonary Embolism Based on Ventilation-Perfusion Scan Interpretation and Pretest Clinical Suspicion

	Clinical Suspicion	
V/Q Scan Findings	High	Low
High probability	90%–96%	56%
Intermediate probability	66%	16%
Low probability	40%	4%

Data from PIOPED Investigators: *JAMA* 263:2753–2758, 1990, and Kelley A et al: *Ann Intern Med* 114:300–306, 1991.

The sensitivity and specificity of the V/Q scan depends on whether the scan is interpreted as high, intermediate, or low probability and on the initial index of clinical suspicion for pulmonary embolism (Table 20–1).

A high-probability scan with a high clinical suspicion has a 90% to 96% probability for pulmonary embolism when compared with pulmonary angiography. If the same high-probability scan is associated with a low clinical suspicion for pulmonary embolism, the probability falls to 56%.

An intermediate-probability scan with a high pretest clinical suspicion has a 66% probability for a pulmonary embolism and 16% probability if there is a low pretest clinical suspicion.

A low-probability scan with a high clinical suspicion has a 40% probability of pulmonary embolism and only a 4% probability with a low clinical suspicion.[1]

A normal scan rules out clinically important pulmonary embolism regardless of the degree of clinical suspicion.

Some authors have proposed using impedance plethysmography of the lower extremities to diagnose deep vein thrombophlebitis (DVT), the major cause of pulmonary embolism, thereby supplementing the value of the V/Q scan results (see Fig 20–2).[2–5] Impedance plethysmography is performed by placing a pneumatic cuff at midthigh and inflating it to 45 cm H_2O. The pressure is maintained for 45 seconds, and then the cuff is rapidly deflated. The changes in blood volume are then measured by an electrode placed on the calf. The rise in pressure is plotted as a function of the fall at 3 seconds into the deflation period. An obstruction of the venous system such as a clot will cause a decrease in the fall of blood volume at 3 seconds. A severe obstruction may also decrease the rate of filling during cuff inflation.[6]

A low-probability scan still carries a probability of pulmonary embolism that is as high as 40%. If clinical suspicion remains high, an intermediate- or low-probability scan should be followed by an angiogram.[2–5]

EVALUATION OF RIGHT UPPER QUADRANT PAIN

CASE 20–2

A 44-year-old female came to the ED because of right upper quadrant and epigastric pain virtually unremitting for the previous 2 days and associated with nausea and vomiting. She denied alcohol use.

On physical examination she was in moderate distress. Her blood pressure was 160/90 mm Hg; pulse, 100/min; respirations, 20/min; and temperature, 100.5° F. There was tenderness in the right upper quadrant and epigastrium with no rebound or guarding. The stool was negative for occult blood. Her complete blood count (CBC) revealed a slightly elevated white blood cell (WBC) count. The amylase and lipase levels were normal.

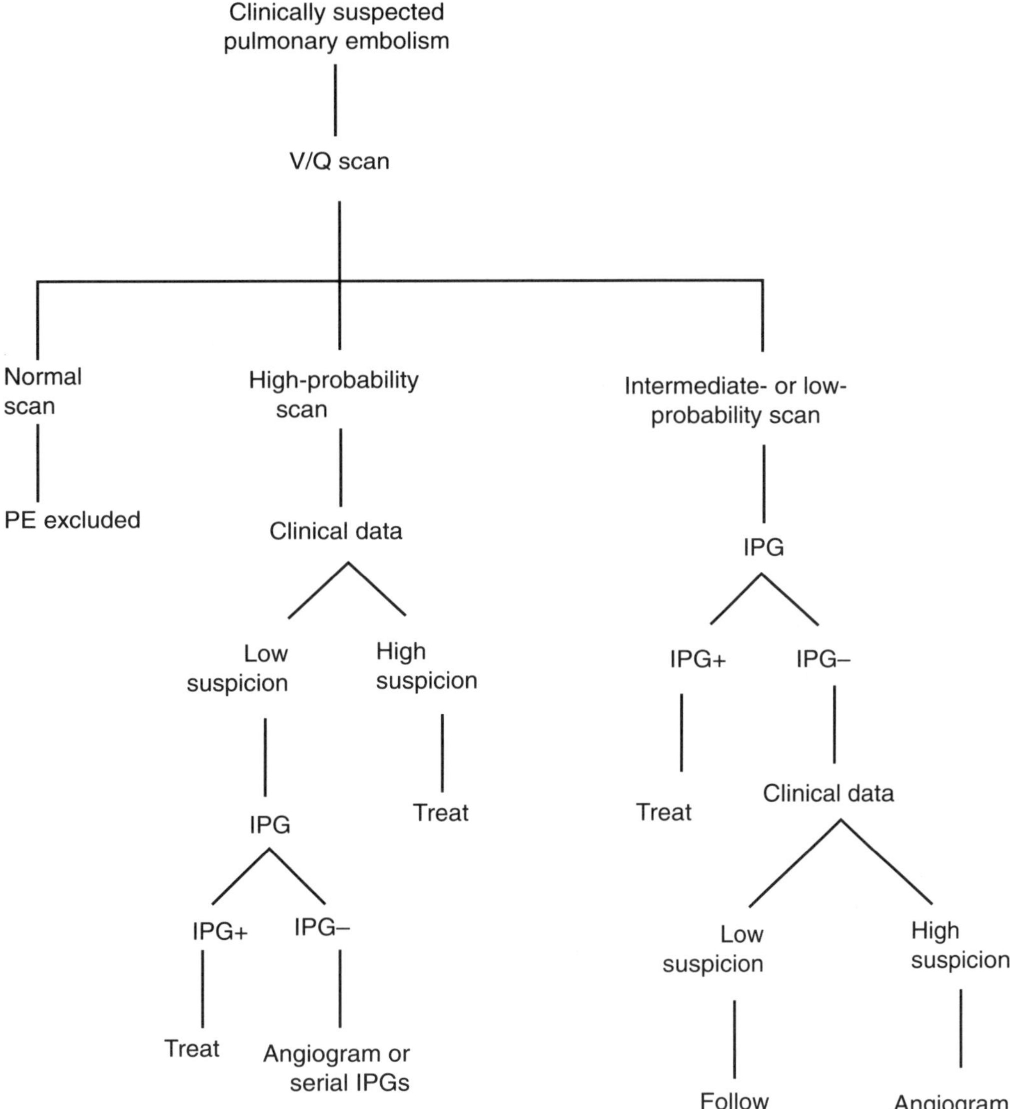

Fig. 20–2. Algorithm for evaluating a patient with a suspected pulmonary embolus *(PE). IPG,* impedence plethysmography.

Comment.—The differential diagnosis in this patient includes pancreatitis, hepatitis, peptic ulcer disease, acute cholecystitis, and Fitz-Hugh–Curtis syndrome.

With these findings the need to rule out gallbladder disease is urgent, and therefore a DESIDA (or HIDA) scan should be ordered.

The DESIDA scan is performed by injecting a technetium-labeled iminodiacetic acid derivative after a minimum of 2 hours of fasting. Images of the hepatobiliary tree are then obtained with a gamma camera. DESIDA is readily taken up by the hepatocytes and excreted into the biliary tree. A normal study reveals isotope in the gallbladder, common bile duct, and small bowel.

Patients with acute biliary colic have obstruction of their cystic duct that allows the common duct to be visualized but not the gallbladder since no isotope enters the gallbladder. Nonvisualization of the gallbladder at 1 hour and 4 hours with delayed images is interpreted as a positive scan. The sensitivity and specificity of the test are nearly 100%, with a 98% accuracy.[7–9]

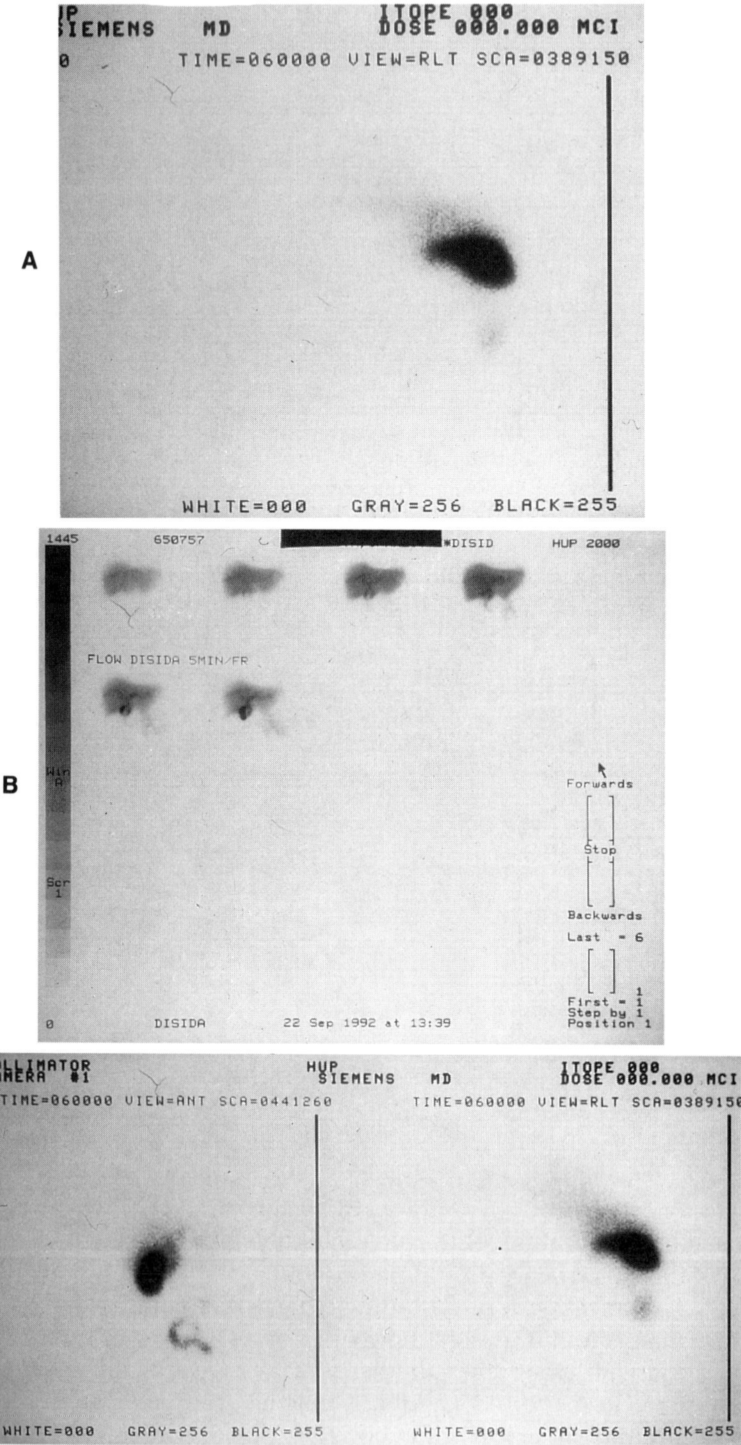

Fig. 20–3. A-D, Gallbladder seen in a normal DESIDA scan. **E-I,** Nonvisualization of the gallbladder in a patient with acute cholecystitis.

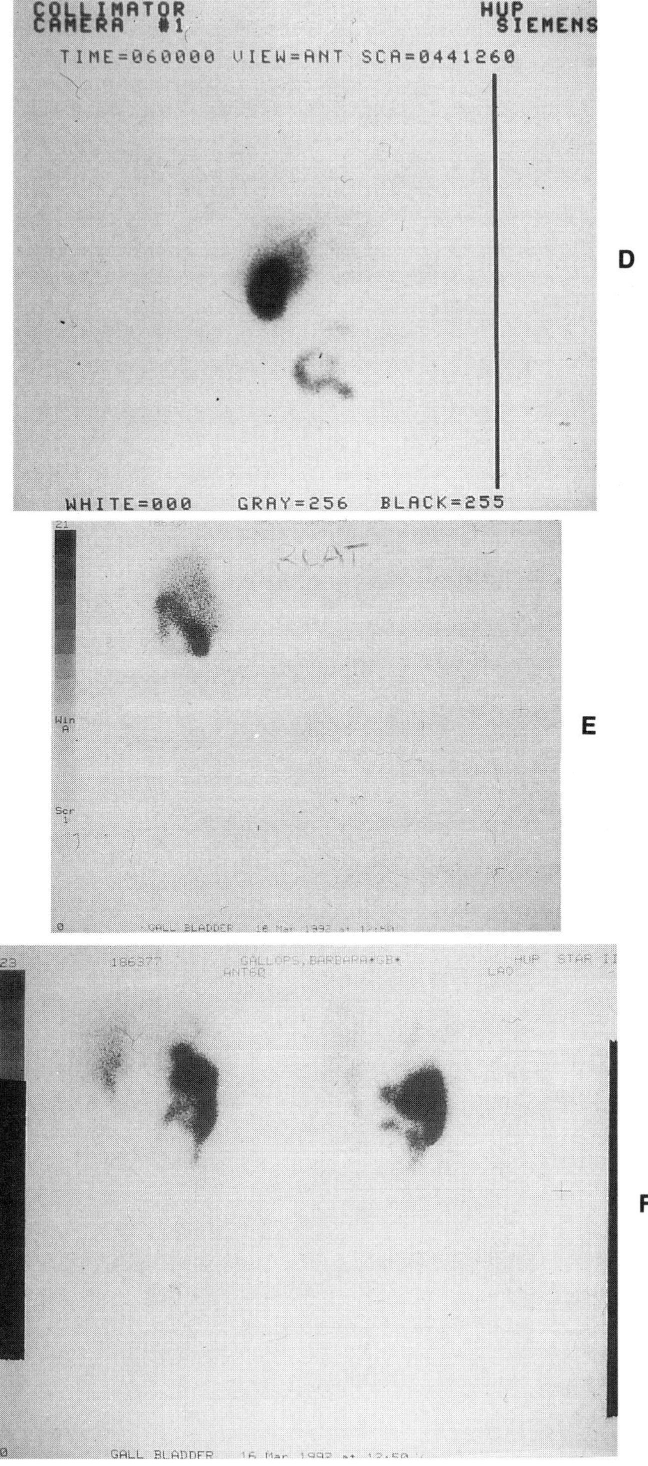

Fig. 20–3, cont'd. For legend see opposite page.

Continued.

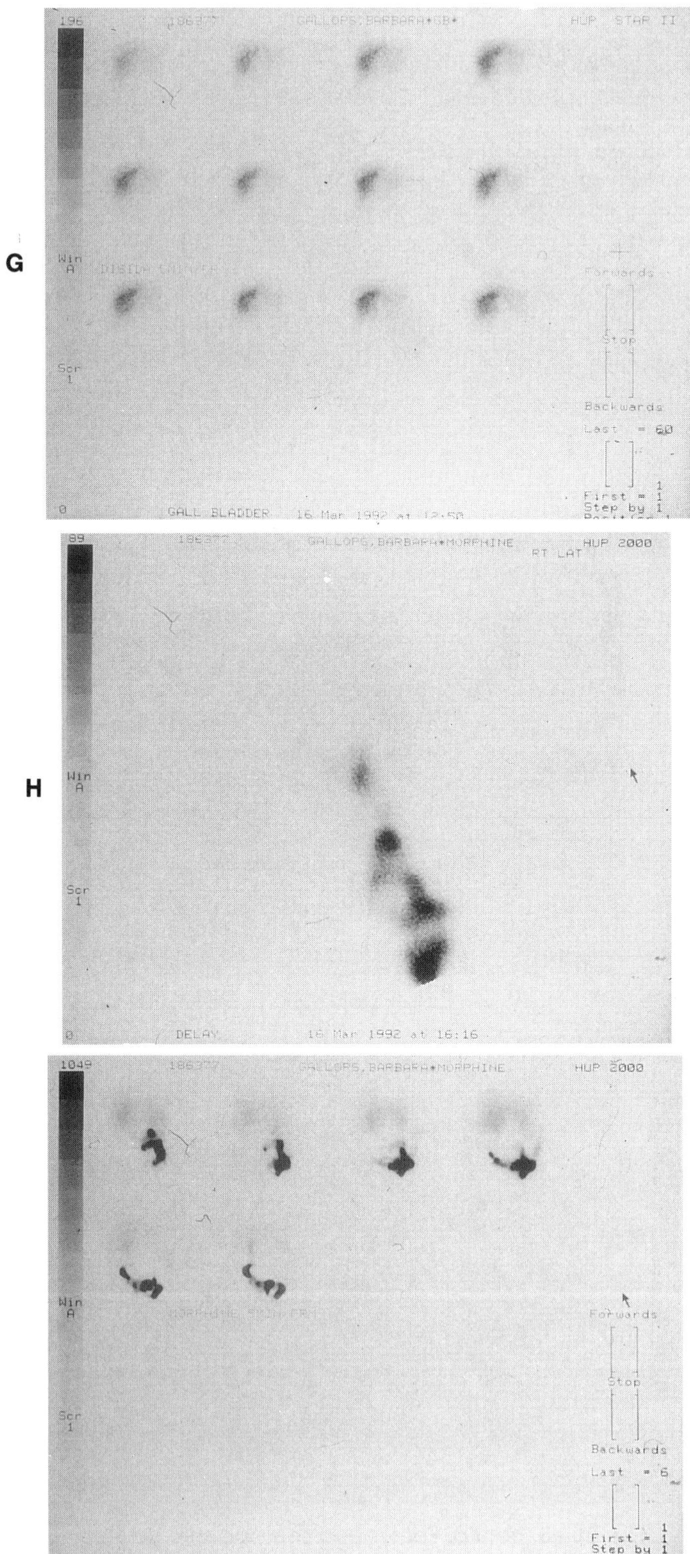

Fig. 20–3, cont'd. E-I, Nonvisualization of the gallbladder in a patient with acute cholecystitis.

Injection of morphine is reported to improve visualization of the gallbladder in patients who have a normal biliary tree by causing contraction of the sphincter of Oddi, thereby increasing the pressure on the common bile duct.

False positive studies may result from a prolonged period of fasting, total parenteral nutrition, pancreatitis, or advanced hepatocellular disease. The major advantage of this test as compared with ultrasonography of the gallbladder is that the HIDA scan is a *dynamic* test of the gallbladder and cystic duct (Fig. 20–3). It is particularly helpful in differentiating patients with silent gallstones from those with biliary colic.

GASTROINTESTINAL BLEEDING

CASE 20–3

A 74-year-old male with a history of hypertension, coronary artery disease, and diabetes mellitus came to the ED because of several episodes of bright red blood per rectum over a 1-week period.

On examination the patient had a blood pressure of 140/80 mm Hg supine and 120/60 mm Hg sitting. His pulse was 80 beats/min supine and 120, sitting. Temperature was 97° F. The abdomen was unremarkable, although old blood was noted in the rectum. Anoscopy revealed no lesions or hemorrhoids, and nasogastric aspirate was normal. The hemoglobin was 8.0 g/dL. Because of this patient's medical problems, the cause and source of his gastrointestinal bleeding had to be established urgently.

Comment.—In a situation such as this, colonoscopy may be helpful, but because the patient is not actively bleeding and because the gastrointestinal tract could not be adequately prepared for the examination quickly, a vascular lesion may be missed. A barium study might also miss a mucosal lesion and would not indicate the rate of bleeding. In addition, the use of barium would opacify the bowel so that subsequent angiography could not be performed to visualize the colonic vasculature.

Mesenteric angiography can detect bleeding rates of 0.5 mL/min or greater and is very specific (slow oozing of blood will not be detected). Radioactively labeled erythrocyte scans are able to detect bleeding rates of 0.1 mL/min, and the patient can continue to be scanned over a 24-hour period to detect the general area of bleeding. Because peristalsis moves the isotope around, the scan is not as precise in localizing the site of bleeding as arteriography and does not give information regarding the vascular anatomy of the bleeding lesion.[10, 11]

The advantages of the erythrocyte scan are that it requires little or no preparation and may localize a lesion well enough to permit endoscopy or arteriography to be more directed, thereby decreasing radiation and dye exposure and reducing the time required for colonoscopy.

The other radionuclide test available is the technetium-labeled sulfa colloid test, which has the same advantages of the labeled red cell test but does not identify intermittent bleeding as well because of its short half-life (less than 2 to 5 minutes) and wide dispersion.

TESTICULAR TORSION

CASE 20–4

An 18-year-old male came to the ED with pain and heaviness in his right testicle for the previous 4 hours. He denied any prior urinary tract symptoms. On exami-

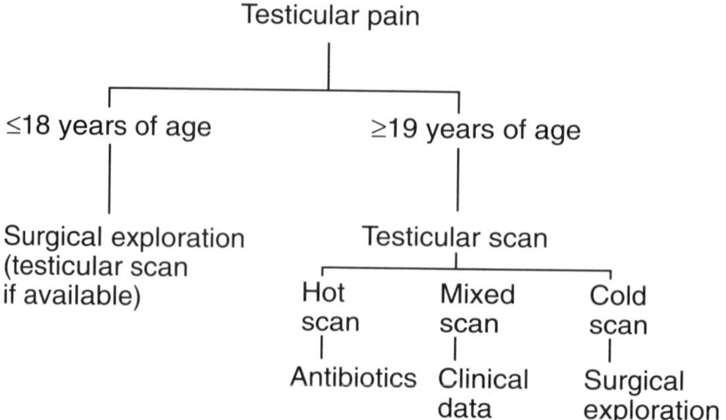

Fig. 20–4. The evaluation of testicular pain.

nation, he had a blood pressure of 120/50 mm Hg, a pulse of 90/min, and an oral temperature of 100.8° F. The right testicle was markedly swollen and tender. The epididymis could not be palpated as a discrete entity. The cremasteric reflex was absent bilaterally, and raising the testicle did not affect the pain. The prostate was not tender on rectal examination, and the remainder of the urogenital examination was normal.

Comment.—The two main diagnoses that must be considered in this patient are torsion of the testicle and epididymitis. Differentiating between these two entities is crucial because torsion requires immediate surgery whereas epididymitis is treated with antibiotics.

A radionuclide scan is very helpful in differentiating the two entities. The scan is performed by administering technetium 99 in the form of sodium pertechnetate injection and then scanning the scrotum. The scanning is divided into two phases: the angiographic or flow phase and the tissue or static phase. The static phase occurs 10 to 15 seconds after the label is injected. The flow phase labels the arteries and spermatic cord followed by the testicular tissue, which is labeled in the late flow phase and early static phase. In a normal scan, a homogeneous uptake is seen throughout the phases.

An increased uptake ("hot scan") in any area suggests inflammation, most commonly caused by epididymitis or epididymo-orchitis. Decreased activity ("cold scan") is most commonly associated with testicular torsion and rarely with an avascular tumor. A mixed scan, meaning areas of increased uptake coupled with areas of poor uptake, may suggest abscess, trauma, tumor, or a late phase of torsion. The sensitivity and specificity of the scan in distinguishing between epididymo-orchitis and torsion approach 100% with an accuracy of a 90% or greater.[12, 13]

Statistically, 80% of males under 19 years of age with testicular pain will prove to have torsion. Conversely, 80% of males 19 years of age or older with testicular pain will have epididymitis (Fig. 20–4).

SUMMARY

The clinical utility of lung, gallbladder, gastrointestinal, and testicular scanning has been discussed. All of these tests provide results with little or no risk to the patient. The images obtained, result from the radioactivity of the structures recorded by a detection device. Interpreting these images, however, is not always easy: there are "gray zones" where the images are indeterminate and open to misinterpretation i.e., low specificity.

None of the aforementioned tests are considered to be the gold standard for imaging the organ system in question. Rather, they help confirm the clinical impression. If the test results are equivocal or contrary to the clinical impression, the diagnostic impression should not be blindly changed but instead, a test should be performed that is considered to be the gold standard. If the two tests are in agreement, it is time to reconsider the clinical impression.

REFERENCES

1. PIOPED Investigators: Value of the ventilation/perfusion scan in acute pulmonary embolism, *JAMA* 263:2753–2758, 1990.
2. Hull RD, Hirsh J, Carter CJ: Diagnostic value of ventilation-perfusion lung scanning in patients with suspected pulmonary embolism, *Chest* 88:819–827, 1985.
3. Hull RD, Hirsh J, Carter CJ: Pulmonary angiography, ventilation lung scanning, and venography for clinically suspected pulmonary embolism with abnormal perfusion lung scan, *Ann Intern Med* 98:891–899, 1983.
4. Hull RD, Raskob GE, Coates G: A new noninvasive management strategy for patients with suspected pulmonary embolism, *Arch Intern Med* 149:2549–2554, 1989.
5. Kelley A, Carson L, Palevsky I: Diagnosing pulmonary embolism: new facts and strategies, *Ann Intern Med* 114:300–306, 1991.
6. Wheeler H et al: Occlusive impedance phlebography: a diagnostic procedure for venous thrombosis and pulmonary embolism, *Prog Cardiovas Dis* 17:199-205, 1974.
7. Bednarz GM, Kalff V, Kelly MJ: Hepatobiliary scintigraphy, *Med J Aust* 145:316–318, 1986.
8. Fink-Bennett D, Freitas JE, Ripley SD, Bree RL: The sensitivity of hepatobiliary imaging and real-time ultrasonography in the detection of acute cholecystitis, *Arch Surg* 120:904–906, 1985.
9. Colletti PM, Ralls PW, Siegel ME, Halls JM: Acute cholecystitis: diagnosis with radionuclide angiography, *Radiology* 163:615–618, 1987.
10. Gupta S, Evangeline L, Kingsley S: Detection of gastrointestinal bleeding by radionuclide scintigraphy, *Am J Gastroenterol* 79:26–30, 1989.
11. Hyams JS, Leichtner AM, Schwartz AN: Recent advances in diagnosis and treatment of gastrointestinal hemorrhage in infants and children, *J Pediatr* 106:1–7, 1985.
12. Eshghi M, Silver L, Smith L, Smith AD: Technetium 99m scan in acute scrotal lesions, *Urology* 30:586–593, 1987.
13. Golimbu M, Florio FE, Al-Askari S: Value of scrotal scanning, *Urology* 25:89–92, 1985.

PART VI

Medicolegal and Forensic Considerations

Chapter 21

Laboratory Evaluation of the Sexual Assault Victim*

Carmen Germaine Warner, M.S.N., R.N.

Emergency physicians frequently become distressed when a sexual assault victim comes to the emergency department (ED) because of the terrible nature of the problem. At times the physician also becomes frustrated because of the exacting nature of the evidence collection requirements. Clearly identified steps in the diagnostic testing and the reasoning behind each procedure will make the entire assessment and intervention easier and provide accurate evidence if the victim decides to prosecute. The ultimate outcome for the victim, the family, and the suspect is predicated on the accurate collection, identification, and preservation of specimens obtained during the examination and documentation of the findings and test results.

THE ADULT FEMALE VICTIM

History and Physical Examination

The initial steps of obtaining a history and performing a physical examination (although not specifically considered diagnostic tests) are of considerable value to the emergency physician who is gathering all the evidence needed for both the medical and the legal aspects of a sexual assault case. The data that need to be included in a history[1] are presented in Table 21–1; it should be used as an assessment tool and can be applied to all victims of sexual assault.

In addition to the history, the information gained through a physical examination is also instrumental in establishing that nonconsensual sexual intercourse occurred. Valuable information to be considered in conducting a physical examination is noted in Table 21–2 (see Appendix 21–1 also).

Diagnostic Tests

Diagnostic procedures that include laboratory tests to provide medical and physiologic information and legal evidence are vital. Whether the legal prosecution is aided or destroyed depends on the conscientious, deliberate, and accurate collection and documentation of the results of these procedures along with the collection and preservation of evidence. It cannot be stressed enough that the accuracy and the com-

*A special note of appreciation is extended to Deborah Kilgore, R.N., S.A.N.C., for her careful review and evaluation of this chapter.

Table 21–1. Sexual Assault Victim History

General Health	Personal History: Female	Personal History: Male and Female	Sexual Assault History	Post Sexual Assault History
Allergies (food, medication, or topical)	Current birth control measures (including sterilization)	Present or past venereal disease	Time, day, date	Bathing
Current immunizations (primarily tetanus)	Estrogen allergies	Present or past rectal bleeding or discharge	Physical surroundings (e.g., sand, grass, leaves, flowers, water)	Washing hair
Medications currently prescribed	Early signs of pregnancy	Present or past lacerations or sores in the mouth	Physical forms of violence If physically assaulted, note what was used (hands, feet, foreign objects, etc.) and where injuries are located	Brushing teeth
Recent illness, injury, or trauma	Past pregnancies		Threats of violence Note which weapons were used or displayed to imply a threat	Gargling
	Live children		Blindfolds used	Changing clothes
	Last menstrual period		Number of perpetrators	Drinking, eating
	Recent consensual intercourse or sexual activity		Forced use of alcohol or drugs	Taking medication
	Recent gynecologic injury or surgery		Loss of consciousness Note length of time	Urinating, douching
	Feelings concerning hormonal pregnancy prevention, abortion, or menstrual extraction		Position of patient during each sexual act Fondling Vaginal entry or approach Oral entry or approach Anal entry or approach Forced to perform lewd acts	Defecating
	Existing or past gynecologic infection		Ejaculation, urination, or defecation on body (be specific)	Taking an enema
			Use of condom or lubricant	Vomiting
			Any information about the perpetrator known to the patient (e.g., perpetrator known to be sterile)	

Modified from Kravis TC, Warner GC, editors: *Rape and sexual assault in emergency medicine: a comprehensive review,* New York, 1993, Raven Press, p. 1247.

Table 21–2. Physical Examination of Sexual Assault Victims

General	Female Genitalia	Male Genitalia	Rectal Area
Note patient's general demeanor and emotional state	Carefully examine the vulva, noting signs of trauma or foreign matter, semen, dirt, grass, pus, or blood	Examine the penis for signs of trauma, foreign material, or infection	Examine the area for signs of trauma
Record vital signs	Gently examine the introitus and hymen for signs of trauma	Examine the scrotum for signs of trauma or foreign material	Assess the presence of lubricant, blood, semen, pus, or any foreign matter
Assess physical appearance	Very carefully assess the vaginal area for trauma, signs of foreign objects, or internal lacerations and bleeding*	Colposcopy	Gently examine the rectum for possible trauma, placement of foreign objects, and internal lacerations and bleeding
Examine skin; collect and label any foreign material such as seminal stains, botanical material, grass, plastic, paper, or blood; also collect a control swab if a swab is taken from skin	Gently inspect the cervix for evidence of parity, signs of pregnancy, presence of menstruation, evidence of trauma, and signs of infection		Colposcopy
Assess the upper trunk, noting breast trauma and sexual maturity	Perform a general pelvic assessment		
Examine the lower trunk noting signs of trauma and sexual maturity	With a Wood's light (ultraviolet), note signs of semen around the perineal area†		
Check the extremities for bruises, fractures, sprains, and scratches	Use a colposcope with a camera (if available) to document any signs of vaginal microtrauma (both external and internal)		
Record head and neck trauma, including the mouth, ears, and scalp; collectible evidence may be secured from the hair and mouth or other orifices			

From Kravis TC, Warner CG, editors: *Rape and sexual assault in emergency medicine: a comprehensive review,* New York, 1993, Raven Press, p. 1247.
*It is critical that water rather than a lubricant be used to lubricate the speculum in order to prevent alteration of the results of the acid phosphatase test.
†Obtain photographs as necessary.

pleteness of medical tests are essential to the victim's well-being. Precision in conducting diagnostic procedures and clarity in case presentation result in a greater likelihood of a correct judgment if the case comes before the courts.

Medical

The medical tests of value to an emergency physician throughout the diagnostic process are listed below:

1. Medical assessment for sexually transmitted diseases (STDs)
   - Purpose: To establish a baseline for the presence or absence of STDs at the time of the victim's initial medical/evidentiary examination (positive results usually indicate an infection before the sexual assault)
     - Gonorrheal cultures (from appropriate sites)
     - Chlamydial cultures (from appropriate sites)
     - Syphilis (rapid plasmin reagin [RPR], Venereal Disease Research Laboratory [VDRL])
   - Human immunodeficiency virus (HIV)/hepatitis
2. Pregnancy assessment
   - Urine/serum testing
3. Total-body assessment (with particular attention to those sites indicated by the victim as being injured or sore)
   - Radiography for any bone or internal injuries and for the presence of foreign objects
   - Tests to assess internal injuries (oral, esophageal, abdominal, vaginal, or rectal)
4. Sperm and semen assessment
   - Location found
   - Motility/nonmotility of sperm (may not be required or recommended in some localities)

Pregnancy after sexual assault is estimated to occur in approximately 1% of all rape victims.[2] Although this percentage may be small, a careful assessment must be made in order to accurately determine whether pregnancy existed before the attack. To make this assessment, the clinician should order a serum test to determine the level of the β-subunit of human chorionic gonadotropin (β-hCG). This test can provide a positive result 1 week after conception.[3] A positive result at the time of the initial visit is essential to reassure a woman later that her pregnancy is not due to the assault.

Emergency physicians should perform a pregnancy test before offering any postcoital therapy. Postcoital treatment should be offered to the victim at the time of the examination. If the patient elects to have ethinyl estradiol, 100 μg, plus norgestrel, 1 mg (Ovral, 2 tablets, the so-called morning-after pill), to disrupt a possible pregnancy resulting from the assault, the treatment must be initiated within 72 hours of the assault and repeated in 12 hours.

The presence of motile and immotile sperm may be detected microscopically in wet mounts of vaginal aspirates and vaginal or rectal washings. Emergency physicians should examine these washings microscopically immediately after the initial assessment in recognition of the fact that a forensic pathologist may not be able to examine samples for hours, days, or even weeks later, when the sperm would be immotile. Some localities, however, discourage inexperienced physicians from performing such an examination. If this examination is improperly performed (if the washings are improperly collected and prepared), "no motile sperm" may be reported, even though actually present, perhaps working against the victim's interests.

The importance of follow-up for medical and psychological care needs to be emphasized to the victim. Medical reexamination should be done approximately 10 to 14 days after the assault. The reexamination should include a vaginal examination to inspect for resolution of any injuries and testing for STDs (repeat VDRL or RPR in 8 weeks). Pregnancy testing should be performed at appropriate times.

Sexual assault results in a major disruption in the victim's physical, emotional, and behavioral reactions. Referrals for psychological support services should be offered immediately. The referrals should include community agencies such as sexual assault centers, women's centers, and victim assistance programs.

New Techniques in Diagnostic Information

A new technology has been developed over the past several years that uses DNA for genetic "fingerprinting." When a significant tissue or body fluid sample is available, a comparison can be made between the DNA collected from the victim and the accused.

Physiologic

The collection of physiologic samples should be a routine part of the ED visit. Protocols may differ slightly, depending on the requirements of the hospital, the laboratory, and the local law enforcement agency. All physiologic evidence becomes the property and the responsibility of the local law enforcement agency, even though it was collected by emergency personnel. All evidence is turned over to law enforcement officials.

Samples of urine and blood are needed for some of the tests that must be performed. Many evidence collection kits provide containers for these specimens (a plastic container for the urine sample and collection tubes for the blood samples). Some localities no longer routinely collect wet blood specimens because of concern for deterioration of the specimen when improperly stored for long periods of time and also because of fear of generating specimens containing infectious agents (hepatitis, HIV, etc.). Also, more information can now be obtained from dry blood specimens, including ABO typing, DNA analysis, etc.

CASE 21–1

A 23-year-old female, married for 3 months and not using any form of birth control, was brought into the ED after being raped in her apartment by a masked male. The woman mentioned that she and her husband had been trying to have a baby, but she did not know whether she was pregnant at the time of the assault.

Comment.—The important fact to determine is whether the woman was already pregnant at the time of the attack. If a β-hCG pregnancy test is obtained on the day of the initial examination and the results are negative, estradiol and norgestrol may be offered to the patient. If the β-hCG test results are positive, the woman can be assured that she was already pregnant at the time of the assault; if the test results are negative, the test should be repeated at the time of the follow-up visit (if the follow-up visit is 1 week or more after the assault). A second test that is positive following a negative first test, would indicate that the patient may have become pregnant as a result of the assault. Suction curettage could be offered to the patient to terminate the pregnancy.

The urine sample is obtained for drug-screening tests and is collected in a single plastic container. Blood is used for a variety of tests and is collected in color-coded tubes:*

- Purple (lavender) top tube —specimen used for blood grouping tests (grouping is compared with those of seminal stains) and also for DNA tests
- Gray top tube —specimen used for blood alcohol and certain drug assays (sedative hypnotics, central nervous system [CNS] depressants) if clinically relevant

*Some states no longer collect "wet" blood specimens as part of the evidence collection kit because of fear of infection potential (HIV) and improper storage and deterioration.

- Yellow top tube—specimen used for determining the ABO and genetic phenotype, phosphoglucomutase, and peptidase A (to determine the race of the suspect).
- Red top tube—miscellaneous testing

Legal

In all cases of sexual assault, information gathered for legal purposes should be collected by the physician caring for the victim. The information that must be gathered includes the following evidence (all items should be properly labeled and sealed):

1. Foreign materials on clothing, body, hair (place in proper containers). Collect, package, and properly label matter found such as seminal stains, blood, any other organic or synthetic materials located and document where found. If foreign material is noted on clothing, the victim should disrobe over a sheet of paper to collect any loose material that might dislodge.
2. Wood's light scan (long-wave ultraviolet). During visual examination of the skin, a Wood's light scan of the body should be done for any evidence of secretions, stains, and fibers that fluoresce under the Wood's light but may not be readily visible in daylight. Semen under the Wood's light is highly fluorescent. Fluorescent areas should be swabbed and collected appropriately. Air-dry samples.
3. Head hairs. Pluck or trim several hairs from various regions of the scalp that represent the range of colors and lengths of the victim's hair.
4. Saliva (for ABO antigens). When collecting saliva samples, obtain the specimens on a paper disk or swab. Do not handle the specimen with fingers, and use forceps. Air-dry samples.
5. Oral swabs. Collect two swabs from the oral cavity. Areas to swab should include the cheek folds, along the gum lines, and from the gums to the tonsillar pillars. Air-dry samples.
6. Nail scrapings (for foreign materials). Obtain skin tissues, blood, or other identifiable material from under the fingernails. Collect scrapings from each hand into a separate envelopes.
7. Perineal area (for foreign material). Collect and properly package all materials obtained. Label foreign material and describe the location from which the specimens were obtained.
8. Pubic hair samples (for foreign materials).
   a. Matted pubic hair. Collect by cutting specimens and placing them in an envelope.
   b. Pubic hair combings. Place a sheet of paper (8″ × 10″) under the victim's perineum and buttocks, and comb the area to collect any loose hairs or foreign material. Place the comb on the paper, fold the paper with the specimens and comb inside, and place in an envelope.
   c. Pubic hair reference. Pluck or trim several hairs from each of several different areas of the pubic region.
9. Vaginal specimens.
   a. External vaginal swabs. With two swabs, collect evidence from the outer vaginal area by wiping in the labial folds, posterior fourchette region, and the urethral and vaginal orifices. Air-dry samples (Fig. 21–1).[4]
   b. Internal vaginal swabs. With four swabs, collect specimens from the vaginal vault. Prepare a saline wet mount slide with these swabs to use for the detection of sperm and sperm motility.
   c. Vaginal aspirates. This procedure involves the collection of evidence from the deepest possible source. Use clear plastic tubing and a 10-mL syringe to collect the fluid directly.

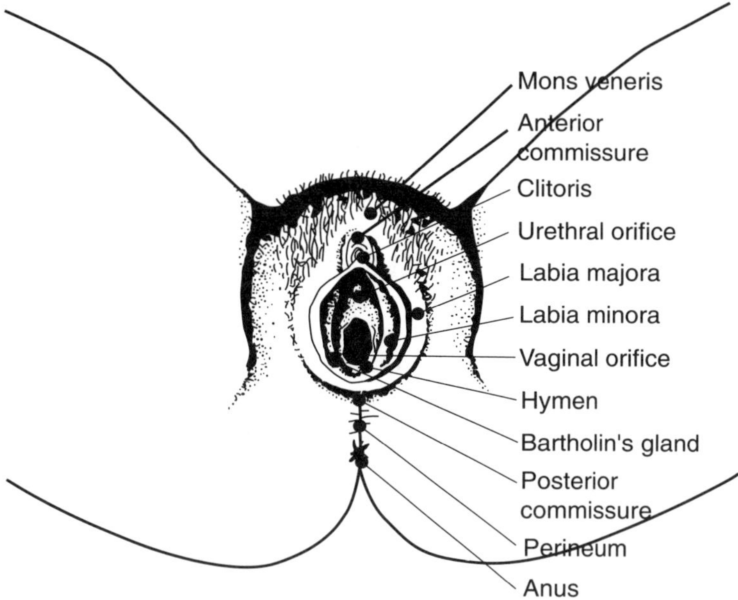

Fig. 21–1. Female external anatomy. (From Warner CG et al: *San Diego County protocol for the treatment of rape and sexual assault victims,* San Diego, Calif, 1978, p 28.)

d. Vaginal washings. Wash the vaginal vault with normal saline (10 mL) if sufficient material is not available.

10. Anal swabs. With two swabs, collect evidence from the anal region both externally and internally (do not use lubricant if inserting an anoscope).
11. Clothing. Examine clothing for foreign matter, semen, blood, or other secretions. (The accompanying box focuses on the orderly handling and accurate preservation of clothing.)
12. Fecal matter. If rectal intercourse has occurred, clinicians should collect both lubricant (if present) and fecal matter as evidence. These specimens can be submitted to the crime laboratory on cotton-tipped swabs. The fecal examination conducted in most crime laboratories assesses undigested food, bacterial species and subspecies, and parasitic constituents (helminths and protozoa).[5]
13. Photography. Signs of physical trauma/injuries can be permanently documented and preserved as evidence with the use of film. All significant injuries including abrasions, bruises, bite wounds, etc., should be photographed. Conventional documentation of genital findings usually describes only 10% to 30% of visible positive genital trauma found in sexual assaults. A colposcopic examination of the genital area at the time of the evidentiary examination can be a valuable tool in detecting microtrauma not visualized with gross inspection. Colposcopic photography provides important medical and legal information obtained by detecting and documenting the injuries seen with colposcopic magnification.

Evidence Collection Kits

Evidence collection kits may vary from facility to facility, but it is extremely important that each staff member be familiar with the particular kit used by the ED and be trained in the use of that kit. A sample evidence collection kit is described in Table 21–3. The steps crucial to the proper collection and preservation of evidence are straightforward once a procedure has been outlined. However, the one area that is frequently mishandled is the preservation of clothing (see the accompanying box).

Preservation of a Sexual Assault Victim's Clothing

1. Note the victim's clothing and record observations on the chart.
2. Examine all clothing for soilage, tears, and the presence of blood or semen.
3. Arrange for fresh clothing to be brought to the emergency department if the patient's clothes need to be collected.
4. Collect the patient's underwear. Do not crumple; place loosely in an ample-sized paper container.
5. Air-dry wet evidence; do not fan dry or use heat.
6. Circle wet marks with a laundry marker to circumscribe the evidence.
7. Place clean paper over the stain and place the item of clothing in a clean container. Do not allow stained areas to come in contact with clean areas.
8. If the patient is menstruating, collect the tampon or sanitary napkin.
9. Place each article of clothing in a separate bag, seal it properly, and mark it with the collector's initials and the date.
10. Record on the chart the name of the person who collected the clothing and the name of the person to whom it was turned over.
11. All clothing used as evidence should be forwarded by law enforcement personnel to the appropriate forensic laboratory.

SPECIAL NOTE: ALL CONTAINERS SHOULD BE PAPER.

From Warner CG et al: *San Diego County protocol for the treatment of rape and sexual assault victims,* San Diego, Calif, 1978, p 14.

Analysis of Evidence

Once the evidence has been collected and preserved, the clinician should submit the materials to law enforcement officials for forensic laboratory evaluation. There the following procedures (which are crucial to any legal case) will be carried out:

1. Determining the presence of sperm.
   a. Examine vaginal slides microscopically for the presence of spermatozoa (manually examine for the presence of motile and nonmotile sperm).
   b. If no sperm are found on the slides, analyze the vaginal swabs and aspirate for the presence of the enzyme acid phosphatase.*
   c. If the acid phosphatase test is positive, confirm the presence of semen by analysis for P_{30}—a protein found only in semen.
   d. An alternate, less reliable method for determining the presence of semen is to subject the sample to acid phosphatase electrophoresis.
   e. If semen is not detected in the vaginal sample, examine the clothing (undergarments, pants, shorts, shirts) for stains. Extract and analyze the stains for the presence of sperm and acid phosphatase.
   f. Examine other samples that may contain semen (such as dried secretions and oral and anal samples) in the same fashion as vaginal samples.
   g. If no sperm are found on vaginal slides, refer to the forensic laboratory procedure.
2. Determining the semen source.
   a. Samples that are positive for the presence of semen are typed in two genetic marker systems—ABO and phosphoglucomutase.
   b. Proper interpretation requires identifying the ABO types of the victim and the suspect, along with their secretor status.
   c. Consequently, blood and saliva from the victim and the suspect are needed.

*If no sperm are found and the test for acid phosphatase is negative, do not assume that intercourse has *not* taken place; semen may have been diluted or destroyed by time, washing, and douching or by subsequent physical activity.

Table 21–3. Victim Sample Evidence Collection Kit*

Examination Item	Material Required
Record of sexual assault and personal history	Appropriate forms
Collection of clothing	Paper bags, butcher paper, labels
Physical examination	Appropriate forms
Urine for pregnancy test and drug test	Two containers, labels
Fingernail scrapings	Fingernail file, envelope, label
Saliva sample	Paper disk or swabs, envelope, label
Blood samples	Tourniquet; gauze pad (nonalcohol); syringe (20 mL); needle (21 gauge); gray-, red-, purple (lavender) and yellow-topped tubes; labels
Pubic hair combings	Plastic comb, towel, envelope, label
Pelvic examination	Gloves, lubricant, speculum, cervical scraper (Ayre stick), two slides, fixative
Vaginal swabs	Four cotton swabs, two plastic containers, saline, two glass slides, labels, pencil
Vaginal washings	Normal saline, 10 mL; aspiration pipette and bulb
Microscopic examination for sperm motility	Microscope, slides, slide covers, vaginal swabs, normal saline
Photography (optional)	Camera, film, flash

*State, municipal, or local law enforcement agencies may suggest or provide specific evidence kits.

   d. Collect the blood and saliva during the examination or at a later time, depending on individual policy.
3. Matching hair types.
   a. The microscopic examination may disclose foreign pubic hairs, which then may be compared with those of the suspect.
   b. If the hair samples are similar, the suspect remains only a suspect; guilt is not established.
4. Special considerations for samples.
   a. Maintain samples in a dry condition until they are delivered to the crime laboratory.
   b. Thoroughly dry all swab, slide, and clothing evidence before packaging them.
   c. Place the evidence in a nonairtight container such as a paper bag.

Sections 2, 3, and 4 are also conducted in accordance with forensic laboratory procedures.

Consent Forms

It is essential to obtain signed consent forms before initiating any procedures. Emergency physicians must realize that a victim does have the right to refuse examination for the purpose of securing evidence and may consent to receive medical attention only. Nevertheless, clinicians should encourage the collection of evidence in the event that the victim decides to prosecute at a later date. The necessary consent forms include those for history, physical examination, collection of evidence, photography, release of information to the authorities, and medical treatment. The forms should be signed only after a thorough explanation has been provided and in the presence of a witness.

THE ADULT MALE VICTIM

History and Physical Examination

The information required from a history and physical examination of a male sexual assault victim is similar to that required of the female. Tables 21–1 and 21–2 identify data needed in the case of the male victim also—except for the data peculiar to female personal history and the female genitalia. Special attention must be placed on

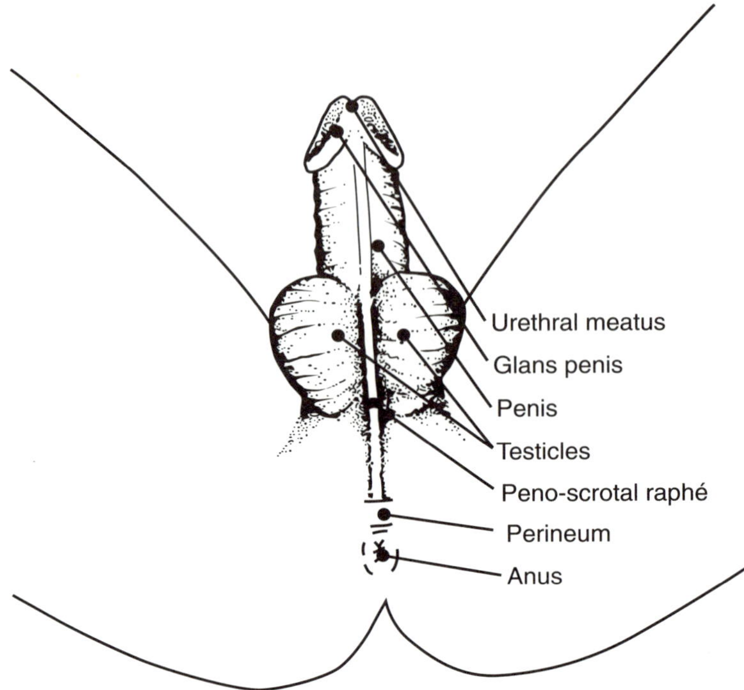

Fig. 21–2. Male external anatomy. (From Warner CG et al: *San Diego County protocol for the treatment of rape and sexual assault victims,* San Diego, Calif, 1978, p 50.)

the assessment and examination of the rectum, the genitals, and the mouth and oropharynx for trauma. Check for bleeding, discharge, soreness, infection, internal injuries, or generalized pain (Fig. 21–2).

Diagnostic Tests

Male victims must also be offered the laboratory tests that provide medical and physiologic information and legal evidence. The tests are described in the section on female sexual assault victims.

CASE 21–2

A 32-year-old married man dressed in a torn business suit was brought into the ED because of multiple cuts, bruises, and a left Colles' fracture. He stated that he was in a car accident but he was unable to recall the location of the car.

Upon further examination, the clinician discovers that the patient's anus appears swollen and tender. Upon further questioning, the patient admits that he had been sexually assaulted by three young men.

Comment.—In addition to the identification procedure already outlined, the emergency physician should insert 10 mL of normal saline into the rectum, aspirate the fluid after 5 to 10 minutes, and save the sample for acid phosphatase and sperm analysis.[2]

Medical

The medical assessment—including evaluation for STDs, identification of sperm, and total-body assessment—is equally important in the case of a male sexual assault victim. Radiography may be invaluable in determining the presence of a foreign object in the rectum or elsewhere.

Physiologic

Physiologic samples—including urine samples for drug screening and blood samples for blood grouping, blood alcohol, venereal disease, and racial determination—are equally crucial in the the case of a male victim. The procedures for collecting, handling, and preserving the evidence are the same as those for a female victim.

Legal

The evidence collection kits are standard for all sexual assault victims, and the method for collecting and preserving the evidence is the same for all victims (except for sex-specific collecting considerations). Although subsequent legal action by a male victim is not as common as in the case of a female victim, the opportunity for such action should be provided, and all phases of diagnostic assessment contribute to the conclusiveness of the evidence (see Case 21–2).

Consent Forms

Signed consent forms should be obtained as outlined in the section on diagnostic procedures for adult female sexual assault victims.

THE CHILD VICTIM

History and Physical Examination

The value of an accurate and specific history and physical examination is no less important in the case of a child sexual assault victim than in the case of an adult victim. Tables 21–1 and 21–2 can be used as a guide for a child victim also—but with increased emphasis on making the following observations:

- The body habitus (including growth of the body parts)
- The distribution of hair on the body
- General signs indicating the degree of sexual maturation
- Signs of trauma or semen deposits on the skin and hair anywhere on the body
- Condition of the back and buttocks
- The apparent degree of maturation of the breasts (female)
- Presence of abdominal tenderness and masses and the presence or the absence of bowel sounds
- Condition of the vulva and the vagina of a small female child, examined in a fashion that ensures comfort for the child (Fig. 21–3)
- Condition of the vulva, vulvar vestibule, hymen, and hymenal orifice by direct exposure through a gentle downward and lateral pressure on each side of the perineum (Fig. 21–4)

Diagnostic Tests

Medical

By using a tube like a vaginoscope, cultures for gonorrhea and saline preparations for trichomonas, sperm, and acid phosphatase can be obtained. Following the female protocol as a baseline for testing, the physician may choose to secure a Papanicolaou smear for purposes of assessing ovarian function and for determining the presence of sperm in suspected cases of penetration and ejaculation. Radiological ex-

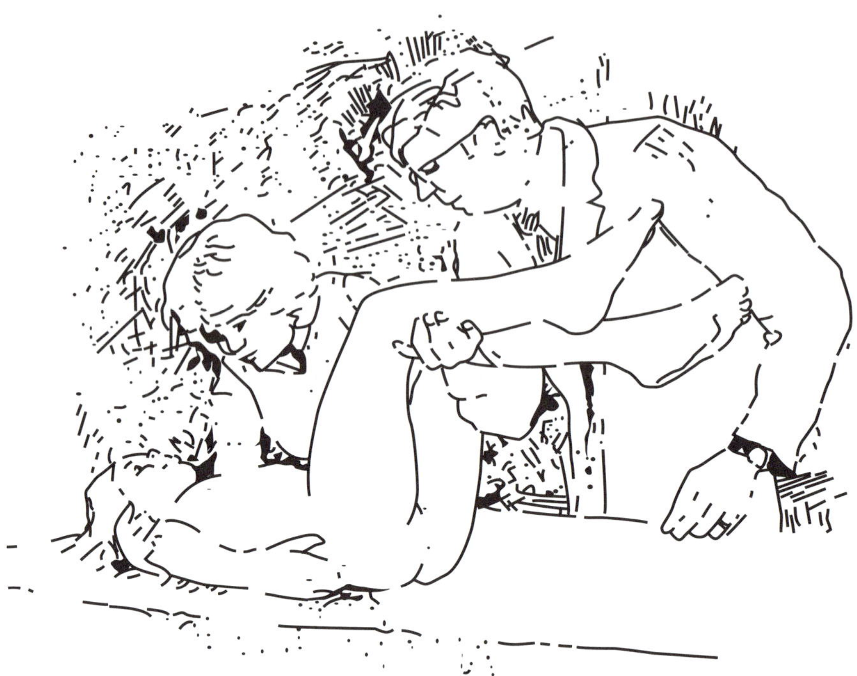

Fig. 21–3. Examination of a young female child. (From Warner CG: *Rape and sexual assault: management & intervention,* Rockville, Md, 1980, Aspen Systems, p 78.)

amination or direct visualization may be useful in determining the presence of foreign objects.

Physiologic

Urine and blood samples listed under physiologic tests recommended in the case of an adult female rape victim are also applicable in the case of a child victim. Nevertheless, the clinician's evaluation of the extent to which those tests are warranted in the case of a child is important. Specific steps pertinent in a laboratory examination protocol are outlined in the accompanying box. The clinician's examination is also discussed in Case 21–3.

Legal

The extent to which legal evidence is required varies with each case, especially when no legal action is contemplated. The physician should take this into account in determining the amount of evidence required in a particular case and then follow the appropriate guidelines listed earlier in this chapter.

Consent Forms

In the case of a minor, the emergency physician must obtain the necessary consent from the parent or guardian in accordance with the laws of the state. In the event that the parent or guardian is a suspect, appropriate legal guidance should be obtained immediately.

CASE 21–3

A 6-year-old female complaining of abdominal pain was brought into the ED by her mother. The girl had been at home under the care of a baby-sitter while the

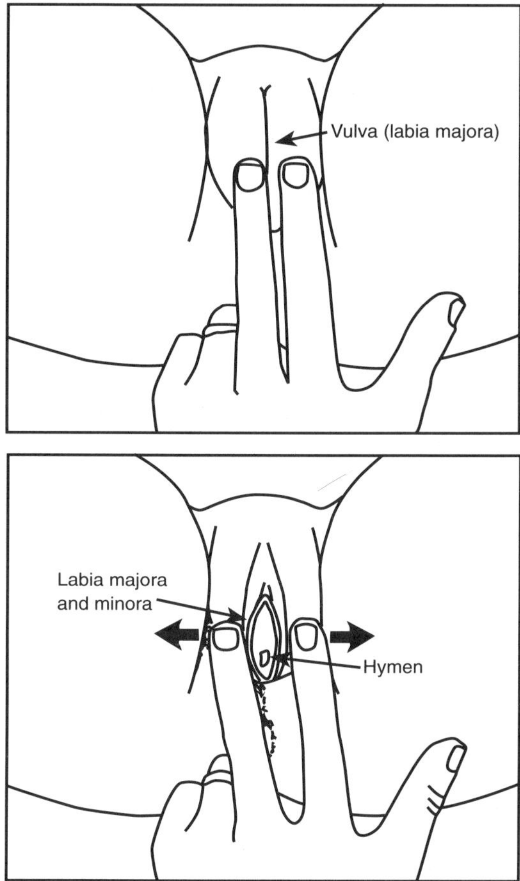

Fig. 21–4. Exposing the hymen in a young female child. (From Warner CG: *Rape and sexual assault: management & intervention,* Rockville, Md, 1980, Aspen Systems, p 79.)

mother was at work. The little girl mentions that the baby-sitter's boyfriend had been playing games with her and had asked her to take down her pants. Upon close examination, the physician finds a lower vaginal vault laceration with an extension of the laceration to the parametrium.

Comment.—To determine the full extent of injury, the emergency physician should request a gynecologic consultation. In addition to the vaginal examination, pelvic radiographs should be requested to determine whether any foreign objects are present.

THE SUSPECT

History and Physical Examination

The medical history obtained from the suspect should include the following information (see Appendix 21–2):

- Previous or current STD
- Whether the suspect is sterile
- Medications currently being taken
- Drug use history

Examining a Sexually Assaulted Child

I. History
   A. From the child alone, if possible
   B. From a parent or guardian (taking into consideration the possibility that child abuse may be involved)
   C. From A and B together
   D. Record direct quotes
   E. Include
      1. History of the event itself
      2. Psychosocial history (helps in establishing a baseline for child's psychological and social adjustment before the examination)
      3. History of other physical or sexual abuse in the family
      4. Immunization history (especially important if tetanus prophylaxis is necessary)
      5. History of medications (include antibiotics and use of alcohol and/or drugs if appropriate)

II. Physical examination
   A. General body survey for signs of violence
   B. Examination of external genitalia for signs of violence
   C. Vaginal examination (if B is positive or if there has been insertion of a foreign object into the vagina) to obtain the following
      1. Samples for motile and immotile sperm
      2. Samples for acid phosphatase
      3. Gonorrhea culture
      4. Samples for trichomonads (if indicated)

III. Laboratory examination
   A. By the physician
      1. Specimen for motile sperm
      2. Specimen for trichomonads
   B. By the forensic laboratory
      1. Sample for acid phosphatase
      2. Sample for sperm
      3. Optional
         a. Sample for seminal blood group antigens
         b. Blood (red top) for determining the patient's blood type
         c. Saliva from the patient to determine secretor status
         d. Fingernail scrapings for foreign material
         e. Samples of any foreign material from hair or body (foreign pubic hairs, etc.)
         f. Clothing samples (if indicated)
   C. By the hospital laboratory
      1. Gonorrhea cultures
      2. VDRL
      3. Pregnancy test (if indicated)
      4. Chlamydia
      5. HIV (with appropriately obtained consent)
      6. Hepatitis

Modified from Warner CG, editor *Assessment and management of adult victims in rape and sexual assault: management and intervention,* Rockville, Md, 1981, Aspen Systems, pp 80–81.

- Past or present allergies
- HIV and hepatitis status

Emergency physicians should refrain from questioning the suspect concerning the alleged attack. Questioning suspects is the responsibility of law enforcement personnel.

The physical examination of the suspect may contribute significantly to the case and should be as accurate as possible. The following items should be determined and recorded:

- The suspect's height and weight
- The suspect's physique and degree of sexual maturity
- The location and size of scratches, scars, tattoos, bites, bruises, and other injuries
- Indications of drug use—including alcohol
- Signs of trauma, venereal disease, or lubrication on the genitals

Diagnostic Tests

Medical

It is crucial for medical and legal purposes that the suspect be examined for venereal disease. A suspect who has chlamydia or syphilis at the time of the examination may have transferred the disease to the victim. Serologic testing for syphilis and appropriate cultures and tests for other STDs must be obtained as a part of the medical diagnostic procedure. Similarly, if the victim has evidence of an STD, the suspect should be examined for it and treated appropriately.

To examine for *Trichomonas,* collect the sample by passing a metal cotton-tipped swab into the urethra (Fig. 21–5). Introduce the swab 2 to 3 cm into the urethra; then mix the sample with a drop of saline, and examine the slide under a microscope.

Physiologic

The tests that should be obtained during the examination of the suspect require the collection of physiologic samples. A urine sample should be collected for urinalysis, culture, and drug screening. Blood samples are collected in four separate color-coded tubes. These specimens are used for the following tests:

- Purple (lavender) top—specimen used for blood grouping tests (grouping compared with seminal stains) and DNA testing

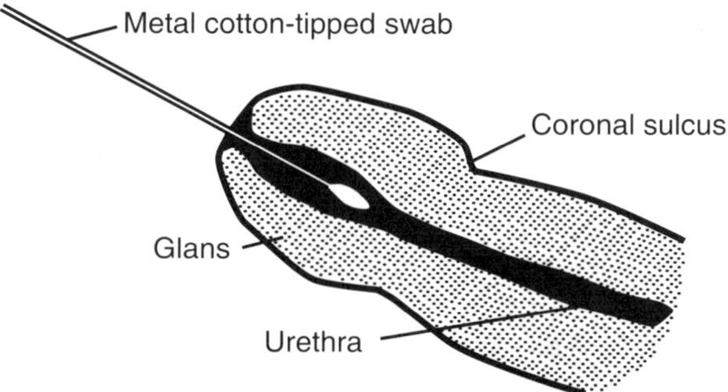

Fig. 21–5. Obtaining a sample from the urethra. (From Warner CG: *Rape and sexual assault: management & intervention,* Rockville, Md, 1980, Aspen Systems, p 89.)

Table 21–4. Suspect Evidence Collection Kit

Procedure	Equipment
Hair combings, body hair, head hair, and pubic hair collection and identification	Comb
	Envelopes (7)
	Labels (7)
	Tweezers
	Scissors
	Paper towels to be placed under the suspect during the clipping, plucking, and combing procedure; submit the towel also to crime laboratory
Saliva sample	Paper disk
	Envelope
	Labels
Penile swabs	Normal saline (50 mL)
	Cotton-tipped swabs (10)
	Containers (2)
	Labels
	Cotton-tipped wire swabs (2)
	Gonorrhea culture media (3)
Blood samples	Tourniquet
	Blood tubes (gray, red, and purple)
	Syringe (20 mL)
	Needle (21 gauge)
	Labels
Chain of evidence, history, physical examination, and consent	Forms
Collection of clothing	Paper bag
Nail scraping	Fingernail file

- Gray top—specimen used for blood alcohol and drug assays
- Yellow top—see the section on physiologic diagnostic tests for adult female victims in this chapter for a description
- Red top—miscellaneous testing

Do not use alcohol swabs in preparing the skin.

Legal

Collecting evidence from a suspect may be difficult even if the person is cooperative. Nevertheless, the evidence is critical for a complete evaluation of the attack and may in fact help exonerate someone who is innocent. The task can be facilitated by use of a kit prepared for collecting the evidence from the suspect. The materials included in most kits are noted in Table 21–4.

Collection Process

Emergency physicians must remember that if the attack occurs within 24 to 36 hours of the ED examination, all specimens listed in Table 21-5 should be collected. If there is a delay of over 36 hours, however, only the items marked with an asterisk should be obtained. Table 21–5 is a complete listing of specimens to be obtained.

Pubic hair may contain other foreign material to be used as evidence in the case. In some cases, vaginal epithelium may adhere to the penis. This should be collected by using a moist cotton swab. The swab should be air-dried and submitted to the police or forensic laboratory as evidence.

The diagnostic procedures required of the emergency physician may not be a pleasant experience for the clinician or the victim. Nevertheless, legally, medically, and psychologically, the procedures must be conducted as carefully, thoroughly, and expeditiously as possible.

Table 21–5. Specimens to be Collected from the Suspect

Specimen	Process
Body hair	
Head*	Obtain at least 25 hairs from different areas of the head
Beard or mustache	Obtain 15 hairs from this area when deemed necessary (optional)
Chest	Obtain 15 hairs
Arm	Obtain 15 hairs when necessary (optional)
Pubic area*	Obtain 15 hairs
Hair combings	Comb loose hairs from the pubic area only (place the suspect on a towel during this procedure and submit the towel along with the combings)
Penile swabs	Using swabs (plain and cotton-tipped metal), collect evidence from the urethra and over the shaft in the glans area
Hair mattings	Any stains or mattings of pubic or other body hairs should be cut off and placed in an extra envelope with correct labeling
Foreign materials	Vegetable matter or stains must be placed in an extra envelope and labeled
Fingernail scrapings*	Collect foreign substances, place in an envelope, and label correctly
Saliva*	Check for secretor status
Clothing*	Collect and preserve clothing in the proper bag after it has dried at room temperature
Blood typing*	Perform the procedure as noted in the physiologic sample section
VDRL or RPR*†	Take a blood serum sample for syphilis

*If there is a delay of over 36 hours between the attack and the emergency department examination, collect only appropriate specimens.
†*VDRL*, Venereal Disease Research Laboratory; *RPR*, rapid plasmin reagin.

REFERENCES

1. Kravis TC, Warner GC, editors: *Rape and sexual assault in emergency medicine: a comprehensive review*, New York, 1993, Raven Press.
2. Warner CG, editor: *Assessment and management of adult victims in rape and sexual assault: management and intervention*, Rockville, Md, 1981. Aspen Systems.
3. Sazena BB: Radio-receptor assay of human gonadotropin: detection of early pregnancy, *Science* 184:793–795, 1974.
4. Warner CG, Koeper JM, et al: *San Diego County protocol for the treatment of rape and sexual assault victims*, San Diego, Calif, 1978.
5. Giertsen JC: Faecal matter in stains: their identification, *J Forensic Med* 8:99–110, 1961.

Appendix 21–1. Examining a Sexual Assault Victim

This following is a condensed version of the procedure for examining sexual assault victims.

A. Label all materials with patient identification. Complete all labels, the examination report, evidence envelope labels, and manila envelopes with patient information in the manner used by the hospital (e.g., addressograph plate). The date, time, and initials of the person collecting the specimens should be included
B. Obtain and record an oral history of the assault, including the following:
   1. The date and time of the assault
   2. The place of the assault, including the address and the physical surroundings
   3. The manner of assault, including the number of assailants, use of weapons and restraints, types of nonconsensual contact, where it occurred, and whether the assailant used a condom or lubricant or stated that he was sterile
   4. The actions subsequent to the assault (change of clothing, douching, toothbrushing, defecating, or vomiting)
C. Obtain a general medical history
D. Obtain the following items:

1. The victim's clothing, placed in separate individual paper bags, sealed with an evidence seal, and marked with the date and the nurse's and the physician's initials
2. The victim's tampon or sanitary napkin if she is menstruating
3. A urine sample to be used for possible drug analysis

E. Perform a physical examination (explain the procedures step-by-step to the victim)
   1. Note the vital signs
   2. Observe and record the victim's general demeanor and emotional state
   3. Observe the victim's physical appearance
   4. Examine the entire body for signs of injury:
      a. Bruises, fractures, sprains
      b. Contusions
      c. Scratches
      d. Blood on clothing or hair
   5. Note sexual maturity—breasts, pubic hair, genitalia
   6. If any foreign material is found on the victim, collect the material in a separate container, label correctly, and note from where the sample was collected

F. Perform a pelvic examination. Do not place the victim in stirrups until the examination is ready to begin; place padding over the metal
   1. Speculum—moisten with only warm water or saline
   2. Mons veneris—examine for tenderness, contusions; note pubic hair distribution
   3. Labia majora—examine for tenderness, contusions, lacerations
   4. Perineum—examine for tenderness, contusions, lacerations
   5. Introitus—examine for abrasions, lacerations, erythema, hymenal morphology
   6. Vaginal vault—examine for the presence or absence of injury, secretion, cervical position
   7. Cervix—examine for morphology injury, color, bleeding
   8. Uterine position and size—observe
   9. Tubes and ovaries—examine

G. Perform a rectal examination. Frequently women are reluctant to state that anal intercourse took place; inquire in *all* cases as to the possibility of rectal penetration
   1. Note any physical trauma
   2. Take anal swabs
   3. Perform rectal examination when indicated

H. Obtain the following specimens and tests from all sexual assault victims:
   1. Comb the pubic area to collect any loose hairs from the suspect
   2. Take vaginal swabs—four deep and two shallow
   3. Take a vaginal aspirate. Make two smears from the swabs taken from the vaginal area. Add saline to the smears to prevent drying out before examining the slides for spermatozoa motility
   4. Obtain saliva swabs on paper disks
   5. Take anal swabs
   6. Take blood samples as follows:
      a. Purple (lavender) top tube (ethylenediaminetetraacetic acid [EDTA]) for forensic laboratory serology blood grouping and DNA testing
      b. Gray top tube (oxalate and fluoride) for alcohol
      c. Yellow top tube (see the section on physiologic diagnostic tests for adult female victims in this chapter)

From Warner CG et al: *San Diego County protocol for the treatment of rape and sexual assault victims,* San Diego, Calif, 1978.

d. Red top tube (no preservative) for (hospital) syphilis serology (VDRL)

7. Examine the slides made of the vaginal swabs to determine whether spermatozoa are detectable and whether they are motile
8. Formulate a diagnostic impression from the history, physical, and laboratory examination
9. Indicate which samples were collected from the victim on the examination report and on the evidence envelopes. Sign the examination report

SPECIAL NOTE: Because the medical chart may become legal evidence, care must be taken to ensure that all statements are objective, accurate, and *legible*. Emphasis on legibility may sound insulting, but a clear report can often save a trip to court. If all persons involved can easily read the report, the court will frequently accept the medical report in lieu of verbal testimony.

Appendix 21–2. Examining a Sexual Assault Suspect

Law enforcement personnel may bring an apprehended rape or sexual assault suspect to the ED for examination. The following procedure should be followed to gather the necessary comparative evidentiary samples.

A. Label all materials with patient (suspect) identification. Complete all labels, the examination report, evidence envelope labels, and manila envelopes with patient (suspect) information in the manner used by the hospital (e.g., addressograph plate)

B. Obtain and record a history, including:
   1. The reason for the examination
   2. The suspect's statement
   3. Previous or current STDs or sterilization
   4. Drugs and medications, including over-the-counter medications currently being taken
   5. Documentation of the time, date, and content of the interview

C. Perform a physical examination
   1. Note the suspect's height and weight
   2. Note vital signs
   3. Examine the suspect for:
      a. Scars
      b. Identifying marks
      c. Tattoos
      d. Injuries
   4. When injuries are observed:
      a. Determine the size and age of any contusions, lacerations, or needle punctures
      b. Determine, if possible, whether the lacerations could have been self-inflicted or are defensive wounds
   5. Note any indications of the use of drugs—the odor of alcohol, needle puncture marks, or physical symptoms (i.e., pupillary size and reactivity)
   6. Check the genitals for trauma, signs of lubrication, and STDs
   7. If any foreign material is found on the suspect, collect the material in a separate container and label it in the same manner as other specimens gathered; note the location from which the sample was collected. Foreign materials may include botanical material, glass, plastic, paper, or blood found in the hair or elsewhere
   8. Comb the pubic area to collect any loose hairs
   9. Take saliva samples, place a paper disk in the suspect's mouth until the disk is saturated with saliva, and then place the disk in the appropriate envelope

10. Take two genital swabs. Moisten both swabs with distilled water
    a. With one swab, swab the urethra
    b. With the other swab, swab the glans and shaft
11. Take the following blood samples after swabbing the arm with a nonalcoholic solution:
    a. Gray top tube (oxalate and fluoride) for alcohol
    b. Red top tube (no preservative) for hospital syphilis serology
    c. Purple (lavender) top tube (EDTA) for forensic laboratory serology
    d. Yellow top (see the section on physiologic diagnostic tests for adult female victims in this chapter)
12. Obtain one urine specimen
13. Obtain hair samples as follows:
    a. Head hairs—obtain at least 25 hairs from different areas of the head
    b. Pubic hairs—obtain at least 15 hairs from the pubic area
    c. Body hairs—obtain at least 15 hairs from the body
    d. Facial hairs—obtain 10 to 15, if possible
14. Determine whether the suspect has any surgical scars or evidence of a vasectomy

D. Indicate which samples were collected from the suspect on the examination report and on the evidence envelopes
E. Collect all clothing in separate individual paper bags, seal with an evidence seal, and mark with the physician's initials and date
F. Sign the examination report

From Warner GC et al: *San Diego County protocol for the treatment of rape and sexual assault victims,* San Diego, Calif, 1978.

Chapter 22

Medicolegal Considerations

Kevin D. Porter J.D.
Michelle A. Merchant J.D.
Mark C. Henry, M.D.

The evaluation and treatment provided in the emergency department (ED) often determine whether an individual will live or die. The appropriate use (and recording) of diagnostic tests in the ED has a similar impact on the ultimate decisions in legal and regulatory cases.

This chapter will examine the significant medicolegal implications of common ED diagnostic tests for clinicians. During the past decade concerns regarding the acquired immunodeficiency syndrome (AIDS) and human immunodeficiency virus (HIV) led to legal activity and state regulation frequently involving the emergency physician and ED. Also during this decade, the federal government has enacted laws and regulations that have led to an examination of the standard of care in ED diagnostic testing. Under the Emergency Medical Treatment and Active Labor Act of 1985, known as the "Federal Anti-Dumping Act," every individual who comes to a hospital's ED for examination or treatment must be provided with "an appropriate medical screening examination within the capability of the hospital's emergency department" to determine whether "an emergency condition" exists.[1] Such a screening exam may include appropriate diagnostic tests as well as a history and physical exam.

Although variations exist among local and state laws and health regulations, guidelines must nevertheless be established for the clinical staff that address the primary legal and regulatory concerns regarding ED diagnostic testing. Indeed, to receive accreditation from the Joint Commission on the Accreditation of Health Care Organizations (JCAHO), EDs *must* have written guidelines on the following topics:

- Informed consent for treatment
- Confidentiality of patient information
- Release of information and materials to police or health authorities
- Handling of alleged or suspected sexual assault and child abuse cases
- Management of irrational and intoxicated patients
- Handling of persons dead on arrival, i.e., performing the legally required collection and preservation of evidence and reporting to proper authorities

All of these topics potentially involve the performance and results of diagnostic testing.

COMMON DIAGNOSTIC TESTS WITH MEDICOLEGAL IMPLICATIONS

Most, if not all, diagnostic tests in the ED are performed to aid the clinician in providing appropriate treatment to the patient. Nonetheless, these same tests are used and relied upon by law enforcement officials, health department inspectors, medical examiners, and other officials with legal and regulatory oversight. Thus, ED diagnostic tests have significant implications beyond the physical confines of the ED or hospital and involve unique legal considerations and concerns for the clinician. The physician should bear in mind the multiple purposes for which ED tests are used and the important and difficult issues that these uses may create.

BLOOD ALCOHOL TESTING

Often, blood tests for alcohol (ethanol) levels are obtained on injured patients because the clinical assessment requires toxicologic testing as part of the medical evaluation. This practice is, however, considerably more complex in terms of legal analysis when the police request a specimen from an automobile driver, for example, for blood-alcohol testing. In some jurisdictions, including New York, there is an implied consent to chemical testing of the blood for the presence of alcohol unless the driver suspected of drunk driving expressly refuses the test.[2] Such a refusal to submit to a blood alcohol test upon the request of the police or other appropriate law enforcement authorities, under New York law, will result in automatic suspension of the driver's license.[3]

The New York law mandates that a chemical test should *not* be performed on an individual under arrest or having a positive breath test who refuses to submit to the requested testing unless a court order has been granted to perform the test.[3] Such a refusal to consent to blood alcohol testing should be clearly documented in the medical record. A patient's willingness or refusal to consent may not always be easy to determine. A review of leading New York case law indicates that if the patient vacillates in the decision to consent by first consenting, then refusing, and eventually consenting, the test should not be performed.[4] The subsequent recantation of the refusal is not valid, and this is an evidentiary rule used to exclude the results of the test from admission into evidence at trial.[5]

Unconscious patients who are unable to give consent may be tested while under arrest.[6] However, chemical testing should never interfere with or supersede provision of necessary immediate medical treatment. Thus, if a police officer attempts to persuade an emergency physician to administer a blood test or provide a blood sample quickly, the clinician may refuse if, in his or her best judgment, necessary medical treatment must first be provided. Having said this, it is important for the physician to understand *why* pressure may be applied to provide a sample early.

Under New York law, in order for the results to be admitted into evidence at the time of trial or court hearing, there is a statutory 2-hour time limit for obtaining a blood sample for alcohol testing that begins from the time of the arrest and/or breath test. Because time is of such great importance to this evidentiary gathering process, an ED protocol should be established that is consistent with local laws and regulations. The development of routine protocols and procedures helps to clarify the relationship between the police and the suspect, the clinician and the patient, and the police and the hospital. Such a procedure may also serve as a defense to a later claim that either the clinician acted against the express refusal of the patient or, conversely, was uncooperative with law enforcement officials. Usually a clinician who obtains a blood sample at the request of the police under these circumstances is granted immunity from liability.[7] As always, all ED protocols and procedures should be a part of the ED policy and procedure manual and periodically updated.

Another key consideration in blood alcohol (ethanol) testing is skin preparation. Ideally a nonalcoholic skin preparation should be used before drawing blood for ethanol levels: if gas chromatography is the method used for analyzing the blood, the separation of ethanol is distinct from isopropanol, but if enzymatic determinations are employed, the use of isopropanol skin swabs may theoretically affect the analysis. In one study, the effect of using alcohol (isopropanol) skin antiseptics on tests for ethanol levels was not found to be statistically significant regardless of the methodology.[8] In any event, whether a determination of ethanol levels is desired for medical evaluation or for law enforcement purposes, skin preparation before venipuncture should reflect awareness of local laboratory procedure.

SEXUAL OFFENSE EVIDENCE

Commonly, the ED treats victims of various sexual offenses such as sexual misconduct, rape, sodomy, sexual abuse, and aggravated sexual abuse. In rendering treatment to patients who have been victims of sexual offenses, various items of evidence are collected and become essential in a subsequent criminal and/or civil trial. Evidence appropriate to injuries includes slides, cotton swabs, clothing, hair combings, fingernail scrapings, photographs, and vaginal washings, etc.

It is imperative that the emergency physician know the current hospital policies and procedures concerning the procurement and maintenance of sexual offense evidence. Similarly, it is necessary for the physician to be aware of relevant local health department regulations that provide specific guidelines for the handling of sexual offense evidence. For example, to establish uniformity in the maintenance and storage of evidence of sexual offenses, the New York State Department of Health has recently promulgated new regulations for hospitals collecting such evidence. Specifically, the regulation requires the following[9]:

> The hospital shall refrigerate items of sexual offense evidence where necessary for preservation and ensure that clothes and swabs are dried, stored in paper bags and labeled, and shall mark and log each item of evidence with a code number corresponding to the patient's medical record.

Furthermore,

> The hospital shall store the sexual offense evidence in a locked, separate and secure area for not less than thirty days unless:
>
> (i) the patient signs a statement directing the hospital not to collect and keep privileged evidence;
>
> (ii) such evidence is privileged and the patient signs a statement directing the hospital to surrender the evidence to the police before thirty days has expired;
>
> (iii) the evidence is not privileged and the police request its surrender before thirty days has expired;
>
> After thirty days from commencement of treatment, the refrigerated evidence shall be discarded and the clothes shall be returned upon the patient's request.
>
> The hospital shall designate a staff member to coordinate the required actions and to contact the local police agency and forensic laboratory to determine their specific needs and requirements for the maintenance of sexual offense evidence.

The primary legal considerations involving sexual offense evidence in the ED are collection technique, storage environment, time of collection, skin or site preparation, and release of the evidence to the local police agency or forensic laboratory (see Chapters 21 and 23).

Proper collection technique is a key concern and may influence a test result.

Site preparation is closely related to collection technique in sexual offense cases. The clinician should be mindful that cleansing of the patient may result in the loss of pertinent evidence. If a patient reports having taken a bath before coming to the emergency department, this information should be documented in the medical record.

When specific handling considerations are required, the technique employed should be carefully documented by the clinician.

The storage of evidence may determine its reliability and usefulness. For example, semen stains on clothing may decompose if stored in plastic bags because moisture accelerates molding. Paper bags should be used to store clothing that is retained as sexual offense evidence. Similarly, acid phosphatase activity deteriorates more rapidly when specimens are not frozen or refrigerated.[10, 11]

Because elapsed time from sampling to testing may modify a test result significantly, the time of collection is especially important when quantitative values are sought and should be routinely documented on labeling slips. In sexual offense cases, testing for the presence of semen is always required. Because spermatozoa do not remain motile for long periods of time outside the body cavity, examination for sperm motility is best done as soon as practicable after specimen collection.

The site from which the specimen is obtained is also an important consideration. In sexual offense cases, the site of sampling is very important and should be clearly recorded on the labels. If the site is not properly noted, this issue will become the subject of considerable controversy in a contested civil or criminal law proceeding. When a sample obtained from the vaginal vault is compared with one from the more favorable environment of the cervix, sperm motility and survival are significantly diminished.[12]

CHAIN OF EVIDENCE

Any material gathered for use as potential evidence must be accounted for from the time of sampling until its introduction in court. For the evidence to be admissible in court, an account must be made of the location and the accessibility of this material until it is turned over to authorities. Documentation of this process is essential. Specimens that need to be refrigerated or held for a time should be kept in a locked area with limited access. Every person who has the sample in his or her possession for any length of time must sign for the acceptance and release of this material until it is formally collected and signed for by the proper authorities. The fewer persons involved, the more likely it is that the material will be acceptable as evidence at the time of a trial.

During trial, allegations are frequently made that the laboratory slide or other test sample produced at trial is not the one originally taken at the time of the ED treatment and that the testimony from the ED or laboratory personnel on the authenticity or validity of the test results should therefore be inadmissable.

A good example of how properly maintaining the chain of evidence may play a critical role in a case is demonstrated by *Missouri v Foster*. This case involved a 17-year-old victim of sexual assault evaluated in an ED. During the medical evaluation a rectal examination was performed and specimens collected for semen analysis. The specimens were placed on slides and in a saline solution by the physician who then requested that the specimens be tested for the presence of sperm. The physician's signature along with the patient's name and date were recorded on the laboratory slips. All of these materials were then given to an ED employee to take to the hospital laboratory for examination. At trial, the defense tried to exclude the evidence. However, the laboratory technician testified that she removed the three slides and saline solution from the laboratory refrigerator, that the slides were labelled with the patient's identification, and that it was these specimens that she tested.[13]

The Missouri court ruled in this case that the chain of evidence rule was amply satisfied and the evidence indicated that proper safeguards were taken to ensure that the specimens examined were the ones taken from the 17-year-old patient by the physician in the ED.[14] The court would be unlikely to have reached the same conclusion if there had been glaring identification discrepancies in specimen samples.[15]

HUMAN IMMUNODEFICIENCY VIRUS TESTING

The HIV status of patients coming to the ED is undoubtedly an important factor both in treatment decisions and with respect to precautions taken by the staff. Universal precautions in hospitals throughout the country are now recommended by the Centers for Disease Control,[16] and New York State[17] mandates their use by all physicians practicing in that state, even those in private practice. In addition to minimizing the risk of transmission of infectious diseases, New York State's requirement creates a standard by which health professionals in that state who fail to follow universal precautions can be deemed guilty of professional misconduct.[17] Despite all of these regulatory requirements, needlesticks and other workplace exposures to patients' blood and body fluids remain a real or potential source of transmission of the AIDS virus to the health care worker.[18] One of the earliest reported cases of HIV transmission to a health care worker in the ED involved a needlestick[18] (see Chapter 17).

Although any ED staff member who sustains a needlestick will understandably become quite concerned and may want to know the HIV status of the patient in whom the needle had been used, in most cases an HIV test may not be performed without the consent of the patient.[19] Under New York law, before an HIV test may be performed, the patient must provide written informed consent and must be counseled about the nature and meaning of AIDS, HIV infection, and discrimination problems that might arise from disclosure of the tests results.[20]

In addition, all HIV-related information must be kept confidential and can be released only under limited circumstances.[21] The only exception to the rule requiring a patient's consent to HIV testing is for blood, tissue, or organ donation.

Whether the HIV status is necessary for diagnosis and treatment or to provide peace of mind to a health care worker, HIV testing may not be performed without the individual's consent. Failure to follow the regulations and laws of any jurisdiction may result in civil or criminal liability.

FEDERAL LAW AND EMERGENCY DEPARTMENT TESTING

Under the federal Emergency Medical Treatment and Active Labor Act (EMTALA) of 1985, commonly referred to as the "Federal Anti-Dumping Act," anyone who comes to an ED for examination or treatment for a medical condition must be provided with an appropriate medical screening examination.[22] The law is violated by any physician who fails to detect an emergency condition because of inadequate screening procedures as defined by the statute.[22]

The challenge for the clinician is to determine which tests and procedures are necessary to provide adequate screening. The increasing statutory scrutiny that patient "screening" is receiving in the ED as a consequence of EMTALA has led to an increasing number of lawsuits. It is therefore even more important for each and every emergency physician to conform to the standard of care at the time that the patient is being screened and treated.[23] In the leading case of *Cleland v Bronson Health Care Group, Inc.,* the court interpreted the terms "appropriate" and "stabilized," as used in the statute, to refer to the motives with which the hospital acts.[24] Thus, the court dismissed the plaintiff's complaint alleging violation of the federal law and ruled that where a hospital acts to screen appropriately and stabilize nonpaying patients with the same efforts and procedures used on paying patients, then there is compliance with the Act.[25]

Other courts, although not all, have followed the *Cleland* decision. In one case the D.C. Circuit Court ruled that "what constitutes an appropriate screening is properly determined not by reference to particular outcomes, but instead by reference to a hospital's standard screening procedures."[26] The important lesson from these cases is that a failure to follow the routine standard of care in ED diagnostic testing could lead to a violation of EMTALA and that it is important for the clinician to ensure that all patients receive the same level of care, based on medical indications and clinical status.

UNPLANNED DISCHARGES AND FOLLOW-UP

An unplanned discharge from an ED against medical advice ("AMA") is a relatively common occurrence. Subsequent attempts to provide follow-up care can be difficult and incomplete if certain basic risk management steps are not taken at the time of such an occurrence.[27] When not managed properly, there is potential liability to the emergency physician. Both Emergency Medicine literature and medical malpractice case law are replete with examples of the problems that confront the physician in the area of unplanned discharges.

A febrile infant who is at risk for bacteremia will probably have a CBC and blood cultures drawn in the course of the clinical assessment in the ED. If the parent insists on taking the child out of the ED before the results of the CBC and blood cultures are available, and the blood cultures are later reported to be positive, aggressive follow-up efforts by the emergency physician are mandated. To ensure maximum protection from medical malpractice liability, the emergency physician must document on the medical record each and every effort made to contact the family, and the follow-up efforts should be charted meticulously. For example, in the hypothetical case above, the telephone number that is used in attempting to reach the family should be charted on the medical record, and if a telegram is sent, a copy of the telegram should be permanently affixed to the ED record. Such specific documentation will enable the physician to later argue effectively in any medical malpractice action that all reasonable efforts were made to call the child back for necessary care in a timely fashion.

Furthermore, if the emergency physician deems the clinical testing information to require immediate patient intervention, the physician should call for police assistance to expedite the patient's return to the ED. The documentation requirement for this latter contingency is equally specific. In such instances, the physician must document which precinct or police station was called, citing the telephone number dialed, as well as the name of the police officer who received the request for assistance. A failure to include such specific information will significantly weaken the physician's position in a court of law if the plaintiff's attorney seeks to prove that both the physician and the ED did not meet an acceptable standard of care with respect to callback requirements.

If a pap smear is performed as part of a pelvic examination in the ED and subsequently reported to be abnormal, attempts to contact the patient *must* be made.[28] Again, the efforts must be documented carefully and performed consistently with the guidelines previously discussed. Appropriate follow-up of pap smears performed in the ED is important not only for medicolegal reasons, but also because there is a high prevalence of cervical dysplasia among women treated in urban EDs. A routine pap smear in conjunction with aggressive, documented follow-up efforts for all abnormal results can be an important component of cervical cancer control programs for women at high risk.

The importance of adequate documentation of "AMA" departures from the ED should be obvious. If the emergency physician has the opportunity to speak to a patient before a medically contraindicated discharge, and the patient has a test result indicating a significantly health-threatening or life-threatening clinical condition, then it is imperative that a note be entered in the record reflecting the discussion with the patient of why the patient should not leave the ED. Furthermore, the time and place of this discussion should be specifically noted. A witness should listen to the conversation and add his or her signature to the medical record. By taking these steps, the emergency physician may preclude any meaningful lawsuit arising out of the patient's visit from being filed. If the patient is clearly able to make a decision, the law permits the patient to decide whether or not to accept medical intervention, even though the underlying medical judgment of the patient may be flawed. However, if the patient is impaired because of mental instability or an alcohol or drug-related problem, the law allows for such a patient with a life-threatening condition to be restrained against his or her will. In such a case, it is imperative that the emergency physician document, with specific references, the actions or statements of the patient that support the diagnosis of impairment.

FAILURE TO OBTAIN INDICATED DIAGNOSTIC TESTS AND RISK MANAGEMENT

Medical malpractice case law demonstrates that nonemergency physicians do not always appreciate the significance of ordering clinical tests before discharging the patient.

In the case of *Atkins v Straghorn*, a California court was confronted with a situation in which an elderly patient appeared at an ED with a history of diabetes; also at that time the toes on his left foot were observed to be purplish in color.[29] A blood test revealed an elevated WBC, with a shift to the left. A staff physician on call responded to the ED and diagnosed a viral infection without noting the foot condition. The staff physician then discharged the patient, and instructed both the patient and his wife to see him on the following day in his private office. However, the unappreciated condition in the left foot worsened, and on the patient's return to the ED the next day, a radiograph demonstrated a piece of glass embedded in his left foot. Blood cultures taken were positive for a streptococcal infection. The patient was then admitted to the hospital but subsequently required an amputation of the leg below the knee. The jury returned an award of $242,000 in favor of the patient; more importantly, the case demonstrates the need to respond to a significant clinical finding in the ED with the appropriate diagnostic test(s) and the need to correlate the results of these tests with observed clinical findings. A hospital policy that mandates responsibility for such patients to the emergency physician, even when a private practitioner is involved, might prevent such an adverse medical and legal outcome.

Failure to perform an indicated diagnostic test is a common, serious problem in the ED and is exemplified by the case of *Brown v North Broward Hospital District, et al.*[30] In this case, a 5-year-old boy who was skateboarding down a street in a prone position slid under a slow-moving vehicle and was pinned by an exhaust pipe for several minutes. The driver of the vehicle jacked up the car, and the boy was removed from under the vehicle by his stepfather. The child was then transferred to a nearby ED and evaluated for a suspected intraabdominal injury. Approximately 2 hours after evaluation in the first ED, the child was transferred to a second ED where he was observed for approximately 5½ hours and then discharged. No spine radiographs were taken at either facility. When the boy awoke the next morning, he was unable to get out of bed and could not move his legs. The failure to perform indicated radiologic testing contributed to a jury finding of $1,100,000 against the hospital defendant.[30]

LEGAL ISSUES

Consent

A basic principle of law holds that every competent adult has the right to make decisions about his or her own medical care. The earliest case on informed consent to treatment was reported in 1914.[31] In *Schloendorff v Society of New York Hospital,* the court stated the following[32]:

> Every human being of adult years and sound mind has a right to determine what shall be done with his own body and the surgeon who performs an operation without his patient's consent commits an assault, for which he is liable in damages, except in cases of emergency where the patient is unconscious and where it is necessary to operate before consent can be obtained.

Thus, before any invasive procedure or care beyond routine medical evaluation and treatment is performed, the informed consent of the patient must be obtained.

As previously noted, documented informed consent is required for HIV testing and blood alcohol testing. In addition, the patient's consent is required to release the results of certain ED diagnostic testing. For example, sexual offense evidence from a competent adult may not be released to the police without the authorization of the patient. In fact, the patient's failure to give consent for the release of such evidence can preclude law enforcement authorities from persuing what might otherwise be a successful prosecution. However, the release of evidence in cases of suspected child abuse does not require parental authorization.[33]

Likewise, the release of evidence such as a recovered bullet from a crime victim usually does not require special authorization from the patient. In such a case, local police and regulatory guidelines set forth the steps necessary to release such evidence. In general, most jurisdictions mandate that gunshot wounds be reported to the local police without regard to the patient's willingness to consent to the release of such information (see Chapter 23).

Reportable Events

To protect public health and safety and to ensure the protection of minors, situations arise that must be brought to the attention of the proper authorities.

Reportable situations encompass some infectious diseases and all poisonings, penetrating wounds caused by violent acts, life-threatening injuries (second-degree assault), child abuse, sexual assaults of a minor or of a mentally incompetent adult, and suspicious or unexpected deaths. While recognizing the confidentiality of the clinical encounter, the statutes nevertheless require that health professionals report these diagnoses and other conditions.

One of the earliest functions of local health departments, for example, was the control of communicable diseases. Early reporting was the first step in controlling the spread of such infections. Poisonings are of similar concern and require notification of authorities.

SUMMARY

Policies and procedures dealing with all aspects of the medical-legal considerations that arise from emergency care should be established in order to provide uniform and consistent service. These policies can serve as a reference source to help the staff adhere to both hospital and community standards. Above all, the protocols must be practical and deal with the common questions that are sure to arise.

Local statutes must be consulted and should be made available for reference. Because emergency physicians must interact with local health departments, medical examiners, and law enforcement personnel, it may be desirable for hospital representatives to meet with members of interfacing agencies. Besides encouraging cooperation among the involved parties, such meetings can serve as forums to discuss practical concerns and problem cases.

Laboratories must also be contacted regularly to elucidate test availability and the methodology used for different determinations. The desired method for collecting and handling evidence and the temperature requirements for specific biological specimens can be delineated. Storage requirements may be a major consideration when the laboratory is not available on a 24-hour basis. The phone numbers of key laboratory contacts and the procedure for specimen delivery to laboratories that are not hospital based should be readily available 24-hours a day.

Hospital representatives may wish to establish consent forms that separate the various levels of interaction. Circumstances requiring the use of specific consents should be clear to the clinical staff. If applicable, the local requirements for consent in the case of controversial tests such as blood alcohol levels should be explored with legal and law enforcement officials so that a consistent procedure can be followed by everyone.

In addition, the ED itself may wish to develop a uniform approach in its policy and procedure manual for reportable situations and medical-legal events. If a stan-

Table 22–1. Medicolegal Considerations for Conditions Treated in the ED

		Consent Required for				
Patient's Condition	Reportable Condition	Medical Treatment	Procurement of Evidentiary Specimen/ Photograph	Release of Information to Authorities	Technical Considerations	Documentation of Chain of Evidence
Tuberculosis	X	X			Isolation	
Food poisoning	X	X				
Poisonings	X	X				
Sexual assault						
Adult victim mentally competent		X	X	X	As per protocol	X
Child victim or person mentally incompetent	X	X			As per protocol	X
Blood alcohol						
Police request		X	X	X	As per protocol	X

dard format is used, answers to frequently asked questions can be quickly ascertained by the staff when the need arises (see Table 22–1). The following questions might be addressed:

- Is consent necessary?
- What type of consent must be obtained?
- What is the time requirement for reporting and which phone numbers can be used 24 hours a day?
- Which laboratory will do the testing and when is it available?
- Are there significant technical considerations for procurement, handling, and storage of a specimen?
- Is a chain-of-evidence form required?

Once these policies and procedures are developed, staff education and continuing medical education conferences can be scheduled to promote consistency and uniformity.

Informed clinicians strive to achieve a balance between the demands of direct patient care and the duty to protect public health and safety. Again, however, the clinician's first and foremost obligation is to the patient.

REFERENCES

1. 42 U.S.C. §1395dd.
2. N.Y. Veh. & Traf. Law §1194 (1) (McKinney's 1986).
3. N.Y. Veh. & Traf. Law §1194 (2).
4. *Nicol v Grant,* 117 A.D.2d 940, 499 N.Y.S.2d 247 (3d Dept. 1986).
5. *Matter of Viger v Passidomo,* 65 N.Y.2d 705, 481 N.E.2d 542, 492 N.Y.S.2d (1985); *Matter of White v Fisher,* 49 A.D.2d 450, 375 N.Y.S.2d 663 (3d Dept. 1975).
6. *People v Dixon,* 149 A.D.2d 75, 543 N.Y.S.2d 993 (2d Dept. 1989).
7. N.Y. Veh. & Traf. Law *Supra* note 2.
8. Goldfinger TM, Schaber DL: A comparison of blood alcohol concentration using non-alcohol and alcohol containing skin antiseptics, *Am Emerg Med* 11:665–667, 1982.
9. 14 N.Y.S. Reg. 27 (1992) (to be codified at 10 N.Y.C.R.R. 405.9, proposed Dec 2, 1992).
10. Findley TP: Quantitation of vaginal acid phosphatase and its relationship to time of coitus, *Am J Clin Pathol* 68:238–242, 1977.
11. Masgood A, Bernhardt HE, Sager N: Quantitative determination of endogenous acid phosphatase activity in vaginal washings, *Obstet Gynecol* 51:33–35, 1978.
12. Gomez RR et al: Quantitative and qualitative determinations of acid phosphatase activity in vaginal washings, *Am J Clin Pathol* 64:423–432, 1975.
13. *Missouri v Foster,* 490 S.W.2d 659 (MO. 1973).
14. *Missouri v Foster,* 490 S.W.2d 660 (MO. 1973).
15. *People v Maurice,* 31 Ill.2d 456, 202 N.E.2d 480, (1964); *People v Resketo,* 3 Ill. App.3d 633, 279 N.E.2d 432, (1972).
16. Centers for Disease Control: Recommendations for prevention of HIV transmission in health-care settings, *MMWR* 36(suppl 2), 1987.
17. 18 N.Y.C.R.R. § 29.2(3).
18. Weiss SH et al: HTLV-III Infection among health care workers; association with needle-stick injuries, *JAMA* 254:2089–2093, 1985.
19. N.Y. Pub. Health Law-Article 27F (many other jurisdiction require informed consent prior to HIV testing, such as AZ, CO, DE, FL, HA, IL, KA, ME, MD, NJ, OR, SD, TX, and WI).
20. N.Y. Pub. Health Law-Article 27F. §2781(2).
21. N.Y. Pub. Health Law-Article 27F. §2782.
22. 42 U.S.C. §1395dd, *Supra* note 1.
23. *Cleveland v. Bronson Health Care Group, Inc.,* 917 F.2d 268 (6th Cir. 1990).
24. *Cleveland v. Bronson Health Care Group, Inc.,* 917 F.2d 272 (6th Cir. 1990).

25. *Cleveland v. Bronson Health Care Group, Inc.*, 917 F.2d 271 (6th Cir. 1990).
26. *Gatewood v Washington Health Care Corp.* 933 F.2d 1037 (D.C. Cir. 1991).
27. Pennycook AG, McNaughton G, Hogg F: Irregular discharge against medical advice from the accident and emergency department—a cause for concern, *Arch Emerg Med* 9(2):2300-2308, 1992.
28. Hogness CG et al: Cervical cancer screening in an urban emergency department, *Ann Emerg Med,* 211(8):933-939, 1992.
29. 273 California Reporter 231 (1990).
30. 521 So.2d 143 (D.C.F1 4th Disst., 1988)
31. *Schloendorff v. Society of New York Hospital,* 211 N.Y. 125, 105 N.E. 92 (1914).
32. *Schloendorff v. Society of New York Hospital,* 211 N.Y. 125, 105 N.E. 93 (1914).
33. N.Y. Soc. Serv. Law §413 (McKinney's Supp. 1992).

Chapter 23

Final Considerations: Interacting with the Medical Examiner

Mark Flomenbaum, M.D., PhD.

Jonathan L. Arden, M.D.

CASE 23–1

A 23-year-old man was brought to the Emergency Department (ED) by an emergency medical service (EMS) ambulance. On admission, he was cold, clammy, tachycardic, hypotensive, tachypneic, and obtunded. His body was covered with a diffuse blotchy purple rash. The neck was supple and there were no focal neurologic signs. There were no abnormal lung or heart sounds. Abdominal examination was normal. Laboratory evaluation included a white blood cell count of 12,500/mm^3; serum was sent for "toxicologic screening." Friends who accompanied the patient to the ED related that the patient had had "flu" (fever, malaise, weakness, and anorexia) for the past 3 days. They knew of no other significant medical history. The patient was employed as a rock musician. Supportive measures were instituted, but during the subsequent evaluation, the patient sustained a cardiopulmonary arrest. Vigorous, prolonged resuscitative efforts were unsuccessful.

What possible diagnoses should be considered here? Do any of the possible diagnoses pose a risk to EMS personnel, ED staff, or outside contacts (intimate or casual)? Are any prophylactic medical interventions appropriate for his contacts at this time? Does diagnostic testing end when the patient dies? What information should be related to the medical examiner (ME)? Should the case be reported to any other government agencies?

CASE 23–2

A 19-year-old man was brought to the ED by an EMS ambulance with cardiopulmonary resuscitation (CPR) in progress. He had five gunshot wounds to the torso and one to the head. While cutting his clothing off in the ED, a bullet fell out and was recovered by a nurse. Another bullet was palpable in the subcutaneous tissues of the chest.

The trachea was intubated, a chest tube placed, and a thoracotomy performed. Another bullet was recovered during these procedures. As a result of the resuscitative efforts, the patient regained vital signs, but he remained in a vegetative state and was declared brain-dead. Permission was sought for harvesting organs and tissues for transplantation.

How should recovered evidence be handled? If the police request it, should the emergency physician perform a postmortem incision, remove the bullet, and hand it to the officer? What agencies need to be notified of this death/injury, and what information must the ED supply? Should the *hospital* seek permission to perform an autopsy? If the ME accepts a case, will the autopsy results be available to the ED for discussion at a mortality conference? Can the hospital proceed with organ harvesting based solely on permission granted by the next of kin?

INTRODUCTION

The ME or coroner* usually takes jurisdiction to certify the cause and manner of deaths that are apparently unknown or unnatural.[1] Unfortunately, the ME is often thought of only as the place to send patients for autopsy when they arrived too late in the ED or when the ED staff is unsuccessful in their resuscitative efforts. Why then is a chapter devoted to this topic in a book on diagnostic testing in the ED?

In many cases the diagnostic evaluation of a patient who ultimately becomes an ME case has begun in the ED. Many physicians, nurses, and others who staff EDs, are unsure of what to do with those test results and with the remaining specimens. Moreover, although the ME is one link between clinical medicine and the criminal justice system, most trauma patients do survive and are not sent to the ME. Certain diagnostic procedures in the ED are necessary for proper documentation of criminality. How does the ED best fulfill its obligation to the criminal justice system and to society at large without compromising its obligation to the patient?

This chapter addresses the interactions between the physician in the ED and the ME (and by extension, other branches of the criminal justice system). Some methods of diagnostic testing and evidence handling that are used in the ME's office are discussed in this chapter, and specific procedural guidelines are provided. The goal is to elucidate what *could* be done in the ED, as well as what *should* be done in the ED and what *should never* be done in the ED. It must be emphasized that what can be done by the *ME* should not be attempted in the ED, but when the injuries are *not* fatal, these procedures and tests should be performed in the ED so that the information is not forever lost.

Much of this chapter is a manual on collecting and handling evidence for forensic purposes. The methods described are standard practice and may have to be somewhat modified for each case. Several books on general principles of forensic medicine and forensic pathology are listed at the end of this chapter.

THE AUTOPSY

The autopsy is the ultimate diagnostic test, although rarely considered in the same light as the other tests and procedures discussed in this book. Because an ED must first and foremost concentrate on caring for living patients (often in large numbers), when a patient arrives dead or dies in the ED, the diagnostic workup typically ceases. But should this be so? Even though the autopsy is not performed in the ED and the procedure does not directly benefit the individual on whom it is performed, the findings may be extremely important to the ED staff and the hospital. For example, the autopsy may reveal an infectious disease such as meningococcal meningitis that poses a public health threat to exposed hospital workers, family, close associates, or the pop-

*For convenience, both will henceforth be referred to as ME.

ulation at large. Other public health concerns (carbon monoxide poisoning, etc.), presumptively identified in the ED, may be confirmed at autopsy and require reporting to local health authorities to prevent further casualties. The reason for an unexpected or unexplained death (carbon monoxide, cyanide, botulism, etc.) may be revealed and may be useful to the ED staff in future clinical encounters under similar circumstances.

Another reason that autopsies are important to the functioning of the ED is that the adequacy of diagnosis and treatment will often be evident at autopsy and in this sense the autopsy may assist the ED in its quality assurance or quality improvement obligations.

Finally, the autopsy may demonstrate why death was the unavoidable result in a given instance, beyond any clinical skills or diagnostic acumen. In this instance, autopsies may help to avoid misunderstanding, embarrassment, or future liability for the physician and/or institution.

Goal of the Autopsy

The circumstances and goals of an autopsy differ significantly depending upon whether the procedure is carried out in the hospital or by the ME. Autopsies done on hospitalized patients are performed by the hospital pathology department or the ME depending on the circumstances of death (age, antecedent illness, etc.). Most commonly, *deaths in the ED* will come under the jurisdiction of the local forensic agency charged with investigating and certifying sudden or unnatural deaths—the ME.

The hospital autopsy is done with family consent on a patient whose death is presumed to be due entirely to natural causes. Permission to perform the procedure should be sought by the clinicians, but the family may also initiate the request. The autopsy concentrates on the extent and manifestations of natural disease (known and unknown), the effects of therapy, and the quality of care. The information derived is vital for quality assurance as well as future clinical management decisions. The results are commonly related to the family to fulfill their desire (or necessity) to know why and how the patient died.

Forensic autopsies are performed under the jurisdiction of the local government agency (ME or coroner) charged with investigating and certifying certain types of deaths defined by applicable statutes.[2] The decision to perform a forensic autopsy is made by the agency defined in these statutes, *not* by consent of the next of kin. Although specific details vary between locations, the ME will usually take jurisdiction over all violent deaths, which are defined as all deaths that are not *entirely* due to natural disease. Included are any instances in which injury causes or *contributes to* the death; these cases may be categorized as homicide, suicide, or accident. The ME also accepts jurisdiction when the cause of death is unknown, when deaths occur in legal custody, and in some instances when therapeutic complications occur. There are differences among jurisdictions in the exact definitions of deaths that are reportable to the ME. Every physician working in an ED should know the local regulations and consult the ME directly if any doubts or questions concerning these definitions arise.

Although the circumstances and focus of the forensic autopsy differ from the hospital autopsy, the findings are also available to the family, clinicians, and hospital. Direct communication between the emergency physician and the ME can be mutually beneficial, and the physician should not hesitate to contact the ME to give or request information.

The forensic autopsy becomes one important link in the chain of information needed to explain a death and may be used as evidence by the criminal justice system. Of course, the ME cannot function in a vacuum; information provided by the ED is often of crucial importance. Conversely, inattention by the ED may significantly hamper a medicolegal investigation.

Autopsy Permission

In general, if a death is being referred to the ME, the hospital physician should *not* request permission to perform an autopsy. If jurisdiction is accepted by the ME, then that agency has the statutory right to perform an autopsy, even over family objections. If the physician seeks permission to perform an autopsy from the family and is refused before consulting the ME, then the family may feel that they have the same right to refuse the ME. This can lead to confusion and unnecessary distress for the family: only *after* the ME declines jurisdiction should the hospital physician seek autopsy permission from the family. It may be useful for the hospital to develop a specific policy for seeking autopsy permission in ED deaths following clearance by the medical examiner.

Traumatic vs. Natural Deaths

Usually deaths due to trauma can be easily separated from those primarily due to a disease process with incidental or secondary injuries (e.g., minor contusions and lacerations from falling *after* loss of consciousness). Violent deaths obviously require special considerations to ensure correct interpretation of injuries, accurate determination of circumstances, and fulfillment of law enforcement needs (such as maintaining the chain of custody over evidence). Some natural deaths also require such considerations. Meticulous procedures for documenting findings and collecting or safeguarding evidence will not only benefit the criminal justice system but can also protect the hospital and ED staff from contagious diseases and perhaps from future liabilities.

Separating natural from unnatural or traumatic deaths may be difficult at the time of death, particularly when trying to distinguish intoxication from natural death, since both typically do not display significant injuries. For example, the laboratory finding of cocaine or its metabolites in blood can be sufficient evidence to certify the death as due to cocaine intoxication. But it is also possible that the mere presence of these substances (on toxicologic analysis) may be only incidental to a fatal anatomic *lesion*. The presence or absence of such a lesion may only be determined by autopsy.

The axiom that a more reliable history allows more accurate diagnosis is just as true in forensic medicine as it is in clinical medicine. Therefore, the emergency physician must provide the ME with as accurate an account as possible of what was discovered, whether by history, physical examination, or laboratory testing. It is imperative that the ED staff leave all catheters in place and document for the record the therapy provided and particularly note the sites where any intravascular punctures were attempted. (At autopsy a stab wound and chest tube incision may be indistinguishable.) The communication should be similar to a brief transfer or admission note and should include a summary of the relevant history, physical examination, procedures, medications, and therapy, including all that occurred during transport to the ED (i.e., the ambulance call report [ACR]). This brief note is not only a courtesy to the physician receiving the body, in most jurisdictions it is also required by law.

Violence and Evidentiary Material

Obviously, not all victims of violence end up in the ME's office; most survive, especially those who reach the hospital. In a court of law the testimony of the surviving victim is often stronger than the "testimony of the cadaver," but in either case evidentiary material that can substantiate the testimony may be present in the ED but be easily overlooked, lost, or inadvertently destroyed.[3] *The following suggestions apply not only to ME cases but to surviving patients as well.* A law enforcement officer assigned to the case will be responsible for physically receiving (and signing for) any evidentiary material recovered in the ED. A knowledgeable emergency physician or staff member can offer suggestions and submit material beyond the minimum ordinarily expected. (In all cases, the ED is responsible for establishing the chain of custody up to this point.)

Evidence External to the Body: Clothing

All of the clothing worn by the victim should be recovered and maintained for evidence. Clothing removed by emergency medical technicians or paramedics on the scene or in the ambulance while in transit to the ED should be kept with the patient. Concern for the clothing should never take priority over patient care; there is nothing of forensic value that could not withstand a reasonable delay. However, contamination due to mishandling can easily destroy the evidentiary nature of the material. For example, blood stains on the clothing may have come from the patient, but they also may have come from the assailant, especially if the violence occurred at close range such as in beatings, stabbings, or sexual assault. Evidence is destroyed by hastily removing clothing and throwing it on the floor in an area where it may become contaminated by blood from *other* ED *patients.*

Semen analysis on clothing from sexual assault victims has been discussed in Chapter 21. Although the usual sampling or collection of evidence in a sexual assault case is from undergarments, it is the outer clothing that may contain the most important evidence. Hairs or fibers and trace material such as paint chips or glass fragments may be present on outer clothing and may be the only link to an assailant. Unfortunately, the preservation of such evidence is too frequently overlooked, and the evidence is lost simply because no one thought to preserve it. Glass is often *deliberately* discarded because it is regarded as a potential hazard for the ED staff; rarely does one think that it may be the only means of identifying the vehicle that injured the patient.[4]

When removing clothing with scissors, avoid cutting through the perforations that were made by the knife or bullet that injured the body. The shape of the knife blade is occasionally better reconstructed from the *clothing* than from the *body,* particularly when the victim survives and there is no autopsy. Multiple gunshot wounds with several exits and reentrances into the body can be difficult to analyze: without the clothing, determining the individual paths may be impossible. Comparing the relationships of clothing perforations with body wounds may reestablish the relative position of the body and limbs at the time that the injuries were inflicted. Well-preserved clothing is often the only means available for determining the range of gunshot fire: the pattern of gun powder residues (particles and powders) deposited around the perforation is used to estimate the muzzle-to-target distance.[5] Even blood-soaked or dark-colored garments, which show nothing to the naked eye, may reveal a residue pattern when analyzed in the crime laboratory. Cutting around these perforations instead of through them when undressing the patient will preserve the accuracy of these ballistic determinations.

HOW TO HANDLE CLOTHING

- Collect all the clothing (at the scene, in the ambulance, in the hospital).
- Do not cut through perforations when undressing a patient.
- Avoid contaminating the clothing with other patients' fluids.

- Hang wet or moist clothing to enable air-drying, if possible.
- Submit the clothing to law enforcement personnel as soon as possible; get a receipt, and attach it to the patient's chart.
- Leave any clothing that is still on the body at the time of death for the ME.

Evidence on the Body: Body Fluids

The following sections describe how the ME handles evidence on the body. When a patient dies or arrives dead in the ED, such evidence should be left for the ME to collect. The procedures are described here to emphasize again that most victims of violent assault who come to the ED will survive and if the evidence is not collected and preserved properly in the ED it may be lost forever.

Virtually any fluid or trace evidence discussed in the previous section on Clothing may be present on the body itself and should be preserved and collected for forensic laboratory analysis. Chapter 21 gives explicit directions for preserving and collecting semen. Other fluids, however, may be equally important not only to establish sexual assault or rape but also to prove other violent acts as well.

Blood.—Dried blood on the body that does not appear to be from the patient is always collected for forensic serology. Not only is ABO and Rh typing possible, but by using current molecular biologic probes, a DNA analysis of the specimen may also be obtained and compared with the DNA analysis of the assailant (or suspect).

HOW TO COLLECT DRIED BLOOD FROM A PATIENT'S BODY

- Moisten a sterile cotton-tipped applicator in saline.
- Wipe the bloodied area until the cotton is pink or red.
- Let the swab(s) air-dry.
- Place the swab(s) in a paper or cardboard *(not plastic)* carrier or an envelope.
- Label the container with the patient's name, the source of the swab, the date, the time, and the physician's name.
- Submit the specimen to the police as soon as possible, obtain a receipt, and attach the receipt to the chart.
- Refrigerate—*do not freeze!*—the specimen if storage is necessary before transport.

Saliva.—*Bite marks* are another possible source of valuable evidence[6, 7] but are often overlooked because dried saliva is not as obvious as dried blood. *Saliva is almost certainly present if there are fresh teeth marks.* The ABO group, type, and secretory status of the biter can be determined. Sloughed oral epithelial cells may be present on the bite mark and can be recovered for polymerase chain reaction methods for DNA analysis.

HOW TO COLLECT DRIED SALIVA FROM A PATIENT'S BODY

- Moisten a sterile cotton-tipped applicator in saline.
- Swab the immediate area around the bite. If the dental arch is visible on the skin, concentrate the swabbing in the center where the tongue would have made contact with the victim's skin.
- Let the swab(s) air-dry.
- Place the swab(s) in a paper or cardboard *(not plastic)* carrier or an envelope. Label the carrier with the patient's name, the source of the swab, the date, the time, and the physician's name.
- Submit the specimen to the police as soon as possible, obtain a receipt, and attach the receipt to the chart.
- Refrigerate—do not freeze!—the specimen if storage is necessary before transport.

Ballistic Evidence

Victims of gunshot injuries may come to the ED with bullet casings (shells) or entire bullets in their clothing, or the bullets may be recovered from their bodies. Bullets are obviously vital for identifying the weapon from which they were fired. Rifling marks, a specific etching pattern on the side of the bullet produced by the inner surface of the gun barrel, will conclusively demonstrate that a bullet was fired from a particular weapon. To preserve the evidentiary nature of bullets it is imperative that metal instruments not be used (if at all possible) when handling them since the instruments may scratch the surface and alter the rifling pattern of the bullet. Police and MEs often mark the bullet for identification (for future court appearances) by inscribing initials or a unique code. (*Never* mark the *sides* of a bullet where the rifling marks are; use the nose or base, and describe in the chart what you have done.) If in doubt, do not make any marks rather than risk destroying evidence.[5]

The only evidentiary value of a bullet lies in its caliber (diameter), weight, and rifling pattern. Specifically, there is no volatile or biological material that may adhere to a bullet that is of any use. (Fingerprints of the assailant are not recoverable.) Therefore, to avoid dissemination of possible blood-borne pathogens to the ballistic laboratory staff, remove all blood and dried tissue by either soaking in alcohol or *gently* scrubbing with a soft (nonmetallic) brush under water. If the victim dies and the body goes to the ME, a note must be included that describes the number of recovered bullets.

Recovered evidence should be transferred to the police department as soon as possible. Many hospitals require that bullets be first sent to their pathology department and then transferred. In either case, the chain of custody must be preserved and documented. The person who finds the bullet must sign and get a receipt to document when and to whom it was transferred. Every person who takes custody of the evidence signs for it, again documenting from whom it was obtained and when the transfer took place—until finally the police department receives it and signs the final receipt. It is essential to familiarize yourself with the hospital policy for custody of evidence and what to do with the receipts.

When describing gunshot wounds in the chart, it is usually best to *use the unmodified term "wound"* rather than to try to characterize the wound as "entrance" or "exit" unless you wish to appear as an expert witness to defend your statement in court.[1] The way to describe a gunshot wound is by *location* (where it is), *size* (dimensions of the perforation), the *shape* and *nature* of the injury *(perforation with a rim of abrasion,* or *perforation with lacerated margins),* and the presence or absence of *fouling* (black/gray powdery soot) or *stippling* (pattern of pinpoint brown dots) on the adjacent skin from gunpowder residue.

The best way to document the appearance of a wound is by taking a close-up photograph. Most hospital ED's keep instant photography (Polaroid) cameras on hand to document sexual assault and abuse lesions. Such a camera with a close-up lens attachment should be used for gunshot wounds as well.

HOW TO HANDLE GUNSHOT WOUNDS

- Do not forget the clothing (see above); preserve them to the best of your ability.
- Do not handle bullets with metal instruments.
- Do not describe gunshot wounds as either "entrance" or "exit" wounds, just "wounds."[8]
- Do not forget to maintain a chain of custody with ballistic evidence.

General Notes Regarding Evidence Collection in the Emergency Department

The ED and hospital should have standing policies and procedures for the collection and transmission of evidence. Since the evidence will be used by law enforcement agencies and many ED deaths will be examined by the ME, prior consultation with the relevant agencies (police, crime laboratory, ME, district attorney) by the chair or director of Emergency Medicine and hospital attorney will facilitate this interaction. Although the hospital is responsible for establishing its own procedures, communication with the other participants in the process will allow for the most mutually beneficial results.

Until the patient is officially pronounced dead, the physician should proceed with any therapeutic procedure or laboratory analysis deemed necessary. However, once that declaration is made, all clinical intervention must cease. Any manipulation, examination, or test done on the cadaver is a postmortem examination and is therefore illegal without proper permission or authority. Even with the best of intentions, drawing a single tube of blood for toxicology or microbiology *after the patient is declared dead* can place that individual at risk for litigation.

If blood or other fluid is drawn for microbiologic study and the patient subsequently dies, continue to handle the specimens as though the patient were still alive, i.e., send them to the hospital laboratory for culture and sensitivity. The *clinical setting* is far more likely to yield uncontaminated *meaningful* bacteriology results and with less delay than a sample drawn in the autopsy room after an indeterminate postmortem interval. Be sure to indicate on the transport form in a brief note that cultures are pending together with the name and/or extension of the laboratory to contact for results.

If specimens were *not* taken and there is concern about contagious disease or other public health emergencies, call the ME's office *yourself*, speak directly to the pathologist on call, explain the nature of the emergency, and document in the chart what you were requested to do (or not do).

If blood or other specimens collected for toxicology, chemistry, or the blood bank are still in the ED when resuscitative efforts end, send them to the ME *instead* of the hospital laboratories. The ME will probably collect additional samples, but the antemortem specimens may be useful for comparison, especially if the hospital samples were taken before therapy was begun.

CASE 23–1 CONTINUED

When the emergency physician called the ME to report the death of this 23-year-old man, she expressed her concern that he might have meningococcal meningitis, and if so, that a number of people involved in his resuscitation might need to receive antibiotic prophylaxis.

The ME arranged to perform the autopsy immediately. As soon as the body arrived, a sample of cerebrospinal fluid (CSF) was taken and rushed to the laboratory for stat latex agglutination. Approximately 30 to 45 minutes after the body arrived, the autopsy revealed a purulent subarachnoid exudate, and the laboratory confirmed that the sample was positive for *Neisseria meningitidis*.

The ME immediately called the emergency physician with the diagnosis. The physician then arranged to contact immediately all the people involved with the initial resuscitation, including a friend of the deceased who had briefly attempted mouth-to-mouth resuscitation. All exposed individuals were given prophylactic antibiotics, and nasopharyngeal swabs were obtained for culture. The Department of Health, Center for Communicable (Reportable) Diseases was also contacted.

If latex agglutination was not readily available, the CSF would have been Gram-stained immediately, and the presence of gram-negative intracellular diplococci would have established the diagnosis.

REQUIRED REPORTING

The specific governmental agencies that must be contacted for criminal injuries differ from state to state. For example, in some states nonfatal gunshot wounds and stab wounds and all forms of homicides must be reported to the police, whereas child abuse and neglect must be reported to child protective services. (In New York City, children who fall out of windows must be reported to the Department of Health, which tracks this as a public health hazard.[9]) Each responsible member of the ED staff must be familiar with the local laws of reporting cases to the ME, the board of health, and the other specific agencies responsible for investigating the nonfatal injuries.

Child Abuse and Neglect

The ED may be the most frequent site where child abuse or neglect is recognized. This places enormous responsibility on the ED staff in protecting children at risk (both the actual patients and any siblings in the household). Not only must the ED staff comply with reporting regulations involving various government agencies, but it is also imperative for the staff to document findings for later use as evidence.

Rules regulating the reporting of injuries and suspected child abuse and neglect vary among states, so emergency physicians must be familiar with their own state and local laws. As described elsewhere in this chapter, many localities require the ED to report criminally violent acts to the police or other agencies, and these general rules include some instances of child abuse. More specifically, however, state laws now universally provide mechanisms for reporting suspected abuse and neglect and *mandate* medical practitioners to report such injuries.[10] Credible evidence of abuse or neglect that must be reported may be limited to those encountered in one's professional duties or may extend further. Again, the ED staff members must be familiar with the applicable statutes to ensure compliance. The intent is to identify children in situations where there is *reasonable suspicion* of abuse or neglect; the physician does not have to prove beyond a reasonable doubt that abuse occurred or determine who abused the child. The emergency physician is not the police, investigator, prosecutor, or judge—but rather the source of the medical recognition that informs the various systems of investigation, social welfare, and criminal justice of the problem.

The task of the emergency physician is to be observant, reasonably interpret observations, and rigorously document these observations. As always, all observations must be carefully recorded in detail and preserved as evidence. Symptoms or signs may not be present later, especially at autopsy, and the *clinical* observations may be the most significant elements on which the ME or court will reach a conclusion.

HOW TO HANDLE CHILD ABUSE AND NEGLECT CASES

- Document the condition of the body (e.g., cleanliness) and clothing on admission; photograph if necessary.
- Be meticulous in documenting vital signs (including body temperature) both on admission and in transport to the ED.
- Photograph all wounds and describe their location, size, shape, pattern, color, and definition of margins. (The color and degree of border distinction of a contusion or bruise may help date an injury.)
- Rigorously document histories. Give details of what was said, by whom, to whom, and when.
- Retain samples of all fluids taken for analysis, especially admission blood samples before extensive therapy begins. (Dehydration and starvation can be documented from the tube of blood in the blood bank and from the urine sample sent for culture.) Ensure that the ME knows how to obtain the laboratory results or the laboratory specimens in cases that become fatalities, i.e., document to whom the specimens were sent.
- Perform a fundoscopic examination to look for the retinal hemorrhages seen in

"shaken babies."[11, 12] The procedure should be performed if there is a high index of suspicion. (If an ophthalmology consultation is necessary, the earlier the examination the better.)

- Swab bite marks for evidence (saliva) (see the procedures detailed earlier).
- Be specific with respect to positive and negative findings; broad statements such as "HEENT WNL" (head, ears, eyes, nose and throat within normal limits) may be interpreted later to indicate no abnormal findings in specific areas that you may not actually have examined (e.g., retinal hemorrhages).
- Avoid editorializing or making emotional statements. A note that begins with *"This poor unfortunate child"* will destroy your credibility as an impartial observer of facts.

ORGAN DONATION

Organs and tissues for transplantation are in high demand and short supply in this country. Under the *Uniform Anatomical Gift Act,* which applies in many localities, hospitals are required to request permission from next of kin for organ and tissue harvesting when a death occurs in the hospital. Although many patients who die in the ED may be good candidates for tissue or organ harvesting, for any death reported to the ME, approval for organ harvesting should be granted only by the ME after permission is obtained from the next of kin. The ME may require a detailed description of the harvesting from the physician or transplant surgeon in order to subsequently evaluate the anatomic findings. Requests for a specific organ or tissue may be denied if that area is necessary for the ME to ascertain the cause of death. However the vast majority of harvesting requests are approved by the ME, who usually aids the transplantation service without compromising the goals of the ME.

Child abuse *deaths* are one of the few sources of pediatric organs for transplantation. A thorny issue is raised when trying to balance the humanitarian need for organs against the necessity of conducting a medical-legal investigation of a criminal death. Often organs can be harvested without destroying the evidence needed to document the cause and manner of death. Again, the clinicians and transplant surgeons must carefully document their findings and communicate these to the ME.

CASE 23–2 CONTINUED

The two bullets that were recovered during resuscitation were kept separate and soaked in alcohol until they were free of organic material. Each was placed in its own envelope and sealed. The envelope was then labeled with the patient's name and chart number, date, physician's name, and a few words describing the location from which the bullet was recovered. (More details of the bullet injury or track were entered onto the chart.) The bullet envelopes were then submitted to the police detective assigned to the case. The detective did not have a receipt book, so he described in the chart the bullets and noted the time he received them, the physician's name, his name and shield number and then he signed his note.

The detective saw one bullet bulging and palpable in the subcutaneous tissue and asked whether the emergency physician could remove it. The physician explained that since the patient was now "brain-dead," he was legally dead and the ME had complete jurisdiction over all matters concerning the body.

The issue of organ harvesting arose at the time the patient was declared "brain-dead" on the respirator. First the family was asked by the emergency physician to sign a release for the organs; then the ME was called and the case discussed to see which organs could possibly be removed without destroying evidence. In this case the shot to the head was the fatal one, and the shots to the torso were all to the chest, with only minor injuries to one lung. The ME gave permission for removal of the kidneys and liver but declined permission to open the chest. The gunshot wound to the head was an occipital perforation, and permission was granted to remove the corneas.

REFERENCES

1. Fisher RS, Platt MS: History of forensic pathology and related laboratory sciences. In *Spitz and Fisher's medicolegal investigation of death: guidelines for the application of pathology to crime investigation,* ed 3, Springfield, Ill, 1993, Charles C Thomas.
2. Curran FJ, McGarry AL, Petty CS: *Modern legal medicine, psychiatry and forensic science,* Philadelphia, 1980, FA Davis.
3. Fierro MF: The pathologist and physical evidence. In Froede RC, editor: *Handbook of forensic pathology,* Northfield, Ill, 1990, College of American Pathologists.
4. Huelke D, Gikas P: Investigations of fatal automobile accidents from the forensic standpoint, *J Forensic Sci* 11:474–484, 1966.
5. Di Maio VJM: *Gunshot wounds: practical aspects of firearms, ballistics and forensic techniques,* Boca Raton, Fla, 1985, CRC Press, pp 275–279, 290, 291.
6. Sopher IM: *Forensic dentistry,* Springfield, Ill, 1976, Charles C Thomas.
7. Sanger RG, Bross DC: *Clinical management of child abuse and neglect: a guide for the dental professional,* Chicago, 1984, Quintessence Publishing.
8. Randall T: Clinicians' forensic interpretations of fatal gunshot wounds often miss their mark, *JAMA* 269:2058-2061, 1993.
9. New York City Health Code, Section 11.03.
10. Besharov DJ: *Recognizing child abuse: a guide for the concerned,* New York, 1990, Free Press.
11. Lambert SR, Johnson TE, Hoyt CS: Optic nerve sheath and retinal hemorrhages associated with shaken baby syndrome, *Arch Ophthalmol* 104:1509–1512, 1986.
12. Caffey J: The whiplash shaken infant syndrome: manual shaking by the extremities with whiplash-induced intracranial and intraocular bleeding, linked with residual permanent brain damage and mental retardation, *Pediatrics* 54:396–403, 1974.

SUGGESTED READINGS

Karch SB: *The pathology of drug abuse,* Boca Raton, Fla, 1993, CRC Press.

Knight B: *Forensic pathology,* New York, 1991, Oxford University Press.

Zumwalt RE: Application of molecular techniques to forensic pathology. In *Molecular diagnostics in pathology,* Baltimore, 1990, Williams & Wilkins.

PART VII

Planning and Cost Considerations

Chapter 24

Designing an Emergency Department Laboratory

Marc R. Salzberg, M.D.

CASE 24–1

A 26-year-old female who had fallen while ice skating came to the emergency department (ED) because of right hip pain. A large contusion over the right greater trochanter was evident, and the patient had moderate pain on passive motion. No shortening or rotation of the leg was noted. Neurovascular findings were normal, as was the remainder of the physical examination. The emergency physician requested a test for the β-subunit of human chorionic gonadotropin (β-hCG), a complete blood count (CBC) and a urinalysis (UA) and informed the patient that he was requesting a hip radiograph. The woman, a famous ice skater, had been having difficulty conceiving and refused to consent to the radiograph unless she was sure that she was not pregnant.

Comment.—This patient's subsequent ED management could follow one of two possible courses:

1. A urine β-hCG test is done in the ED by the physician, nurse, or dedicated laboratory technician; the results are available in less than 15 minutes and are negative. Radiographs are taken and are negative. The CBC and urinalysis results are available soon thereafter; the patient is discharged less than 1 hour after arrival.
2. The β-hCG test is performed by the central hospital laboratory, and the laboratory results are available in 1 hour. β-hCG testing is negative. Radiographs are taken, and the patient is discharged 2 to 3 hours after arrival.

Although the ultimate outcome will be the same, the first course will obviously make a more positive impression on the patient as well as help to reduce the number of patients waiting in the ED for laboratory results. In this case, it is clear that a small laboratory in the ED where a rapid pregnancy test could be performed would result in a significant reduction in the time required to evaluate and manage patients.

In this chapter we will consider some of the laboratory options available to EDs. In particular, we will examine (1) the physicians' "teaching laboratory," its characteristics and equipment, and the role it may play in a comprehensive laboratory testing program and (2) the ED satellite laboratory or ED stat laboratory, its relation to (1), and the regulations under which it is required to operate.

THE PHYSICIANS' TEACHING LABORATORY

Space Requirements

The diagnostic tests listed in the following section can be accommodated in a relatively small space: a work counter that is 24 in deep and 8 ft long with a sink on either end and a hood above and storage below (see Fig. 24–1). This space can be located in a small room designated as the "Emergency Department Physician (Staff) Laboratory." If possible, more space than currently is necessary should be allocated so that expansion or perhaps conversion to a satellite laboratory may be accomplished easily in the future. Whatever testing is done in the ED must be done in accordance with Joint Commission on the Accreditation of Healthcare Organizations (JCAHO) standards, state and local regulations, and quality control guidelines. The accuracy of the testing and qualifications of the testers will generally be the responsibility of the chairman of pathology or the director of laboratories. Alternatively, in a teaching facility, the laboratory may be designated strictly as a teaching laboratory with a mechanism in place to ensure that the results of such resident physician and student testing and microscopy be used solely for educational purposes. In this situation, the regular hospital laboratory facilities (including perhaps a professionally staffed and equipped satellite laboratory), will perform all official testing.

TESTS TO BE PERFORMED IN THE PHYSICIANS' LABORATORY

- Hematocrit
- Erythrocyte sedimentation rate
- Urinalysis by (leukocyte esterase) dipstick
- Gram stain
- Acid-fast stain
- Methylene blue stain
- KOH wet mount for fungi
- Crystal analysis (by compensated polarized microscopy)
- Quantitative analysis of cells found in cerebrospinal fluid and joint fluid (by hemocytometer)
- Dipstick analysis of blood (glucose and ketones) and urine (pH, protein, glucose, ketones, blood, bilirubin, and urobilinogen)
- Rapid urinary β-hCG pregnancy test

EQUIPMENT NECESSARY TO PERFORM TESTS

- Binocular light microscope with polarizing components and a red compensator
- Slides and coverslips
- Centrifuge
- Hemoglobinometer (the use of microhematocrit centrifuges should be avoided to prevent accidental deep innoculation with a patient's blood if the tube shatters in the physician's fingers)
- Pipette (no specimen should be suctioned by mouth)
- Sink and small Bunsen burner
- Stain equipment—slides, coverslips, gentian or crystal violet, Gram's iodine, 95% ethanol, safranin red; Kinyoun carbolfuchsin; methylene blue; potassium hydroxide (KOH)
- Erythrocyte sedimentation rate racks and tubes
- Alcohol
- Acetone

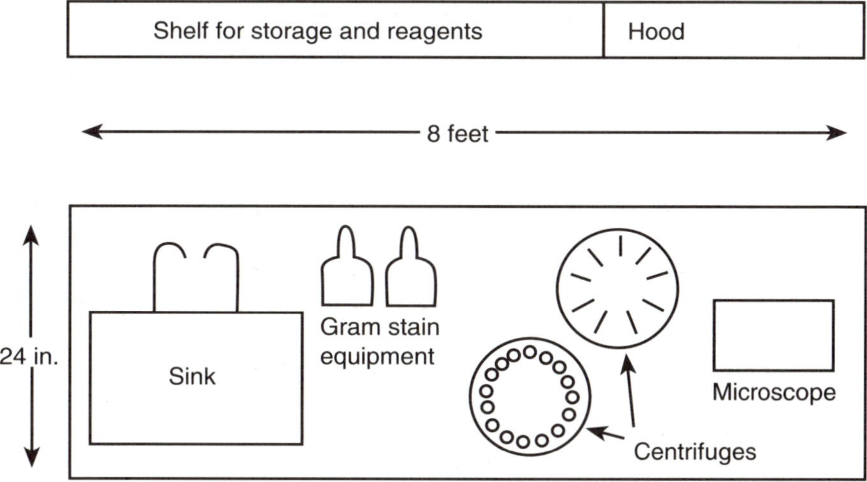

Fig. 24–1. Laboratory space requirements.

- Sterile swabs
- Hemocytometer
- Urine reagent and leukocyte esterase dipstick
- Blood reagent tablets
- Commercially available pregnancy test
- Rapid mono-spot test
- Rapid streptococcal antigen assay
- Gonococcal assay
- Chlamydial assay
- Disposable needle (sharps) container
- Disposable gloves

THE SATELLITE "STAT" LABORATORY

In the past the physicians' teaching laboratory in the ED and the ED stat laboratory were often one and the same. Today, however, any satellite laboratory outside the main hospital laboratory that performs one or more tests is considered an ancillary laboratory and as such must be run under strict guidelines to ensure adherence to JCAHO regulations as well as those of state and local accrediting agencies. All ED protocols describing laboratory activities within the ED also must comply with these regulations (see Appendix 24–1) and, more importantly, make clear the differences between the physicians' teaching laboratory and the satellite stat laboratory when both are present in a particular ED.

Defining "Stat" Testing

Stat is an abbreviation for the Latin *statim,* or "immediately."[1] There is no universally accepted time frame for the word *"stat."* It must be defined by each department and for each test, for example, "CBC, within 30 minutes"; "amylase, within 60 minutes." To be fair to the laboratories, the "clock" for their portion of the process should begin only when the specimen actually arrives in the laboratory, and not from the time that the test was requested and sent; phlebotomy, labeling, and transportation are the responsibility of the ED. Thus, if a requested test requires 20 minutes for samples to be drawn and the specimen then remains on the shelf for 15 minutes until it is finally carried to the laboratory by hand, 40 minutes may be lost in a process over which the laboratory has no control. It is therefore essential to look at the entire process and analyze each step along the way to identify delays that may easily be corrected. In this example, a point-to-point pneumatic tube from the ED to the laboratory might be a partial solution. Effectively analyzing the problem and monitoring the solution is an area that has received considerable attention from JCAHO and state regulatory agencies.

By establishing effective communication with the chairman of pathology or the director of laboratories and by employing continuous quality improvement (CQI),* many of the common problems involving laboratory testing in the ED can be alleviated. As noted above, the first step is to jointly analyze the entire process beginning with the decision to request a test and ending when the provider has the information required. This type of flow analysis will often identify roadblocks to a quick turnaround time, which can then be remedied. Some examples include simple agreement as to the definition of "stat" as it relates to ED patients. Because almost all tests done in the ED are considered "stat" by that department, laboratory personnel often ignore the stat nature of the request and process the specimens on a routine basis. To correct this, most laboratories have established separate accessioning areas and dedicated analyzers for samples from the ED rather than waiting to batch the ED sample with other specimens. Another solution isto use point-of-care or point-of-source testing (POST) equipment (see Chapter 1). Each hospital has unique characteristics, so a flow analysis must be unique to the institution. The challenge is to work together to analyze the flow, critique it objectively, make suggestions for improvement, implement those changes, and then monitor the results with continuous feedback to the group that has been charged with the responsibility. CQI is an ongoing process that, if conducted correctly, never ends.

SUMMARY

The key to successful "stat" testing for ED patients is to formulate the goals of ED laboratory testing with representatives from clinical pathology and hospital administration. How this goal is reached in a particular institution will depend on a host of variables including patient volume, structure of the present clinical laboratory, and a careful analysis of the process as it exists in the institution. Because many systems are available, time spent analyzing which system is best for a particular institution along with site visits to similar existing facilities will aid immeasurably. In the future, as point-of-care testing in the ED becomes more widespread (see Chapter 1) it will be even more important for emergency physicians to be aware of and adhere to the requirements governing each type of laboratory facility in the ED.

REFERENCES

1. *Dorland's Illustrated Medical Dictionary.*
2. Deming WE: *Out of crisis,* Cambridge, Mass, 1986, MIT Press.
3. Juran JM: The quality triology, quality progress 19, No. 8. In *Juran on planning for quality,* New York, 1989, Free Press, pp 19–24.

*In the late 1970s, Japanese industry, led by the Americans Deming[2] and Juran,[3] adopted the management tool of CQI (or TQM—total quality management) to improve both the quality and production of goods. U.S. industry incorporated the concepts of CQI in the 1980s, and subsequently hospitals also recognized its value. CQI and TQM have now become widely used management techniques for all aspects of hospital care.

Appendix 24–1. **Joint Commission on Accreditation of Healthcare Organizations (JCAHO) Standards**

PA.6.4 Decentralized Laboratory testing*

PA.6.4.1 If diagnostic clinical laboratory testing for the organization's patients is done within the organization, outside a central laboratory,

PA.6.4.1.1. personnel responsible for test performance and those responsible for direction/supervision of the testing activity are identified;

PA.6.4.1.2. personnel performing tests demonstrate satisfactory levels of competence;

PA.6.4.1.3. current written policies and procedures are readily available and address;

P.A.6.4.1.3.1. specimen collection

P.A.6.4.1.3.2. specimen preservation

P.A.6.4.1.3.3. instrument calibration

P.A.6.4.1.3.4. quality control and remedial action

P.A.6.4.1.3.5. equipment performance evaluation and

P.A.6.4.1.3.6. test performance

PA.6.4.1.4. quality control checks are conducted on each procedure each day the procedure is performed, and identified problems are resolved; and

PA.6.4.1.5. appropriate quality control and test records are maintained.

*From Joint Commission on Accreditation of Healthcare Organizations: *1993 Joint Commission accreditation manual for hospitals*, vol 1, *Standards*, Oakbrook Terrace, Ill., 1993, the Organization.

Appendix 24–2. **Suggested Guidelines for Establishing a Satellite Laboratory in the ED**

- *Ancillary Laboratory—Definition:*
  A laboratory that performs tests used for patient care is an ancillary laboratory.
- *Classification of Laboratories:*
  A laboratory that performs one or more laboratory tests used in the diagnosis or treatment of patients is classified as having "ancillary" status.
- *Organization:*
  Ancillary laboratories report for all technical purposes to the Director of Laboratories.
- *Materials, Supplies, Equipment:*
  All materials, supplies and equipment purchased for use by an ancillary laboratory must be approved by the Director of Laboratories.
- *Operations:*
  All technical operations active in ancillary laboratories must have the approval of the Director of Laboratories.
- *Technical Procedures:*
  All technical procedures used for patient care must meet laboratory standards as required by state and accrediting agencies. Standardization and quality assurance of these techniques must also meet required state and accrediting agency standards. It is the responsibility of the Director of Laboratories to ensure that these standards are met.
- *Assigned Staff:*
  Staff assigned to perform technical procedures relating to patient care must be trained properly and designated by the medical director of the service that

the laboratory functions in, and a record of such staff must be forwarded to the Director of Laboratories.

- *Hours of Operation:*
  Operating hours are optional for each ancillary laboratory depending upon needs of the department it services. Hours of operation must be confined to those during which trained staff are available for test performance.
- *In-Service Training:*
  Staff assigned to perform laboratory tests used in patient care must have available to them adequate in-service training for technical procedures, quality assurance, laboratory safety and infection control, and proficiency testing.
- *Manuals:*
  Policy and Procedure Manuals must be available on site at all times in each ancillary laboratory. Manuals must contain required information as designated by state and accrediting agencies. The Department of Laboratories provides such manuals with necessary updates and required review and revisions. The staff in ancillary laboratories must have this manual available to them for reference during all operating hours.
- *Record Keeping:*
  Each laboratory is required to maintain a "log." This log contains patient information, identification, and test results as per state and accrediting agency standards.
- *Quality Control:*
  Each ancillary laboratory is required to participate in quality control testing on each shift in which laboratory tests are performed. Protocols for quality control testing are provided by the Department of Laboratories. Laboratories failing to maintain proper quality control testing are not permitted to continue laboratory tests used for patient care. Materials and documentation forms are provided by the Department of Laboratories. Results are reviewed by the Director of Laboratories or his or her designee. Corrective actions required are discussed with the Medical Director of the ancillary laboratory. Documentation of all corrective actions taken is also required.
  Records of all ancillary laboratory quality control testings must be kept in the main laboratory for inspection by state and accrediting agencies. Quality control records must be stored and available for inspection for 2 years.
- *Preventive Maintenance:*
  Preventive maintenance must be performed in each ancillary laboratory as required by state and accrediting agency standards. Records of preventive maintenance must be maintained in the main laboratory and reviewed by the Director of Laboratories or his or her designee. Where stipulated, the main laboratory performs preventive maintenance.
- *Repairs:*
  All instrument failures must be reported to the main laboratory concerned. The reports include the inability to recover quality control values. Records of repairs must be maintained by the laboratory area servicing the complaint.
- Specimens:
  All specimens collected must use methods and materials as prescribed by the Department of Laboratories. See Technical Procedures for requirements.
- *Safety-Infection Control:*
  Staff members in each ancillary laboratory must comply with safety and infection control methods as required. Disposing of specimens must meet required standards.
- *Proficiency Testing:*
  All ancillary laboratories are required to participate in proficiency testing pro-

grams. The Department of Laboratories provides program, materials, and reporting mechanisms for this purpose. Failure to participate in proficiency testing must be reported to the Medical Board. Laboratories failing to comply are not permitted to continue laboratory tests for patient care purposes. All records of proficiency testing results must be maintained in the main laboratory and reviewed by the Director of Laboratories. Corrective actions required are discussed with the Medical Director of the ancillary laboratory concerned. Records must be maintained for 2 years and be available for inspection by state and accrediting agencies. The College of American Pathologists Survey Program is used for proficiency testing purposes.

- *Quality Assurance:*

  All staff performing laboratory tests must simultaneously perform quality controls. Technical procedures performed without controls are invalid. Controls must be run in both normal and abnormal ranges on each shift in which the laboratory tests are performed.

  Ancillary laboratories performing hematology tests are provided controls in both normal and abnormal ranges by the main hematology laboratory.

  These controls must be used by the ancillary laboratory before the expiration date specified by the manufacturer.

  Additionally, a chart for documentation must be posted that includes the usual ranges of recovery. Documentation of all quality control testing must be collected and maintained for review by the main laboratory.

Chapter 25

Decision Analysis and Cost Containment

Stephen V. Cantrill, M.D.

CASE 25 1

A 29-year-old female with a history of asthma comes to the Emergency Department (ED) complaining of increased wheezing. Her initial vital signs include a blood pressure of 128/85 mmHg, a pulse rate of 80/min, a respiratory rate of 22/min, and a temperature of 98.6° F. She is able to speak in full sentences without difficulty. Initial physical examination of the chest reveals moderate inspiratory and expiratory wheezes bilaterally. The treating physician's initial requests include an arterial blood gas determination. The blood gas specimen is drawn, and the following results are reported: pH 7.33, pCO_2 48 mmHg, pO_2 50 mmHg.

DECISION ANALYSIS

Decision making in emergency medicine may be viewed as a series of feedback loops involving data gathering, hypothesis formation, and hypothesis testing. As a clinician evaluates a patient, one or more hypotheses are generated (with varying degrees of specificity) concerning the diagnostic entity or entities that may be affecting the patient. These diagnostic hypotheses are then "tested" through the performance of diagnostic studies. The results of these studies are evaluated in light of the entire clinical picture to better define the patient's problem. In the best case, the clinician is able to refine the patient's initial complaint to a specific diagnostic entity. Diagnostic testing is important in this process, but it may also cause confusion and result in incorrect conclusions.

Requesting a diagnostic test is easy; however, requesting the *right* diagnostic test and properly interpreting the results may be quite difficult. Many physicians fall into the bad habit of "shotgunning"—requesting a rash of diagnostic tests without carefully determining what would be the most appropriate evaluation plan. This is often done in the hope that an abnormality will turn up to steer them to the patient's underlying problem. Even worse, this technique is sometimes employed instead of taking a careful history and performing a thorough physical examination. This approach is not only wasteful but also often leads to inadequate and misguided care.

The decision of which diagnostic test(s) to request is multifactorial. Certainly, there should be a significant clinical reason to obtain the test, i.e., the results of the test will assist in either the diagnostic or therapeutic aspects of the patient's care. The operative form of this question is "How will the results change what I do for the patient?" If the answer is that the results will not change the physicians's care of the patient, the value of requesting the diagnostic test must be questioned.

Other important considerations in requesting a diagnostic test are how sensitive and how specific the test is. That is, how often could the patient have a suspected disease entity and the test still give a negative result (false-negative—poor sensitivity) or give a positive result when the patient does not have the disease in question (false-positive—poor specificity). Unfortunately, these data are often not available to the clinician. Alternative forms of evaluation are also factored into this decision, as well as test costs (if they are appreciated by the physician). Often a more expensive test may be more specific and/or more sensitive for a diagnostic entity than a less expensive test and may therefore be the more appropriate test to request (pulmonary ventilation-perfusion scan vs. arterial blood gas to diagnose pulmonary embolism). However, sometimes the less expensive test may actually be more appropriate than the more expensive test (streptococcal screen vs. full throat culture in an attempt to exclude streptococcal pharyngitis). The risk to the patient and potential side effects of performing the test must also be considered.

Although test sensitivity (the percentage of patients who actually have a suspected disease vs. all who have a positive test result) and test specificity (the percentage of patients who have a negative test result vs. all who do not have the suspected disease) are helpful, the real questions are (1) if the test result is positive, how likely is it that the patient has the disease? and (2) if the test result is negative, how likely is it that the individual does not have the disease?[1] These numbers will be different, based upon the pretest probability that the patient has the suspected disease, which in turn is based upon the prevalence of the disease. Unfortunately, these numbers cannot be known because although the prevalence of a disease in the population may be known, it is difficult to know what the disease prevalence is for the subpopulation of which the patient is a member (e.g., all middle-aged females with abdominal pain).

Diagnostic tests with a quantifiable result usually have a "normal" range for the result. However, it is sometimes unclear exactly what these values mean. Clinical laboratories use many (different) methods to establish these ranges. Some will establish a range that will include a large fraction of the normal population, often 95%. This may cause difficulties for clinicians who request excessive tests. Assume that 12 tests are done, each with normal ranges that include 95% of the normal population. The chance that the patient will have 1 or more "abnormal" results of the 12 tests (and yet still be "normal") is

$$1.0 - 0.95^{12} = 0.46$$

or nearly 1 chance in 2. If we do 20 tests, the chance the patient will have one or more abnormal results is 0.64, or almost 2 chances in 3. Tests whose normal values are even more tightly constrained will have an even greater chance of producing "abnormal" results for a "normal" patient. These spurious "abnormal" results may stimulate additional inappropriate evaluation, further complicating the care of the patient and incurring additional unnecessary costs.

For the clinician to make the best judgment concerning the utilization of diagnostic tests, the following characteristics of any diagnostic test should be considered before the test is requested[2]:

- Reproducibility: How similar would the results be if a specific test was repeated multiple times on the same patient at the same time?
- Accuracy: How closely do the results of a specific test measure the desired observed phenomena in the patient? How close is this measurement in the clinical setting vs. the ideal experimental setting?

- Normal: What percentage of the disease-free population will have test results within the defined range of normal for this test?
- Abnormal: What percentage of the diseased population will have the results outside of the established range of normal?
- Disease definition: What is the "gold standard" for the definition of a patient having the disease in question? How accurate is this so-called gold standard in actually including those who have the disease and excluding those who do not have the disease?
- Test sensitivity: How often is the test positive in those individuals who have the disease in question?
- Test specificity: How often is the test negative in those patients who do not have the disease?
- Disease prevalence: How prevalent is the disease entity in question in the population at large? How prevalent is it in the subpopulation of which the patient is a member?
- Predictive value: Given the prevalence of the disease in the population of which the patient is a member, how well does a positive result predict that the patient will have the disease in question? How well does a negative result predict that the patient will *not* have the disease in question?

CASE 25 1 CONTINUED

The physician suspects that the ABG results represent venous blood values and repeats the test. Essentially normal values are reported.

COMMENT: An arterial blood gas determination in this setting will provide little, if any, useful information. This patient is not in respiratory extremis, so the possibility of using these data as a guide for intubation is not a consideration. The first attempt at an accurate arterial blood gas determination resulted in a venous sample being obtained, forcing the physician either to repeat this (inappropriate) test, or to ignore the apparent abnormal values.

Assessment of pulmonary function by measuring peak flow rates provides better "baseline" and prognostic information. Moreover, measuring peak flow rates is less invasive and usually less costly.

As can be seen, requesting a test and dealing with the results can often confuse matters rather than clarify the patient's disease process. Of the many pitfalls in this process, one that is particularly dangerous in emergency medicine is the concept of premature closure. In this situation, the physician "labels" a patient with a diagnosis (such as gastroenteritis in a patient with abdominal pain) that when carefully analyzed is not supported by the data. The major problem (other than being wrong) is that such a diagnostic label, when it is made known to a subsequently treating physician, often causes that physician to shut his or her "diagnostic hypothesis creation process" down, thus making it even more difficult to properly diagnosis and care for the patient. Although it may not be as intellectually satisfying for the physician to define the patient's problem at the actual level of understanding (e.g., "abdominal pain, etiology unknown" in the example above), such a practice is much safer for both the physician and the patient and is to be encouraged.

COST CONTAINMENT

Why Contain Costs?

There are multiple reasons to attempt to contain costs in the practice of emergency medicine. First and foremost is improved patient care. No one supports the concept of requesting tests that are not indicated. Therefore, we owe it to our patients to look carefully at our test-ordering habits. Although not carefully studied, logic would lead us to believe that lower health care charges would result in improved patient satisfaction, a better competitive position, and improved public relations.

The other major factor, of course, is the enormous cost of medical care in the United States. The rate of rise of this expenditure is of significant concern to all. The current cost of medical care is almost 14% of the gross national product. Governmental concern is now so intensely focused on this area that significant government involvement is almost certain. In the interest of both fiscal responsibility and good medicine, every physician should attempt to constrain excessive spending on health care. Clearly, if we do not exercise restraint ourselves, the government will step in and "assist" us in this process. One area of health care expenditures over which we, as emergency physicians, have complete control is diagnostic testing in the emergency department (ED). After all, we are the ones making the decisions to requests the diagnostic tests.

Expenditures on diagnostic testing represent a significant proportion of ED charges. Karras[3] found that diagnostic testing charges accounted for 44% of all ED charges, more than any other class of expenditure (e.g., professional charge, institutional charge). This finding has been validated by other studies. Because of our direct control over these charges, our efforts to become more precise in our testing can have a direct impact on overall health care costs.

Causes of Excessive or Inappropriate Diagnostic Testing

Unfortunately, little is taught during medical training about appropriateness in diagnostic testing. Traditionally medical students and house officers were criticized for *not* ordering a certain test. Rarely was anyone criticized for requesting an unneeded test or praised for limiting test requests. These influences have probably resulted in a mind-set of "more is better" in terms of diagnostic testing. Several other forces encourage diagnostic test abuse:

- Physician ignorance: It has been well (and repeatedly) documented[4, 5] that we physicians frequently have little knowledge of the incurred costs of care. Certainly, not considering the cost of a specific test is not considering one of its major "side effects."
- Peer pressure (real and imagined): "The consultant will want this test" is a common refrain in justifying test ordering, even if the test has little merit. Certainly, pleasing the consultant is easier than trying to educate him or her as to the appropriateness or inappropriateness of specific diagnostic tests.
- "Defensive medicine": Requesting a diagnostic test only out of fear of a malpractice suit is inappropriate, especially when the results in turn cause the physician to pursue specious (false positive) test results. The concept of "good medicine is good law" should prevail.
- Hospital policies: Although less of a problem than previously, inappropriate "routine admission test orders" can drive up health care costs. Routine ordering policies should be periodically reviewed and evaluated in terms of cost and yield (see Chapter 1).
- Old ordering practices: Unfortunately, when a new test is introduced in medicine, we are quick to request the new test but slow to cease requesting the test that it was meant to replace. We should periodically reexamine the logic of our test request patterns.
- Patient expectations: We have unconsciously convinced most (if not all) outpatients that some diagnostic testing is *necessary* for a complete evaluation of any

complaint. Although often true, when it is not, we must educate our patients that *not* requesting unnecessary tests is also appropriate care. This type of patient education may be a major undertaking but is necessary if we are ever to change patients' inappropriate expectations of the health care system.

- Intellectual curiosity: The temptation is very strong to engage in excessive testing to satisfy our curiosity. Requesting a test for only this reason is obviously inappropriate.
- "Insurance will pay": Even if this were true, it would be inappropriate. Although many patients (and physicians) are under the illusion that all care in the ED is covered by some form of health insurance, many policies have significant deductibles for outpatient care that result in large out-of-pocket expenses for the patient. Also, the marked increase in the number of health maintenance organizations (HMOs) has resulted in many more denials of claims for ED care, again resulting in patient expense. Many HMOs consider the clinical laboratory a resource to be managed rather than a resource to be used freely and in these situations, the participating treating physician has a vested interest in limiting expenditures. Pending health care reform may increase the number of physicians practising in this manner by encouraging HMO membership or imposing a capitation form of reimbursement.

Strategies to Contain Costs by Reducing Inappropriate Diagnostic Testing

Significant cost savings can be realized through minimizing inappropriate test requests by emergency physicians. A demonstration project done by the American College of Emergency Physicians showed a 10.0% decrease in overall costs from test ordering following an educational program targeted at practicing emergency physicians.[6] This project involved 20 hospitals and included public, private, teaching, and nonteaching hospitals with small and large EDs. For cost containment in diagnostic testing to be successful, physicians must be educated about basic strategies that are helpful in reducing inappropriate test requests:

- Be aware of the charges for diagnostic tests: Awareness alone encourages more thoughtful and reasoned decisions about test ordering.[5]
- When research into diagnostic testing has demonstrated high-yield criteria for a specific test, attempt to use these criteria in clinical practice: Unfortunately, this area of medical research has received too little attention except for isolated examples—such as Lowe's[7] work on electrolytes—that have established acceptable guidelines for diagnostic test ordering.
- Always consider the golden question of test ordering: "How will the results of this test have an impact on the patient's care?"
- Avoid reflexive ordering: Carefully consider which tests the patient truly needs before requesting them. Ordering diagnostic studies for "baseline" values is rarely indicated.
- Avoid requesting tests only for the sake of intellectual curiosity: Request a test if you would be willing to (1) pay for it yourself if you were a patient and (2) have it done on yourself.
- Periodically reevaluate health care protocols: Protocols, once established, often continue forever unquestioned. All protocols involving diagnostic testing should be reviewed and revised on a regular basis.
- Establish guidelines for the use of new technologies: As new diagnostic tests become available, thoughtful guidelines should be established for their use. Often in medicine we are quick to adopt the latest in diagnostic testing without carefully evaluating which tests should be replaced by the new test. Instead,

both tests are requested, with a subsequent increase in health care expenditures.

- Avoid requesting tests for "medicolegal" reasons: In the broad scope of malpractice problems in emergency medicine, the potential for lawsuits solely because a specific test was not requested is extremely low. On the other hand, we create many more problems by not educating patients, not following up on the tests we *do* request, not documenting what we have done in the ED, not giving adequate discharge instructions, and not having functional systems in place to deal with patient complaints and radiologic follow-up. Many of these factors at the very least will alienate a patient, and it is in *these* areas that we need to focus our risk management efforts.
- Use patient education to reshape patient expectations: Often the patient's insistence on a test demonstrates only a lack of knowledge of what constitutes appropriate medical care. Patient education by the physician can often bridge this gap.
- Avoid "stat" abuse: Most clinical laboratories impose an additional "stat" charge on requests to perform a test immediately. "Stat" tests are appropriate in many situations in the ED but are inappropriate when the results are to be used for follow-up, instead of immediately.
- Cancel unnecessary tests: Often after requesting a diagnostic test, additional history or other data become available that make the previously requested test unnecessary or redundant. In these cases, if the test has not yet been completed, it may often be canceled with no charge to the patient.
- Establish continuous quality improvement (CQI) projects to evaluate appropriate test ordering: Often by evaluating test ordering patterns and frequencies, areas of inappropriate use may be discovered. This may focus on specific tests or specific individuals and may help target an educational program to improve the appropriateness of test ordering. When a specific test is found (or felt) to be misused, specific suggested guidelines for requesting that test can be developed and agreed upon by the physicians in the ED.

Experience with Cost Containment

The cost containment demonstration project mentioned above proved that an educational model is effective in decreasing physician requests for diagnostic tests.[6] In this program, 17 tests and groups of tests were targeted for specific attention because they were thought to be overordered. The educational program consisted of general aspects of cost containment and test-specific suggested guidelines for the targeted tests. When compared with a preeducational control sample of 3 months of test request data, total charges for the targeted tests decreased an average of 12.5% (32% in one hospital), whereas total charges for nontargeted tests decreased by 4.6% for an overall decrease in total charges of 10.0% for all tests. The highest dollar savings were seen for extremity radiographs, chest radiographs, electrolyte panels, abdominal radiographs, and complete blood counts. The largest percent decrease in tests ordered was seen in rib radiographs (35%), urine cultures and sensitivity (34%), throat cultures (31%), blood products (24%), and blood alcohol levels (20%). If these savings were extrapolated to national scale, the savings would be billions of dollars. These positive efforts in cost containment were accomplished without diminishing the quality of care provided. Moreover, among the 20 hospitals in the program, there were no malpractice suits related to a lack of diagnostic testing.

Cost containment achieved by more careful diagnostic testing is easily within the grasp of any ED. All that is required is a commitment by the physicians to critically review their own diagnostic test request habits and a willingness to change those patterns when they can be demonstrated to be inappropriate. Cost containment in the ED is the emergency physician's responsibility.

REFERENCES

1. Sackett DL, Haynes RB, Guyatt GH, et al: *Clinical epidemiology: a basic science for clinical medicine,* ed 2, Boston, 1991, Little, Brown.
2. Riegelman RK, Hirsh RP: *Studying a study and testing a test,* ed 2, Boston, 1989, Little, Brown.
3. Karas S: Cost containment in emergency medicine, *JAMA* 243:1356-1359, 1980.
4. Skipper JK, Smith G, Mulligan JL, et al: Physicians' knowledge of cost: The case of diagnostic tests, *Inquiry* 13:194-199, 1976.
5. Tierney WM, Miller ME, McDonald CJ: The effect on test ordering of informing physicians of the charges of outpatient diagnostic tests, *N Engl J Med* 322:1524-1525, 1990.
6. Cost Containment Task Force: *Guidelines for cost containment in emergency medicine.* Dallas, Tex, 1983, American College of Emergency Physicians (available from ACEP, PO Box 619911, Dallas, TX, 75261-9911; Phone: 214-550-0911).
7. Lowe RA, Wood AB, Burney RE, et al: Rational ordering of serum electrolytes: development of clinical criteria, *Ann Emerg Med* 16:260-269, 1987.

Appendices

Appendix 1. Representative Normal Values*

A. Blood

1. Chemistry

A/G ratio	1.5–2.5
Albumin	4.0–5.5 g/dL (Biuret) (40–55 g/L)
	3.5–5.0 g/dL (electrophoresis)
Ammonia	30–70 μg/dL (17.6–41 μmol/L)
Bilirubin	
Total	0.2–1.5 mg/dL (3.42–25.7 μmol/L)
Direct	0.1–0.5 mg/dL (1.71–8.56 μmol/L)
BSP (45 min)	0%–5%
BUN	10–20 mg/dL (3.57–7.14 mmol/L)
Calcium	8.5–10.5 mg/dL (2.12–2.62 mmol/L)
Chloride	98–109 mEq/L (mmol/L)
Cholesterol	
Total	150–200 mg/dL (3.87–5.17 mmol/L)
Esters	65%–75%
CO_2 (combining power)	20–30 mEq/L (mmol/L)
Cortisol, plasma	5–20 μg/dL (138–552 mmol/L)
Creatinine, serum	0.8–2.0 mg/dL (70.1–176.8 μmol/L)
Folic acid (serum)	3–15 ng/mL (6.80–3.40 nmol/L)
α-Glutamyl transferase	
Males	0–30 mU/mL at 25° C (0–0.5 μkat/L)
Females	0–20 mU/mL at 25° C (0–0.33 μkat/L)
Globulin	1.2–3.0 g/dL
Glucose (fasting)	70–110 mg/dL (3.89–6.11 mmol/L)
Iron, serum	60–150 mg/dL (10.7–26.9 μmol/L)
Iron-binding capacity	250–350 mg/dL (44.8–62.7 μmol/L)
% TIBC solution	16%-N50%
Lipids	
Total	400–1000 mg/dL (4.0–10.0 g/L)
Phospholipids	200–300 mg/dL
Triglycerides	30–190 mg/dL
Magnesium	1.5–2.5 mEq/L (0.62–1.03 mmol/L)
Osmolality, serum	278–295 (lit. range, 257–305) mOsm/L (mmol/kg)
Phosphorus (inorganic)	2.5–4.5 mg/dL (0.81–1.45 mmol/L)
Potassium	3.6–5.5 mEq/L (mmol/L)
Sodium (serum)	135–145 mEq/L (mmol/L)
Total protein	6–8 g/dL (60–80 g/L)
Triglyceride	<200 mg/dL (<2.26 mmol/L)
Uric acid	
Male	3.0–8.5 mg/dL (178–506 μmol/L)
Female	2.5–7.0 mg/dL (149–416 μmol/L)
Vitamin B_{12}	200–1000 pg/mL (147–738 pmol/L)

2. Thyroid tests

BEI or T_4 by column	3–7 μg/dL
PBI	4–8 μg/dL
RAI uptake	10%–35%
T_3 uptake	Below 0.87, hyperthyroid; above 1.13, hypothyroid (Res-O-Mat)
	25%–35% (Triosorb)
	39%–64% (Trilute)
	90%–110% (Thyopac)
T_3-RIA	100–200 ng/dL
T_4 by immunoassay	4–100 μg/dL (Murphy-Pattee)
	5.5–14.5 μg/dL (Tetrasorb) (70.8–186.6 nmol/L)
	5.3–12.2 μg/mL (Tetralute and Res-O-Mat)
TSH	1.5–9.0 μU/mL (mU/L)

From Ravel R: *Clinical laboratory medicine: clinical application of laboratory data,* ed 6, St Louis, 1994, Mosby.

*Abbreviations: *A/G,* albumin/globulin; *BSP,* Bromsulphalein; *BUN,* blood urea nitrogen; *TIBC,* total iron-binding capacity; *BEI,* butanol-extractable iodine; T_4, thyroxine; *PBI,* protein-bound iodine; *RAI,* radioactive iodine; T_3, triiodothyronine; *TSH,* thyroid-stimulating hormone; *SMA,* Sequential Multiple Anaylzer; *HBD,* 3-hydroxybutyric dehydrogenase; *LAP,* leucine aminopeptidase; *LDH,* lactate dehydrogenase; *SGOT,* serum glutamic-oxaloacetic transaminase; *AST;* aspartate aminotransferase; *SGPT,* serum glutamate pyruvate transaminase; *ALT,* alanine aminotransferase; *BE,* base excess; *TRP,* tubular reabsorption of phosphate; *PRI,* phosphorifase isomerase; *Hgb,* hemoglobulin; *RBC,* red blood cell count; *MCH,* mean corpuscular hemoglobin; *MCHC,* mean corpuscular hemoglobin concentration; *MCV,* mean corpuscular volume; *WBC,* white blood cell count; *PT,* prothrombin time; *PTT,* partial thromboplastin time; *aPTT,* activated partial thromboplastin time; *CSF,* cerebrospinal fluid; *VMA,* vanillylmandelic acid; *17-KS,* 17-ketosteroid; *17-OHCS,* 17-hydroxycorticosteroid; *17-KG,* 17-ketogenic steroid; *5-HIAA,* 5-hydroxyindoleacetic acid; *HPF,* high-power field.

Appendix 1. Representative Normal Values*—cont'd.

3. *Serologies*	
Antistreptolysin O	0–200 U
Febrile agglutinins (Weil-Felix)	0–1:40
Cold agglutinins	0–1:32
4. *Enzymes*	
Amylase	60–180 U/dL (Somogyi)
Acid phosphatase	0.5–2 U/dL (Bodansky)
	0.1–5 U/dL (King-Armstrong)
	0.1–0.8 U/dL (Bessey-Lowry)
	0.1–2 IU/L (Babson) (1.67–13.3 μkat/L)
	0.1–2 U/dL (Gutman)
Alkaline phosphatase	1–4 U/dL (Bodansky)
	4–13 U/dL (King-Armstrong)
	0.8–2.5 U/dL (Bessey-Lowry)
	30–110 mU/mL (SMA 12/60) (0.5–1.8 μkat/L)
CPK	1–12 IU/L (Okinaka—activated)
Males	5–50 mU/mL (Oliver-Rosalki) (0.08–0.83 μkat/L)
Females	5–30 mU/mL (Oliver-Rosalki)
	0–12 U (sigma)
	0–1.5 IU/L (Tanzer-Gilvarg—nonactivated)
	1–12 IU/L (Tanzer-Gilvarg—activated)
Males	5–70 IU/L (Hughes—activated)
Females	5–45 IU/L (Hughes—activated)
	25–145 mU/mL (SMA 12/60)
HBD	
Males	150–300 U/dL (Rosalki-Wilkerson)
Females	95–210 mU/mL (Rosalki-Wilkerson)
	55–125 U (Sigma)
LAP	
Males	75–230 U (Goldberg-Rutenberg)
Females	80–210 U (Goldberg-Rutenberg)
	70–200 U (Sigma)
LDH, total	200–500 U/mL (Wroblewski-LaDue)
	200–600 OD units (Teller)
	25–80 IU/L Babson)
	5–50 IU/L (Wacker UV)
	30–100 mU/mL (Wacker UV)
	100–225 mU/mL (SMA 12/60) (1.67–3.75 μkat/L)
LDH, heat stable	20%–40% of total
Lipase	0–1.0 Sigma units
SGOT (AST)	8–40 U/dL (Reitman-Frankel)
	1–12 IU/L (Reitman–Frankel)
	15–36 U/mL (Henry)
	9–36 IU/L (Babson)
	5–40 U/dL (Karmen UV)
	5–20 mU/mL (Kamen UV)
	10–40 mU/mL (SMA 12/60) (0.17–0.67 μkat/L)
SGPT (ALT)	5–35 U/mL (Reitman-Frankel)
	1–12 IU/L (Reitman-Frankel)
	12–55 U/mL (Henry)
	5–25 mU/mL (Wroblewski) (0.08–0.42 μkat/L)
5. *Blood gases (arterial)*	
pH	7.38–7.42
pCO_2	35–45 mm Hg
pO_2	80–90 mm Hg (<65 yr)
	75–85 mm Hg (>65 yr)
O_2 saturation	96%–97% (room air)
BE	0 ± 2 mEq/L

Appendix 1. Representative Normal Values*—cont'd.

6. *Clearances*	
Urea	
Standard	40–65 mL/min
Maximum	60–100 mL/min
Creatinine	90–120 mL/min (1.5–2.0 ml/sec)
Phosphate reabsorption (TRP, PRI)	Over 80%
7. *Hematology and coagulation*	
Hgb	
Males	14–18 g/dL (140–180 g/L)
Females	12–16 g/dL (120–160 g/L)
Hematocrit	
Males	40%–54%
Females	37%–47%
RBC	
Males	4.5–6.0 million (4.5–6.0 × 10^{12}/L)
Females	4.0–5.5 million (4.0–5.5 × 10^{12}/L)
MCH	26–34 pg
MCHC	31%–37%
MCV	80–100 μm^3 (fL)
Platelets	150,000–4,000/mm^3 (150–400 × 10^9/L)
WBC	4,500–11,000/mm^3 (4.5–11.0 × 10^9/L)
Differential lymphocytes	20%–40
Segmented neutrophils	50%–70%
Band neutrophils	0%–7%
Eosinophils	0%–5%
Monocytes	0%–7%
Sedimentation	
Males	0–15 mm/hr (>60 yr, 0–25)
Females	0–20 mm/hr (>60 hr, 0–30)
Fibrinogen (quantitative)	200–400 mg/dL (2.0–4.0 g/L)
Coagulation time (Lee-White)	5–15 min
PT	Control ± 2 sec
PTT	40–100 sec (nonactivated)
aPTT	30–45 sec
Bleeding time	2.5–10 min (Simplate method)
PRT	90–130 sec
8. *Protein electrophoresis (cellulose acetate)*	
Albumin	3.5–5.0 g/dL (50%–65%)
α_1-Globulin	0.2–0.4 g/dL (2.5%–5.5%)
α_2-Globulin	0.6–1.0 g/dL (7%–12%)
β-Globulin	0.6–1.0 g/dL (7%–15%)
α-Globulin	0.7–1.3 g/dL (11%–21%)
B. Spinal fluid (CSF)	
Glucose	40–70 mg/dL (2.22–3.89 mmol/L)
Protein	20–45 mg/dL (0.20–0.45 g/L)
WBC	0–5 monocytes
RBC	0
Colloidal gold	No number more than 1
Chloride	20 mEq/L higher than serum

Appendix 1. Representative Normal Values*—cont'd.

C. Urine	
1. *Adrenal chemistry*	
Aldosterone	2–26 μg/24 hr (Kliman and Peterson)
Catecholamines	5–150 μg/24 hr
	5–100 μg/25 hr (Lund)
Metanephrines	0.3–0.9 mg/24 hr (Pisano)
VMA	0.5–12 mg/24 hr
	0.5–7 mg/24 hr (Pisano)
17-KS	
Male	10–25 mg/24 hr (34.7–86.7 μmol/day)
Female <50 yr	5–15 mg/24 hr
Female >50 yr	4–8 mg/24 hr
17-OHCS	
Male	3–12/24 hr (8.3–33.1 μmol/day)
Female	3–10 mg/24 hr
17-KG	
Male	8–25 mg/24 hr (27.7–86.7 μmol/day)
Female	5–18 mg/24 hr
2. *Miscellaneous urine chemistry*	
Amylase	Up to 300 U/hr
Amylase clearance/creatinine clearance ratio	1%–4%
Calcium	Less than 250 mg/24 hr (regular diet) (6.23 mmol/day)
	Less than 150 mg/24 hr (low-calcium diet)
Creatinine	1.0–1.8 g/24 hr (8.84–7.07 mmol/day)
Glucose	0–0.3 g/24 hr
Phosphate (phosphorus)	400–1300 mg/day (varies greatly with diet) (12.9–42.0 mmol/day)
Potassium	25–120 mEq/24 hr (mmol/day)
Protein	0–0.1 g/24 hr (0.0–0.01 g/day)
Sodium	30–90 mEq/L
	40–200 mEq/24 hr (mmol/day)
Urea nitrogen	6–17 g/day (normal BUN) (214–607 mmol/day)
Uric acid	250–800 mg/24 hr (normal diet) (1.49–4.76 mmol/day)
	Less than 600 mg/24 hr (low purine diet) (<3.57 mmol/day)
5-HIAA	1–7 mg/24 hr (Goldenberg)
3. *Urinalysis*	
Protein	0–30 mg/dL (random)
	0–0.1 g/24 hr
WBC	0–5/HPF
RBC	0–1/HPF
Urobilinogen	0–1 Ehrlich unit
	0–1:20
Sugar	Negative
Acetone	Negative

Appendix 2. Conversion of Traditional Units to SI Units*

	Current Unit	SI Unit	Conversion Factor
Albumin	g/dL	g/L	10
Aspartate aminotransferase	U/L (mU/ml)	μkat/L	0.0167
Ammonia	μg/dL	μmol/L	0.587
Bicarbonate (HCO_3)	mEq/L	mmol/L	1.0
Bilirubin	mg/dL	μmol/L	17.1
Blood urea nitrogen (BUN)	mg/dL	mmol/L	0.357
Calcium	mg/dL	mmol/L	0.25
Chloride	mEq/L	mmol/L	1.0
Cholesterol	mg/dL	mmol/L	0.026
Cortisol	μg/dL	μmol/L	0.0276
Creatinine	mg/dL	μmol/L	88.4
Creatinine clearance	mL/min	mL/s	0.0167
CSF protein	mg/dL	g/L	0.01
Folic acid	ng/mL	nmol/L	2.27
Glucose	mg/dL	mmol/L	0.0555
High-density lipoprotein	mg/dL	mmol/L	0.0259
Iron	mg/dL	μmol/L	0.179
Lithium	mEq/L	μmol/L	1.0
Magnesium	mEq/L	mmol/L	0.44
Osmolality	mOsm/kg	mmol/kg	1.0
Phosphorus	mg/dL	mmol/L	0.323
Potassium	mEq/L	mmol/L	1.0
Sodium	mEq/L	mmol/L	1.0
Thyroxine (T_4)	μg/dL	nmol/L	12.9
Total protein	g/dL	g/L	10
Triglyceride	mg/dL	mmol/L	0.0113
Uric acid	mg/dL	mmol/L	0.0595
Vitamin B_{12}	ng/mL	pmol/L	0.0738
pCO_2	mm Hg	kPa	0.133
pC_2	mm Hg	kPa	0.133
Hemoglobin	g/dL	g/L	10
Hematocrit	vol%	None	0.01
Mean corpuscular volume (MCV)	μm^3	fL	1.0
WBC count	mm^3	$10^9/L$	0.001
Platelet count	mm^3	$10^9/L$	0.001

From Ravel R: *Clinical laboratory medicine: clinical application of laboratory data,* ed 6, St Louis, 1994, Mosby.
*Current unit × conversion factor = SI unit; SI unit ÷ conversion factor = current unit.

INDEX

N

O

P

R

T